Technique Systems in Chiropractic

Technique Systems in Chiropractic

Robert Cooperstein, MA, DC

Professor, Coordinator of Technique and Research,
Palmer Chiropractic College West, San Jose, California, USA

Brian J. Gleberzon, DC

Associate Professor, Canadian Memorial Chiropractic College,
Toronto, Canada

Foreword by
Dr Robert D. Mootz DC

Associate Medical Director of Chiropractic,
State of Washington Department of Labor and Industries,
Olympia, Washington, USA

Publisher: Robert Cooperstein and Chiropraxis Publishing
539 Elsie Avenue, San Leandro CA 94577 USA

Second printing 2018
ISBN-13:
ISBN-13: 978-1983577543

Library of Congress Cataloging in Publication Data
A catalog record for this book is available from the Library of Congress

Notice
Medical knowledge is constantly changing. Standard safety precautions must be
followed, but as new research and clinical experience broaden our knowledge,
changes in treatment and drug therapy may become necessary or appropriate.
Readers are advised to check the most current product information provided by the
manufacturer of each drug to be administered to verify the recommended dose, the
method and duration of administration, and contraindications. It is the responsibility
of the practitioner, relying on experience and knowledge of the patient, to determine
dosages and the best treatment for each individual patient. Neither the Publisher nor
the authors assume any liability for any injury and/or damage to persons or property
arising from this publication.

The Publisher

Disclaimer
Every effort has been made by the Author and the Publisher to ensure that the descriptions of the
techniques included in this book are accurate and in conformity with the descriptions published
by their developers. The Publishers and the Authors do not assume any responsibility for any
injury and/or damage to persons or property arising out of or related to any use of the material
contained in this book. It is the responsibility of the treating practitioner, relying on independent
experience and knowledge of the patient, to determine the best treatment and method of
application for the patient, to make their own evaluation of their effectiveness and to check with
the developers or teachers of the techniques they wish to use that they have understood them
correctly.

Contents

Foreword

WHAT'S IN A NAME-BRAND?

Name-Brand Chiropractic Techniques: Gonstead, Upper Cervical Specific, Cox, Sacro-Occipital Technique, Applied Kinesiology, Activator Methods, Chiropractic Biophysics, Pettibon, Diversified, Logan Basic, Motion Palpation, Network, Thompson Terminal Point, Toftness, Grostic, Pierce-Stillwagon, Meric, BEST, and the list could go on for dozens more. These are the bread and butter of the chiropractic profession. When you set your politics, your research, and your philosophy at the door and step inside, clinical techniques are where the rubber meets the road between the patient and the doctor of chiropractic.

Patients often search out doctors who use the same technique as a previous chiropractor they had success with. Chiropractic students seek out off-campus seminars to learn the wisdom of technique entrepreneurs' experience in the "real world" of patient care. Insurance companies hire chiropractors to decipher the lingo of chiropractic techniques to assist in determining appropriateness of care and medical necessity. Some techniques are even banned from the scope of chiropractic practice by governmental regulatory bodies. The culture of chiropractic techniques is firmly imbedded in every aspect of the chiropractor's existence; and the carry-over of chiropractic technique culture extends to our patients and our non-chiropractic colleagues, not to mention those pesky payers and regulators.

The aura of chiropractic techniques is fraught with uncertainty and questions. Why so many different techniques? What makes a technique system a technique system? Where did they all come from

and what makes one technique approach so different from another? What systems are similar? Should some techniques be used on some patients but not on others? How should one determine when a particular technique is appropriate? What are the clinical and scientific foundations upon which different techniques are based? Why do some techniques approach patients with similar problems in such different ways and with such varied interventions, frequencies, and durations of care?

At long last, a thorough inventory of popular chiropractic techniques has been compiled to begin systematically to satisfy just such inquiries. Throughout chiropractic history, technique knowledge has been in many ways an experiential, hierarchical, and word-of-mouth kind of process. You had to "go to the mountain" to really learn what it was all about. Yet, name-brand technique knowledge has often been proprietary and entrepreneurial. As a result, many techniques have simply faded away with their developers, their use and popularity more dependent on the marketing savvy of proponents than on demand from the benefited healthcare consumer.

The world is now a different place; healthcare in the information age relies as much on the guidance of science and skeptics as it does on the ruminations of enlightened innovators. In recent decades, chiropractic has embraced the tools of science in order to study, document and understand what our work does, but we are just on the cusp of using these tools to refine our ability to make chiropractic techniques better, more efficient and perhaps even safer.

Even though clinical studies to assess and refine chiropractic procedures are just in their infancy, the book you hold in your hands demystifies much of the jargon and lingo inherent in chiropractic techniques. It is the first scholarly chiropractic work that tackles head-on the status of evidence regarding specific commonly used chiropractic techniques. It is not a "promotional" vehicle for any particular technique proponent, so lots of sacred cows get challenged. Neither is it a strawman caricature of procedures developed with the shoestring resources of an historically ostracized profession, so esoteric techniques are not dismissed out of hand. A reasoned discussion of each technique's evolution is presented, with both strengths and weaknesses delineated. That means the time you spend delving into these pages will be stimulating, enjoyable and rewarding.

This text is not a "how to" book for performing different techniques. It does not attempt to replace the innovations and training that come from technique developers in practice or the technique departments within chiropractic colleges. However, the theoretical foundations and clinical approaches are assessed from both scholarly and pragmatic perspectives, alongside a critical exploration of materials and literature about chiropractic techniques. It is refreshing to explore these pages, which are written in an accessible style that simply makes it hard to put them down. Perhaps some will consider Drs Cooperstein and Gleberzon's discussions of the state of scientific evidence for the effectiveness of procedures used by each "name-brand" technique to be provocative, but truly this is the very discussion that goes on in the hallways of academia and science in every healthcare field. The difference is that the scholarship here provides a roadmap for the journey to develop and enhance evidence-informed chiropractic practice.

The book is obviously written for chiropractors, particularly those in training, but anyone who ever works with chiropractors and their care decisions will find it to be an essential tool. For students, this survey lays a critical foundation upon which to build one's clinical skill set. For the scholars and developers within chiropractic, this text provides a much-needed mirror that establishes a framework upon which the future must be built. Although objective introspection of our own fabric is likely to involve some discomfort (didn't a well-know chiropractic mentor encourage us to teach our patients to embrace their "recovery symptoms"?), an accurate assessment is essential for sustaining our growth as profession. More importantly, inventory, appraisal and refinement allow us to improve the care we provide to our patients. For non-chiropractors, context and clarity for chiropractic procedures can now be found within these pages.

Although you, dear reader, will undoubtedly have even more questions than you receive answers for as you explore each topic, this is the kind of scholarly work that becomes a classic reserve, updated and revised regularly as new information becomes available, turned to as a resource for both clinical and reference purposes. Yes, you will want to buy the second edition, and the third. And perhaps it will even be singled out as a lightning rod for vigorous discussion, debate and refinement of our theory and who we are as chiropractors. Exactly the kind of book you want to read.

Dr Robert D. Mootz

Preface

Technique Systems in Chiropractic has been written with several different target audiences in mind. We expect our readers to be students of chiropractic, but not necessarily individuals currently enrolled in a chiropractic college. Field practitioners, irrespective of their philosophical perspective and current practice patterns, will find easy access to information on other forms of chiropractic practice, whether they are thinking of making changes in their own practice procedures or simply need to know what other chiropractors are doing. In addition, government and private sector healthcare policy makers, healthcare benefits administrators, insurance claims adjustors, attorneys, allied health professionals, non-chiropractic faculty at chiropractic colleges, individuals interested in complementary and alternative medicine, current and prospective chiropractic patients, academicians interested in chiropractic, and other stakeholders will also find this information valuable.

This textbook is not a chiropractic practice manual designed to teach readers how to perform the described procedures or chiropractic technique systems. It describes how chiropractic is done, rather than explaining how to do it. *Technique Systems in Chiropractic* may best be thought of as a "Traveler's Guide" through the landscape of different chiropractic technique systems. To continue with the analogy, each of the techniques' historical sites, landmarks, and major cities is discussed, but we do not describe their quaint towns and villages. We can help you get around town, but we are not a removals company.

Technique Systems in Chiropractic is divided into four sections. In addition to a general overview of the textbook, Section 1, "An Overview", confronts the question of chiropractic terminology, whose lack of standardization and proprietary nature often confounds discussion and comprehension of different forms of chiropractic technique. Many of the terms used by chiropractors take on vastly different meanings depending upon the context in which they are used. Moreover, many terms would be unfamiliar to persons outside of the chiropractic profession, and such individuals can easily get lost in the world of unknown semantics. We have included a brief discussion of the core adjustive methods used in chiropractic, many of which cut across and show up in several different technique systems.

Section 2, "Core Chiropractic Diagnostic/ Assessment Procedures", discusses diagnostic/ assessment procedures that cut across multiple technique systems. Many of the dozens of technique systems we describe use these core diagnostic/assessment procedures, such as leg checks, X-ray line marking, thermography, etc., albeit in somewhat different ways, both from a procedural and interpretive point of view. It would be unnecessary to repeatedly describe the same or similar diagnostic/assessment procedures for each technique that uses it. By avoiding that, we could more easily focus on differences in usage in the separate discussions of each technique system. Where a diagnostic/assessment method is used primarily or exclusively by one technique system, for example, arm fossa testing in Sacro-Occipital Technique, it is described in the relevant chapter rather than in Section 2.

There are many, many diagnostic/assessment procedures commonly used in chiropractic, but luckily for the purposes of this text, most find common application across a large number of technique systems. The generic examination procedures included in Section 2 are: leg checking, static and motion palpation, manual muscle testing, radiography and X-ray line marking, thermography, and instrumentation. The reader will find additional, less broadly applied examination procedures described in the individual chapters on named technique systems.

Section 3, "Chiropractic System Techniques", is the heart of the book. In alphabetical order, each of the most commonly used chiropractic technique systems is described using a template that we adapted from one used originally by the Council of Advisors to the ACA Council on Technique. Here we had to make choices that are guaranteed to offend various technique mavens, by putting their technique into a chapter with closely related techniques, for example, Upper Cervical Techniques, or by leaving it out of the book altogether, for example, the Total Body Modification technique of Victor Frank. It would have been impossible to cover the 97 technique systems listed by Bergmann,[1] but, more importantly, it would have been counterproductive to do so. Many of them are too obscure or little practiced to be of more than historical interest, and would have taken space better used in covering the more mainstream techniques.

We also had to decide what to call the technique systems, since some of them have descriptive names but are also commonly known by the surname of the associated technique developer. As a convention, we alphabetized Section 3 by the descriptive names where one existed; hence "Receptor Tonus Technique," not "Nimmo Technique." We also had to choose among alternative names for the techniques that the technique developers themselves had come up with in different times and places; for example, we elected to use Flexion Manipulation, rather than Flexion-Distraction Technique or the Cox Technique. In some cases we had to resist the temptation to collapse some system techniques, such as the Thompson and Pierce-Stillwagon techniques.

Finally, in many ways, we have adopted the same approach to describing the chiropractic technique systems that is used when describing a literary character. That is, if we were charged with describing Hamlet, we would synthesize what he says about himself, what he does, and what others say about him. In much the same way, we combine the following information:

- how the technique is described by its developers or proponents
- how practitioners actually perform the technique in a clinical setting
- how others describe the technique.

We have also undertaken an extensive review of the evidence base for each technique, where it exists, and provided a detailed discussion of the clinical effectiveness and safety of each technique, based on that literature.

Section 4, "Issues in Chiropractic Technique", discusses many of the topics that underpin the world of chiropractic technique. We explore some historical matters pertaining to chiropractic technique, focusing on some of the forces that have fragmented the profession and led to the development of so many different and often mutually exclusive technique systems. A discussion of the utilization rates of the technique systems is provided, as well as a broad discussion of the utilization of chiropractic care in general. We also briefly discuss the position of chiropractic in the complementary and alternative medicine (CAM) world, since the determination of the profession's identity and its role in the healthcare delivery system impacts on the future role of technique systems. We next turn to the allure of technique systems to both chiropractic practitioners and patients.

Where chiropractic practice leads, issues of jurisprudence follow. With this in mind, Section 4 continues with a description of some of the challenges facing the profession's regulators regarding the use of different technique systems. Since much of the debate within legal circles often distills down to which techniques have a broad evidence base and which do not, we briefly discuss evidence-based medicine or, evidence-based chiropractic. This chapter discusses the historical establishment of research in the chiropractic profession, what constitutes "evidence", and the challenges facing the chiropractic research community.

The first appendix is an article we originally published in *Topics in Clinical Chiropractic*,[2] establishing the concept of the "subluxation-equivalent" and contributing toward the development of a chiropractic technique taxonomy. The second appendix is an article originally reprinted in the *Journal of Chiropractic Humanities*, clarifying the ambiguities involved in characterizing that most ubiquitous of chiropractic techniques, Diversified Technique. Finally, we gather the definitions of technique-specific terms that are included within the technique system chapters and a few other terms from elsewhere in the book, to comprise a master glossary of terms pertinent to chiropractic name techniques. It differs from other chiropractic glossaries that one finds in that generic terms, like subluxation and adjustment, do not appear.

We hope you will find *Technique Systems in Chiropractic* a useful resource in making sense of the abundance of chiropractic techniques that are commonly used.

Toronto and   Brian Gleberzon
San Jose 2003   Robert Cooperstein

REFERENCES

1. Bergman T F 1993 Various forms of chiropractic technique. Chiropractic Technique 5(2): 53–55

2. Cooperstein R, Gleberzon BJ 2001 Toward a taxonomy of subluxation-equivalents. Topics in Clinical Chiropractic 8(1): 49–60

Acknowledgments

Writing a textbook is a daunting task, and cannot be done without the help of others. We would like to thank the editors at Elsevier for their patience and professionalism with respect to preparing this manuscript. We also acknowledge Glenda Wiese, co-author of *Chiropractic: An Illustrated History*, for her assistance with some of the photos used in this book. The many individuals who served on the Panel of Advisors to the ACA Council on Technique, and its descendent organization, the ACC Technique Consortium, have left an indelible mark on this book.

Brian thanks his parents, William and Ann Gleberzon, as well as his in-laws, Nathan and Shirley Rosenberg, for their continued and ongoing support; and especially his two sons, Jared and Andrew, and wife Anita, who is always there when he needs her most. Robert's parents, Sam and Hilda, although no longer with us, were graduates of The School of Hard Knocks, and were always generous with their support. Robert's two sons, Sam and Lucas, currently enrolled, have made it all worthwhile and mean the world to him. Robert also extends his thank to EM, OH, MH and JG.

The following four chapters are edited versions of articles originally published in the former journal *Chiropractic Technique*: Activator Methods Chiropractic Technique, ch. 10; Chiropractic Biophysics Technique (CBP), ch. 14; Sacro-Occipital Technique, ch. 25; and Thompson Terminal Point Technique, ch. 29. We thank National University of Health Sciences (NUHS) for permission to reprint these articles. Chapter 20, Gonstead Chiropractic Technique, is an edited version of an article published in the Journal of Chiropractic Medicine, and we once again thank NUHS for granting permission to reprint.

Some of the chapters in this book were developed in part out of technique and procedure summaries prepared by Dr. Cooperstein for American Specialty Health Plans (ASHP) in February, 2000. These chapters are: Applied Kinesiology spinoff techniques (ch. 11), Bioenergetic Synchronization Technique (ch. 13), Directional Non-Force Technique (ch. 18), Network Spinal Analysis (ch. 22), Spinal Stressology (ch. 28), Tottness Technique (ch. 30), and Upper Cervical (NUCCA) technique (chs. 32–33). We thank ASHP for granting us permission to draw upon this material in writing this book.

Chapter 34, Genesis of System Techniques in Chiropractic, contains edited passages originally published as a book chapter in *Advances in Chiropractic, Volume* 2, and we thank Elsevier for granting permission to utilize parts of this chapter. Chapter 36, Allure of System Techniques; Appendix on Medicine vs. Chiropractic, contains edited passages from an article originally published in the Journal of Chiropractic Education, Brand name techniques and the confidence gap, and we thank DataTrace Publishing for permission to reprint.

Appendix 1, Toward a Taxonomy of Subluxation-Equivalents, originally published by Aspen, is reprinted in its entirety with permission of Lippincott Williams & Wilkins, to whom we extend our thanks. Appendix 2, The Special Case of Diversified Technique, was originally published as *Diversified technique: Core of chiropractic or "just another technique system"?*, and is once again reprinted with the permission of National University of Health Sciences, which we gratefully acknowledge.

1. Cooperstein R 1997 Technique system overview: Activator Methods Technique. Chiropractic Technique 9 (3): 108–114

2. Cooperstein R 1995 Technique system overview: Chiropractic Biophysics Technique (CBP). Chiropractic Technique 7 (4): 141–146.

3. Cooperstein R 1996 Technique system overview: Sacro Occipital Technique. Chiropractic Technique 8 (3): 125–131.

4. Cooperstein R 1995 Technique system overview: Thompson Technique. Chiropractic Technique 7 (2): 60–63.

5. Cooperstein R 1995 Contemporary approach to understanding chiropractic technique. In: Lawrence D, editor. Advances in Chiropractic Volume 2. Chicago IL: Mosby Year Book, Inc. p. 437–459.

6. Cooperstein R 1990 Brand name techniques and the confidence gap. The Journal of Chiropractic Education 4 (3): 89–93.

7. Cooperstein R, Gleberzon BJ 2001 Toward a taxonomy of subluxation-equivalents. Topics in Clinical Chiropractic 8 (1): 49–60.

8. Cooperstein R 1995 Diversified technique: Core of chiropractic or "just another technique system"? Journal of Chiropractic Humanities 5 (1): 50–55.

An overview

Although we were tempted to plunge into the core of this book, the 24 chapters on named chiropractic technique systems (Section 3), we thought it best to lay down some of the groundwork and characterize the context from which they draw their sustenance. Chapter 1 explains why this book needed to be written, and further explains why *we* wrote it instead of inviting the technique system developers to describe their techniques. Chapter 2, on terminology, provides readers inside and outside chiropractic with a glimpse into representative usages, as well as the historical basis for the huge variation in usage of terms. We are aware of the exemplary work done by the Association of Chiropractic Colleges just a few short years ago in having the college presidents reach consensus on the term "subluxation" and some other terms, but we expected this laudable effort to eventually run into problems – and it has. We have already witnessed grumbling and unilateral reinterpretations of some of the concepts upon which "consensus" was supposed to have been reached. Chapter 3, concluding Section 1, provides thumbnail sketches of the core treatment methods used in chiropractic, many of which cut across and appear in several different technique systems.

Introduction to *Technique Systems in Chiropractic*

I have never considered it beneath my dignity to do anything to relieve human suffering.

(DD Palmer: quote on the statue at Palmer Memorial Park, Port Perry, Ontario, Canada; Fig. 1.1)

Technique Systems in Chiropractic is about those technique systems, also referred to in this book as "named techniques," "brand-name techniques," or "proprietary techniques." A technique system amounts to a step-by-step protocol for diagnosing and treating just about any patient that walks through a clinician's door. It is a blend of standalone rules, practical tips, and patient care algorithms that often originate from the practice experience of an individual practitioner. Although the metaphor is probably overdone, the comparison of a technique system to a cookbook is not unfair. Although some technique systems specialize in treating a specific type or range of patient problems, most claim to address more or less any patient complaint imaginable, either directly (condition-based care) or indirectly (subluxation-based care). Oddly enough, new technique systems, as they are created, do not usually replace existing techniques, but rather stand alongside them. That is why the several lists of chiropractic technique systems that have been compiled can number in the hundreds; there are several historical reasons for this great proliferation of technique systems in chiropractic (Ch. 34).

TECHNIQUE SYSTEM DIVERSITY IN CHIROPRACTIC

Chiropractic currently occupies a mainstream position in the western healthcare delivery system,

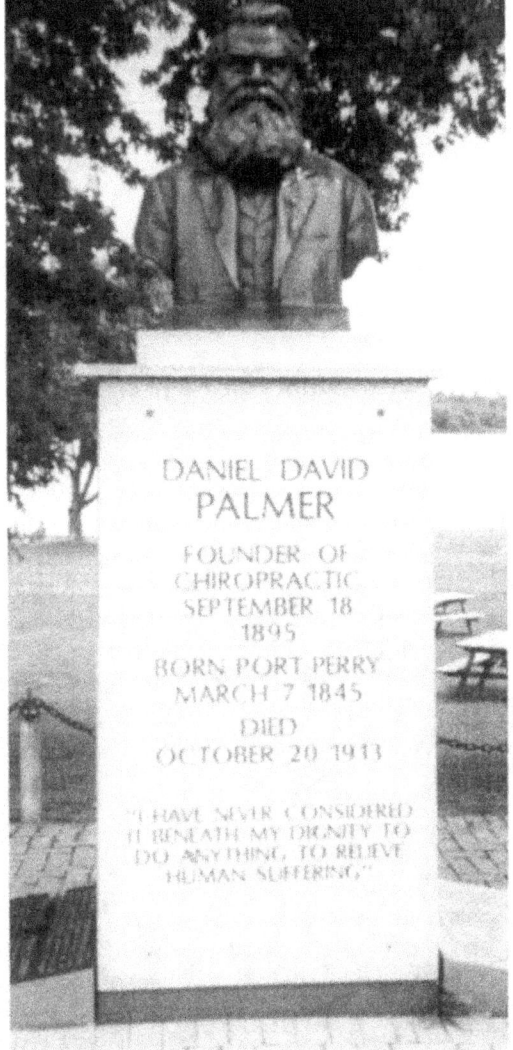

Figure 1.1 Statue of DD Palmer at Palmer Memorial Park, Port Perry, Ontario, Canada.

irrespective of whether chiropractic is regarded as complementary or alternative to the medical profession (Ch. 37). In actuality, unique among all the other complementary and alternative medicine professions, chiropractic is comfortably situated as both alternative and complement to modern medicine, deriving substantial benefits from this dual existence. However, this has not always been the case, and some areas of chiropractic still display the properties of a profession that developed at the fringes of healthcare, not at its center. It shows just the sort of methodological diversity that one would expect of a discipline that developed on the edge. It is always at the margins of society that freedom of experimentation commingles with reckless adventurism, that lack of regulation can breed simultaneously bold innovation and abject quackery. In the case of chiropractic these forces contributed to the development of different theoretical approaches to healing, and eventually to different technique systems. The ameliorating impact of the passage of time tends to tip the scales from the side of quackery toward that of innovation. Other reasons for the popularity and proliferation of technique systems are given in Chapter 36.

There have been both good and bad consequences of this technique proliferation, worthy of some discussion, and we do explore some of these wider issues in Section 4. However, the primary focus of *Technique Systems in Chiropractic* remains the characterization, classification, comparative description, and critical evaluation of the technique systems. Although in conceiving this book we did not intend to insert very much of our own opinions into this text, preferring at first that the evidence and the technique innovators speak for themselves, we cannot at this time claim neutrality. The temptation to editorialize on these techniques was irresistible, and we thought it necessary and beneficial to indulge that temptation from time to time, mostly in the conclusions of each of the technique chapters in Section 3. That stated, our primary focus has been more one of technique description than technique criticism.

There is an important statement of intent that needs to be made perfectly clear. This book is *not* meant to serve as an instruction manual for the different technique systems that are described. It is intended to offer an overview of the different technique systems, some or many of which may be unfamiliar to the readers: chiropractic students, field doctors, third-party payers, patients, college faculty and administrators, government agencies, allied health professionals, and other constituencies. A reader who wishes to learn more about a particular technique, or perhaps to utilize a technique's diagnostic or therapeutic protocols, is encouraged to attend an instructional seminar, access internet websites, or consult any one of a number of technique system textbooks to achieve the desired level of competence.

A rather obvious question is posed: why didn't we simply invite the technique innovators to describe their own technique systems, and make ourselves available as editors to facilitate their work? The answer: in our view, technique descriptions written by technique advocates run the risk of becoming glorified advertisements. Indeed, we have seen previous works of this nature; even the most cursory glance at some of these anthologies and articles confirms that mixed with accurate technique description can be silly and baseless claims of superiority and originality compared with other techniques; grandiose claims for clinical effectiveness; non-interpretable, technique-specific jargon; and much else of spectacle value only. We, who take pride in being "technique guys" – meaning we love chiropractic technique – thought we could best show our respect for our profession and for the techniques we describe, including some that contain elements about which we are dubious, by describing them fairly using a systematic and evenly applied approach.

We do not suppose this textbook will be met with approval from all the stakeholders and other interested parties in the chiropractic profession. On the one hand, some academics, faculty members, and administrators in pedagogical and research circles may believe we were not objective enough, that we were too tactful to deconstruct rigorously the oftentimes weak foundational science, philosophy, or theory upon which some of these techniques are built. On the other hand, some technique developers or their partisans may feel we were unfair in addressing their favored technique, that we erred in not simply endorsing it. After all, "all techniques work," don't they? (Chapter 38 addresses evidence-based chiropractic care.) The answer is yes and no: all techniques work according to the criteria for success defined by individuals for their favored technique system, but the chiropractic profession does not currently entertain a universally agreed-upon standard of clinical success. As an example, one chiropractor may rejoice in having eliminated a patient's terrible pain, while another scolds this chiropractor for not having effected a change in the patient's X-rays. Was this a "successful" clinical outcome or not?

This situation clearly invites constructive criticism by technique non-partisans. We believe it necessary that non-participants in the world of competing technique systems describe chiropractic techniques and subject them to critical commentary. Indeed, the chiropractic profession is obliged to provide a forum for this type of scrutiny, as a matter of social responsibility and in the interests of patients' welfare. In short, the authors felt that it was important, indeed necessary, to have a textbook written on technique systems by independent reviewers.

AVOIDING THE ETHNOCENTRIC TRAP

The authors adopted somewhat of an anthropological approach during the writing of this book. A textbook on anthropology defines culture as: "A set of rules or standards shared by members of a society, which when acted upon by the members produce behavior that falls within a range of variation the members consider proper and acceptable."[1] We believe that each of the technique systems described in this textbook, in this sense, manifests a distinct culture. Anthropologists, unlike researchers in most other social sciences, often participate in a culture's activities in order to obtain a better understanding of that culture from an insider's perspective, in a process known as ethnography.[1] We are no different: as technique guys describing technique systems, we simultaneously practice and observe these techniques. Although one is always subject to ethnocentric bias, the belief that one's personal approach is

somehow superior, it can get in the way of accurate description.

For our purpose, in order to accomplish immersion into the cultural context of each of the chiropractic technique systems, we tried temporarily to set aside (although not entirely shed) our ethnocentric views and opinions. Again, borrowing from anthropology, we proceeded from the perspective of cultural relativism, meaning we tried to suspend judgment on other people's practice procedures in order to understand them on their own terms.[1] In this manner, we avoided trying to fit the square peg of each technique's unique approach into the round hole of our own world-view. In cases where, despite our relativistic approach, we felt critical commentary was warranted, we did not hesitate to make our views known in the conclusions of each chapter.

We have each been involved for many years in intercollegiate chiropractic technique groups such as the Technique Consortium of the Association of Chiropractic Colleges[2] and its predecessor group, the Panel of Advisors to the American Chiropractic Association Council on Technique. Given the diversity of views represented in such organizations, we know not to equate chiropractic technique with chiropractic philosophy. Some technique systems focus on pain reduction, whereas others eschew patients' symptoms, in favor of subluxation correction. (These opposite poles of care have most recently been rendered by the pair of terms condition-based versus subluxation-based care.) From the standpoint of technique relativism, when it comes to a technique system, we do not dwell on its therapeutic intent, nor even if it has one. From a strictly operational view, we simply ask: how is the patient examined, what does the doctor do, how are outcomes measured, and what evidence do we have on the technique's safety and effectiveness? We are not unaware that some of the technique systems we review have some rather strange views on how the body works, but we did not find it difficult to look the other way, nor separate such views from matters of ethics and principles, except in so far as such views impact upon the technique procedures that are applied. A recent article emphasized that using the terms "rational" and "principled" when contrasting different groups of chiropractors is a destructive process, adding very little to the advancement of the profession.[3]

Although this book is about the practice of chiropractic in the field, it all begins with what students learn in the chiropractic colleges. Not surprisingly, they exhibit much the same differences from one another as these doctors in the field, although private practitioners are permitted more freedom to take up procedures that would have a hard time flourishing in the core curriculum, and even within the elective curriculum, of any of the accredited chiropractic colleges. Students and alumni are often ingrained with the philosophical slant under which they are taught, and often develop ethnocentric technique perspectives.

Chiropractic college graduates often believe that what they were taught is not only the best method to use for patient care, it's the only way. However, it is an intriguing fact that ethnocentrism within chiropractic circles works both ways. For example, the group of chiropractors who consider themselves to be rationalists and evidence-based may think the other group of chiropractors who expose a more orthodox view of chiropractic (innate, vitalism, the subluxation) are archaic and antiquated. For their part, the latter group (who often refer to themselves as principled chiropractors) may, in turn, believe the former to be too concerned with appeasing the medical community and at risk of losing their chiropractic identity.

The authors have observed this phenomenon several times, often during intercollegiate chiropractic technique conferences. At one of these meetings, which took place at one of the more traditional colleges (one with more confidence in those chiropractic examination procedures that purport to identify subluxations), the authors were provided a description of the spinal assessment tools used at that college. This assessment included thermography, supine leg checks, and radiography. One of the authors, a representative from a more modernist chiropractic college (one that purports to use only those procedures with a strong evidence base), puzzled by this unabashed and unapologetic use of methods that can be traced back to the time of BJ Palmer, squinted like the proverbial deer caught in the headlights of an oncoming car. He expressed his confusion and surprise that a scientifically minded clinician could advocate relatively unproven diagnostic methods. The representative from the traditional college asked if the puzzled modernist used prone or supine leg checks at his college. The answer: "No." Does it use thermography? "No." Well, how about X-rays to get listings? Again, "No." The traditionalist, awestruck by the modernist college's omissions, following a moment of stunned silence and contemplation, declared: "Things are worse there than I thought!" The modernist, wistfully lacking the unbridled confidence so typical of chiropractic traditionalists, was left to stew on the disquieting phenomenon of dueling technique paradigms. Could it be, could it just be, he thought, that ignorance is bliss?

REFERENCES

1. Haviland W A 1997 Anthropology, 8th edn. Harcourt Brace College Publishers, Orlando, FL
2. Gleberzon B J, Cooperstein R 2002 The Technique Consortium of the Association of Chiropractic Colleges: the first twenty years. Journal of Chiropractic Education 16 (1): 12–13
3. Gatterman M, Dobson T P, Lefevbre R 2001 Chiropractic quality assurance: standards and guidelines. Journal of the Canadian Chiropractic Association 45 (1): 11–17

2

Technique systems terminology

Terminology has always been important to chiropractors, ever since the days when using the word "diagnosis" could have meant a trip to jail for practicing medicine without a license. These issues are important, because professional identity, and even professional survival, may hinge on the use of a shared lexicon. For example, some chiropractors profess to perform *spinal analysis*, following which they *adjust* the spine to *correct subluxations*.[1] Others are more likely to say they *diagnose* back complaints, following which they *treat* spinal conditions with spinal *manipulation* or other methods acting, in essence, as neuromusculoskeletal specialists.[2] Of course there is a middle ground, like chiropractors who *diagnose* and *treat subluxations*. We have italicized all the words that are controversial, and stipulate our intention not to get involved in any of these controversies, except as required to characterize chiropractic technique systems. In essence, in writing this book, we did not want to get bogged down using too many words separated by dashes and hyphens (e.g., "diagnosis and/or analysis"). We ask the reader in advance to be patient with our usage of various terms, which is context-sensitive and most likely will not suit all of the readers all of the time. That said, we do need to offer a few comments on several key terms.

TECHNIQUE, TECHNIQUE, AND TECHNIC

Chiropractic is a profession, not a treatment modality. It is commonly stated that chiropractic is an art, science, and philosophy. Chiropractic technique can be understood as the integration of all three components: the thoughtful application of scientific understanding to chiropractic patient care. It combines the practice of chiropractic theory and the theory of chiropractic practice. Chiropractors historically used the word "technic" to describe adjustive procedures and their rationales, such as in "rib subluxation technic" or "sacroiliac technic." A few years ago, the American Chiropractic Association's Council on Technique decided to modernize the spelling, so that these generic, mainstream treatment methods are now referred to as "techniques," with a lower-case "t" for reasons to be discussed in a moment. A chiropractic technique is thus a clinical intervention or method, as well as a supporting rationale, that belongs to the chiropractic common domain, and the totality of these generic treatment methods is what we mean by chiropractic technique.

Now we turn to Technique with an upper-case "T." Chiropractic has been around more than a century. It is no exaggeration to state that, during that time, hundreds of technique systems have been devised, such as Gonstead Technique, Logan Technique, and so on. Most of these technique systems claim to be superior to the others, and to treat a great variety of (if not all) health problems without needing treatment methods that would be found in a different technique system. These, then, are Techniques, with a capital T.

Some chiropractors use the term "Diversified Technique" to refer to the body of generic technique procedures, the sum total of many, if not most, chiropractic techniques.[3] To them, "diversified" just means eclectic, or integrated. On the other hand, some chiropractics use the term

"Diversified Technique" to refer to a standalone system technique, with unique attributes, that we describe in Chapter 17. We take up the special case of Diversified Technique in Appendix 2.

SUBLUXATION

The word "subluxation" is and always has been central to most chiropractors, who have adopted the simplifying assumption that patients suffer at root from the same type of disorder, no matter how extreme the differences in manifestation. Although there are profoundly different definitions from one technique system to another, almost all chiropractors who use the term "subluxation" have in mind that there is something wrong with the spine, that has had negative consequences for human health, and is amenable to manual and other conservative treatments. We have included as Appendix 1 of this book an abstract of our previously published article "Toward a taxonomy of subluxation-equivalents,"[4] in which we amplify this point in great detail. In this book, our usage of "subluxation" is context-sensitive, and derives its full meaning from the entire chapter in which it appears. We chose not to include long discussions in each of the chapters in Section 3 on how each technique system uses the term "subluxation," since readers can obtain our fully developed views in Appendix 1.

According to some scholars, the term "subluxation" can be traced back as far as Hippocrates and Galen,[5] although the word makes its first appearance in the English language in 1746 in the works of Joannes Henricus Hieronymi.[6] In that definition, the term "subluxation" is more in keeping with the use of the word in medical circles, denoting a joint that has limited motion, is painful, and has changed position with respect to other articulations.

The first use of the word subluxation within chiropractic circles can be found in the profession's first textbook, written by Smith, Langworthy and Paxson, (Figs 2.1–2.3) and entitled *Modernized Chiropractic*.[7] In their use of the word, Smith and his colleagues referred to a subluxated vertebra as differing from a normal vertebra in terms of its field of motion, that could be either too

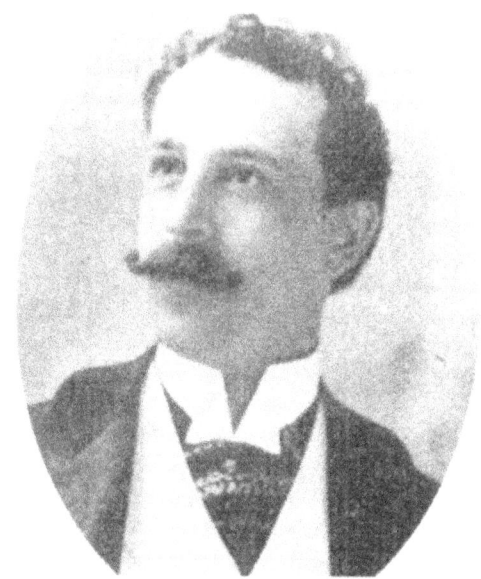

Figure 2.1 Solon M Langworthy, one of the most influential of early chiropractors, was a 1901 graduate of DD Palmer's. He established the American School of Chiropractic in Cedar Rapids, IA, in 1903 and published the first chiropractic textbook, *Modernized Chiropractic*, in 1906. Courtesy of Palmer College of Chiropractic Archives, Davenport, IA.

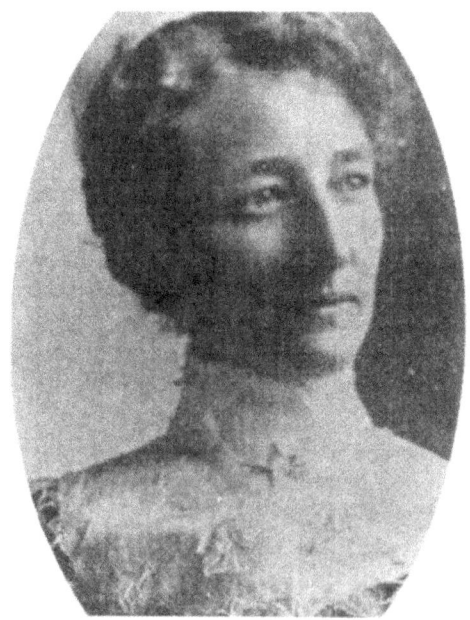

Figure 2.2 Minora C Paxson, an 1899 graduate of DD Palmer's, in 1905 received the first license in the nation to practice chiropractic and coauthored the 1906 *Modernized Chiropractic* with Oakley Smith and Solon Langworthy, then seemed to disappear from the profession. Courtesy of Palmer College of Chiropractic Archives, Davenport, IA.

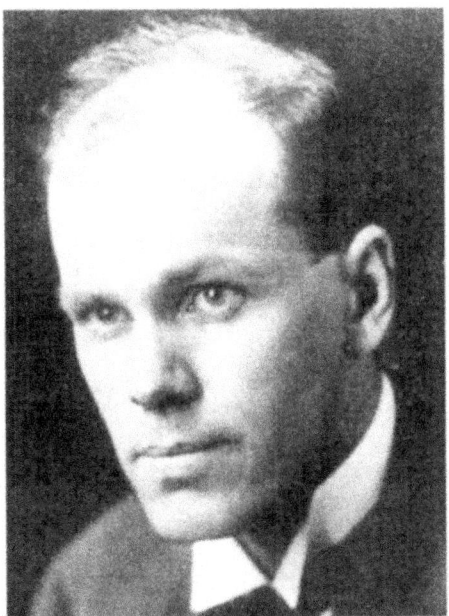

Figure 2.3   Oakley G Smith, an 1899 graduate of DD Palmer's Chiropractic School and Cure, studied at the University of Iowa Medical School from 1899 to 1901. In 1906, he established the American School of Chiropractic in Cedar Rapids, IA, and coauthored *Modernized Chiropractic* with colleagues Minora Paxson and Solon Langworthy. In 1907, he moved to Chicago and founded the Chicago College of Naprapathy. Courtesy of Palmer College of Chiropractic Archives, Davenport, IA.

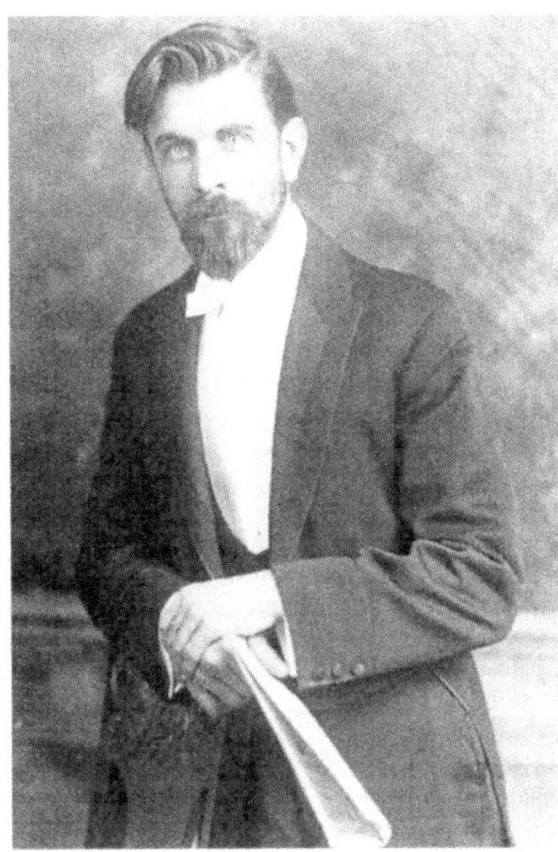

Figure 2.4   Formal photograph of BJ Palmer *c.* 1910. Courtesy of Palmer College of Chiropractic Archives, Davenport, IA.

great or too limited. This definition differed from the one favored by the profession's developer DD Palmer, who saw subluxation as an intervertebral malalignment less than a full-blown joint dislocation. DD Palmer's son, BJ Palmer (Fig. 2.4), added to the definition that there should be an element of nerve interference (Ch. 34). The malalignment concept eventually culminated in a system of radiographic classifications of subluxations, to address reimbursement matters under Medicare and Medicaid in the USA, a finding no longer required after the year 2000.[6] In her textbook, Gatterman[6] describes the debate that eventually required the differentiation between those subluxations amenable to manipulation and subluxations for which manipulation would be contraindicated, a topic beyond the scope of this book.

It should also be mentioned that, although many in the chiropractic profession reject the concept of "subluxation" and shun the use of this term as a diagnosis, the presidents of at least a dozen chiropractic colleges of the Association of Chiropractic Colleges developed a consensus definition of "subluxation" in 1996. It reads:

Chiropractic is concerned with the preservation and restoration of health, and focuses particular attention on the subluxation. A subluxation is a complex of functional and/or structural and/or pathological articular changes that compromise neural integrity and may influence organ system function and general health. A subluxation is evaluated, diagnosed, and managed through the use of chiropractic procedures based on the best available rational and empirical evidence.[8]

It should be noted that several national chiropractic organizations, including the American Chiropractic Association, the International Chiropractic Association and the World Federation of

Chiropractic, have adopted this Association of Chiropractic Colleges paradigm.[4]

MANIPULATION AND ADJUSTMENT

Technique systems often draw careful distinctions between "manipulation" and "adjustment." Although pages can be and have been written on the subject, the gist is that an adjustive thrust is usually said to use a short lever (such as a transverse or spinous process) to correct a segmental misalignment associated with nerve interference (see below), whereas a manipulation uses longer leverage to increase range of motion, usually in a non-specific sense. In this book, we use the term "manipulation" to refer to a high-velocity, low-amplitude (HVLA) thrust, sometimes simply described as a dynamic thrust, that moves a joint into the paraphysiological space, beyond what is accessible through active and passive movements.

We used the term "adjustive thrust" above to convey the notion that, unlike manipulations, some adjustments are performed using low, even minimal, force. Some chiropractors would add that an adjustment corrects "nerve interference" or in some other way normalizes the nervous system, whereas manipulation is intended only to affect musculoskeletal structures, perhaps to improve range of motion. It may be high-force or low-force, manually applied, or instrument-assisted, but in the end the sine qua non of the adjustment is that it corrects the subluxation to eliminate nerve interference. Adjustment for subluxation is the cornerstone of chiropractic technique; barring that, there would be nothing left that is uniquely chiropractic.

Some chiropractors reserve the word "adjustment" for vertebral segments only, while other chiropractors are comfortable stating that they can adjust any osseus articulation from the atlas to the sphenoid to the talus. To complicate matters further, some chiropractors state they do not "treat" the spine to relieve pain or ameliorate diseases, but "adjust" or "correct" it to remove or reduce subluxations. The general public frequently equates the chiropractic adjustment with an HVLA thrust (the type that makes "popping noises" in the spine), most often directed on the spine.

In this book the term "adjustment" is used broadly, referring to any chiropractic procedure aimed at correcting specific joint dysfunction, or, simply put, subluxation. An adjustive procedure may use low or relatively higher forces; it may be delivered by hand or by instrument. A recent article by Meeker and Haldeman[5] emphasized that the underlying principle separating a generic non-chiropractic manipulation from a chiropractic manipulation or adjustment is the *intent* of the practitioner. Of course, this "therapeutic intent" varies greatly between practitioners and much depends on the subluxation-equivalent the clinician purports to be correcting.

NERVE INTERFERENCE

A concept central to many chiropractic Techniques described in this textbook, innate intelligence,[9] has been both a source of inspiration and derision within the chiropractic profession (Figs 2.5[10] and 2.6[11,12,10]). It was first described by DD Palmer, who began his career as a magnetic healer and combined that approach with his interest in other disciplines, namely Christian Science, faith cure, mind cure, metaphysics, and osteopathy.[9] According to Morgan,[9] Palmer seemed to blend these beliefs into what would become Innate Intelligence, which he described as "a segment of that Intelligence which fills the universe, this universe, all wise, is metamerised, divided into metemeres as needed by individual being." Innate, in Palmer's view, was eternal and had a dual existence as both physical reality and a spiritual being. By contrast, the mind only existed during the person's lifetime.[9]

It is tempting to look up this hallowed expression in someone's glossary of chiropractic terms, and there are certainly several excellent ones among which to choose. However, rather than provide an answer that is technically "correct" and properly referenced, we might better explain how this controversial expression has been used by most chiropractors, from an operational point of view. First, most technique systems believe that the central goal of chiropractic care is to eliminate or reduce as much as possible any

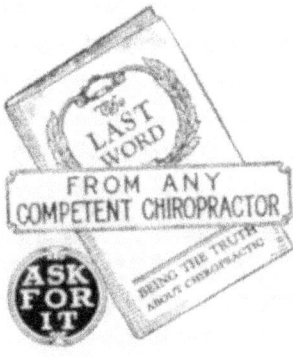

Figure 2.5   A 1923 advertisement from *Photoplay* magazine features Innate Intelligence. Reproduced from Keating J C Jr 2002 The meaning of innate. Journal of The Canadian Chiropractic Association 46(1): 4–10.[10]

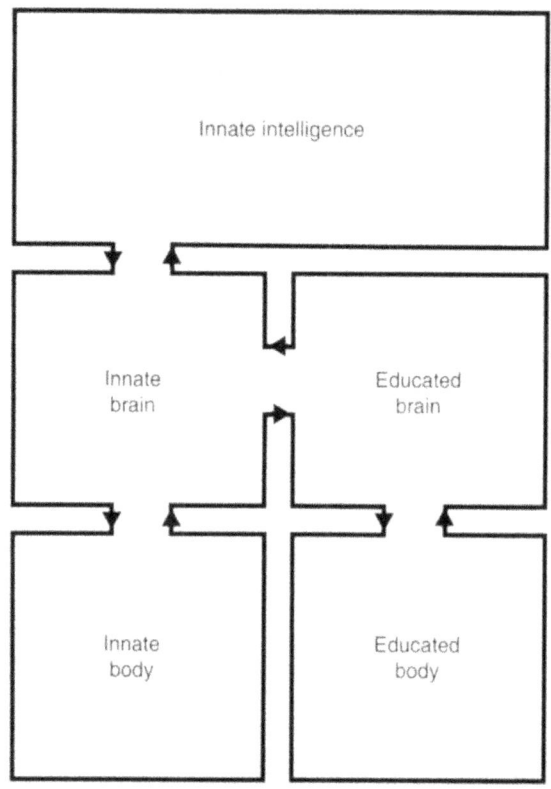

Figure 2.6 "The most valuable drawing in the world – for it solves all the problems of man" (BJ Palmer, quoted in *Digest of Chiropractic Economics*[11]): the diagram originally appeared in Stephenson's *Chiropractic Textbook*.[12] Reproduced from Keating J C Jr 2002 The meaning of innate. Journal of The Canadian Chiropractic Association 46(1): 4–10.[10]

impediment to the normal functioning of the nervous system, to maximize the body's ability to recover from the noxious effects of any threat to health and heal itself. Nerve interference distorts not only the central nervous system's control of effector organs, such as muscles and glands, but also the information flow from the periphery back to the central nervous system, upon which it depends for proper regulation of effector organs and muscles. The appropriateness of control mechanisms is therefore dependent on the accuracy of the incoming afferent information.

The concept of a supposed non-verbal communication between the innate intelligence of the doctor and that of the patient can be found in Van Rumpt's Directional Non-Force Technique

(DNFT; Ch. 18). In DNFT, the doctor mentally asks the patient's innate intelligence to indicate where the subluxation of the patient is located while he or she is prone. The doctor then inspects for leg-length changes (Ch. 4); this is thought to manifest a communication from the innate intelligence of the patient. Morter, developer of Bioenergetic Synchronization Technique (BEST; Ch. 13) defined Innate by stating that there is "irrefutable evidence of the functioning of an intelligent plan that was placed in and put in operation in that fertilized egg at the moment of conception. Conscious thought was in no way involved in the process."[13]

That there exists great divisiveness in the profession surrounding the use of the term "Innate Intelligence" and its place in conventional chiropractic care became abundantly clear from the reaction to an article published in the *Journal of the Canadian Chiropractic Association* (JCCA) in 1998 by Lon Morgan.[9] Morgan's article spawned dozens of angry letters to the editor which were published in subsequent issues of the JCCA. Many of these letters vehemently defended the concept of innate intelligence while viciously attacking Morgan himself, accusing him of being "antichiropractic." Perhaps little would be lost if chiropractors started using more modern terms, such as neuropathy or radiculopathy, in place of nerve interference. On the other hand, this somewhat antiquated term retains the essential flavor of the cornerstone of chiropractic philosophy: chiropractic technique doesn't so much heal the body as remove interference to the nervous system's control over the body's ability to heal itself.

DIAGNOSIS AND SPINAL ANALYSIS

Some would say the medical doctor *diagnoses* conditions, eventually to *treat* symptoms; whereas the chiropractor *analyses* the spine to *identify* and *correct* subluxations, irrespective of the presence or absence of symptoms. Again, our usage of these terms is context-sensitive, since not all technique systems place equal emphasis on these distinctions, and some place none. We will often use the terms "examination," "diagnostic," or "assessment" procedure in place of these controversial terms, in order to steer clear of chiropractic philosophical matters, which are not our primary concern in writing this book.

WCA POSITION STATEMENT

In July 2002, the World Chiropractic Alliance (WCA) issued a position statement on the issue of chiropractic care for asymptomatic patients, comparing "asymptomatic" subluxations to high blood pressure (the silent killer) and dental cavities (often detectable only by radiographs). This statement was prompted by the suspension of a New York chiropractor who, according to one article, was suspended for treating patients without symptoms earlier in the year.[14] In part, it was the position of the WCA that:

the presence of symptoms and/or a medical diagnosis should not be a factor in determining the need for or appropriateness of chiropractic adjustments, nor should the presence of symptoms be required by any chiropractic board, insurance company or court of law to justify the rendering of chiropractic care to any patient.[15]

REFERENCES

1. Owens E 2000 Theoretical constructs of vertebral subluxations as applied by chiropractic practitioners and researchers. Topics in Clinical Chiropractic 7 (1): 74–79
2. Nelson C F 1993 Chiropractic scope of practice (commentary). Journal of Manipulative and Physiological Therapeutics 16 (7): 488–497
3. Cooperstein R 1995 On Diversified Chiropractic Technique. Journal of Chiropractic Humanities 5 (1): 50–55
4. Cooperstein R, Gleberzon B J 2001 Toward a taxonomy of subluxation-equivalents. Topics in Clinical Chiropractic 8 (1): 49–60
5. Meeker W C, Haldeman S 2002 Chiropractic: a profession at the crossroads of mainstream and alternative medicine. Annals of Internal Medicine 136: 216–227
6. Gatterman M 1995 Advances in subluxation terminology and usage. In: Gatterman M (ed.) Advances in chiropractic, pp. 461–469 Mosby-Year Book, St Louis, MO
7. Smith O G, Langworthy S M, Paxon M C 1906 Modernized chiropractic, vol. 1, p. 26. Lawrence Press, Cedar Rapids, IO
8. Association of Chiropractic Colleges 1996 The ACC chiropractic paradigm. Journal of Manipulative and Physiological Therapeutics 19 (9): 634–637
9. Morgan L 1998 Innate Intelligence: its origins and problems. Journal of the Canadian Chiropractic Association 42 (1): 35–41
10. Keating J C Jr 2002 The meaning of innate. Journal of the Canadian Chiropractic Association 46 (1): 4–10
11. Frigard T L 1994 How the elite one percent use the innate factor to achieve noble goals. Digest of Chiropractic Economics (September/October): 36–37
12. Stephenson R W 1927 Chiropractic Textbook. Palmer School of Chiropractic, Davenport, IA
13. Morter M T 1984 Innate friend or foe? Digest of Chiropractic Economics July/August: 133, 491
14. WCA 2002 WCA fights for right to care for asymptomatic patient. Chiropractic Journal 16 (10): 36
15. WCA 2002 Position paper on chiropractic for asymptomatic patients. Reprinted in Chiropractic Journal July 16 (10): 37

3

Core chiropractic adjustive methods

Not surprisingly, the same adjustive methods seem to come up over and over again among the various technique systems. Some of these methods belong so much to a given technique system that the latter is essentially defined by it, e.g., flexion–distraction adjusting defines the Cox Technique (Ch. 16). Others, such as side-posture manipulation, are commonly used in many if not most of the technique systems. We thought it best to describe briefly the primary adjustive methods in this chapter, to avoid redundancy in Section 3, which describes the technique systems.

In the early 1990s, the Panel of Advisors to the American Chiropractic Association Council on Technique produced a detailed algorithm for the categorization of chiropractic technique procedures,[1,2] one that is frequently cited. Treatment procedures are first classified as either manual or non-manual. The manual procedures are divided into articular and extra-articular procedures. The articular procedures are further characterized as specific or non-specific, and as either using a manual force that is mechanically assisted or a mechanical force that is manually assisted. Finally, all the articular procedures are characterized according to their leverage (long, short, long and short), their velocity, and their amplitude. Although we find this algorithm useful in some ways, we elected to take a more descriptive approach in preparing this chapter, the purpose of which is less to categorize and more to make readers aware of how chiropractors apply adjustive procedures.

HVLA, WITH DROP-TABLE ASSIST

A drop table (Fig. 3.1) has one or more table sections, underlying different regions of the patient, that are designed to fall through a small distance when the doctor applies a thrust to a part of the patient's body. The droppable section of the table is held aloft by a cam mechanism until the thrust is applied. The doctor is able to adjust the amount of force it takes to set the table section in motion. Drop tables may be used with the patient prone (Fig. 3.2), supine, or lying on the side (in side-posture).

Drop tables are sometimes thought to allow the application of high-velocity, low-amplitude (HVLA) forces in a relatively safe manner, since

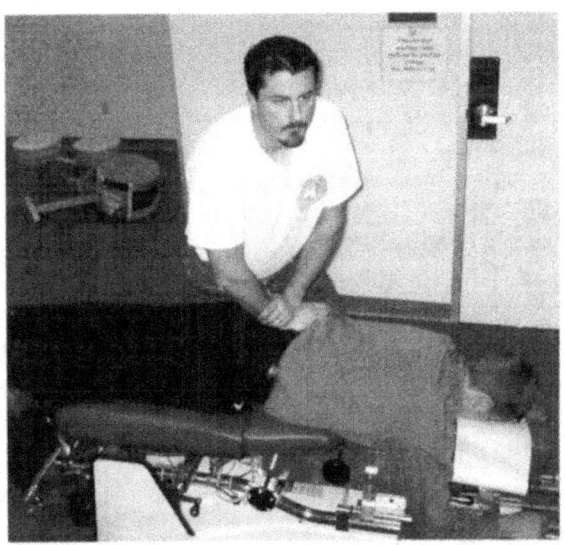

Figure 3.1 Drop-table manipulation.

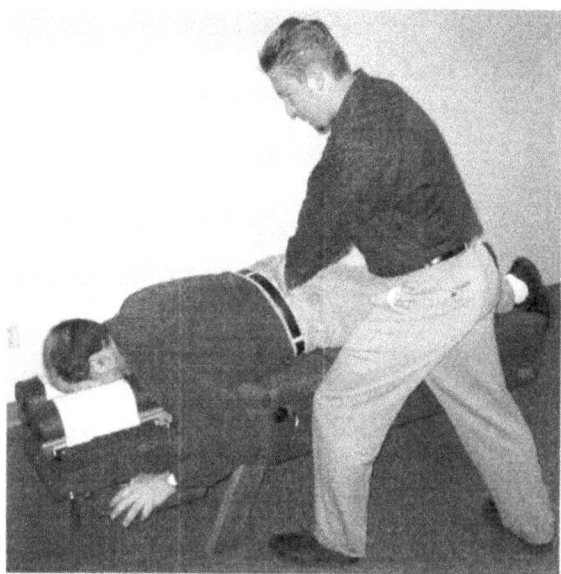

Figure 3.2 Prone drop.

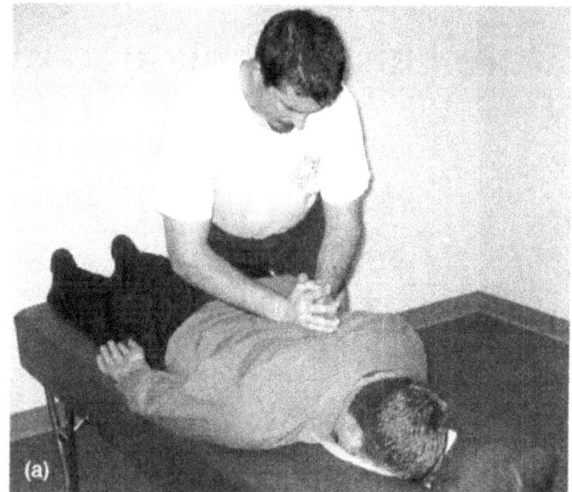

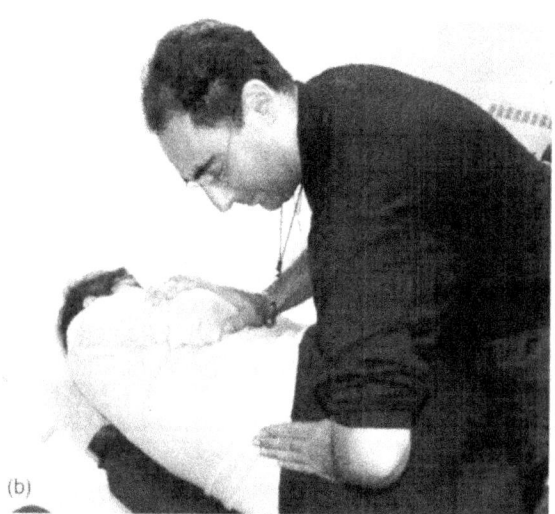

Figure 3.3 Patient receiving HVLA/thrust (a) prone; (b) in side-posture.

the distance through which the patient's body is moved is limited by the design of the cam mechanism. The term "high-velocity" speaks for itself; by "low amplitude," it is meant that the part of the patient which is contacted moves through a short distance. Drop-table techniques are relatively doctor-friendly, at least compared with side-posture adjusting (see below), in that the height of many drop tables can be adjusted in accordance with the doctor's height. In a sense (although the comment is often abused), the "table does the work." In other words, even a doctor with a back injury can apply an HVLA thrust using a drop table. Chapters 23 and 29 on the Pierce– Stillwagon and Thompson Techniques, respectively, are largely about drop-table adjustive methods.

HVLA, NO DROP TABLE

An HVLA thrust is applied with the patient lying supine, prone (Fig. 3.3a), or in side-posture (Fig. 3.3b) on an adjusting table. None of the table's drop pieces, if it has any, are deployed during the adjustment. In a side-posture adjustment, the patient's upside knee is brought towards his or her abdomen, while the doctor stabilizes the patient's torso by placing a hand upon either the patient's upside shoulder or forearms in front of the abdominal area. The doctor applies a manual

thrust to the lumbopelvic area, to which this method is largely restricted, on either a lumbar vertebra or one of the pelvic bones. There are infinite variations on the theme, having to do with how specific is the contact on the patient, whether the prestress on the patient uses rotation or not, whether leverage is applied to the patient's downside leg, and so on. Joint cavitation is typical but not mandatory. Chapters 17 and 20 on Diversified and Gonstead techniques, respectively, are largely about side-posture adjustive methods.

HVLA methods may also be applied to supine (Fig. 3.4a) and prone patients (Fig. 3.4b), in the

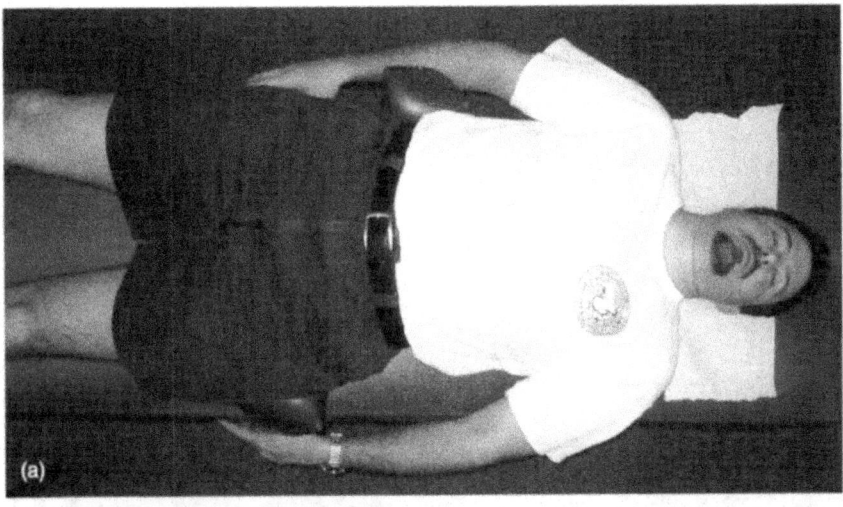

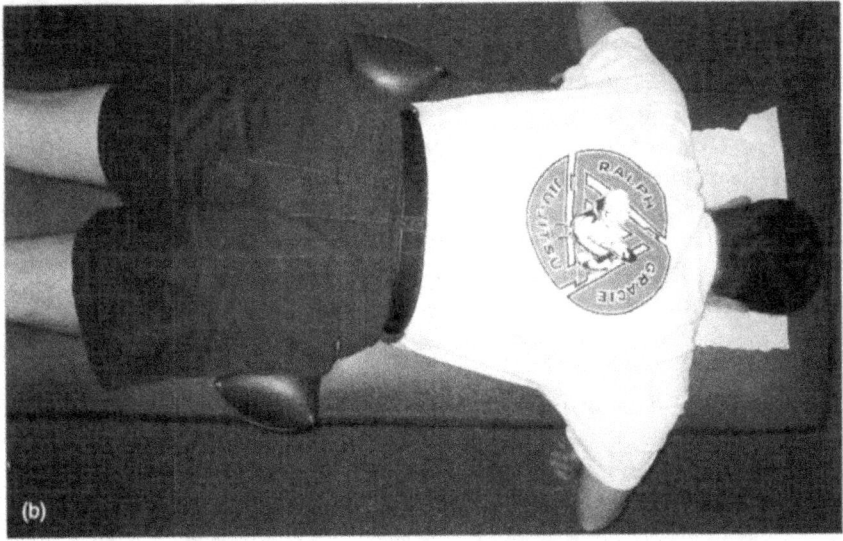

Figure 3.4 (a) Supine patient; (b) prone patient.

cervical, thoracic, and lumbar regions. The prone moves are usually applied to the cervical and thoracic spines, but may be applied to the lumbar spine as well. The supine moves are usually applied to the thoracic spine, but may be applied to the upper lumbar vertebral levels as well, as anterior thoracic and anterior lumbar maneuvers, respectively.

PELVIC BLOCKING PROCEDURES

A pair of padded wedges (blocks) are inserted under the patient's pelvis for various periods of time, one under each hemipelvis, in a position thought to be appropriate for that patient's condition. The patient may be either prone or supine, and the precise direction in which the padded wedges are inserted varies according to the patient's examination findings. The patient is kept on the wedges for 2 min or less if supine, and possibly for longer periods of time if prone. The adjustment is accomplished by means of gravity applied across asymmetrically placed fulcrums, and must be considered a relatively low-force method. Chapter 25 on Sacro-Occipital Technique describes the system technique most likely to deploy padded wedges.

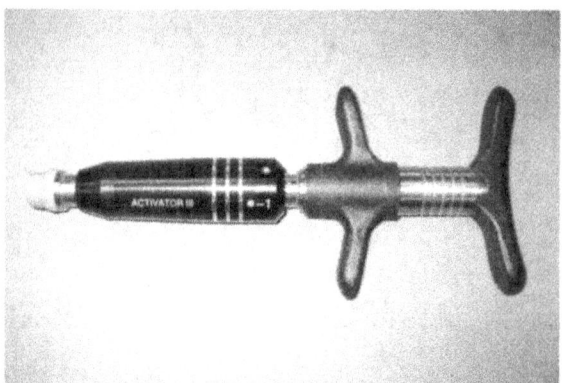

Figure 3.5 Activator adjusting instrument.

INSTRUMENT ADJUSTING

The adjustive force is applied by a percussive device that features a stylus tip that is in direct contact with the chosen segmental contact point of the subject. Although instrument adjusting developed within the Upper Cervical Technique milieu, it has become popular as a full-spine adjustive method during the last two decades. Several mechanical means have been devised to deliver the adjustive force, using, for example, cockable cams or solenoids. Some adjusting instruments are handheld (Fig. 3.5), some are mounted on the adjusting table, and some are integrated into devices that stand on the floor. Most have the capacity to adjust the force level, and some are designed to effect complex motions, such as turning during the thrust. Chapters 10, 31, and 32 on Activator, Torque Release Technique, and Instrumented Upper Cervical Techniques, respectively, include discussion on instrumented adjusting. To a lesser extent, Chapters 14 and 27, Chiropractic Biophysics and Spinal Biomechanics, also involve instrumented adjusting.

DISTRACTION MANIPULATION

A y-axis distractive force is applied to the axial skeleton, manually assisted and segmentally specific, possibly coupled with either flexion or, more rarely, extension (Fig. 3.6). Although distraction methods were originally designed to treat the low back, they are now being used to treat the cervical

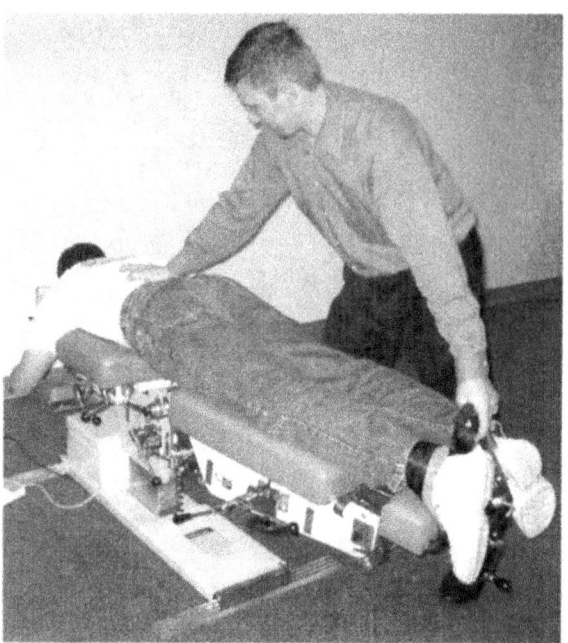

Figure 3.6 Flexion–distraction.

spine as well. This technique generally involves using special tables designed to combine safely flexion and traction of the spinal region being treated. Chapter 16 on flexion–distraction is the most immediately relevant chapter.

MOBILIZATION

The adjustive force is applied singularly or repetitively within or at the end of a joint's physiological range of motion, without imparting a thrust or impulse (Fig. 3.7). Although mobilization is more common outside chiropractic, such as in osteopathy and physical therapy, we thought it commonly enough used in chiropractic to warrant inclusion in this chapter. Even techniques that favor HVLA methods, such as Gonstead or Diversified, adapt their manual methods to the patient's condition, which may require a less forceful technique, such as mobilization. In a sense, the mobilization procedures may be thought of as including blocking procedures and flexion–distraction procedures, as described above, differing only in that mobilization is purely manual, rather than mechanically assisted.

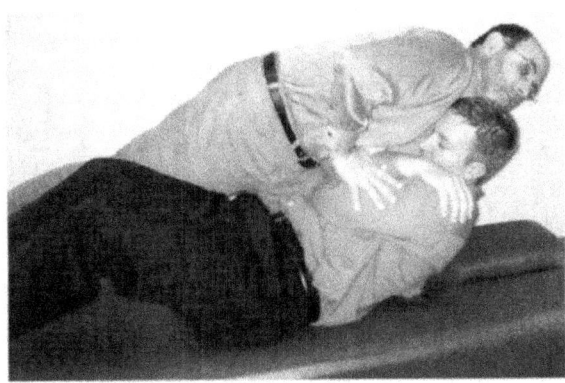

Figure 3.7   Anterior thoracic.

LOW-FORCE ADJUSTIVE TECHNIQUES (REFLEX TECHNIQUES, SOFT-TISSUE TECHNIQUES)

There is no simple way to render the thought here. Many chiropractic techniques use very low forces, although the system technique that describes itself as "non-force" (DNFT, Ch. 18), protestations notwithstanding, does use force – as any must, to bring about a mechanical effect. Some individuals would say that instrumented adjusting is a low-force method, and it is probably true that no mechanical percussive device has ever been designed to deliver a force in excess of those that can be achieved through hand adjusting. On the other hand, the substantial acceleration that can be achieved by such devices does bear on the forces that they may develop, since force equals mass times acceleration ($F = ma$). The use of padded wedges (Ch. 25) qualifies as a low-force adjustive method, and no doubt there are ways of using drop tables (Chs. 23 and 29) and distraction equipment (Ch. 16) that would constitute low-force methods, again, in comparison to some times of purely manual adjusting.

Then there is the world of reflex technique. A chiropractic reflex technique purports to examine or treat the patient by means of speculative physiological pathways that *tend to* lie outside what has been established by normal science. Such techniques often, but not always, claim undocumented connections between body parts and functions, such as a specific point on the thumb

that would relate to cardiac function, or a tender point in the trapezius muscle that would influence uterine function. We should not confuse such reflex techniques with other, proven usages of the word "reflex," as in "deep tendon reflex" or "pathological reflex." Reflex techniques tend to be less forceful than other techniques, although nothing prevents a reflex practitioner from using a highly accelerated thrusting technique.

Sacro-Occipital Technique (Ch. 25) and Applied Kinesiology (Ch. 11) and its spinoff kinesiologies (Ch. 12) are probably the leading (in terms of numbers of practitioners) chiropractic reflex technique systems. Other examples, although we are not certain in each case that the technique developers would concur, include: Bioenergetic Synchronization Technique (Ch. 13), Cranial procedures (Ch. 15), Directional Non-Force Technique (Ch. 18), Network Spinal Analysis (Ch. 22), Spinal Stressology (Ch. 28), and Toftness Technique (Ch. 30). It is debatable whether the Logan Technique (Ch. 21), which claims many practitioners, is truly a reflex technique, since the founder, Hugh Logan, argued that it was not. About the same can be said of Receptor-Tonus Technique (Ch. 24), since founder Nimmo felt that his trigger point work effected mechanical results directly, even if mediated by subtle neurological pathways.

The use of diagnostic measures like compression and isolation testing may qualify Activator Methods Chiropractic Technique (Ch. 10) as to some degree a reflex technique (Fig. 3.8), although some individuals may argue that the use of instrumented adjusting is a more important justification for such a classification, a point with which we do not agree. The use of a mechanical instrument to deliver force does not automatically qualify a technique procedure as proceeding through a reflex mechanism, at least not in our sense of reflex mechanisms, as discussed above. Torque Release Technique (Ch. 31) may be similarly regarded.

Finally, there is a great variety of soft-tissue methods used in chiropractic (Ch. 26), some more or less borrowed from other professions (e.g., the osteopathic strain–counterstrain technique of Jones), some developed concurrently with other professions (e.g., the trigger point work of

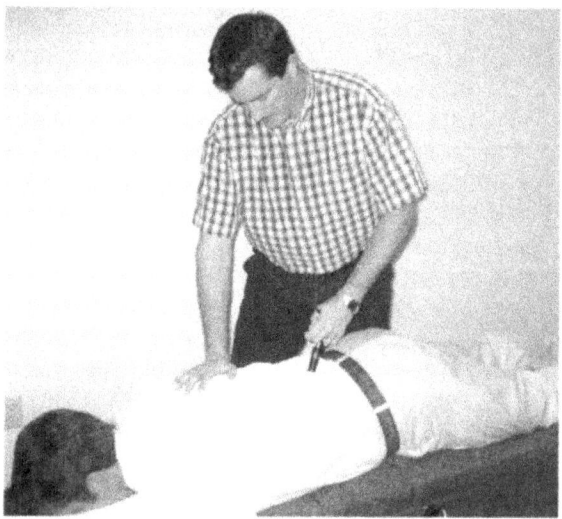

Figure 3.8   Activator Methods Chiropractor Technique.

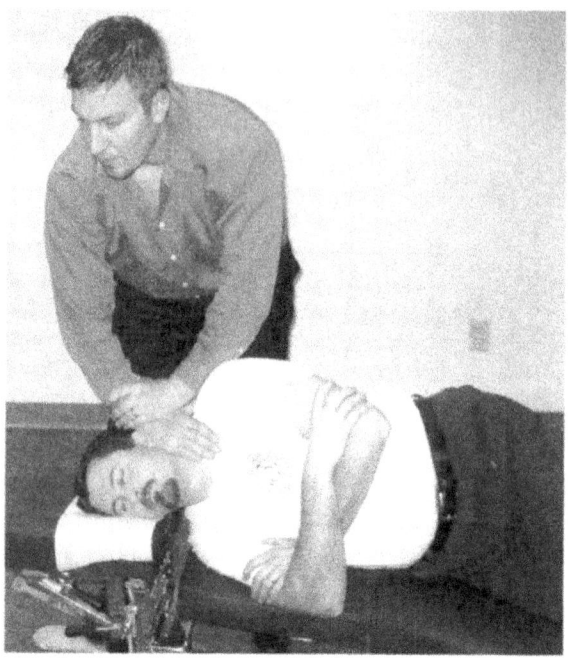

Figure 3.9   Toggle recoil.

Nimmo, Ch. 24), and others almost uniquely chiropractic (e.g., Chiropractic Manipulative Reflex Technique, Ch. 25). Some of these soft-tissue methods are seen and deployed as rehabilitative methods, more or less adjunctive to adjustments, whereas others are seen as adjustive procedures in themselves, in that they are thought to confront nerve interference directly (Receptor-Tonus Technique, Ch. 24).

UPPER CERVICAL

Unlike all the other adjustive methods described in this chapter, Upper Cervical methods (Fig. 3.9) are defined by the location of force application, not their mechanical properties. Upper Cervical adjustments are delivered by a variety of means, including high-force and low-force techniques.

Upper Cervical adjustive methods can be classified as part of a larger category that might be called "extraregional;" these have in common that the impact on the body is thought to occur somewhere other than the point application. A technique that concentrates on the foot, to impact upon the locomotor system, and therefore effect changes within the entire spine, would also qualify as an extraregional technique, parallel to Upper Cervical technique in that regard. From this point of view, Upper Cervical and other extraregional techniques would also qualify as reflex techniques, but only to the extent that the mechanism by which the remote effect unfolds is speculative.

REFERENCES

1. Bartol K M 1992 Algorithm for the categorization of chiropractic technique procedures. Chiropractic Technique 4 (1): 8–14

2. Bartol K M 1991 A model for the categorization of chiropractic treatment procedures. Chiropractic Technique 3 (2): 78–80

Core chiropractic diagnostic/assessment procedures

Section 2 covers, in turn, leg checking, static and motion palpation, manual muscle testing, radiography as assessed through X-ray line marking, thermography, and selected instrumentation procedures. The rationale for Section 2 is quite straightforward. Although each of the technique systems is distinct enough from the others to warrant its own chapter, in many cases they share similar core assessment methods. Our short descriptions of mainstream diagnostic and assessment methods in this section avoids the composition of redundant discussions in various chapters, and also spares the readers the repetitive task of having to read such discussions. This allows Section 3 to more easily focus on the differences among the technique systems in their diagnostic and assessment methods.

Leg checking, manual

INTRODUCTION

Manual leg checking is typically used by Upper Cervical techniques, Diversified, Pierce–Stillwagon, Thompson, Sacro-Occipital Technique, Activator Methods, Directional Non-Force Technique, and many others.

I remember my first out-patient visit very well. I was standing around about half an hour before the clinic closed on a Friday afternoon, when an old man showed up for an unscheduled visit. His regular intern wasn't there. As the office manager's forefinger began its inexorable rise and aim in my direction, I felt my soul possessed of an angst I had previously supposed confined to death row inmates. Yes, they wanted me to see this patient! Having apparently managed to introduce myself to the old man – but only "apparently," since he was too hard of hearing to make any sense of my pseudo-confident assortment of mumbled expressions of good will – I laid him down. (Prone, so he couldn't see the blank look in my eyes and the rivulets of sweat pouring down my face.) Seemingly interminable moments raced by as a stuporous paralysis yielded to a dreadful solipsism. And then it happened. From somewhere deep within the words arose, and I thankfully knew what to do – "check the legs"! As I reached for the old man's ankles, a flood of technique maxims chased the fog from my mind. I checked those legs for a very long period of time, until one or two arbitrarily chosen things-to-do had prevailed over the less-favored options. I know now that the main reason why most of us check the legs is to stall for enough time to figure out what to really do...[1]

We are certain that every chiropractor who has ever done a leg check, whether he or she admits it or not, has at least once experienced a moment of doubt in which the entire procedure suddenly seemed, well, silly. After all, peering down at the patient's feet, what rational adult would *not* wonder whether the legs appear of different length due to subluxation (or something like that), or whether they just happen to be of really different lengths?

The respect afforded leg checking by those who have grown accustomed to its use is exceeded only by the scorn of the skeptics, who find it bizarre that any thinking person, let alone a doctor, would find it useful to inspect the feet carefully, when the patient, after all, complains of neck or back pain. Strong opinions notwithstanding, very little quantitative or qualitative information is available as to what precisely is being measured, what creates the putative functional short leg, how stable it might be, how it may be distinguished from an anatomical short leg, or what pathological significance it may have.

Neither outright rejection nor uncritical faith in leg checking makes sense if leg checking is seen for what it is: a single component of what could be a full-fledged, bilateral determination of non-weight-bearing foot posture. The foot, like any other segment of the body, is capable of deviating from a neutral postural position (however defined) in any of six degrees of freedom: three of translation and three of rotation. The conventional leg checker, in focusing on y-axis "shortening" of the leg as evidenced by foot position, mostly ignores the other five degrees of freedom, to the point that he or she usually regards their variations as mere noise confounding the signal. This error of omission is easily corrected.[2–4]

As for the future of leg checking, we think leg checking, like rock'n'roll, is here to stay.

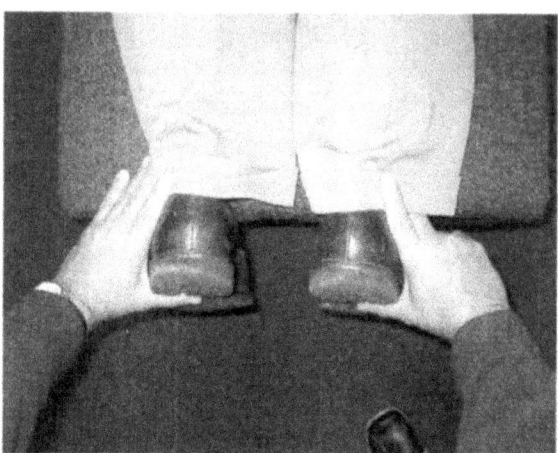

Figure 4.1 Leg-length inequality.

OVERVIEW

Chiropractic leg checking involves determining the relative "length" of the legs – more precisely, determining the relative position of the distal legs – in either a supine or prone patient, by careful observation of the location of the feet. In the Derifield variation of the prone leg check, the feet are also carefully observed with the knees flexed to 90°.

Asymmetry in distal foot positions may be the result of an actual discrepancy in the length of the lower extremities, i.e., structural leg-length inequality (LLI; Fig. 4.1), or may result from a postural imbalance, i.e., functional LLI.[5] Many chiropractors and allied health professionals feel that LLI, whether structural or functional, may contribute to musculoskeletal pain and degenerative changes, and requires treatment. Moreover, chiropractors believe that functional LLI has diagnostic significance as well, providing evidence of subluxation, generally either intrapelvic (pelvic torsion) or upper cervical (atlas). That granted, reduction of functional LLI serves as an outcome measure, providing evidence of more symmetry in body function and structure.

HISTORY

We do not know who first checked the legs, nor even in what profession, given that chiropractors,

physical therapists, and osteopaths all have versions of leg-checking procedures. We do know that one of the most venerable of leg-checking procedures, what is now called the Derifield leg check, was developed by Dr. Weldon Derifield, a 1936 graduate of the Palmer College, and his father, Dr. Romer Derifield.[6,8] According to the late J Clay Thompson, a leading proponent of leg checking, Romer Derifield, having pioneered prone leg checking, later discovered quite fortuitously that leg lengths occasionally changed when the patient rotated the head. This led to the concept of "cervical syndrome" (Ch. 29). As Thompson recounts the story,[9] Derifield, who worked for a railroad in Detroit at the time, was having trouble treating a difficult case. One day the phone rang for the patient while his legs were being checked. As he turned his head to speak, the legs suddenly and unexpectedly evened. Further investigation by Derifield into this case and others revealed that thrusting into tender nodules in the (mostly upper) cervical spine would not only reduce patients' symptomatology but ameliorate prone LLI. Thompson credits a Dr. Alvin Niblo with the discovery of the negative Derifield.[9]

Other leading proponents of leg-checking procedures have included Fuhr of Activator Methods Chiropractic Technique (Ch. 10), Van Rumpt of Directional Non-Force Technique (Ch. 18), and DeJarnette of Sacro-Occipital Technique (Ch. 25), and many Upper Cervical practitioners, including Grostic and Gregory (Chs 32 and 33). An extremely thorough literature review on LLI was prepared by Donna Mannello in conjunction with the Seventh Annual Conference on Research and Education, 1992.[10] Mannello also published a review article, looking at various concepts of the structural and functional short leg, and how they are measured, in a journal setting.[11]

COMMONLY ASSOCIATED TERMS AND CONCEPTS

- Leg-length inequality (anisomelia, leg-length discrepancy, etc.): asymmetry in distal foot positions, due to anatomic or functional factors
- Leg checking: a procedure usually, but not always, manual and visual, for assessing LLI

- Anatomical short leg (or structural short leg): a leg which is demonstrably shorter than the other leg, due to fracture, deformity, or uneven growth rates
- Functional short leg (or physiological short leg, apparent short leg, etc.): a leg which is actually even in length with the other leg, but which appears shorter due to a postural imbalance that draws up the hip in the non-weight-bearing position
- Supine leg check: leg-checking procedure commonly employed by Upper Cervical practitioners, thought to identify atlas subluxation
- Prone leg check: leg-checking procedure commonly employed by Full-Spine practitioners, usually thought to identify pelvic torsion, with posterior innominate rotation on the short-leg side
- Derifield leg check: a prone leg-checking protocol involving two primary components: (1) assessment of relative leg lengths with the knees extended compared to knees flexed to 90°, identifying pelvic syndrome; and (2) assessment of change in relative leg lengths as the head is turned in either direction, identifying cervical syndrome.

MODE OF USE

Although there are numerous styles of non-instrumented (manual) leg checking, a few common elements can be described. The doctor must standardize how the patient mounts the table, to prevent an arbitrary, artifactual result in leg checking. Often, a Hi-Lo table, which is mechanized so as to allow a standing patient to be gently lowered to the prone position, is used for this purpose. Alternatively, the doctor tries to neutralize the patient's starting position by lifting and tugging on the legs, having the patient try to force them apart, or some other method thought to provide an honest baseline condition. The prone or supine patient must be centered on the table, parallel to the long axis of the table (Fig. 4.2). The doctor usually removes any resting asymmetry in the foot posture as gently as possible, prior to looking for y-axis translatory asymmetry of the distal feet

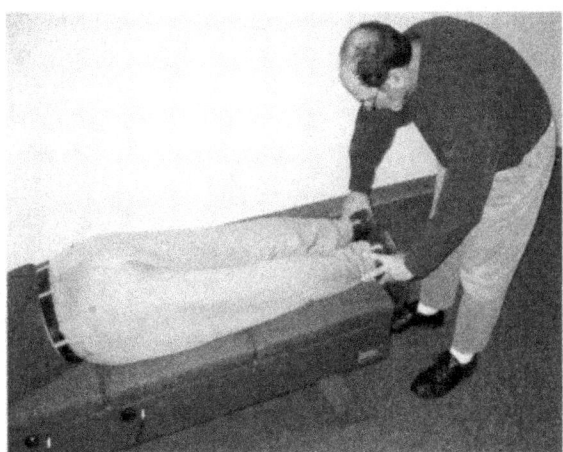

Figure 4.2   The prone leg check.

(a torturous way of saying looking for a short leg). This means removing any or all of the following triaxial rotations: dorsiflexion/plantarflexion, internal/external rotation, inversion/eversion. Finally, often with mild cephalad pressure, the doctor carefully observes the relative position of an anatomic or external landmark, such as the medial malleolus, calcaneus, or union of the heel and shoe if the patient has not removed the shoes.

The Derifield subtype of the prone leg check would go on to assess relative foot elevation from the table with the knees flexed, and with the knees extended as the head is rotated. Finally, sometimes the doctor looks for changes in relative distal leg positions as mild clinical interventions (usually called challenges) are executed, such as applying mild pressure to a vertebral segment thought to be subluxated, or having the patient touch a suspected level of involvement with the fingers. The Derifield leg check, owing to its historical association with the Thompson Terminal Point Technique, is further discussed in Chapter 29.

Instrumented leg checking is beyond the scope of this review. Suffice it to say that chiropractors have introduced a number of devices to measure the legs, some manually assisted, including a friction-reduced table,[12] the Chiro-Slide,[13,14] the Anatometer,[15,16] modified surgical boots with indicators,[17] and no doubt many others. Methods used by other professions to measure structural LLI include X-ray, advanced imaging, tape measure methods, a measurement screen, iliac crest palpation, and the indirect method. The indirect method involves placing shims of known dimension under the foot of a standing patient until the iliac crests become even in their distance from the floor.

PHYSIOLOGICAL RATIONALE

Although it seems obvious at first glance that the clinical imperative to identify and possibly correct anatomic LLI is straightforward, in fact this has been very controversial. Some authorities find anatomic LLI an important cause of low-back pain, whereas others do not. As representative studies, we may cite Friberg,[18] who found that about 50% of an asymptomatic population had uneven anatomic leg lengths, and about 75% of the low-back-pain patients had LLI of 5 mm or more; Nourbakhsh and Arab[19] found no such correlation. Compounding the matter is the difficulty in distinguishing functional and structural LLI.[20] Assuming, none the less, that there is some relationship between LLI and back pain, the probable mechanism would be through its effect on the postural mechanism, the resulting asymmetric loads borne by joints, and the increased metabolic expense of maintaining balance.

Turning to the functional (physiological) short leg, the existence of which was confirmed using a special friction-reduced table optimized for that purpose,[21] two primary types of explanation exist, one based on pelvic torsion and the other based on muscle imbalance. Turning first to the pelvic torsion explanation, some authorities[22,23] and probably many practitioners believe that posterior rotation of the innominate bone shortens the ipsilateral leg, presumably by rotating around the sacroiliac joint relative to the other innominate bone and swinging the hip up (Fig. 4.3). This model of the prone short leg was criticized by Cooperstein[24] as being anatomically impossible in the absence of symphysis luxation. Simply put, if innominate rotation about the sacroiliac joint were to hoist the hip up, it would also have to elevate to an even greater extent the symphysis pubis, which is anterior to the hip. This would luxate the symphysis. Strange models like this

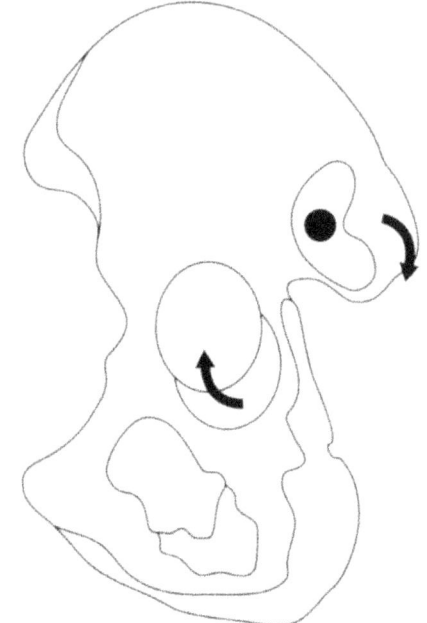

Figure 4.3   Pelvic torsional model of leg-length inequality. Posterior swing of innominate bone thought to raise hip.

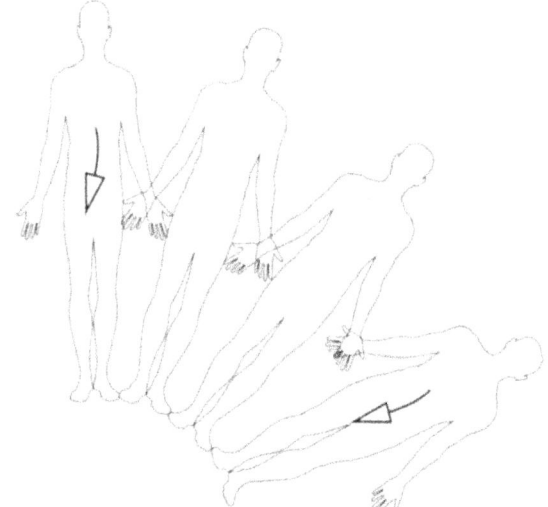

Figure 4.4   Muscle imbalance explanation of leg-length inequality. Increased suprapelvic muscle tone flexes pelvis on trunk.

can also be found in the physiotherapy literature, e.g., Manheimer and Lampe's textbook on transcutaneous electrical nerve stimulation.[25]

The alternative muscular model of the prone short leg (Fig. 4.4) posits that suprainnominate muscle hypertonus and/or soft-tissue contractures hoist up the ipsilateral hip, knee, and foot of the prone patient.[24,26,27] This, of course, does not address the question as to what has caused the putative suprainnominate muscle imbalance and soft-tissue asymmetries, but that is mostly beyond our scope here. Cooperstein hypothesizes[28,29] that if the standing patient carries a hemipelvis low compared to the other, whether due to an anatomic short leg or posterior innominate rotation, postural reflexes would attempt to elevate that ilium via the quadratus lumborum and sacrospinalis muscles. Of course, this cannot succeed in the weight-bearing position, since this would be tantamount to picking up one's leg by the bootstraps, but the only resistance to these muscles pulling the ilium cephalad, and thus creating a short leg, in the prone position would be the friction at the patient–table interface.

As a special variation on this muscular type of explanation for the prone short leg, the Upper Cervical practitioners would add that the underlying mechanism for the pelvic imbalance is due to atlas subluxation. In that context, we frequently see various brain and spinal cord structures said to be involved in this, but we will resist the temptation to go through them.

More recently, less typical leg checks have been described, including the triaxial leg check[2–4,30] and the compressive leg check.[29,31] The significance of the triaxial foot, which shows relatively increased plantarflexion, inversion, and abduction, remains obscure, although it seems to predict an ipsilateral low-standing hip. The compressive leg check seems to identify anatomic LLI, but that is not proven.

Confounding any simple explanation of prone or supine LLI is the finding that, in standing subjects, structural LLI may result in pelvic torsion,[32–36] that could affect the relative acetabular positions, reducing the correlation of radiological parameters with leg-checking results.

EVIDENCE

There have been many studies on the intra- and interexaminer reliability of prone and supine leg checking, and very few on the validity of leg-checking procedures, which has to do with determining to what extent they are accurate, and provide information about the patients that is clinically useful. Lawrence[37] and Mannello[10,38] have provided very useful review articles, mostly on the reliability studies, which are equivocal in their findings. These studies tended to find intraexaminer reliability superior to interexaminer reliability. Although these reviews did not find much support for the reliability of leg checking, a few studies since then have been more encouraging, for both prone[39–41] and supine[42] leg-length assessment procedures. A paper by Cooperstein et al, in press at the time of this writing,[17] summarizes the little that has been published on the validity of prone leg checking.[13,14,40,41,43] Cooperstein et al show the accuracy of compressive leg checking to be ±2 mm;[17] these investigators believe, but have not proven, that compressive leg checking is more likely to detect structural LLI than functional LLI.

Several studies pertaining to the Derifield leg check procedure[44] have been performed. Researchers have attempted to assess the interexaminer reliability of the Derifield pelvic leg check,[45–52] but have failed to demonstrate consistent results. Fuhr and Osterbauer did find a measure of reliability,[45] but Haas and Peterson[46] had methodological criticisms of the study. DeBoer et al[50] found good interexaminer reliability in both the knees-extended and knees-flexed positions, but their interpretation of the data was later questioned by Danelius.[48] By comparison, Rhudy and Burk[52] were unable to obtain significant interexaminer reliability in any of four different evaluations of the Thompson leg-check system, with Thompson himself participating in part of the study. Shambaugh et al[47] reported good interexaminer reliability for the knees-extended position, but this study also has been criticized for improper statistics.[53,54] Falltrick and Pierson[51] failed to find leg reactivity in response to head rotation, but were criticized for failing to exert cephalad pressure on the feet during the test.[55] Cooperstein[56] provides a kinesiological interpretation of the Derifield pelvic leg check, but this otherwise interesting work is data-free.[57]

CONCLUSIONS

- About 50% of an asymptomatic population and 75% of low-back-pain patients may have anatomic LLI of 5 mm or more.[18] Therefore, an examiner finding LLI should not leap to the conclusion that this reflects subluxation or any other type of somatic dysfunction, without first having attempted to rule out anatomic LLI.
- Although the trend is for examiners, at least in laboratory settings, to improve their reliability (concordance) in detecting LLI, this by itself does not bring us closer to discriminating anatomical from functional LLI. Indeed, although it is easy to define and characterize an anatomic short leg, it is more challenging (although not impossible) to prove the existence of and explain the physiological mechanism for a functional short leg.
- Granted there is some evidence that anatomic LLI of some magnitude can result in back pain and other somatic problems, there is little evidence that the putative functional short leg is related to common patient complaints and physical examination findings.
- The prevailing explanation of the functional short leg, which has a posterior rotation of the innominate bone around a sacroiliac axis hoisting up the hip, needs to be withdrawn, unless

we are willing to assume the average patient with a few millimeters of LLI has a dislocated symphysis pubis. The alternative hypothesis of suprapelvic muscle hypertonus and other soft-tissue functional asymmetries, although largely unstudied, results in fewer logical contradictions and thus is preferred from a purely Aristotelian point of view. Occam's razor, you know: don't make up anything more than you need to!

- This hypothesis of non-weight-bearing postural imbalance accounting for functional LLI does not in any way contradict Upper Cervical theories that atlas subluxation may be reflected in such postural imbalance.
- If, indeed, the functional short leg reflects non-weight-bearing postural imbalance, it remains to be seen what specific joint misalignments and/or restrictions (i.e., subluxations) may be related to the overall process. At the present time, theories to the effect that the short leg equals a posterior-inferior ilium, although not without merit, are quite speculative. Studies linking pelvic examination findings, such as posterior superior iliac spine locations or radiological benchmarks, with leg-check findings, are virtually non-existent, although a few may be cited.[31,40-43]

REFERENCES

1. Cooperstein R 1990 Brand name techniques and the confidence gap. Journal of Chiropractic Education 4 (3): 89–93
2. Cooperstein R, Pigg J 1998 Triaxial measurement of foot loading responses as related to pelvic biomechanics. In: Herzog W (ed.) CCCRC 98: Proceedings of the Inaugural Conference, p. 36. Walter Herzog, Calgary, Canada
3. Cooperstein R, Fitzpatrick A 2000 Triaxial assessment of end-range foot posture: a novel and reliable leg checking method. In: FCER 2000 International Conference on Spinal Manipulation, pp. 184–186. Foundation for Chiropractic Education and Research, Northwestern College of Chiropractic, Bloomington, MN
4. Cooperstein R, Pigg J 1999 Triaxial assessment of extreme end-range foot posture: a novel method of leg checking. In: National Vertebral Subluxation Conference, p. 1. Journal of Vertebral Subluxation Research, Spartanburg, SC
5. Cooperstein R, Grunstein J 2002 Interdisciplinary assay of literature pertaining to leg length inequality.

In: Owens E (ed.) 10th Annual Vertebral Subluxation Conference; Sherman College of Straight Chiropractic, Hayward, CA
6. Zemelka W H 1992 The Thompson Technique. Victoria Press, Bettendorf, IA
7. Staff editor PCC presents special awards during homecoming. Dynamic Chiropractic http://www.chiroweb.com/archives/11/22/20.html
8. Jackson D R 1987 Thompson terminal point technique. Today's Chiropractic 16 (3): 73–75.
9. Thompson J C 1977 Thompson Terminal Point Technique. In: Kfoury P W (ed.) Catalog of chiropractic techniques, pp. 89–92. St Louis, MO Logan College of Chiropractic
10. Mannello D 1992 Leg length insufficiency: a review of the literature. In: Proceedings of the 7th Annual Conference on Research and Education, pp. 67–89. Consortium for Chiropractic Research, Palm Springs, CA
11. Mannello D M 1992 Leg length inequality. Journal of Manipulative and Physiological Therapeutics 15 (9): 576–590

12. Cooperstein R, Jansen P 1996 Technology description: the friction-reduced segmented table. Chiropractic Technique 8 (3): 107–111

13. Russo R A 1998 Instrumentation for leg length discrepancy. Today's Chiropractic 27 (3): 92–95

14. Russo R A 1998 Quantifying leg length analysis. Today's Chiropractic 26 (1): 42–44

15. Seemann D C 1990 Exploring the relationship between anatometer measurements and x-ray listings. Upper Cervical Monograph 4 (9): 1–2

16. NUCCA/NUCCRA 2002 NUCCA-NUCCRA historical highlights. http://www.nucca.org/histhigh.html

17. Cooperstein R, Morschhauser E, Lisi A, Nick T G N 2003 Validity of compressive leg checking in measuring artificial leg length inequality. Journal of Manipulative and Physiological Therapeutics (in press)

18. Friberg O 1987 Leg length inequality and low back pain. Clinical Biomechanics 2: 211–219

19. Nourbakhsh M R, Arab A M 2002 Relationship between mechanical factors and incidence of low back pain. Journal of Orthopedic Sports and Physical Therapy 32 (9): 447–460

20. Knutson G A 2000 The functional "short leg"; physiological mechanisms and clinical manifestations. Journal of Vertebral Subluxation Research 4 (1): 22–25

21. Jansen R D, Cooperstein R 1998 Measurement of soft tissue strain in response to consecutively increased compressive and distractive loads on a friction-based test bed. Journal of Manipulative and Physiological Therapeutics 21 (1): 19–26

22. Bergmann T, Peterson D H, Lawrence D J 1994 Chiropractic technique. Churchill Livingstone, New York, NY

23. Gatterman M I 1990 Chiropractic management of spine-related disorders. Williams & Wilkins, Baltimore, MD

24. Cooperstein R 1993 Functional leg length inequality: geometric analysis and an alternative muscular model. In: 8th Annual Conference on Research and Education, pp. 202–203. Consortium for Chiropractic Research, Monterey, CA

25. Manheimer J, Lampe G 1984 Clinical transcutaneous electrical nerve stimulation. F A Davis, Philadelphia

26. Schneider M 1993 The "muscular" short leg. American Journal of Clinical Chiropractic 3 (3): 8

27. Travell J G, Simons D G 1992 Myofascial pain and dysfunction: the trigger point manual, vol. 2. Williams & Wilkins, Baltimore, MD

28. Cooperstein R 1997 The reverse double whammy leg check. Dynamic Chiropractic 15 (16): 35–38

29. Cooperstein R 2000 Integrated chiropractic technique: chiropraxis. Self-published, Oakland, CA

30. Knutson G A 2002 Incidence of foot rotation, pelvic crest unleveling, and supine leg length alignment asymmetry and their relationship to self-reported back pain. Journal of Manipulative and Physiological Therapeutics 25 (2): 110E

31. Cooperstein R, Lisi A 2001 Correlation of PSIS measurements and ankle-joint complex ROM. In: 4th Interdisciplinary World Congress on Low Back and Pelvic Pain, pp. 353–354. Montreal, Canada

32. Cummings G, Scholz J P, Barnes K 1993 The effect of imposed leg length difference on pelvic bone symmetry. Spine 18 (3): 368–373

33. Drerup B, Hierholzer E 1987 Movement of the human pelvis and displacement of related anatomical landmarks on the body surface. Journal of Biomechanics 20 (10): 971–977

34. Young R S, Andrew P D, Cummings G S 2000 Effect of simulating leg length inequality on pelvic torsion and trunk mobility. Gait Posture 11 (3): 217–223

35. Beaudoin L, Zabjek K F, Leroux M A, Coillard C, Rivard C H 1999 Acute systematic and variable postural adaptations induced by an orthopaedic shoe lift in control subjects. European Spine Journal 8 (1): 40–45

36. Pitkin H, Pheasant H 1936 Sacrarthrogenetic telalgia. Journal of Bone and Joint Surgery 18 (2): 365–375

37. Lawrence D 1985 Chiropractic concepts of the short leg: a critical review. Journal of Manipulative and Physiological Therapeutics 8: 157–161

38. Mannello D M 1992 Leg length inequality. Journal of Manipulative and Physiological Therapeutics 15 (9): 576–590

39. Nguyen H T, Resnick D N, Caldwell S G et al 1999 Interexaminer reliability of activator methods' relative leg-length evaluation in the prone extended position. Journal of Manipulative and Physiological Therapeutics 22 (9): 565–569

40. Rhodes D W, Mansfield E R, Bishop P A, Smith J F 1995 Comparison of leg length inequality measurement methods as estimators of the femur head height difference on standing X-ray. Journal of Manipulative and Physiological Therapeutics 18 (7): 448–452

41. Rhodes D W, Mansfield E R, Bishop P A, Smith J F 1995 The validity of the prone leg check as an estimate of standing leg length inequality measured by X-ray. Journal of Manipulative and Physiological Therapeutics 18 (6): 343–346

42. Hoiriis K T, Hinson R H, Elsangek O et al 2000 Baseline characteristics of chiropractic patients: correlation of anatometer readings with supine leg length inequality. Journal of Vertebral Subluxation Research 3 (3): 2–3

43. Venn E K, Wakefield K A, Thompson P 1983 A comparative study of leg-length checks. European Journal of Chiropractic 31: 68–80

44. Thompson C 1984 Thompson technique reference manual. Thompson Educational Workshops, Williams Manufacturing, Elgin, IL

45. Fuhr A E, Osterbauer P J 1989 Interexaminer reliability of relative leg-length evaluations in the prone, extended position. Chiropractic Technique 1 (1): 13–18

46. Haas M, Peterson D 1989 Interexaminer reliability of relative leg-length evaluations in the prone, extended position [letter, comment]. Chiropractic Technique 1 (4): 150–151

47. Shambaugh P, Scolfani L, Fanselow D 1988 Reliability of the Derifield–Thompson test for leg-length inequality, and use of the test to determine cervical adjusting efficacy. Journal of Manipulative and Physiological Therapeutics 11 (5): 396–399

48. Danelius B D 1987 Letter to the editor: inter- and intra-examiner reliability of leg-length measurement: a preliminary study. Journal of Manipulative and Physiological Therapeutics 10 (3): 132

49. DeBoer F F 1987 In reply: inter- and intra-examiner reliability of leg-length measurement: a preliminary study. Journal of Manipulative and Physiological Therapeutics 10 (3): 133

50. DeBoer K F, Harmon R O, Savoie S, Tuttle C D 1983 Inter- and intra-examiner reliability of the leg-length differential measurement: a preliminary study. Journal of Manipulative and Physiological Therapeutics 10 (3): 61–66

51. Falltrick D R, Pierson D S 1989 Precise measurement of functional leg length inequality and changes due to cervical spine rotation in pain-free subjects. Journal of Manipulative and Physiological Therapeutics 12 (5): 369–373

52. Rhudy T R, Burk J M 1990 Inter-examiner reliability of functional leg-length assessment. American Journal of Chiropractic Medicine 3 (2): 63–66

53. DeBoer F F, Wagnon R J 1989 Letter to the editor. Journal of Manipulative and Physiological Therapeutics 12 (2): 151

54. Haas M, Nyiendo J 1989 Reliability of the Derifield-Thompson test for leg length inequality, and use of the test to demonstrate cervical adjusting efficacy [letter; comment]. Journal of Manipulative and Physiological Therapeutics 12 (4): 316–320

55. Osterbauer P J, Fuhr A W 1990 The current status of Activator Methods Chiropractic Technique, theory, and training. Chiropractic Technique 2 (4): 168–175

56. Cooperstein R 1991 The Derifield pelvic leg check: a kinesiological interpretation. Chiropractic Technique 3 (2): 60–65

57. Hestbaek L, Leboeuf-Yde C 2000 Are chiropractic tests for the lumbo-pelvic spine reliable and valid? A systematic critical literature review. Journal of Manipulative and Physiological Therapeutics 23 (4): 258–275

5

Palpation, static and motion

INTRODUCTION

Virtually all chiropractors, using any technique system, employ static and motion palpation.

Motion palpation is taught within the core curriculum of probably every chiropractic college, in spite of the abundance of studies showing it to be very unreliable. This means two examiners examining the same patient are not likely to come to the same conclusions as to where and to what degree motion is asymmetric or otherwise abnormal. Since examination findings that are not reproducible are generally discounted, we are left scratching our heads trying to rationalize the continued popularity of motion palpation, a conundrum with which we deal in our closing comments below.

Cooperstein once had the misfortune of being cast as a character in a motion palpation study, in which his findings were compared with those of another examiner. As is usually the case in such a study, the two examiners' findings were not concordant above chance levels, and this is what was appropriately reported.[1] On the other hand, data were also collected (although not reported) on Cooperstein's *intraexaminer* reliability: his ability to agree with himself in examining each of 25 subjects twice. In each of two data collection sessions, Cooperstein showed 90% agreement between his first and second examinations of 25 subjects. Therefore, although Cooperstein could not agree with a second examiner as to what cervical joints were restricted, he was able to agree with himself. This finding is not unrelated to why Cooperstein continues to use some version of motion palpation, innumerable negative studies

notwithstanding. The other palpator must have been wrong ....

Of course, when two examiners agree, or when one examiner agrees with him- or herself, there is no guarantee that the findings are correct. Both examiners could be wrong, and the one examiner agreeing with him- or herself might simply be consistently wrong. Reliability is just a way station on the way to validity: necessary, but not sufficient, to confirm clinical utility.

OVERVIEW

Palpation is an examination method by which the hands can be used to feel the patient's body, to explore visceral and somatic structures (Fig. 5.1). In the context of chiropractic technique, palpation is mostly used to assess the character, position, and movement capacity of cutaneous and somatic structures: skin, bones, joints, muscles, tendons, ligaments, bursa, etc. Palpation may be static, where structures are assessed in their neutral position, or dynamic, in which active and passive movements are evaluated. Dynamic palpation is usually called motion palpation. Among the possible findings, the doctor may feel textural and motility differences in the skin overlying suspected vertebral subluxations, muscle hypertonus or flaccidity, changes in other soft tissues, abnormal or clinically variant osseous structures, abnormal joint alignment, and abnormal active or passive joint movement capacity. Any or all of these findings form part of the clinical impression, leading to a diagnosis and treatment plan.

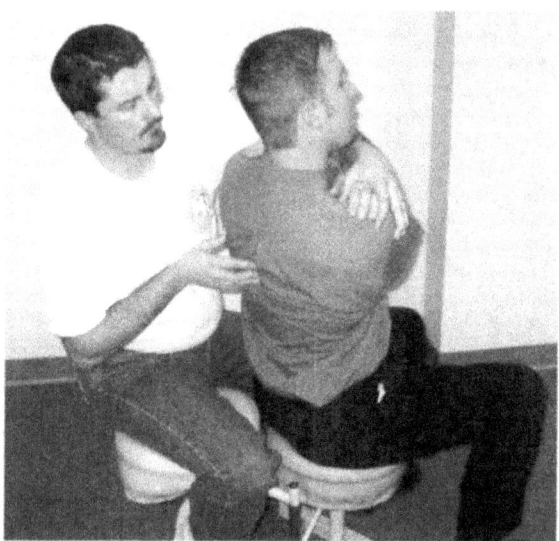

Figure 5.1 Motion palpation.

Intrinsic to the palpatory method is the possibility of assessing the patient's response to the examination, which may include muscle spasm or twitching, tissue tenderness, or perceived apprehension. These patient responses, as bona fide examination findings, may be just as important to the diagnosis as the doctor's palpatory impression in a more limited sense. Sometimes subtle clinical phenomena cannot be easily detected unless and until they are perturbed, during the process of examination.

HISTORY

Static palpation was present at the very beginning of chiropractic, when DD Palmer, describing his first adjustment, said: "An examination showed a vertebra racked from its normal position. I reasoned that if that vertebra was replaced, the man's hearing should be restored."[2] Motion palpation is almost as old, having been described as early as 1906 by Smith et al:[3] "A simple subluxated vertebra differs from a normal vertebra only in its field of motion and the center of its field of motion; because of its being subluxated, its various positions of rest are differently located than when it was a normal vertebra ... its field of

motion may be too great in some directions and too small in others" (cited by Leach[4]).

Although motion palpation may find its roots early in the profession's history, it traditionally received far less emphasis than models of subluxation based on vertebral misalignment. None the less, the European Gillet was a leading proponent of dynamic analysis throughout his career,[5,6] and strongly impacted on the practice and teaching of an influential American exponent of motion palpation, Leonard Faye.[7,8]

At this time, the motion palpation paradigm seems more popular than the more traditional emphasis on static vertebral alignment. Improper motion (too much, too little, or improper coupling patterns) is now seen as a vitally important component of the vertebral subluxation complex.[9]

COMMONLY ASSOCIATED TERMS AND CONCEPTS

- Misalignment: refers to a joint in which the contiguous bones are not in normal alignment when the subject is attempting to remain within a neutral position
- Range of motion: the amount of translatory and rotatory movement available to a joint
- Static palpation: somatic structures are assessed in their neutral, stationary position
- Motion palpation (also known as dynamic palpation): somatic structures are assessed for active and passive movement capacity
- Motion segment: according to Lantz,[9] the motion segment (previously known as the spinal motor unit, motor segment, functional spinal unit, or basic spinal unit) is the basic unit of spinal mobility. It consists of two adjacent vertebrae, the intervening intervertebral disk, the two posterior joints, and various ligaments (capsules, interspinous, and intertransverse)
- Active and passive range of motion: the active range of motion is what can be accessed by the unassisted patient, whereas passive motion is the range that can be

accessed by the doctor taking the joint some distance beyond this active limit

- Paraphysiological joint space: incremental movement beyond the elastic barrier that is attained at the end of passive range of motion, accessed by means of a high-velocity, low-amplitude thrust[10]
- Fixation: a state in which a vertebra has become immobilized in a position it could normally occupy during physiological movement, including an aligned position
- Restriction: a limitation of joint movement, named by the direction in which the patient exhibits limitation, in either translatory or rotational movement. For example, a patient restricted in left lateral flexion has difficulty bending toward the left. The term "restriction" is currently preferred in situations where the less specific term "fixation" had been formerly used
- Accessory joint movements: joint movements that cannot be performed voluntarily (unassisted) by a patient. These are necessary for the normal function of joints and may include such actions as rolls, slides, spins, distractions, and compressions
- Hard vs soft end-feel: a hard end-feel to passive joint movement is thought to be due to articular (structural) degenerative changes, while a soft end-feel would be associated with contractured muscles and other soft tissues
- Joint play: movements not under voluntary control, but necessary to achieve full painless joint function; a springiness and rebound in the joint movement, that occurs at the end of this passive range of motion, thus inaccessible to the unassisted patient.

MODE OF USE

Palpation procedures may be done with the patient standing, sitting, supine, or prone, and the doctor's position directly follows from the patient's position. *Static palpation* is a rather straightforward procedure, although differences in how the touch is executed will vary depending on the structure being palpated, the information that is sought, and the status of the patient. For example, palpation for tissue textural changes may require a very light touch, whereas palpation for tenderness necessarily requires pressing firmly enough to generate a patient response. Likewise, the pressure that is required for identifying a skeletal landmark may differ markedly from that required to identify the margins of a soft-tissue structure, such as a muscle.

To accomplish *motion palpation*, the examiner introduces motion into one or more joints with one hand while palpating with the other, in order to assess the range, pattern, and quality of movement. Perhaps the broadest distinction that might be made is between the motion palpation of intersegmental range of motion, as compared with unisegmental motion.[11] In palpation of intersegmental range of motion, usually, but not always, the examiner contacts elements of two or three vertebrae, using the fingers of the palpating hand to assess intersegmental movements while the other hand imparts motion into the articulation(s): rotation, flexion–extension, and lateral flexion. This is quantitative analysis, and the results are interpreted in terms of intersegmental range of motion, or joint excursion. The examiner decides whether the motion units are hypermobile, normal, or hypomobile.

In palpation of unisegmental motion, the examiner contacts a single segment, using the fingers of the palpating hand to apply overpressure into rotation, flexion–extension, and lateral flexion, while the other hand either stabilizes or assists in imparting motion. This is qualitative analysis, and the results are interpreted in terms of unisegmental movement, presumably in relation to the segments above and below (even though, as a semantic convention, the restriction listing will be in reference to the segment below). Thus, both dynamic palpatory methods represent dynamic analysis, but their methods and interpretation are quite different.

PHYSIOLOGICAL RATIONALE

According to Lantz,[9] the dominant model for joint restriction descends from the work of Gillet, in which there are three stages of joint fixation: muscular hypertonicity, ligamentous shortening, and articular adhesions. These are well-described by RC Schafer[12] in a recent monograph, and also by Gatterman.[13]

Although one commonly thinks of muscles as effecting movement, it is also true that muscles complement ligaments in preventing excessive movements. If a muscle, or group of muscles, becomes hypertonic or even undergoes spasm, whether due to injury, patient apprehension, neurologic insult, or inflammation, then the joint spanned by these muscles will become restricted. This *muscular fixation* tends to be self-perpetuating, as the contracted muscle undergoes vascular stasis and enters into a pain–spasm–pain cycle. Long-standing muscle hypertonus would be expected to result in the shortening of other soft tissues that span the involved joints, including the ligaments, thus entering the patient into Gillet's second phase of fixation, that of *ligamentous shortening*. Schafer believes that these fixations may be the only chronic fixations found in many elderly spines, or those with a history of severe joint trauma.[14] Finally, the patient may progress to Gillet's third phase, that of *articular adhesion*, with associated fibrosis, the ultimate result of which would be complete joint fusion, or ankylosis. Any event that requires immobilization of the involved joint, such as trauma, increases the likelihood of articular fixation development. In addition to fibrotic changes, other mechanisms that have been suggested as contributory to articular fixation include meniscoid fragments incarcerated in the synovial joints, disk herniations, and mechanical joint locking.[13]

Theories abound as to how musculoskeletal injuries can result in reflex muscle hypertonus, starting from the simple observation that muscle and joint injuries lead to protective, splinting spasm to immobilize the affected tissues. The more subtle theories mostly date back to the work of osteopaths Denslow and Korr. In their view, when a spinal segment is in a state of *somatic dysfunction* (a chiropractor would say "subluxation"), it is more easily stimulated, or activated by pressure or irritation from other apparently normal segments, even some distance

above or below it. It could be said to be in a state of facilitation, or perhaps a central excitatory state. Due to afferent bombardment related to subluxation (somatic dysfunction, musculoskeletal injury), there is reflex neural activity involving the anterior, posterior, and lateral horns of the spinal cord at the involved level. This leads to muscle hypertonus (causing or perpetuating fixation), hyperalgesia, and increased autonomic function, respectively.

EVIDENCE

There have been several comprehensive reviews on the reliability of motion palpation, all of which draw the same conclusion: motion palpation is not a reliable (reproducible) procedure. Troyanovich and Harrison[15] not only reviewed the primary studies, but some of the other comprehensive reviews as well: Keating,[16] Haas,[17] and Jensen and Gemmell.[18] Hestbaek and Leboeuf-Yde's subsequent review[19] came to the same conclusion, after reviewing 15 studies of motion palpation for the lumbar spine, and six for the sacroiliac joint: "the esteem chiropractors have for motion palpation in particular has not been substantiated by scientific data."[19] Panzer came to a similar conclusion,[20] as did Russell,[21] in their reviews.

Although the palpatory procedures of Jull et al[22,23] are sometimes regarded to be valid, their interpretation has been questioned because in their work the examiner's finding of restriction is commingled with other findings, such as pain and soft-tissue textural changes. Thus, it is not clear that the finding of fixation is central to their identification of dysfunctional spinal segments (see Troyanovich's reply to Lewit[24]). Since there is no disagreement that palpation for tenderness is reliable,[25] Jull's procedure may say a lot more about pain reproduction than it does about joint movement assessment.

CONCLUSIONS

- Motion palpation may be the most universally accepted chiropractic examination procedure, occupying a place in the core curriculum of virtually every chiropractic college. In addition, motion palpation may be more studied than any other chiropractic examination method, partially because it has also been studied by allied practitioners in physical therapy and osteopathy. One would suppose that the popularity of motion palpation would follow from validation through research, but on the contrary, the popularity of motion palpation remains high in spite of little validation by the many studies that have been done.

- Both Troyanovich and Hestbaek come to the same conclusion, that widespread enthusiasm for motion palpation is not justified by research into its reliability and validity. They both agree that part of the explanation is that motion palpation has high "surface validity,"[19] or "face validity."[15] In other words, the procedure just seems to make sense. Letters to the editor complaining about Troyanovich's call for rejecting the procedure reflect that very point.[24,26]

- Since most of the motion palpation reliability studies find that intraexaminer reliability (the ability of an examiner to agree with him- or herself) surpasses interexaminer reliability, we must consider the possibility that motion palpators might be using different methods, their stated intentions notwithstanding. Clearly, there would be no reason to expect appreciable interexaminer concordance in motion palpation studies if there were no guarantee that the examiners were using the same methodology.[11]

- It may be theoretically difficult, if not impossible, to determine the reliability of motion palpation.[27,28] Examiner 1, in motion palpating a research subject, most likely alters that subject so that we should not be surprised, nor excessively disheartened, to find that examiner 2 does not come up with the same result. The first examiner may have attenuated spinal restrictions, since the palpatory procedure resembles mobilization; which is, after all, a treatment modality. Or, and this is less commonly pointed out, the first examiner may leave the subject with aggravated restrictions, the result of stirring up guarding reactions

from injured joints. To use words that we learned during the OJ Simpson trial, motion palpation is a destructive test: it partially or completely destroys the evidence it is designed to detect.

- Although the fact that the patient is altered by the examination procedure may subtract from motion palpation's value as a diagnostic test, this may be clinically offset by the fact that the examination procedure may help patients, by in effect mobilizing their joints. Thus, perhaps the outcome of care is made better by its use, although not necessarily for the reason its most strident defenders might invoke.

- Byfield and Clancy[29] offer another important perspective to this issue. Perhaps motion palpation finds its greatest utility not in the ability to assess a joint quantitatively (that is, its excursion, how many degrees of rotation or lateral flexion are lost or present in excess), but rather as a qualitative assessment tool.[25] As they suggest, perhaps the perception of motion is more important to appreciate than the degree of motion.[25] Simply put, as one of the authors is fond of saying to chiropractic students, perhaps the best use of motion palpation is for a clinician to follow the advice of his youthful Sesame Street mentors and determine which "one of these things is not like the other ...."

- This approach to motion palpation sheds light on hotly contested arguments swirling around the concept of specificity. Some chiropractors vehemently defend the notion that they are able to detect specific joint movements, and that this identification requires that the practitioner choose a uniquely appropriate adjustment to correct the restriction.[30] Other chiropractors exhibit a less stringent approach to restoring lost joint motion, in which the choice of the particular adjustment strategy has little differential impact on the patient.

- With motion palpation, as with any other procedure of equivocal value, it is important to make sure that the test is supplemented by a combination of other diagnostic procedures, so as to allow the preponderance of clinical evidence to guide treatment.

REFERENCES

1. Nansel D D, Peneff A, Jansen R D, Cooperstein R 1988 Interexaminer reliability with respect to the detection of joint-play asymmetries in the cervical spines of otherwise asymptomatic subjects. In: Coyle B (ed.) CCA Convention, pp. A6-1–A6-8. Pacific Consortium for Chiropractic Research, San Diego, CA

2. Palmer D D 1910 The chiropractor's adjuster, the science, art and philosophy of chiropractic. Portland Printing House, Portland, OR

3. Smith O G, Langsworthy S M, Paxson M C 1906 Modernized chiropractic. Lawrence Press, Cedar Rapids

4. Leach R 1997 Stephenson's principles revisited in 1997. Dynamic Chiropractic. http://www.chiroweb.com/archives/15/08/18.html

5. Gillet H, Liekens M 1981 The different types of fixation. In: The Belgian chiropractic research notes, pp. 13–16. Motion Palpation Institute, Huntingon Beach, CA.

6. Gillet H 1952 Belgian chiropractic research, 10th edn. Self-published, Brussels, Belgium

7. Faye J 1987 Motion Palpation Institute course notes. Motion Palpation Institute, Huntington Beach, CA

8. Faye L J 1999 The subluxation complex. Journal of Chiropractic Humanities 9 (1): 1–4

9. Lantz C 1989 The vertebral subluxation complex – part I: an introduction to the model and the kinesiological component. Chiropractic Research Journal 1 (3): 23–36

10. Sandoz R 1976 Some physical mechanisms and effects of spinal adjustments. Annals of the Swiss Chiropractic Association 6: 91–141

11. Brown J, Cooperstein R 2001 Why motion palpation is so confounding. Journal of the American Chiropractic Association 38 (10): 34–36

12. Schafer R C 2002 The art of pioneer chiropractic technic: reflections from an era in which miracles were taken for granted. http://www.chiro.org/LINKS/RC_SCHAFER/mono-b1.htm

13. Gatterman M I 1990 Chiropractic management of spine-related disorders. Williams & Wilkins, Baltimore, MD

14. Shafer R C The art of pioneer chiropractic technic: reflections from an era in which miracles were taken for granted. http://www.chiro.org/LINKS/RC_SCHAFER/mono-b1.htm

15. Troyanovich S J, Harrison D D 1998 Motion palpation: it's time to accept the evidence. Journal of Manipulative and Physiological Therapeutics 21 (8): 568–571

16. Keating J C Jr 1989 Inter-examiner reliability of motion palpation of the lumbar spine: a review of the literature. American Journal of Chiropractic Medicine 2 (3): 107–110

17. Haas M 1991 The reliability of reliability. Journal of Manipulative and Physiological Therapeutics 14 (3): 199–208

18. Jensen K J, Gemmell H 1993 Motion palpation accuracy using a mechanical model. European Journal of Chiropractic 41: 67–73

19. Hestbaek L, Leboeuf-Yde C 2000 Are chiropractic tests for the lumbo-pelvic spine reliable and valid? A systematic critical literature review. Journal of Manipulative and Physiological Therapeutics 23 (4): 258–275

20. Panzer D M 1992 The reliability of lumbar motion palpation [published erratum appears in Journal of Manipulative and Physiological Therapeutics Nov–Dec; 15 (9): following table of contents]. Journal of Manipulative and Physiological Therapeutics 15 (8): 518–524

21. Russell R 1983 Diagnostic palpation of the spine: a review of procedures and assessment of their reliability. Journal of Manipulative and Physiological Therapeutics 6 (4): 181–183

22. Jull G, Bullock M 1987 A motion profile of the lumbar spine in an aging population assessed by manual examination. Physiotherapy Practice 3, 70–81

23. Jull G, Bogduk N, Marsland A 1988 The accuracy of manual diagnosis for cervical zygapophysial joint pain syndromes. Medical Journal of Australia 148 (5): 233–236

24. Lewit K 1999 Motion palpation: it's time to accept the evidence. Journal of Manipulative and Physiological Therapeutics 22 (4): 260–261

25. Hubka M J 1994 Palpation for spinal tenderness: a reliable and accurate method for identifying the target of spinal manipulation. Chiropractic Technique 6 (1): 5–8

26. Lucas N P 2000 Motion palpation: it's time to accept the evidence. Journal of Manipulative and Physiological Therapeutics 23 (1): 60–62

27. Cooperstein R 2001 The chiropractic technique–research interface: when neither loyal ignorance nor enlightened despair will do. The Bartlett 9 (2): 7–8, 23

28. Breen A 1992 The reliability of palpation and other diagnostic methods. Journal of Manipulative and Physiological Therapeutics 15 (1): 54–56

29. Byfield D, Clancy M, Kelly V 2002 Diagnostic palpation and anatomical landmark location: clinical concepts and the evidence. In: Byfield D, Kinsinger S (eds) A manual therapist's guide to surface anatomy and palpation skills, pp. 1–33. Butterworth-Heinemann, Oxford, UK

30. Gleberzon B J 2003 Chiropractic name techniques: a continued look. (in press)

6

Muscle testing, manual

INTRODUCTION

Manual muscle testing is typically used by Applied Kinesiology and its spinoffs (see Ch. 12 for discussions of Clinical Kinesiology, Contact Reflex Analysis, Neuroemotional Technique, Total Body Modification, and Neural Organization Technique). Manual muscle testing is also closely related to *mind language*, as described by Sacro-Occipital Technique (Ch. 25).[1]

The chiropractor shows a group of onlookers that the outstretched arm of a standing patient is strong, as demonstrated by his inability to push it down. Then, sweeping his own arm in front of the patient's eyes, retesting of the patient's arm now shows it to be weak. This is always something of a spectacle. Some among the onlookers declare the doctor to be a fraud; he is either pressing more firmly on the patient's outstretched arm, or he has recruited a shill who secretly allows the arm to go down when the muscle test is repeated. The chiropractor explains that no fraud has been perpetrated, that it is all a question of using muscle testing to read the body's nervous system directly. What does it all mean?

Manual muscle testing, as performed by chiropractors, does not necessarily differ in its execution and interpretation from manual muscle testing as performed and interpreted by the standards of orthopedic medicine. To either practitioner, a weak muscle might suggest a primary muscular or neurological pathology. That stated, manual muscle testers generally invoke altogether different *reflexes* (in the sense of reflex technique, as described in Ch. 3) to explain how and why muscles respond to provocative challenges. The finding of a weak muscle may be thought to identify a disease or a chiropractic subluxation, even a repressed emotion or a vitamin deficiency. To put it mildly, that does not happen in orthopedic medicine.

Manual muscle testing can be and has been used as a primary exhibit by those interested in disestablishing the chiropractic profession. Serious efforts at muckraking in chiropractic often take the form of showing a manual muscle tester explaining how muscle weakness confirms a vitamin deficiency, allergy, or organ disease. One of the reasons for the failure of the attempted affiliation of York University with the Canadian Memorial Chiropractic College was the mere existence of the technique system known as Applied Kinesiology, despite the fact the college does not teach this technique. This serves as an interesting measure of just how reprehensible some members of the medical community find manual muscle testing to be, for the purpose of identifying diseases, chiropractic subluxations, and whatever else. On the other hand, we are aware of many medical practitioners, including many Europeans, who have become very interested in manual muscle testing, and made Applied Kinesiology a focal point of their practices. Whatever else can be said about muscle testing, it is a practice about which no one in or out of chiropractic is neutral. It is high time we separated fact from fiction, and hyperbole from either camp will not do.

OVERVIEW

Chiropractors and other kinesiologists use manual muscle testing as a window into a broad range of purported pathologies: segmentally related or more distant subluxations, allergies, nutritional deficits or needs, learning disabilities, emotional problems, and other entities too numerous (and sometimes too eccentric) to mention. In this context, the strength of a muscle is thought to increase or decrease in response to *challenges* (diagnostic clinical interventions) of various types and during the course of care, thus providing information on the status of the body's subsystems. The practitioner believes, in assessing muscle strength under a variety of clinical conditions, that he or she is directly communicating with the body's nervous sytem.

HISTORY

Manual muscle testing – again, as an indirect indicator of reflexively related primary pathology – appears to be the invention of George Goodheart. He himself states that manual muscle testing is his central and unique contribution to chiropractic, the defining core of his Applied Kinesiology. This seminal technique system inspired several spinoff technique systems, which we call kinesiologies in Chapter 12. Goodheart claims to have originated Applied Kinesiology in 1964,[2] after having observed that postural distortion, in the absence of congenital pathology, is often associated with weak muscles. The original case was one of winging of the scapula.[2]

COMMONLY ASSOCIATED TERMS AND CONCEPTS

- Previously strong indicator muscle (PSIM): the muscle tester, in order to undertake muscle testing as a diagnostic procedure, must first identify a muscle that is strong (of normal strength) when *in the clear*. This muscle may be any in the body, and is not specifically related to the subluxation or other clinical problem being investigated

- Reflex: the word "reflex" in this context specifically does not refer to the types of reflexes one could read about in an orthopedics or neurology textbook, such as a deep tendon or pathological reflex. It refers to a hypothetical, often unstudied cause-and-effect physiological relationship between two phenomena. As an example, a mild thrust on a spinous process may cause a reflex weakening of a PSIM, or thyroid disease may produce weakness in the infraspinatus muscle by some sort of reflex

- Challenge: a challenge amounts to some sort of mild clinical intervention, such as a mild thrust on a spinous process, or placing a nutritional substance under the tongue, in order to assess its effect on the strength of a PSIM. It usually refers to the weakening, but could refer to the strengthening, of a PSIM

- Rebound challenge: a muscle which is specifically inhibited by a vertebral subluxation may strengthen when a challenge is applied that would correct that subluxation; this is called a rebound challenge

- Therapy localization (TL): muscle strength may change when a patient touches his or her own hand to a part of the body, indicating a non-specific problem with that part of the body. The muscle tester must then identify the reflex associated with that positive TL

- Mind language: although developed by Sacro-Occipital Technique practitioners, mind language bears an obvious resemblance to TL as utilized by Applied Kinesiologists. According to DeJarnette,[1] the right arm is used as the testing mechanism and the left index finger as a pointer or finder. The patient touches the point of pain or complaint area while the doctor tests the arm for strength or weakness. Weakness identifies a problem area

- Doctor-initiated and patient-initiated muscle testing: different physiological mechanisms may be involved according to the timing, depending on whether the test is begun by the examiner first applying force (eccentric testing, doctor-initiated); or the patient first bracing by exerting resistance (concentric testing, patient-initiated).[3]

MODE OF USE

There are many variations among the various techniques that employ muscle testing, having to do with the force involved, the timing (e.g., doctor- vs patient-initiated resistance), the preferred muscles that are used, and of course, in the interpretation of what constitutes a positive finding.

In manual muscle testing, the examiner applies force to a muscle or group of muscles while the patient exerts resistance (Fig. 6.1). It is thought by some that different physiological mechanisms are involved according to whether the test is begun by the examiner applying force, before the patient has had a chance to resist (doctor-initiated testing), or the patient first braces by exerting resistance (patient-initiated).[3] This concept was studied by Hsieh and Phillips, using a dynamometer as a surrogate for manual muscle testing.[4]

The muscle test amounts to a one-shot, pre–post assessment of a change in muscle strength following a diagnostic intervention, either patient- or doctor-initiated. For example, the patient may rotate the neck and head to the left, or touch a point on his or her abdomen; or the doctor may place a vitamin under the patient's tongue or push a spinous process from right to left. Usually, the baseline muscle is strong and a positive test involves a weakening of the muscle, although sometimes the baseline muscle is weak and a positive test involves strengthening.

Since manual muscle testing is a diagnostic procedure, it must be combined with a thorough history and physical examination to arrive at a clinical impression. It is usually necessary first to identify a PSIM, which may in principle be any muscle in the body. The particular muscle chosen happens to be convenient, more than anything else, for the part of the body being diagnosed and the position in which the patient happens to be. For example, the hamstring muscles are very convenient for testing the sacroiliac joints of a prone patient, and the arm flexor group (there is no requirement that one muscle be isolated to be used) for testing points in the inguinal ligament of a supine patient.

PHYSIOLOGICAL RATIONALE

Again, there are as many explanations of what is at play in manual muscle testing as there are technique systems that employ it. None the less, what all these explanations have in common is the simple thought that the manual muscle test is some sort of direct dialogue with innate intelligence, or shall we say, "the body." The test amounts to some sort of question, and some examples follow:

- Would this line of drive be an appropriate correction of this suspected subluxation?
- Is the joint I am touching the source of the patient's problem?
- Is there allergy to the scent I have placed under the patient's nose?
- Is there a problem with the left side of the brain, that is manifested when the patient is asked to recite a multiplication table?
- Or with the right side of the brain when the patient is asked to sing a tune?

Muscle weakening in response to any of these clinical interventions (pardon our very general usage of the term "clinical intervention") amounts to the body's way of saying "yes." If muscle function changes with diagnostic intervention, something

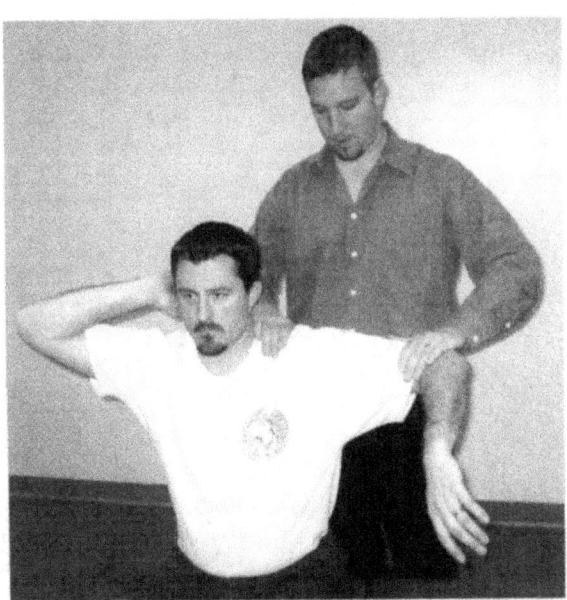

Figure 6.1 Manual muscle testing.

may be going on which is worthy of further diagnostic work-up.

As for the physiology involved, Walther provides the most succinct explanation of which we are aware. Suppose a hypertonic muscle has pulled a spinous process into subluxation. An exploratory push on that spinous process in the direction that would correct the misalignment would also stretch that hypertonic muscle. Whatever the reason for that muscle's hypertonicity, this push provokes a stretch reflex that pulls the spinous process into a state of greater misalignment. This in turn causes a weakening of the PSIM, or a strengthening of a previously weak, inhibited muscle, confirming the wisdom of that particular exploratory push. Then, the changes in muscle strength would amount to the body's way of saying "Yes, adjust me that way!" Walther hypothesizes that this reflex results from "temporary general confusion in the nervous system".[5]

EVIDENCE

Klinkoski and LeBoeuf[6] examined 50 scientific papers published by the International College of Applied Kinesiology between 1981 and 1987, 20 of which were classified as research papers, several of which had to do with the core procedure of manual muscle testing. These were evaluated on the basis of criteria considered crucial in research methodology: clear identification of sample size, inclusion criteria, the use of blind and naive subjects, reliable test methods, blind assessors, and statistical analysis. None satisfied all seven of these criteria, and a letter to the editor estimated the average study to have achieved a score of 2.3 out of 7.[7] Klinkoski and LeBoeuf concluded that no valid conclusions could be drawn from these studies[6] about manual muscle testing or anything else.

A pair of more recent review articles[8,9] summarized research on manual muscle testing, and its neurophysiological basis respectively, emphasizing research conducted within the Applied Kinesiology milieu. Motyka and Yanuck[5] find the research equivocal, sometimes confirmatory of reliability and validity, other times disconfirmatory, and often simply irrelevant due to various design flaws.

More recently, Caruso and Leisman[10,11] investigated the force/displacement characteristics of manual muscle testing, finding that a relatively steep slope – meaning that the distance through which the tested limb moves as a function of force application is large – predicts with 98% accuracy that an experienced manual muscle tester would find a weak muscle. A less experienced muscle tester would get it right, under the assumption that the force/displacement curve is definitive, only 64% of the time. The authors conclude: "The experiment lays the groundwork for studies of the objectivity of muscle-strength assessment in applied kinesiology".[10]

Seven patients with proven allergy to wasp venom were tested by four trained muscle testers, to see if there was a difference in deltoid strength (a PSIM) when challenged with venom as compared with placebo.[12] Both patients and muscle testers were blinded. Analysis showed that muscle testing was not superior to guessing in discriminating venom from placebo, meaning the test was not valid. On the other hand, an earlier study found that manual muscle testing could identify food allergies in 19/21 cases, when its results were compared with immunological assays.[9] Likewise, Schmitt and Leisman[9] used manual muscle testing to identify 19 subjects as having 21 food allergies, as demonstrated by muscle weakening when the suspected allergen was placed in the mouth. Immunological serum testing, including both a radioallergosorbent test (RAST) and immune complex test for immunoglobulin E (IgE) and IgG, tested positive in 19 of the 21 suspected allergens. According to the investigators, the results of this pilot study warrant further investigation of whether manual muscle testing can provide a means to predict the clinical utility of using nutritional supplements.

Eleven subjects were examined by three trained muscle testers for their need for four different nutrients (zinc, vitamin C, thiamin, and vitamin A).[13] The examiners did not agree with one another, nor did any of their individual results correlate with laboratory testing, nor was there any correlation of manual and mechanical measures of muscle strength. Another study, on the other hand, found some correlation of manual muscle testing and standard laboratory testing for thyroid function.[14]

Although Jacobs failed to find much relation between sugar ingestion and muscle strength,[15] Rybeck and Swenson found that manual muscle testing, but not mechanical muscle testing, was able to discriminate between sugar and no sugar being placed under the tongue, using the latissimus muscle as the PSIM.[16] (It should be noted that the subjects were not blinded.) Triano, testing the putative relationship between the strength of latissimus dorsi and pancreatic extract, found the muscle to be affected about 20% of the time no matter what nutritional extract was placed under the tongue.[17] Leisman et al found significant differences in electromyogram between muscles found to be weak and strong.[18] Some degree of interexaminer reliability was found for manual muscle testing of the pectoralis and piriformis muscles, but not for the hamstrings or the tensor fascia lata muscles.[19]

The so-called *arm-fossa test*, a manual muscle-testing method used in Sacro-Occipital Technique, was evaluated in 45 subjects tested by an examiner blinded as to their treatment status.[20] One group received "correct" supine blocking, another received "incorrect" prone blocking, and the third group was not treated at all. The muscle test was unchanged in 86% of the controls, became negative in 73% of the "correctly" treated group, and was mixed in the "incorrectly" treated group.

CONCLUSIONS

- Muscle testers believe that manual muscle testing reveals sources of chronic symptoms that are often overlooked by more conventional medical evaluation.
- In drawing conclusions about it, we must consider both the reproducibility of the test itself, and what manual muscle testing might tell us about body function. Although we may be willing to accept the poor correlation of manual muscle testing results with mechanical testing, we are less patient with lack of interexaminer reliability.
- Since there is very little information on the reproducibility of manual muscle testing, we must take studies that attempted to correlate findings of weak and strong muscles with other variables, such as laboratory tests, with a big grain of salt. If we are not certain that a muscle tester gets the right answer, presuming there is one, we cannot easily interpret correlation of a muscle test or lack thereof with another physiological variable.

- The poor correlation of instrumented and manual muscle testing hardly invalidates the latter, as some investigators and commentators have suggested, owing to the substantial differences in the way the tests are performed[16] and the likelihood that differences in outcome would be expected. We believe the work of Caruso and Leisman[10,11] to be the best evidence yet for the accuracy of manual muscle testing, and probably a better barometer of its validity than studies comparing the results of manual muscle testing with instrumented muscle testing.
- The extensive use of manual muscle testing by many of chiropractic's most esoteric practitioners is noted. Clearly, any diagnostic method placed by its developers in the common domain is capable of being used and *abused*; and that in and of itself is not automatically incriminating of the technique system. On the other hand, it certainly gives one pause.
- The primary explanations offered, by kinesiologists and by Sacro-Occipital Technique practitioners, represent a rather creative blend of normal and paranormal physiology, so that a less than careful reader or seminar attendee may easily fail to realize where and to what degree the science has been stretched.
- In the short term, it would be clinically unsound to base diagnoses on the results of manual muscle testing alone, or even weight it significantly in comparison to validated laboratory and orthopedic–neurological testing.
- It is quite simply unfair that patients be told, on the basis of manual muscle testing, that they are allergic to this or that, have some organ weakness or another, or need some nutritional supplement, *in the absence of other clinical findings*. If manual muscle testers believe their methods can detect preclinical or subclinical findings, then they had best validate their methods. The entire chiropractic profession is negatively judged when dramatic diagnoses are made on the basis of such equivocal findings.

REFERENCES

1. Delarnette M B 1983 Sacro-occipital technic: 1983. Self-published, Nebraska City, NE

2. Goodheart G J 1989 Applied Kinesiology – the beginning. Digest of Chiropractic Economics (May/June): 15, 17–20, 22–23

3. Schmitt W H Jr, Yanuck S F 1999 Expanding the neurological examination using functional neurologic assessment: part II. Neurologic basis of applied kinesiology. International Journal of Neuroscience 97 (1–2): 77–108

4. Hsieh C Y, Phillips R B 1990 Reliability of manual muscle testing with a computerized dynamometer. Journal of Manipulative and Physiological Therapeutics 13 (2): 72–82

5. Walther D S 1981 Applied Kinesiology, vol. I, p. 55. Systems DC, Pueblo, CO

6. Klinkoski B, LeBoeuf C 1990 A review of the research papers published by the International College of Applied Kinesiology from 1981–1987. Journal of Manipulative and Physiological Therapeutics 13: 190–194

7. Morgan L G 1990 A review of the research papers published by the International College of Applied Kinesiology from 1981 to 1987. Journal of Manipulative and Physiological Therapeutics 13 (9): 553

8. Motyka T M, Yanuck S F 1999 Expanding the neurological examination using functional neurologic assessment part I: methodological considerations. International Journal of Neuroscience 97 (1–2): 61–76

9. Schmitt W H Jr, Leisman G 1998 Correlation of applied kinesiology muscle testing findings with serum immunoglobulin levels for food allergies. International Journal of Neuroscience 96 (3–4): 237–244

10. Caruso W, Leisman G 2000 A force/displacement analysis of muscle testing. Perception and Motor Skills 91 (2): 683–692

11. Caruso W, Leisman G 2001 The clinical utility of force/displacement analysis of muscle testing in applied kinesiology. International Journal of Neuroscience 106 (3–4): 147–157

12. Ludtke R, Kunz B, Seeber N, Ring J 2001 Test – retest-reliability and validity of the Kinesiology muscle test. Complementary and Therapeutic Medicine 9 (3): 141–145

13. Kenney J J, Clemens R, Forsythe K D 1988 Applied kinesiology unreliable for assessing nutrient status. Journal of the American Dietary Association 88 (6): 698–704

14. Jacobs G E, Franks T L 1984 Diagnosis of thyroid dysfunction: applied kinesiology compared to clinical observations and laboratory tests. Journal of Manipulative and Physiological Therapeutics 7: 99–104

15. Jacobs G E 1981 Applied kinesiology: an experimental evaluation by double blind methodology. Journal of Manipulative and Physiological Therapeutics 4 (3): 141–145

16. Rybeck C H, Swenson R 1980 The effect of oral administration of refined sugar on muscle strength. Journal of Manipulative and Physiological Therapeutics 3: 155–161

17. Triano J J 1982 Muscle strength testing as a diagnostic screen for supplemental nutrition therapy: a blind study. Journal of Manipulative and Physiological Therapeutics 5: 179–182

18. Leisman G, Zenhausern R, Ferentz A, Tefera T, Zemcov A 1995 Electromyographic effects of fatigue and task repetition on the validity of estimates of strong and weak muscles in applied kinesiological muscle-testing procedures. Perception and Motor Skills 80 (3 Pt 1): 963–977

19. Lawson A, Calderon L 1997 Interexaminer agreement for applied kinesiology manual muscle testing. Perception and Motor Skills 84 (2): 539–546

20. Leboeuf C, Jenkins D J, Smyth R A 1988 Sacro-occipital technique: the so-called arm fossa test. Intraexaminer agreement and post-treatment changes. Journal of the Australian Chiropractors' Association 18 (2): 67–68

7

Radiography and X-ray line marking

INTRODUCTION

Radiography and X-ray line marking are used by Gonstead, Pierce–Stillwagon, Upper Cervical techniques, Diversified, Spinal Stressology, Applied Spinal Biomechanical Engineering, Spinal Biomechanics, Chiropractic Biophysics, Logan, and other technique systems to varying degrees.

The heated opinions of detractors notwithstanding, chiropractic adjustive care is by all accounts extraordinarily safe. The incidence of adverse reactions worse than minor, self-resolving problems appears to be very low. On the other hand, there is a serious issue regarding the overall safety of chiropractic care which remains unresolved: it is very difficult to assess the health hazards of X-ray examinations. Debate on this issue is ongoing, having constituted a major and most contentious issue in the area of public health policy for many decades; the debate shows no signs of letting up. Since by all accounts X-ray examinations are frequently performed by chiropractors, we are unable to state, compared with adjustive care, that chiropractic examination methods are equally safe.

According to the National Board of Chiropractic Examiners,[1] (p. 119) chiropractors frequently obtain X-rays on new patients (2.93 on a 1–4 scale). We also have a survey conducted by the American Chiropractic Association[2] in which survey respondents reported that a substantial 60% of their new patients received X-rays, although this represents a decline from the 69% reported in 1997 and 75% reported in 1995. About 13% of patients received post X-rays during the course of their care, a figure that is consistent with data from previous surveys.

In addition to the ongoing debate on the X-ray safety question, a companion debate has raged within the chiropractic profession on the clinical utility of X-rays, as is discussed below. X-ray is not the only commonly performed chiropractic examination procedure that has been controversial; we still argue about the clinical utility of leg checking (Ch. 4), thermography (Ch. 8), and other methods. However, there is a big difference: these other examination procedures, although at worst they may steer the patient towards inappropriate care, cannot be held to injure the patient *directly*. X-ray is another matter altogether, in that we remain unable to rule out a direct hazard to the patient. Whatever patience we may have for using non-invasive examination methods that are not validated, demonstrably unreliable, or even unstudied, we do not exhibit that same patience when it comes to X-ray examination, owing to its potentially invasive character. This double uncertainty – health hazards unknown, clinical utility unknown – entirely explains the stormy history of X-rays in chiropractic, both within and without the profession. Nothing makes for a vaguer risk/benefit assessment than not having good estimates for either the numerator or the denominator!

OVERVIEW

X-rays (radiographs) may be taken either for diagnostic purposes, to determine if *pathology*, including contraindications to adjustive care, is present, or for analytic purposes, to determine *listings*. By listings, we mean identification of that most traditional of chiropractic pathologies: misalignment – that is, subluxation – of skeletal structures. Analytic X-rays are taken to identify spinal, pelvic, and extremity joint subluxations, as well as to determine reduction or progression of misalignments over time. X-ray line-marking methods have been devised to measure distances and angles on radiographs – what MacRae called *roentgenometrics*.[3]

Many of the technique systems have developed proprietary patient-positioning protocols, X-ray series, and line-marking procedures. These are customized relative to each technique system's particular concept of subluxation. Static X-rays of patients neutrally positioned are taken to assess both segmental misalignments and regional disturbances, such as sagittal plane curve abnormalities (hypo- and hyperlordosis, hypo- and hyperkyphosis), and frontal plane lateral curvatures (e.g., scoliosis). Dynamic or stress X-rays are taken with the patient flexed or extended in the sagittal plane, or side-flexed in the frontal plane, to assess for segmental hypomobility (restriction) or hypermobility (instability). Static and dynamic radiographs, as evaluated by roentgenometric analysis, are thought to help determine appropriate vectors for subluxation correction.

HISTORY

Roentgenology and chiropractic originated in the same year, 1895, when Wilhelm C Roentgen discovered X-ray and DD Palmer performed the first adjustment. BJ Palmer, the "developer of chiropractic," introduced *spinography*, as he called it, to the chiropractic profession in 1911, stating it was necessary to X-ray the spine to find vertebral misalignment on a scientific basis. He imported the fifth X-ray unit into the USA, and the first west of the Mississippi river. His immediate endorsement of the technology may have sparked Loban's break with the Fountainhead and the founding of the rival Universal Chiropractic College.[4,5]

By the late 1920s and early 1930s, most of the chiropractic colleges included radiology in their curricula. X-ray was important to the development of Upper Cervical Specific Technique at the BJ Palmer Clinic in the early 1930s, providing the basis for its listings and for research. Sausser took the first successful upright full-spine film in 1935.[5] According to practitioners of the Atlas Orthogonality upper cervical technique, Dr. John F Grostic introduced post X-rays in 1946, taken immediately after the atlas adjustment in order to compare them to the pre X-ray. He claimed that post X-rays should show that the subluxation had been reduced, improved, or was a non-reducible subluxation. The American Chiropractic Board of Radiology was founded in 1958, and by 1995 had credentialed 235 chiropractic radiologists.[5]

Throughout its history, the routine use of radiology to obtain subluxation listings has been controversial, given that the risk–benefit ratio for this use of ionizing radiation has been unknown. Kato questions whether doctors of chiropractic need to take routine X-rays on every new patient.[6] As a barometer of current trends in X-ray utilization as of 1999, we provide a section from a recent report[2] on a survey conducted by the American Chiropractic Association:

Survey respondents reported 60 percent of their new patients received X-rays, a decline from the 69 percent reported in 1997 and 75 percent reported in 1995. About 13 percent of patients were X-rayed again during the course of treatment, which is consistent with data from previous surveys. It appears that the number of new patient X-rays is declining, while the number of established patients who were X-rayed again during the course of treatment remains the same. Seventy percent of new Medicare patients received X-rays.

COMMONLY ASSOCIATED TERMS AND CONCEPTS

- X-ray line marking: the practice of marking anatomical landmarks on plain radiographs, in order to measure distances between them, the angles created by intersecting lines connecting these landmarks, or where these landmarks lie in relation to true horizontal or vertical lines
- Lines of mensuration: although the word "mensuration" simply means measurement, it is generally used in the chiropractic profession to refer to roentgenometrics. These include not

only special measures unique to chiropractic technique systems, but measures commonly taken by medical radiologists. Common "medical" cervical lines of mensuration include the horizontal line of the atlas, horizontal line of the axis, lordotic curve angle, Chamberlain's line, physiological stress lines, and George's line. Common lumbar lines of mensuration include the angle of curvature, Ferguson's line, George's line, McNabb's line, the lumbosacral disk angle, Ullman's line, and grades of spondylolisthesis

- Roentgenometrics: mensuration of X-ray films, either done by hand, or using computerized radiographic digitization procedures
- Plain film studies: simple use of X-ray, as opposed to advanced imaging (computed tomography (CT), magnetic resonance imaging (MRI), etc.) methodologies
- Stress film: films acquired in which the patient holds a posture at end-range of motion (lateral flexion, extension, forward flexion), taken to identify hypomobility or hypermobility
- Radiographic series: a set of plain films considered adequate for the area under investigation, including at least two films taken at right angles
- Full-spine radiograph: standing plain film, anteroposterior view taken on 14" × 36" (35 × 90 cm) film; sometimes called a scoliogram in orthopedic medicine
- Videofluoroscopy: technology that permits dynamic motion X-rays, consisting of an X-ray generator capable of operating at low (1/4 to 5) milliamperage settings, an X-ray tube assembly, an image intensifier tube, a television camera, a video tape recorder, and a monitor. The image intensifier tube permits imaging at very low radiation levels, and is used instead of intensifying screens and film as an image receptor
- CT: advanced imaging procedure in which cross-sectional pictures or tomographic slices of the body are made by X-ray. A series of X-ray beams from many different angles are used to create cross-sectional images of the patient's body, that can be reconstructed by a computer into a three-dimensional picture displaying organs, bones, and tissues in great detail
- MRI: advanced imaging procedure in which a powerful magnetic field and radio signals

provide a detailed picture of structures and organs inside the body. It does *not* require X-rays or the injection of dyes or other substances.

MODE OF USE

We must point out that the aim of this section is not to describe how chiropractors take X-rays, but how they make use of the information provided by radiological examination. There are certain indications for taking *diagnostic* X-rays upon which all chiropractors, and all technique systems, would agree: ruling out fractures, infections, and tumors. X-rays not only help render the differential diagnosis, but rule out contraindications to manipulation and other forms of chiropractic treatment. Where it becomes problematic is whether *analytic* X-rays should be taken for the purpose of obtaining listings. We deal with this issue below. In the meantime, we may note that plain X-rays are commonly subjected to mensuration (roentgenometric analysis) in as many different ways as there are technique systems that use analytic X-ray analysis. These include Pierce–Stillwagon, Gonstead, Chiropractic Biophysics, Pettibon Spinal Biomechanics, Logan, Applied Spinal Biomechanical Engineering, Spinal Stressology, Diversified, and a myriad of Upper Cervical techniques. Not surprisingly, the radiological protocols (patient positioning, tube distance, views obtained) also vary from technique to technique.

PHYSIOLOGICAL RATIONALE

The physiological rationale for taking diagnostic films is straightforward. Sometimes there are red flags in the history or physical examination that warrant radiographic follow-up. This may result in absolute or relative contraindications to certain types of adjustive procedures, to further diagnostic studies, or referral for concurrent or alternative care by an allied healthcare provider.

The physiological rationale for taking *routine* radiographs (i.e., as a general screening procedure for patients, irrespective of clinical findings) is controversial, and cannot even be discussed without becoming involved in thorny questions about chiropractic philosophy and related practice patterns.

Chiropractors who might classify themselves as "subluxation-based" take X-rays in order to identify subluxations. They have no problem with taking routine radiographs, as defined above, because they do not emphasize whether a subluxation is symptomatic or not. More broad-based practitioners, many of whom are less confident that clinically significant subluxations even show up radiographically (for example, a vertebral restriction that occurs in a joint that exhibits neutral alignment), do not take routine radiographs. They tend to support guidelines for the use of X-ray like those suggested by Gatterman,[7] writing on behalf of the American Chiropractic College of Radiology (ACCR), as reviewed by Kato.[6]

In its current guidelines, the ACCR states: "Imaging is used to characterize the components at the VSC [vertebral subluxation complex] when such characterization is necessary to render chiropractic care, [sic] imaging may be indicated if less hazardous or less expensive alternative examinations are not available or conclusive."[8] This conservative language makes it clear that radiological examination for the purpose of identifying the vertebral subluxation complex may be undertaken *if necessary to render chiropractic care*, and only when *safer alternative examination procedures* are not available. By comparison, the subluxation-based chiropractors consider the information provided by radiographic examination inaccessible by alternative examination procedures, and almost always necessary to render appropriate chiropractic care. As one group put it, "It should be obvious that X-rays are taken for biomechanical and pathological analysis, not to determine the presence or absence of pain."[9]

Stress X-rays are taken to evaluate how the spine behaves under gravitational stress, in a non-neutral position. Although in the medical field such films are generally taken to diagnose vertebral instability, either post-traumatically or in cases of suspected congenital hypermobility, chiropractors are quite interested in using stress films to identify vertebral hypomobility: segments that do not participate as fully as adjacent segments in gross flexion and extension movements.

Those whose definition of subluxation includes a component that is at least potentially seen on radiographs, meaning it involves either segmental or regional misalignment, or hypomobility as seen on stress films, naturally regard the taking of pre and post films as justified.

EVIDENCE

A huge number of studies have been conducted on the *reliability* of line-marking procedures: how likely are independent evaluators to obtain concurrent results? In spite of the almost folklorish sentiment common in chiropractic circles that line marking is an unreliable procedure, Harrison et al wrote a review article presenting abundant evidence to the contrary.[10] (For a dissenting view, see Haas et al).[11] Indeed, X-ray line marking for spinal displacement tends to be very reliable, with intraclass correlation coefficients (ICCs) in the 0.8–0.9 range, compared with ICCs in the 0.40–0.75 range for the determination of pathology.[10] These investigators evaluated the ICCs for both selected "medical" lines of mensuration (e.g., Cobb angles, endplate lines, stress X-rays), and chiropractic technique system-specific lines (e.g., Upper Cervical, Gonstead, and Chiropractic Biophysics). Owens[12] came to a similar conclusion for Upper Cervical technique X-rays, but concluded: "It is not known how much of the changes that are seen in pre/post-radiograph sets are due to positioning changes of the patient between radiographic procedure, and how much are due to actual changes of skeletal relationships brought about by adjustment."[12]

In other words, even if X-ray line marking can be performed reliably, there remains the possibility that variations in between-office and within-office patient-positioning procedures would render pre and post X-rays non-interpretable. To address this criticism, Plaugher et al showed, in an $n = 37$ study, that they could obtain essentially the same radiograph taking a repeat X-ray either 1h or 18 days after the initial X-ray.[13] This study was not designed to address the larger questions: (1) Are the patient-positioning protocols that are used in the chiropractic profession sufficiently standardized to permit proper interpretation by those practicing different techniques? (2) Are field practitioners and X-ray technicians trained well enough, and/or are they careful enough, to use their patient-positioning protocols in a consistent manner?

In addition to knowing if X-rays can be reliably obtained and analyzed, we need to know if X-ray analysis is valid; that is, if such analysis provides accurate information about the patient. Owens[12] stated: "The accuracy of the analysis methods has not been ascertained to establish the extent to which angular measurement of vertebral relationships actually reflects three-dimensional movement." Even if chiropractors can agree on what they measure on radiographs, and position patients in a reproducible manner, there is still no guarantee that what is seen on the film corresponds to a real, anatomical parameter of the flesh and blood patient. To put it simply, the question of the *concurrent validity* (i.e., accuracy) of the radiograph still needs to be explored.

Very little is known about the validity of X-ray line marking. We may cite the work of Janik et al,[14] who found that line marking correlated well with a plastic specimen that served as a reference standard for "misalignment" of a C3 model. Zengel et al[15–17] performed similar work. We also note the work of Jeffery,[18] whose doctoral dissertation at the Anglo-European College of Chiropractic characterized three general methods of radiometry for pelvic torsion. Adapted versions of these methods were then used to calculate innominate tilting of a dry specimen tilted to varying known degrees and radiographed. Although the work is not entirely satisfactory, Jeffery found the pelvic line-marking methods of Reinert and Hildebrandt more sensitive for hemipelvic rotation than the method of Gonstead. Cooperstein also tested the validity of the Gonstead line-marking rule for pelvic torsion by modeling the procedure in a computer simulation,[19–21] trigonometrically calculating projected changes in innominate vertical lengths by performing experiments on a digitized pelvis, assuming a pubic symphysis axis for torsion. He concluded that the Gonstead "rule" is not really a rule, since it is valid only some of the time and under certain circumstances.

Finally, there is the question of *clinical validity*, to what extent the information provided by X-ray line marking is associated with other clinical findings, and beyond that, improves the outcome of care. Here the evidence is very equivocal. Haas and Peterson found in a series of studies[22–24] that lateral flexion malalignment was not correlated with lumbar pain. Phillips et al came to a similar conclusion using stress X-rays in patients with low-back pain.[25,26] Li et al[27] had similar findings for the cervical spine, where they failed to find a significant relationship between radiological signs and clinical findings. Reinert's study[28,29] finding a correlation of lumbar radiographic findings with patient complaints, was strongly criticized by Cassidy.[28,29] Chiropractors who are not very concerned with pain reduction as a goal of care do not find the lack of association of pain and X-ray findings a problem. On the other hand, owing to the growing tendency to expect diagnostic findings to be patient-centered, and have relevance to the daily life of a patient, we would expect this lack of association of pain and X-ray findings to become increasingly problematic.

CONCLUSIONS

- It is hard to argue against the following simple thoughts concerning plain film radiography: (1) it provides information concerning the structural integrity of the spine, skull and pelvis; (2) it may help visualize the misalignment component of the vertebral subluxation; and (3) it may help us assess the postural status of the spinal column.

- Although some believe that analytic X-rays represent an unnecessary expense more likely to turn up red herrings than valuable clinical information, others remain dumbfounded as to how a chiropractor could profess to do well without them. Plaugher makes the case that arguments against routine radiography in chiropractic often confound medical and chiropractic indications for taking X-rays.[30]

- Although line marking seems to be a reproducible procedure, and patient positioning is at least a soluble problem in theory, the clinical relevance is still unknown. There is scant evidence that improvements in patients' symptoms track changes in their X-rays, or that the outcome of care is made better by the practice of taking X-rays to establish listings.

- Although some chiropractors would counter by claiming that subluxation analysis, including radiography, should not be symptom-driven, the unique situation of radiographic examination, unlike other chiropractic examination procedures, is that it poses a risk to the patient. While we continue to debate the clinical utility of X-ray line marking, we must address the very real possibility that there are some good reasons to consider exposure to ionizing radiation a bio-hazard. (For a particularly sobering view of the risks, the reader is advised to consult virtually any of the writings of the controversial John Gofman, such as his very detailed discussion of X-ray risks in *X-rays: Health Effects of Common Exams*,[31] or *Preventing Breast Cancer*.[32])

- The standing full-spine radiographic has had a contentious history of its own: some chiropractors are very much for and others very much against it. Taylor's review[33] finds that full-spine radiography is an effective diagnostic and analytic procedure with an acceptable risk–benefit ratio.

- Despite any proof that radiographic examination improves the outcome of care, it is still reasonable for a clinician to obtain radiographs if doing so is likely to influence the course of treatment. The Canadian chiropractors put it well in their Glenerin practice guidelines document: "The critical issue is *need* for the study. The practitioner considering imaging, from plain film to MRI, must consider this question: 'Will the results of this study have an impact on the treatment I propose to deliver?' If this question is asked and answered objectively in every case, there will be proper acquisition of imaging studies."[34]

REFERENCES

1. Christensen M G 2000 Job analysis of chiropractic. A project report, survey analysis and summary of the practice of chiropractic within the United States. National Board of Chiropractic Examiners, Greeley, CO
2. Jackson P 2001 Summary of the "2000 ACA professional survey on chiropractic practice." http://www.chiroweb.com/archives/19/06/17.html: Dynamic Chiropractic
3. MacRae J E 1974 Roentgenometrics in chiropractic. Canadian Memorial Chiropractic College, Toronto, Canada
4. Keating J C 1992 Shades of straight: diversity among the purists. Journal of Manipulative and Physiological Therapeutics 15 (3): 203–209
5. Yochum T R 1995 1895–1995: diagnostic imaging in its first century. Journal of Manipulative and Physiological Therapeutics 18 (9): 618–625
6. Kato J-D 2002 Do DCs need to take routine X-rays? Journal of the American Chiropractic Association 39 (12): 28–30
7. Gatterman B Guidelines in the use of radiography in chiropractic. http://www.chiroweb.com/archives/08/12/01.html: Dynamic Chiropractic
8. ACCR 2002 Diagnostic imaging in chiropractic for general and specialty practice. http://www.accr.org/ACCR_advanced_imaging_guidelines.rtf: American Chiropractic College of Radiology
9. WCA. Position paper on The guidelines for chiropractic quality assurance and practice parameters (Mercy guidelines). http://www.worldchiropracticalliance.org/positions/mercy2.htm: WCA
10. Harrison D E, Harrison D D, Troyanovich S J 1998 Reliability of spinal displacement analysis on plain X-rays: a review of commonly accepted facts and fallacies with implications for chiropractic education and technique. Journal of Manipulative and Physiological Therapeutics 21 (4): 252–266
11. Haas M, Taylor J A, Gillette R G 1999 The routine use of radiographic spinal displacement analysis: a dissent. Journal of Manipulative and Physiological Therapeutics 22 (4): 254–259
12. Owens E F Jr 1992 Line drawing analyses of static cervical X-ray used in chiropractic. Journal of Manipulative and Physiological Therapeutics 15 (7): 442–449
13. Plaugher G, Hendricks A H, Doble R W Jr et al 1993 The reliability of patient positioning for evaluating static radiologic parameters of the human pelvis. Journal of Manipulative and Physiological Therapeutics 16 (8): 517–522
14. Janik T, Harrison D E, Harrison D D et al 2001 Reliability of lateral bending and axial rotation with validity of a new method to determine axial rotation on anteroposterior cervical radiographs. Journal of Manipulative and Physiological Therapeutics 24 (7): 445–448
15. Zengel E, Davis B P 1988 Biomechanical analysis by chiropractic radiography: part III. Lack of effect of projectional distortion on Gonstead vertebral endplate lines. Journal of Manipulative and Physiological Therapeutics 11 (6): 469–473
16. Zengel E, Davis B P 1988 Biomechanical analysis by chiropractic radiography: part II. Effects of X-ray

projectional distortion on apparent vertebral rotation. Journal of Manipulative and Physiological Therapeutics 11 (5): 380–389

17. Zengel F, Davis B P 1988 Biomechanical analysis by chiropractic radiography: part I. A simple method for determining X-ray projectional distortion. Journal of Manipulative and Physiological Therapeutics 11 (4): 273–280

18. Jeffery K R 1981 X-ray analysis of differential leg length and pelvic distortion. Anglo-European College of Chiropractic dissertation, Bournemouth, UK

19. Cooperstein R 1990 Innominate vertical length differentials as a function of pelvic torsion and pelvic carrying angle. In: Jansen R D (ed.) Proceedings of the 5th Annual Conference on Research and Education, pp. 1–14. Consortium for Chiropractic Research, Sacramento, CA

20. Cooperstein R 1992 Roentgenometric assessment of innominate vertical length differentials. In: Proceedings of the 7th Annual Conference on Research and Education, pp. 273–277. Consortium for Chiropractic Research, Palm Springs, CA

21. Cooperstein R, Lisi A 2000 Pelvic torsion: anatomical considerations, construct validity, and chiropractic examination procedures. Topics in Clinical Chiropractic 7 (3): 38–49

22. Haas M, Peterson D 1992 A roentgenological evaluation of the relationship between segmental motion and malalignment in lateral bending. Journal of Manipulative and Physiological Therapeutics 15 (6): 350–360

23. Haas M, Nyiendo J 1992 Lumbar motion trends and correlation with low back pain. Part II. A roentgenological evaluation of quantitative segmental motion in lateral bending. Journal of Manipulative and Physiological Therapeutics 15 (4): 224–234

24. Haas M, Nyiendo J, Peterson C et al 1992 Lumbar motion trends and correlation with low back pain. Part I. A roentgenological evaluation of coupled lumbar motion in lateral bending. Journal of Manipulative and Physiological Therapeutics 15 (3): 145–158

25. Phillips R B 1992 Plain film radiology in chiropractic. Journal of Manipulative and Physiological Therapeutics 15 (1): 47–50

26. Phillips R B, Howe J W, Bustin G et al 1990 Stress X-rays and the low back pain patient. Journal of Manipulative and Physiological Therapeutics 13 (3): 127–133

27. Li Y K, Zhang Y K, Zhong S Z 1998 Diagnostic value on signs of subluxation of cervical vertebrae with radiological examination. Journal of Manipulative and Physiological Therapeutics 21 (9): 617–620

28. Reinert O C 1988 An analytical survey of structural aberrations observed in static radiographic examinations among acute low back cases. Journal of Manipulative and Physiological Therapeutics 11 (1): 24–30

29. Cassidy J D 1988 An analytical survey of structural aberrations observed in static radiographic examinations among acute low back cases. Journal of Manipulative and Physiological Therapeutics 11 (4): 329–330

30. Plaugher G 1992 The role of plain film radiography in chiropractic clinical practice. Chiropractic Journal of Australia 22 (4): 153–161

31. Gofman J W, O'Connor E 1985 X-rays: health effects of common exams. Sierra Club Books, San Francisco, CA

32. Gofman J W 1995 Preventing breast cancer: the story of a major, proven, preventable cause of this disease CNR Book Division, Committee for Nuclear Responsibility, San Francisco, CA

33. Taylor J A 1993 Full-spine radiography: a review. Journal of Manipulative and Physiological Therapeutics 16 (7): 460–474

34. CCA 1994 Clinical guidelines for chiropractic practice in Canada. http://www.ccachiro.org/client/CCA/CCAWeb.nsf/web/ClinicalGuidelinesMain?OpenDocument: Canadian Chiropractic Association

8

Thermography

INTRODUCTION

Thermography is typically used by Upper Cervical techniques, Gonstead, Thompson, Pierce–Stillwagon.

While still a chiropractic student, one of us volunteered to serve as a subject in a classroom demonstration of how thermography is done. The instructor, unhappily noting the superabundance of hair on the volunteer's back, agreed to use him, but only under the condition that the back hair first be shaved. That did not happen, although this subject has more recently consented to have his chest hair partially shaved for an electrocardiogram procedure. The reader may safely conclude that many years ago, the author (rightly or wrongly) did not regard dual-probed thermography as valid as electrocardiography.

Some chiropractors regard *instrumentation*, as it is called, essential to the objective demonstration of a state of vertebral subluxation. Without instrumentation, so they say, we would be left with little beyond the patient's subjective account of the pain that has brought him or her to the chiropractor. And if the patient has come in without symptoms, let's say for a spinal checkup, it becomes even more important to use instrumentation, to demonstrate the existence of asymptomatic subluxation pathology and in so doing document the need for chiropractic care.

Thermography may have been the first among the forms of instrumentation that have been developed over the years. (We review a few other selected forms of instrumentation in Ch. 9.) Patients tend to be very impressed with thermographic results, especially when they can be printed out and attached to the patient's chart. On the other hand, as we discuss below, the interpretation of such findings has been controversial over the years, both with technical objections to the various forms of thermographic technology that have been devised, as well as the underlying assumption that thermal symmetry is the norm.

OVERVIEW

Thermography is a procedure by which the surface temperature of the body can be measured, recorded, and depicted. Although the physiological rationale has been subject to reinterpretation over the years, the prevalent underlying premise is that a difference in surface temperature reflects a difference in vascular flow through the skin, which in turn reflects the state of the nervous system. Specifically, in a state of subluxation, there may be asymmetric left–right paraspinal temperature; or abnormal variation in the temperature of the spinal levels between the sacrum and the atlas; or there may be an abnormal *pattern* in paraspinal surface temperature as measured over the course of several days.

HISTORY

Although D D Palmer himself believed that nerve pressure would create "an increased amount of heat," the first measuring device was not built until 1924 by Dossa Evins. The early chiropractors thought thermographic devices directly measured the "heat of nerves." Evins took his thermographic device, the neurocalometer, to the Palmer College where it was used before and after adjustments to show that nerve pressure had been present and eliminated. BJ Palmer was so enamored with the device that he came to the conclusion that it was not possible to practice as a true chiropractic without using the device. Apparently, the majority of the profession did not agree, and those who did see value in using thermography tended to object strongly to BJ Palmer's attempted monopolization of the market: the only way to get one was to lease it from Palmer for an exorbitant fee. The débâcle was so extreme that BJ Palmer lost much of his influence over the profession for decades, even though thermography continued to interest many practitioners.

In the 1930s, Otto Shiernbeck developed technology that allowed the original neurocalometer to produce a printout of the result, that could be attached to the patient file and used for research purposes. The improved unit was termed the neurocalagraph. Since then, many other thermographic devices have been developed, inside and outside chiropractic. Although medicine has lost much confidence in thermography as a diagnostic procedure capable of detecting pathology, many chiropractors continue to feel comfortable with it. Both the dual-probe and infrared technologies (described below) claim practitioners today, even though they are increasingly challenged to demonstrate that the technology can discriminate between injured and non-injured, or sick and well patients, let alone identify specific subluxations, as chiropractors since the time of BJ have hoped it could.

COMMONLY ASSOCIATED TERMS AND CONCEPTS

- Dual-probe thermography: the thermographic device has two sensors that measure the temperature *differential* between the two points of application; examples: the Nervo-Scope, the neurocalometer
- Single-probe thermography: the thermographic device has one sensor that measures

the temperature at the point of application; example: the DT-25
- Infrared thermography (telethermography device): the thermographic device measures infrared radiation (heat) emitted from the body surface, essentially taking a colorized photo of skin temperature; example: the Tytron C-3000
- Liquid crystal thermography: an elastomeric latex sheet contacts the body, with embedded organic crystals that change color in relation to skin temperature
- Thermocouple thermography: measures skin temperature by direct contact of a thermal sensor composed of dissimilar wires; example: the Nervo-Scope
- Break analysis: interpretation of a rapid deflection of the device pointer, back and forth, believed to be within one dermatome
- Heat swing: interpretation of a deflection of the device pointer to the left and right over one or more apparent dermatomes
- Pattern system of analysis: it is believed that, under normal circumstances, the body is able to adapt to its changing environment in such a manner that there is a constant fluctuation of its thermal pattern
- Sick pattern: a relatively constant thermographic pattern, seen for 2–3 days, thought to reflect the body's inability to adapt to environmental changes and thus subluxation
- Mean heat line: slow and gradual drift of the indicator, thought to reflect some degree of normal bilateral thermal asymmetry
- Reading: rapid deflection and return of the indicator to the mean heat line.

MODE OF USE

Each of the two thermographic devices commonly used in chiropractic, the dual-probe and the infrared thermographic instruments, are not only used differently from one another, but are available in a number of forms that are used somewhat differently. Notwithstanding this variation in their mode of use, we can still provide a thumbnail sketch of how a typical unit is used.

Dual-probe thermography device

Practitioners emphasize the importance of exposing the patient's skin to the examination room ambient temperature for 10–12 min prior to the examination. The examiner draws the device along the entire length of the spinal column, moving at the rate of about 2–3 s per level. The examiner tries to exert a constant and firm pressure each time, use a steady speed, and remain parallel to the intervertebral disk planes. The sensors must be firmly pressed into the muscle, to prevent "air leaks." If and when the indicator swings toward a relatively warm side of the spine, the examiner confirms the finding by repeating the stroke several times at that same level. Any heat breaks that occur on the third pass are noted and thought to represent spinal subluxation (Fig. 8.1).

Infrared thermography devices

Since these devices in essence photograph the temperature of the back, they not only provide information on left–right thermal asymmetry, comparable to the dual-probe units, but also level-specific variations in absolute temperature from the sacrum to the head. Key to the proper use of these devices is maintaining a constant distance from the spine, since the amount of heat energy stimulating the reader varies inversely with the distance of the device from the source of the heat. Some devices (e.g., the DTG, or Dermo-Thermo-Graph) are lightly rolled along the spine, using a spacer to maintain a uniform distance from the skin. Thus, these thermographic devices share the property of patient contact with the thermocouple devices.

PHYSIOLOGICAL RATIONALE

The dual-probe devices employ two thermocouples, one per sensor, and a galvanometer, thus allowing the measurement of left–right paraspinal thermal asymmetry as the unit is applied to the various spinal levels. The single-probe devices sense infrared radiation from the skin and produce a digital readout of the temperature at any number of locations, paraspinally and elsewhere.

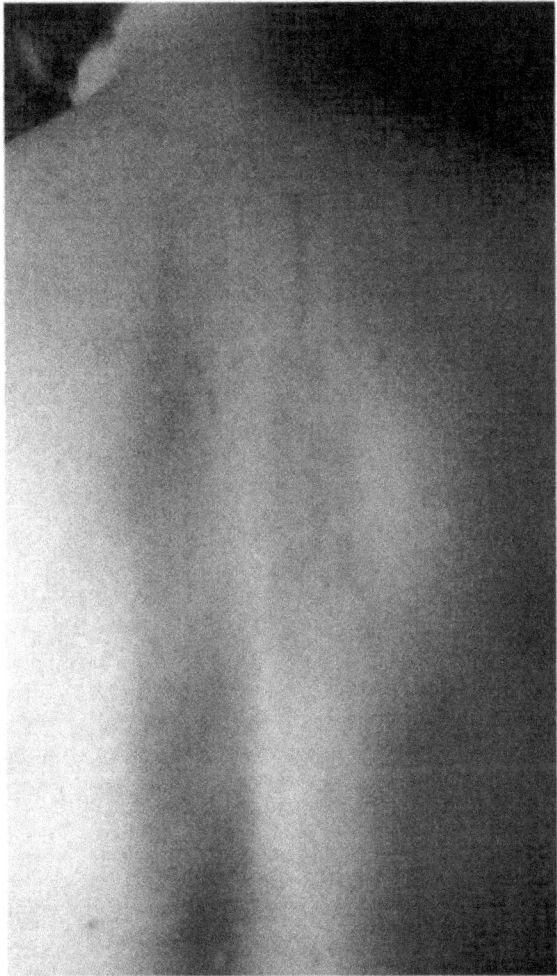

Figure 8.1   Triple response: acute inflammation produced by examination.

A roller device allows the unit to be kept at a constant distance from the spine. Liquid crystal thermography, in which a thin plastic film placed in contact with the body changes color in proportion to the surface temperature, is not used much anymore and will not be further described.

In the early days of the chiropractic use of thermography it was thought that temperature variation *directly* reflected nerve interference, in the sense that blockage to the flow of nerve impulses would create heat in body tissues, just as increased resistance raises the temperature of an electrical conductor. This theoretical rationale is completely invalidated by our contemporary understanding of the physiology of the nervous system, as most chiropractors are likely to acknowledge. Nevertheless, a more viable interpretation of thermal asymmetry and abnormal variation has been developed over several decades, which centers around the concept that thermal patterns reflect skin vascular flow, which in turn provides a window into the function of the nervous system, as affected by spinal subluxations.

Sir Thomas Lewis, in 1927, described the triple response to a blunt instrument, such as the handle of a reflex hammer, being pulled firmly across the skin: a relatively narrow red streak develops in the path of the instrument, followed by a red flare extending several centimeters out, and finally there is elevation of the skin (wheal formation). The elements of the triple response involve respectively capillary dilation, arteriolar dilation, and exudation into the extravascular space, as histamine is released from mast cells and basophils. In so many words, the firm pressure on the skin produces an acute inflammatory response. Some, but not all, chiropractors believe that skin temperature *indirectly* reflects spinal subluxation and resultant nerve interference, as it affects the autonomic nervous system. Chiropractic thermographers are quick to point out that thermal asymmetry should not be interpreted as a stand-alone finding, but should rather be correlated with the results of various other examination procedures in forming the clinical impression.

Those using dual-probe devices, given the finding of left–right thermal asymmetry, are likely to find the warmer side diagnostic of recent subluxation – in essence, evidence of an acute inflammatory response to local tissue damage. By comparison, the cold side may be thought to identify a chronic subluxation, one in which long-term tissue damage has resulted in diminished vascularity and blood flow. Given the finding of thermal asymmetry, deciding whether one side is abnormally warm or the other side is abnormally cold must depend on other information, such as the patient's history and other physical examination findings.

Since the infrared devices provide more information, it is possible to elaborate more complex physiological explanations. The bottom line is the assumption that, under normal circumstances, there should be not only right–left thermal symmetry (skin surface temperature) but also no abrupt level-specific changes in skin temperature.

In pattern analysis, the central hypothesis is that it is normal for skin surface temperature to fluctuate on a daily basis, from region to region. When a patient stays *in pattern* for 3 consecutive days, a state of subluxation is presumed to exist, in which abnormal spinal structure and/or function results in abnormal nervous system operation, conserving a given thermal pattern day after day.

EVIDENCE

There is a vast literature on thermography, both inside and outside chiropractic. (For a broad selection of references involving chiropractic alone, see sources).[1-41] Plaugher et al provide a comprehensive review article.[24] They conclude that infrared thermography seems to be sensitive for several disorders, including back pain, radiculopathy, and intervertebral disk lesions. They also believe it compares well with the results of reference technologies like computed tomography (CT) and myelogram. On the other hand, Plaugher et al report the dual-probe thermocouple devices to be less reliable than infrared devices, and moreover, largely unstudied in terms of their sensitivity for clinical conditions and correlation with more studied forms of thermography (infrared and liquid crystal).

Most research on the sensitivity and specificity of thermography pertains to the infrared technology. Although the conclusions are controversial, there is some evidence that it correlates with CT, magnetic resonance imaging, and electromyography; and can be used to evaluate conditions such as disk herniation, radiculopathy, and reflex sympathetic dystrophy. (For an interesting interchange, see online sources).[42-44] On the other hand, we must understand that, whatever physiology is measured by dual-probe thermography, there has been very little research on how well it correlates with infrared technology or to what degree its findings predict demonstrated pathologies like disk herniation or radiculopathy, let alone less verified "subluxation" findings.

Hoffman et al[45] executed a well-known meta-analysis (which pools the data from multiple studies in order to increase their collective power) that found little support for the routine use of thermography in the diagnosis of lumbar radiculopathy. It must be noted that the methodology of meta-analysis is itself controversial, and that the extreme rigor often used in this methodology in selecting studies to include is sometimes criticized as misleading. As Hoffman et al describe,[45] most studies show high true-positive rates (high sensitivity), but also high false-positive rates (low specificity). The best study showed sensitivity = specificity = 0.48, meaning that thermography was unable to discriminate between having and not having radiculopathy.

CONCLUSIONS

- The dual-probe devices, because of the firm pressure that is commonly used, produce a very visible reddening of the skin – in other words, acute inflammation.[1,10] This invalidates any assumption that these devices detect baseline skin thermal asymmetry. However, the amplitude and symmetry of the acute inflammation produced by dual-probe devices may be affected by subluxation states. If so, then the thermographic examination would detect not static skin vascularity, but the skin's dynamic evoked response to a clinical intervention, in this case a firm stroke across the skin. This possibility seems to be unstudied at this time.
- Whatever physiology is measured by dual-probe thermography, there has been very little research on how well it correlates with infrared technology or to what degree its findings predict demonstrated pathologies like disk herniation or radiculopathy, let alone less verified "subluxation" findings.
- Moreover, there is another comment to be made about diagnostic testing in general. Sometimes we want to measure what is, and other times we want to measure what happens. Clearly, to measure what is, our measuring device had best not alter the target phenomenon very much. Dual-probe thermography without doubt violates that stipulation, because it cannot measure a baseline condition.
- By comparison, to measure what happens, we necessarily alter the system, sometimes to a state of maximal perturbation. Therefore, in principle, dual-probe thermography may be used to assess a clinical intervention, firm skin pressure that evokes histamine response and a triple response. But even then, this clinical endpoint could not be compared with a baseline condition, unless we had obtained it beforehand using infrared technology. Since we can use the infrared device to measure the post-intervention skin temperature as well, after stroking the skin with any blunt instrument, we are not certain what need is filled, even putatively, by the dual-probe devices.
- The central problem with thermography over the years has been less a question of poor reliability, and more one of validity. In other words, although some studies show some level of inter-examiner agreement in heat readings, not everyone is convinced that thermography devices can distinguish symptomatic from asymptomatic, and injured from non-injured subjects.

REFERENCES

1. Amalu W C, Tiscareno L H 1994 The evolution of modern paraspinal thermography. Today's Chiropractic 23 (3): 38–41
2. BenEliyahu D J 1992 Infrared thermographic imaging in the detection of sympathetic dysfunction in patients with patellofemoral pain syndrome. Journal of Manipulative and Physiological Therapeutics 15 (3): 164–170
3. BenEliyahu D J, Silber B A 1990 Infra-red thermography and magnetic resonance imaging in patients with cervical disc protrusion. American Journal of Chiropractic Medicine 3 (3): 57–62
4. BenEliyahu D J, Duke S G 1991 Pathoneurophysiology assessed by infra-red thermography in patients with lumbar facet syndrome. Chiropractic: The Journal of Chiropractic Research and Clinical Investigation 8 (1): 3–9
5. BenEliyahu D J, Silber B A 1991 Infra-red thermographic imaging of lumbar dysautonomia owing to lumbar disc

protrusions: an observational single blind study. Manual Medicine 6: 130–135

6. BenEliyahu D J 1991 Infrared thermographic assessment of chiropractic treatment in patients with lumbar disc herniations: an observational study. Chiropractic Technique 3 (3): 126–133

7. Brand N E, Gizoni C M 1982 Moire contourography and infrared thermography: changes resulting from chiropractic adjustments. Journal of Manipulative and Physiological Therapeutics 5 (3): 113–116

8. Cannon L 1987 The validation of thermography. The American Chiropractor (February): 12, 14, 16–17, 21–22, 24, 26

9. Cockburn W 1986 Erroneous information is hurting thermography. California Chiropractic Journal (November): 12, 13

10. Cooperstein R 2002 Dual probe thermography: constructive test par excellence. Journal of the American Chiropractic Association 39 (9): 32–34

11. DeBoer K F, Harmon R O, Chambers R, Swank L 1985 Inter- and intra-examiner reliability of paraspinal infrared temperature measurements in normal students. Research Forum (Autumn): 4–11

12. Diakow P R, Oullet S 1988 Correlation of thermography with spinal dysfunction: preliminary results. Journal of the Canadian Chiropractic Association 32 (2): 77–80

13. Diakow P R 1992 Differentiation of active and latent trigger points by thermography. Journal of Manipulative and Physiological Therapeutics 15 (7): 439–441

14. Ebrall P S, Iggo A, Farrant G 1994 Preliminary report: the thermal characteristics of spinal levels identified as having differential temperature by contact thermocouple measurement (Nervo Scope). Chiropractic Journal of Australia 24 (4): 139–146

15. Harris W, Wagnon R J 1987 The effects of chiropractic adjustments on distal skin temperature. Journal of Manipulative and Physiological Therapeutics 10 (2): 57–60

16. Hart J F 2000 Toward a guideline for quantifying pattern analysis. Chiropractic Research Journal 7 (2): 79

17. Hart J F 2001 Analyzing the neurological interference component of the vertebral subluxation with the use of pattern analysis: a case report. Journal of Chiropractic Education 15 (1): 30–31

18. McClean J D 1999 Peripheral neuropathies: a guide to diagnostic imaging. Topics in Clinical Chiropractic 6 (4): 33–38

19. McConekey C, Patterson S, Waddel M, Steffen R 1990 Pre and post thermographic evaluation of chiropractic adjusting: a case report. ACA Journal of Chiropractic (July) 27 (7): 73–74

20. Owens E F, Stein T 2000 Computer-aided analysis of paraspinal thermographic patterns: a technical report. Chiropractic Research Journal 7 (2): 65–69

21. Perdew W, Jenness M, Daniels J et al 1976 A determination of the reliability and concurrent validity of certain body surface temperature-measuring instruments. Digest of Chiropractic Economics (May/June): 60–64

22. Pierce W V 1982 Instrumentation. Digest of Chiropractic Economics (September/October): 41–44

23. Ping Z, You F T 1993 Correlation study on infrared thermography and nerve root signs in lumbar intervertebral disk herniation patient: a short report. Journal of Manipulative and Physiological Therapeutics 16 (3): 150–154

24. Plaugher G, Lopes M A, Melch P E, Cremata E E 1991 The inter- and intraexaminer reliability of a paraspinal skin temperature differential instrument. Journal of Manipulative and Physiological Therapeutics 14 (6): 361–367

25. Plaugher G 1992 Skin temperature assessment for neuromusculoskeletal abnormalities of the spinal column. Journal of Manipulative and Physiological Therapeutics 15 (6): 365–381

26. Rademacher W J 1994 A premise for instrumentation. Chiropractic Technique 6 (3): 84–94

27. Reynolds C 1995 Thermogaphy in chiropractic. International Review of Chiropractic (May/June): 45–51

28. Sawyer C E, Meeker W C, Phillips R B 1992 Module summaries from consensus conference 2. Chiropractic Technique 4 (2): 37–45

29. Spector B, Fukada F, Kanner L, Thorschmidt E 1981 Dynamic thermography: a reliability study. Journal of Manipulative and Physiological Therapeutics 4 (1): 5–9

30. Stewart M S, Riffle D W, Boone W R 1989 Computer-aided pattern analysis of temperature differentials. Journal of Manipulative and Physiological Therapeutics 12 (5): 345–352

31. Stillwagon G 1985 Visi-therm: non-contact computerized infrared thermography. American Chiropractor (May): 63–67

32. Selko R, Stillwagon G, Stillwagon K 1985 Early observations of the Visi-Therm. Today's Chiropractic 14 (5): 38–40

33. Stillwagon G, Stillwagon K L 1986 Adjust or not to adjust. Digest of Chiropractic Economics 28 (5): 49

34. Stillwagon G, Stillwagon K L 1986 Thermography: an evaluation tool. Today's Chiropractic 15 (3): 59

35. Stillwagon G 1989 Thermography: is chiropractic ready for it? American Chiropractor (April): 28–31

36. Stillwagon G, Stillwagon K L, Stillwagon B S, Dalesio D J 1992 Chiropractic thermography. ICA International Review of Chiropractic 48 (1): 8–13

37. Stillwagon G, Stillwagon K L 1993 Objective chiropractic model for research. American Chiropractor 15 (5): 20–24

38. Stillwagon G, Delesio D 1998 Chiropractic thermography for outcomes measurement of the vertebral subluxation complex. Today's Chiropractic (May/June): 96–102

39. Stillwagon G, Stillwagon K L 1998 Vertebral subluxation correction and its effect on thermographic readings: a description of the advent of the Visi-Therm as applied to chiropractic patient assessment. Journal of Vertebral Subluxation Research 2 (3): 137–140

40. Wallace H, Wallace J, Resh R 1993 Advances in paraspinal thermographic analysis. Chiropractic Research Journal 2 (3): 39–52

41. Thompson C 1992 Paraspinal thermography. American Chiropractor (July/August): 32

42. Croft A C Thermography in soft tissue trauma: does it have a place? http://www.chiroweb.com/archives/11/10/01.html

43. Croft A C Rebuttal on thermography. http://www.chiroweb.com/archives/11/18/01.html

44. BenEliyahu D J Thermography in clinical practice: the rebuttal. http://www.chiroweb.com/archives/11/14/03.html

45. Hoffman R M, Kent D L, Deyo R A 1991 Diagnostic accuracy and clinical utility of thermography for lumbar radiculopathy. A meta-analysis. Spine 16 (6): 623–628

9

Instrumentation in chiropractic

INTRODUCTION

Instrumentation is the use of measuring equipment to demonstrate a parameter of the chiropractic subluxation. Although it is tempting to declare X-ray the ultimate example, chiropractic usage has tended to regard instrumentation as exclusive of X-ray. It would also be tempting to include relatively common devices, such as goniometers and inclinometers, as examples of chiropractic instrumentation, were it not for the fact that some in the chiropractic profession would consider such devices to be medical, or common-domain devices. They would be considered incapable of demonstrating a *segmental subluxation*. In the end, usage is usage, and we discuss a few devices that have been considered at various times and places examples of chiropractic instrumentation. They satisfy two primary criteria: (1) they provide objective measurements; and (2) they are thought to identify a segmental problem.

Some chiropractors regard instrumentation to be essential to the objective demonstration of a state of vertebral subluxation. Without instrumentation, it is said, we would have nothing but the patient's subjective account of the pain that probably brought him or her to the chiropractor. Moreover, if the patient is asymptomatic, instrumentation may demonstrate the existence of asymptomatic subluxation pathology and in so doing document the need for chiropractic care.

In Chapters 4–8 we covered what we regard as the five primary examination procedures common to many chiropractic technique systems and individual practitioners: leg checking, muscle testing, palpation, thermography, and X-ray line marking.

There are other examination procedures, mostly instrumented, that are utilized widely enough to warrant description, although not in separate chapters. We describe some of these in this chapter, although our relative brevity for each procedure precludes implementation of the examination procedure template that we used for the other four procedures. We use the term *instrumentation* less rigorously than Kyneur,[1] who reserves the term for electrical devices applied to the spine to detect vertebral subluxation.

TISSUE COMPLIANCE METER (TCM)

The tissue compliance meter was devised by Fischer[2,3] in the 1980s, and had some currency into the 1990s. The device, resembling to some extent a handheld adjusting instrument, measures the depth of penetration of a rubber-tipped stylus for a given force applied. The more kilograms of force it takes to penetrate a standard depth, say 6 mm, then the stiffer (or less compliant) the tissue is. Although Fischer's intent was that the tool be used to detect changes in soft-tissue consistency that occur in muscle spasm, spasticity, swelling, tumors, lumps, and hematomas, most investigators and clinicians who took up the use of the TCM thought it would be most useful as a barometer of muscle tonus. Muscles could then be determined to be hypertonic or hypotonic through TCM readings, or found responsive or not to clinical interventions.

Although Waldorf et al[4] in 1989 and Jansen et al[5] in 1990 found too much temporal variability in subjects for the TCM to be clinically useful, Sanders and Lawson in 1992[6] came to a different conclusion, finding great stability in subjects' findings. In 1993 Nansel et al,[7] to some extent reversing Nansel's previous finding of excessive subject temporal variation in TCM measurements, concluded that "test–retest measures obtained from the same subjects initially, and again 15 min or 2 wk later indicated fairly low short-term as well as long-term temporal variabilities for the measure."

The TCM was used as a clinical outcome measure by Vernon and Gitelman[8] in a headache case report. It was also used for basic science research by Kawchuk et al,[9] to show that multiple thrusting procedures increased soft-tissue compliance; and by Nansel et al[10] to show that lower cervical manipulation had a robust impact in increasing the compliance of the lumbar paraspinal musculature.

On the negative side, in 1992 Lawson and Sanders[11] found the TCM not to correlate well with electromyographic (EMG) findings, which they considered to be the gold standard. By 1994, Kawchuck, having previously used the tool in a research setting, had come to the conclusion that its accuracy and reliability had not been adequately studied. (One of us, Cooperstein, having been present at the 1994 scientific meeting where the TCM was criticized,[12] recalls that the symposium participants afforded the data much skepticism.) In 1995, Kawchuk and Herzog[13] executed a well-designed study in which a TCM was tested on four surfaces (one of which was perfectly rigid) with five different input forces, resulting in 20 different surface/force combinations. For each combination, 10 trials were obtained in a random order by each of five examiners, for a total of 1000 separate measurements of surface compliance. When all the statistics were done, the TCM was judged unreliable and inaccurate. Even the perfectly rigid surface was found penetrable up to 2 mm. Haas,[14] commenting on the study, felt that the statistical methods used were erroneous and that several of the study's conclusions were in doubt, although the investigators did not accept any of the criticisms.

That appears to have been the end of the TCM, in that we are unable to find very much published about it since 1995. We are somewhat amazed that the TCM, despite its great construct validity – in other words, despite the fact that its design and intended use make a great deal of sense – even granted the equivocal nature of research on it, has just about dropped off the face of the earth! By comparison, the popularity of thermography seems to be impervious to negative studies. At the time of this writing, we were unable to find a TCM for sale anywhere.

SOFT-TISSUE ALGOMETER (STA)

Manual palpation to identify tissue tenderness is already *pressure algometry*, just non-instrumented, and not very useful for the purpose of documentation. The soft-tissue algometer, sometimes called a *dolorimeter*, is a spring-loaded gauge attached to a rod with a soft rubber cap, resembling a handheld adjusting instrument. When the device is slowly pushed against the body, so that it depresses the soft tissue, the gauge measures how much force is applied, in either pounds or kilograms. The doctor applies progressively greater pressure until the patient reports that the sensation of pressure has changed to one of pain, at which point the number is recorded. Higher numbers (e.g., 5 kg or greater) indicate that the patient can tolerate a lot of pressure, meaning that area of the body is relatively pain-insensitive (non-tender) whereas lower numbers (e.g., 2 kg or less) mean that body part is relatively more prone to tenderness. At the pain–pressure threshold, as it is called, the algometer quantifies when the firm pressure becomes painful; it specifically does not measure how much pain the patient can tolerate. This is an important distinction in pressure algometry.

The STA, having been subjected to several reliability and validity studies,[15–19] is used to identify tender points and monitor their changes during treatment and over time. In addition to fairly generic use in uncomplicated musculoskeletal pain cases, it has also been used in more special circumstances, to identify malingerers and to document fairly nebulous syndromes such as fibromyalgia[20] and myofascial[2,21] trigger point syndromes. Moreover, it has been used as an outcome measure in the chiropractic research setting.[22–24] One of us (Cooperstein) has participated in a study that used an STA to measure changes in subjects' pain–pressure thresholds while lying on padded wedges (SOT blocks) arranged in various ways.[25]

Despite the better research record of the STA, compared with the TCM, at the time of this writing we were unable to find an STA for sale anywhere.

GALVANIC SKIN RESPONSE (GSR)

Many devices, the GSR unit and others, have been devised over the years to measure the resistance of the skin to the passage of an electrical current, by several professions and for several reasons. To put the matter simply, increased sudomotor activity (sweating) increases skin conductivity.

- Psychiatrists are interested in using this technology to evaluate emotional states, e.g., "Compared with controls, psychopaths were characterized by decreased electrodermal responsiveness."[26]
- Polygraphers make use of this physiology as part of a lie detector test, which contains other components, e.g., "GSR peak latency … responses corresponded to deception."[27]
- Neurologists are interested in monitoring the extent of spinal cord injury through its effect on sudomotor activity: "Somatosympathetic reflex was studied in 29 patients with definite multiple sclerosis (MS) by the non-invasive sympathetic skin response (SSR) method."[28]
- Acupuncturists believe that skin conductance measurements can help identify acupuncture sites: "Reports on the anatomy and electrical properties … of these sites indicate that many are significant local skin resistance minima."[29]
- According to Plaugher et al, osteopaths like Korr and his associates did extensive research in the 1940s on whether spinal lesions could be detected or confirmed by their effects on sympathetic activity and thus skin conductivity.[30]
- Chiropractors, finally, have also been using such devices for many decades; in a letter to the editor, Johnston[31] claimed in 1989 to have been using a GSR unit for 28 years, although he doesn't really say for what purpose.

Certainly by the 1980s some chiropractors were claiming they could diagnose certain spinal conditions, such as subluxations, through the use of the GSR unit. Their idea was that spinal subluxations that caused nerve root impingement were likely to have an impact on autonomic function that could in principle be detected by skin conduction studies. Nansel and Jansen,[32] in a particularly meticulous study in 1988, found tremendous instability in the location of such points of lowered resistance. They also found they tended to coincide with known acupuncture loci, that the tool seemed actually to *cause* increased skin conduction, and finally that the results for live research subjects were very similar to those obtained on eight embalmed cadavers! Plaugher et al[30] found unacceptably low interexaminer reliability in using the GSR unit, and in essence called for discontinuing its use, as least for identifying spinal musculoskeletal problems.

In retrospect, it seems obvious that since emotional factors heavily influence sweat secretion, and since sympathetic activity is rapidly affected by environmental influences (including testing procedures), it is not surprising that the vertebral levels identified in the Nansel and Jansen study[32] were unreliable, both temporally and in terms of interexaminer reliability. The magnitude of electrical resistance is affected not only by the subject's general mood, but also by immediate emotional reactions. Moreover, it seems to require a fairly significant spinal cord or nerve injury to impact on sudomotor activity, so it is not surprising that such impacts fail to show up on typical chiropractic or osteopathic patients, let alone the asymptomatic chiropractic students that usually enter into studies like those of Plaugher et al,[30] and Nansel and Jansen.[32]

Finally, the following words of Nansel and Jansen are particularly chilling: "The observation that the GSR unit itself can significantly lower the resistance at these acupuncture loci suggests that it may create, in a matter of seconds, the very low resistance points that it is designed to detect. The likelihood of this occurring would increase if the operator is led by previous diagnostic tests or impressions to even marginally prolong 'search' time in any given area."[32]

As of this writing, although skin electrical conductance readers remain in widespread use in other professions, including neurology and polygraphy, we are not aware of any significant use being made in the chiropractic profession.

NERVE FUNCTION TESTS

EMG, sensory evoked potentials, nerve conduction velocity, and electroencephalography

Only the primary neurodiagnostic examination procedure likely to be performed by a chiropractor, the EMG, warrants discussion. It is used to discern differences between an injured or symptomatic patient, or to monitor changes in a patient. EMG produces a graphical record of electric currents associated with muscle contractions, and is used to diagnose neuromusculoskeletal disorders. It can, for example, distinguish between problems with the nerves that stimulate a muscle (as in multiple sclerosis) and primary muscle pathology, as in muscular dystrophy. Medical practitioners use needle EMG, in which a fine needle is placed in a muscle belly for recording purposes, whereas chiropractors perform scanning EMG, in which surface electrodes are used.

The reliability, validity, and indications for using scanning EMG remain controversial. A review article in 1994[33] did not identify substantive support in the literature, a view that received further support from Triano.[34] Danneels et al[35] did not find the interexaminer reliability of scanning EMG to be acceptable. On the other hand, Herzog et al[36] used surface electrode EMG to show reflex responses associated with spinal manipulation. More recently, Lehman[37] used scanning EMG in three separate studies, one of which showed the technology to have "excellent repeatability"

on tests conducted on three separate days. For an account of the growing tendency of chiropractors to specialize in neurology, we refer you to an article published in the Journal of The American Chiropractic Association.[38]

CONCLUSIONS

Let's face it, every one of us chiropractors would love to get our hands on a safe and effective *subluxometer*. The problem is, once we deploy any definition of subluxation beyond vertebral misalignment, and once we go beyond the tried and true X-ray technology that measures vertebral misalignment, the possibility of a universally accepted subluxometry erodes quickly.

Equipment entrepreneurs have attempted to assuage our thirst for a subluxometer by devising an endless stream of gadgets, some of rather dubious nature, and others that actually make a lot of sense. The better tools do not purport to measure the subluxation per se, the original dream of chiropractic instrumentation (such as the Toftness Radiation Detector, Ch. 30) but rather some aspect of spinal dysfunction: reflex activity, manipulation-related audibles, other vibrations, joint fixation, and more. Time will tell if any of the newer devices catch on. One thing is certain: as the adherence of chiropractic to the standards of contemporary technology assessment solidifies, the time is past when any such devices could be marketed and find widespread use in the absence of any correlation with patient-relevant other examination findings. In other words, patients, insurers, and researchers are not likely to be impressed with measurements that do not predict symptoms.

REFERENCES

1. Kyneur J S 1992 Lost technology: the rise and fall of chiropractic instrumentation. Chiropractic History 12 (1): 31–35
2. Fischer A A 1988 Documentation of myofascial trigger points. Archives of Physical Medicine and Rehabilitation 69 (4): 286–291
3. Fischer A A 1987 Tissue compliance meter for objective, quantitative documentation of soft tissue consistency and pathology. Archives of Physical Medicine and Rehabilitation 68 (2): 122–125

4. Waldorf T, Paiso A, Devlin L, Nansel D 1989 The assessment of paraspinal tissue compliance at different vertebral segments in otherwise asymptomatic male subjects. In: Coyle B (ed.) 4th Annual Conference on Research and Education, pp. A4-1–A4-6, Pacific Consortium for Chiropractic Research, Belmont, CA
5. Jansen R D, Nansel D D, Slosberg M 1990 Normal paraspinal tissue compliance: the reliability of a new clinical and experimental instrument. Journal of

Manipulative and Physiological Therapeutics 13 (5): 243–246

6. Sanders G E, Lawson D A 1992 Stability of paraspinal tissue compliance in normal subjects. Journal of Manipulative and Physiological Therapeutics 15 (6): 361–364

7. Nansel D D, Waldorf T, Cooperstein R 1993 Effect of cervical spinal adjustments on lumbar paraspinal muscle tone: evidence for facilitation of intersegmental tonic neck reflexes. Journal of Manipulative and Physiological Therapeutics 16 (2): 91–95

8. Vernon H, Gitelman R 1993 Pressure algometry and tissue compliance measures in the treatment of chronic headache by spinal manipulation: a single case/single treatment report. Journal of the American Chiropractic Association 34 (3): 141–144

9. Kawchuk G, Zhang Y K, Conway P, Herzog W 1993 Sequential manipulations to the thoracic spine and their effect on achieving cavitation. In: Seater S R (ed.) International Conference on Spinal Manipulation, p. 16. FCER, Montreal, CA

10. Nansel D, Waldorf T, Cooperstein R 1992 Effect of cervical adjustments on lumbar paraspinal tissue compliance – evidence for facilitation of intersegmental tonic neck reflexes. In: Callahan D L (ed.) International Conference on Spinal Manipulation, p. 149. Foundation for Chiropractic Education and Research, Chicago, IL

11. Lawson D, Sanders G 1992 A comparison of measurements between the tissue compliance meter and surface electromyography. In: Callahan D L (ed.) International Conference on Spinal Manipulation, p. 105. Foundation for Chiropractic Education and Research, Chicago, IL

12. Kawchuk G, Herzog W 1994 Tissue compliance measurement: wishful thinking? In: Seater S R (ed.) International Conference on Spinal Manipulation, p. 26. FCER, Palm Springs, CA

13. Kawchuk G, Herzog W 1995 The reliability and accuracy of a standard method of tissue compliance assessment. Journal of Manipulative and Physiological Therapeutics 18 (5): 298–301

14. Haas M 1996 The reliability and accuracy of a standard method of tissue compliance assessment (letter and response). Journal of Manipulative and Physiological Therapeutics 19 (1): 60–61

15. Antonaci F, Sand T, Lucas G A 1998 Pressure algometry in healthy subjects: inter-examiner variability. Scandinavian Journal of Rehabilitative Medicine 30 (1): 3–8

16. Kosek E, Ekholm J, Nordemar R 1993 A comparison of pressure pain thresholds in different tissues and body regions. Long-term reliability of pressure algometry in healthy volunteers. Scandinavian Journal of Rehabilitative Medicine 25 (3): 117–124

17. List T, Helkimo M, Falk G 1989 Reliability and validity of a pressure threshold meter in recording tenderness in the masseter muscle and the anterior temporalis muscle. Cranio 7 (3): 223–229

18. Nussbaum E L, Downes L 1998 Reliability of clinical pressure-pain algometric measurements obtained on consecutive days. Physical Therapy 78 (2): 160–169

19. Ohrbach R, Gale E N 1989 Pressure pain thresholds, clinical assessment, and differential diagnosis: reliability and validity in patients with myogenic pain. Pain 39 (2): 157–169

20. Lautenschlager J, Bruckle W, Schnorrenberger C C, Muller W 1988 [Measuring pressure pain of tendons and muscles in healthy probands and patients with generalized tendomyopathy (fibromyalgia syndrome)]. Zeitschrift für Rheumatologie 47 (6): 397–404

21. Reeves J L, Jaeger B, Graff-Radford S B 1986 Reliability of the pressure algometer as a measure of myofascial trigger point sensitivity. Pain 24 (3): 313–321

22. Schiller L 2001 Effectiveness of spinal manipulative therapy in the treatment of mechanical thoracic spine pain: a pilot randomized clinical trial. Journal of Manipulative and Physiological Therapeutics 24 (6): 394–401

23. Haas M, Peterson D, Panzer D et al 1993 Reactivity of leg alignment to articular pressure testing: evaluation of a diagnostic test using a randomized crossover clinical trial approach. Journal of Manipulative and Physiological Therapeutics 16 (4): 220–227

24. Haas M, Peterson D, Hoyer D, Ross G 1994 Muscle testing response to provocative vertebral challenge and spinal manipulation: a randomized controlled trial of construct validity. Journal of Manipulative and Physiological Therapeutics 17 (3): 141–148

25. Lisi A, Cooperstein R, Morschhauser E 2003 An exploratory study of provocation testing with padded wedges: can prone blocking demonstrate a directional preference? in press.

26. Herpertz S C, Werth U, Lukas G et al 2001 Emotion in criminal offenders with psychopathy and borderline personality disorder. Archives of General Psychiatry 58 (8): 737–745

27. Dollins A B, Cestaro V L, Pettit D J 1998 Efficacy of repeated psychophysiological detection of deception testing. Journal of Forensic Science 43 (5): 1016–1023

28. Gutrecht J A, Suarez G A, Denny B E 1993 Sympathetic skin response in multiple sclerosis. Journal of the Neurological Sciences 118 (1): 88–91

29. Reichmanis M, Becker R O 1978 Physiological effects of stimulation at acupuncture loci: a review. Comp Med East West 6 (1): 67–73

30. Plaugher G, Haas M, Doble R W Jr et al 1993 The interexaminer reliability of a galvanic skin response instrument. Journal of Manipulative and Physiological Therapeutics 16 (7): 453–459

31. Johnston R J 1989 Concordance between galvanic skin response and spinal palpation findings in pain-free males. Journal of Manipulative and Physiological Therapeutics 12 (5): 402–404

32. Nansel D D, Jansen R D 1988 Concordance between galvanic skin response and spinal palpation findings in pain-free males. Journal of Manipulative and Physiological Therapeutics 11 (4): 267–272

33. Meyer J J 1994 The validity of thoracolumbar paraspinal scanning EMG as a diagnostic test: an examination of the current literature. Journal of Manipulative and Physiological Therapeutics 17 (8): 539–551

34. Triano J J 1995 The validity of thoracolumbar paraspinal scanning EMG as a diagnostic test: examination of the current literature. Journal of Manipulative and Physiological Therapeutics 18 (7): 482–484

35. Danneels L A, Cagnie B J, Cools A M et al 2001 Intra-operator and inter-operator reliability of surface

electromyography in the clinical evaluation of back muscles. Manual Therapy 6 (3): 145–153

36. Herzog W, Scheele D, Conway P J 1999 Electromyographic responses of back and limb muscles associated with spinal manipulative therapy. Spine 24 (2): 146–152; discussion 153

37. Lehman G J 2002 Clinical considerations in the use of surface electromyography: three experimental studies. Journal of Manipulative and Physiological Therapeutics 25 (5): 293–299

38. Staff 2000 Neurology: heart of the profession. Journal of the American Chiropractic Association 37 (6): 8–10, 12–14

Chiropractic system techniques

Section 3 consists of 24 chapters on named technique systems presented in alphabetical order, making up the core of this book. As simple a task as alphabetizing the technique systems presented us with some difficult choices, as some technique systems are known by more than one name depending on the context. Therefore, if, as the reader, you have been unable to find a technique system under the name you were expecting, please look through the table of contents to see if we listed it under a different name.

No doubt there are some who will think that we have left out an important technique, and others who will think that we have included a technique which we should not have, but we do think if anything it is best to err on the side of inclusiveness. More importantly, we had choices to make about how to cover closely related techniques: whether to collapse them into one chapter or provide each in a separate chapter. We elected to collapse techniques in chapter 12 on Kinesiologies, and chapters 32 and 33 on manual and instrumented Upper Cervical techniques. We hope that proponents of the various technique systems realize that our personal feelings about the safety and effectiveness of individual techniques had nothing to do with our decisions to group the material in the way we have done.

10

Activator Methods Chiropractic Technique (AMCT)

This chapter is partially based on previously published material, and is printed with the permission of the National University of Health Sciences

INTRODUCTION

When people experience or hear of Activator Technique, the first thing they think of is the handheld adjusting tool – the "clicking thing," as patients sometimes put it. However, it's not that simple. AMCT, like most other technique systems, cannot be reduced to the adjustive intervention alone. Technique systems deploy distinctive analytic procedures, terminology, and practice patterns. The possibility of distinguishing a technique's analytic protocol from its adjustive style creates a situation where a practitioner might partially use a technique. This is true of all technique systems in chiropractic, but it is especially obvious in the case of Activator Methods technique, owing to the very distinct method by which the adjustive force is applied.

A chiropractor could conduct an examination procedure according to the protocol described in an Activator textbook or seminar manual (leg checks, isolation, and compression testing), and then adjust the patient from head to foot using high-velocity, low-amplitude thrusts. In a very limited sense, deriving listings "the Activator way" constitutes a kind of Activator practice. A different chiropractor might derive listings without relying on any typical Activator protocols, say, depending entirely on X-ray examination, and then adjust the patient using the handheld adjusting instrument. That also, in a limited sense, would constitute a type of Activator practice. Since the tool is more characteristic of an Activator practice than the more generic analytic protocol, that "clicking thing" continues to define the Activator doctor more than any other practice characteristic.

OVERVIEW[1]

According to Fuhr and Osterbauer,[2] AMCT is a synthesis of several analytic systems and low-force adjustive procedures, including Logan Basic, Derifield–Thompson leg checking, and Van Rumpt's Directional Non-Force Technique (DNFT), featuring thumb thrusts and a system of leg-length analysis. Subluxations as detected primarily by the leg check and reflex procedures are addressed using a mechanical percussive tool called the Activator adjusting instrument, AAI, or simply, "Activator." The leg-checking procedure also serves to establish correction of the subluxations.

AMCT seeks to conduct a systematic analysis of basic body biomechanics, with the understanding that disturbed mechanics leads to disturbed function. Using a series of diagnostic provocative maneuvers and leg checks to identify the location of subluxations, the therapeutic goal is to restore proper body mechanics through the application of low-force adjustments. The use of the Activator adjusting instrument is thought to promote both increased patient and doctor safety.

HISTORY

Arlan Fuhr, cofounder of AMCT, and a 1961 graduate of the Logan College of Chiropractic, always felt himself qualified in the study of basic body mechanics, but perceived both a personal and profession-wide weakness in terms of the systematic clinical application of these biomechanics. He decided to develop a "step by step procedure ... a system of analysis"[3] that would fill this void.

Drs Arlan Fuhr and WC Lee founded Activator Methods Technique in 1967, in Redwood Falls, MN.[1] Both doctors, having been practitioners of the low-force Logan Basic Technique, saw this as a logical extension of their previous work. They stated from the outset that "force is not the key to moving bones."[5] Fuhr stated later on: "My philosophy of practice has been to use as little force as possible on patients ... My views have been colored by my Logan training ... I have been very careful to only adjust segments which show-up on analysis and correlate with the patient's symptoms."[6]

Originally, AMCT used a thumb thrust similar to that used by Van Rumpt in DNFT, but later on introduced instrument adjusting, a practice that is central to the technique as it is perceived by the profession. Osterbauer et al claim[7] that instrument adjusting originated as an attempt to emulate the effect of a manual toggle-recoil adjustment, which he dates to the introduction of the Hole-In-One (HIO) upper cervical technique by BJ Palmer in the early 1930s. (We note that the toggle-recoil adjustment had already been described by Stephenson in his 1927 *Chiropractic Textbook*.[8] Furthermore, it has been traced by Carl Cleveland III to the earliest years of chiropractic.[9]) The idea was to invest the thrust with "a greater degree of controllable and repeatable speed, depth and direction."[7] According to Osterbauer and Fuhr, "The AAI is the most widely used thrusting device among chiropractors, and has been in use for approximately 20 years."[10]

In addition to presumed greater patient safety, doctor safety is another important consideration for having adopted instrument adjusting: "We used a [thumb thrust] for 3 years, until our elbows and thumbs started to hurt more than the patients we treated. It was because of our own physical discomfort that the Activator instrument was designed."[5] The percussive device was awarded a patent and is recognized under the Food and Drug Administration Medical Devices Act. It has also been qualified as a method of manual manipulation, which permits practitioners to be reimbursed under the Medicare program.

Although Fuhr was instructed in the Derifield leg-check procedure by Dr. Mabel Derifield herself, a member of the family that devised the system, he has never referred to his own leg-check methodology as a "Derifield leg check." He states that he has added enough "additional correlations to Derifield's methods to justify the term 'Activator Methods leg check'."[4]

Activator Methods has been conducting seminars since 1967, and claimed there were 8000 practitioners worldwide in 1986.[1] AMCT is taught (usually as an elective or continuing education course) in several of the chiropractic colleges, and was the first chiropractic group to receive a Small Business Innovative Research grant from the National Institutes of Health.

DEFINITION OF TECHNIQUE-SPECIFIC TERMS

- Activator: the term "activator" originated from the concept that it does not take much force to move a bone; muscles do the work, provided the bone has been "activated" in the correct direction[3]
- AAI: activator adjusting instrument, "a manually manipulatable instrument capable of providing a dynamic thrust that includes a controlled force of adjustment at a precise and specific line of drive at high speed."[11] It has also been described as a handheld, manually assisted, spring-activated device which delivers a maximum of 0.3 J of energy under controlled conditions (Fig. 10.1)[7]
- Isolation testing: "prone observations are made of straight and flexed LLs [leg lengths] while the patient's extremities are positioned so as to exacerbate muscular imbalance at specific spinal segments."[10] The isolation test is a specific, active movement of the patient, aimed at detecting facilitated segments through leg reactivity
- Pressure testing: this has been described as "light pressure applied in the direction of the correction,"[11] as it determines the result of the leg-checking procedure. It is a brief application of provocative pressure to a body structure under investigation, typically the spinous process of a vertebra. The outcome of the test is determined by responsiveness or lack thereof in relative leg positions

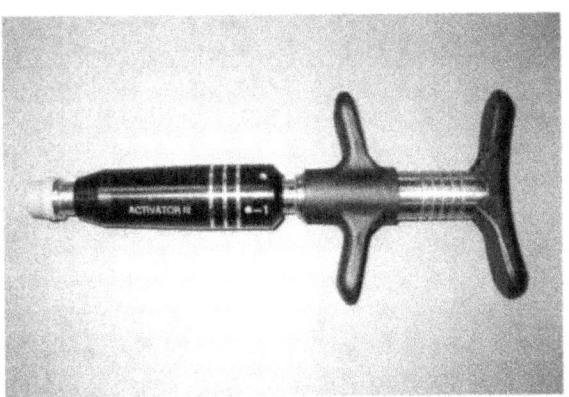

Figure 10.1 Activator adjusting instrument.

- Pelvic deficiency (PD) leg: the leg that appears short in performing a prone leg check, or which "gives, shortens or feels soft and spongy" in the prone leg check;[3] not to be confused with an anatomically shortened lower extremity
- Reactive leg: the leg that relatively shortens response to a provocative, diagnostic procedure
- MFMA: mechanical force, manually assisted, short lever adjustment
- Stress test: this has been described as "light pressure applied into the direction of the subluxation."[11]

PHYSIOLOGICAL MECHANISMS AND RATIONALE

Bearing witness to its Loganesque roots, AMCT generally posits a primary anterior–inferior subluxation of the sacrum, which eventually leads to a state of interinnominate pelvic torsion. AMCT also believes that biomechanical and postural asymmetry present in the weight-bearing position is at least to some extent preserved in the prone patient. In particular, pelvic torsion is associated with neurological irritation and muscular imbalance that produce a physiological short leg in the prone patient. Changes in relative leg length during diagnostic and therapeutic procedures are thought to assist identification and localization of subluxations.

According to Osterbauer and Fuhr,[10] "Apparent differences in leg lengths (LLs) are suggestive of segmental dysfunction of the spine, pelvis, and/or extremities. Pelvic torsional stress and/or unilateral muscular hypertonus (due to facilitation) are thought to be manifested by the presence of a functional short leg." The isolation test is thought to identify the presence of vertebral subluxation; the putative (hypothetical) mechanism is that passive movement of a subluxated and therefore hyperirritable segment results in muscle contraction that causes a change in leg length.[12] Slosberg[13] describes how the theoretical rationale follows from the original work of Denslow and Korr.

Duell[14] speculated that the effect of the Activator thrust (and the DNFT thumb toggle as well) might well resemble what is seen in "hold/relax" proprioceptive neurofacilitation (PNF) technique. That is, the thrust dramatically elongates a shortened muscle, provided the AAI is used to prestress it. The result would be relaxation of that muscle through activation of the Golgi tendon organ reflex.

DIAGNOSTIC/ANALYTIC PROCEDURES

The measurement of relative leg length constitutes the primary AMCT-specific diagnostic procedure, at least for somatic dysfunction (Fig. 10.2). Fuhr claims to have introduced enough modifications into the Derifield leg-checking procedure to warrant the term "Activator leg check" (Fig. 10.3). Indeed, there are significant differences between the AMCT leg-check procedure and that of other practitioners using an otherwise similar Derifield-like procedure. Thompson and Stillwagon Technique doctors, for example, do not use changes in relative leg lengths following provocative procedures (like pressure testing) as an outcome measure.

Leg checking in AMCT serves at least two roles:

1. Relative leg lengths may change in response to isolation testing, turning the head, or possibly other provocative maneuvers, providing evidence of subluxation.

2. Relative leg length differentials, as detected in a Derifield-like leg-check procedure, provide evidence of pelvic torsion and associated lumbopelvic dysfunction, including muscle imbalance.

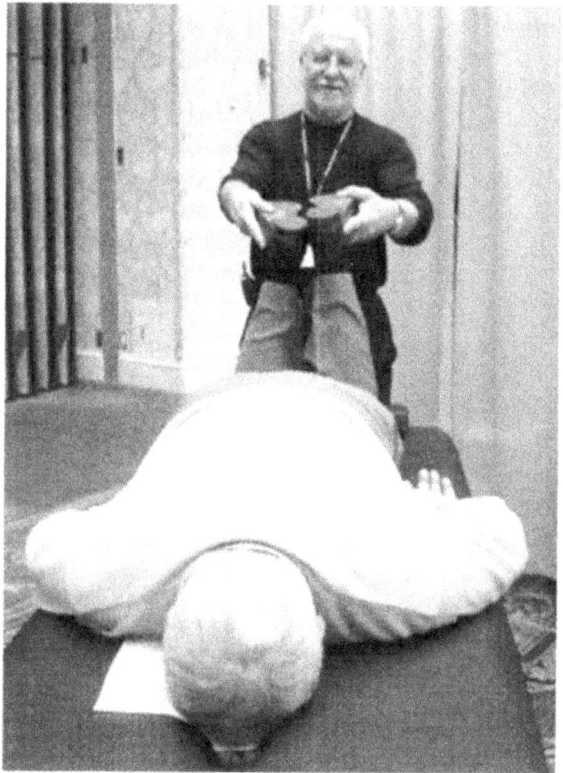

Figure 10.2   Dr. Fuhr performing an Activator leg check.

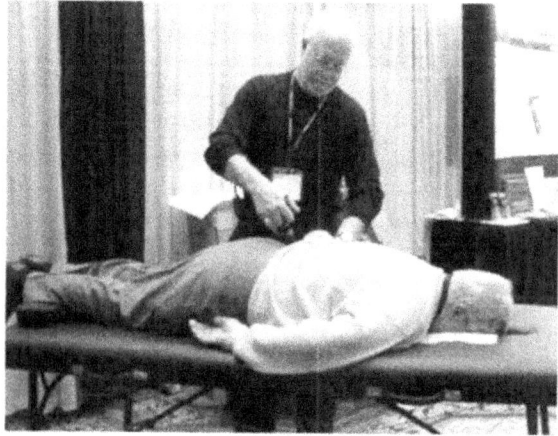

Figure 10.3   Fuhr adjustment.

Isolation testing, as defined above, is the primary screen for subluxation detection, in that changes in relative leg length in response to provocative positioning of the extremities are thought to indicate segmental dysfunction. Suspected segments would then be systematically subjected to pressure testing and palpation as confirmatory procedures.

Henningham[15] describes a hybrid Sacro-Occipital Technique–AMCT analysis of torticollis, coming to the conclusion that the misalignment involved is generally a laterality of atlas (to either side) coupled with a posterior rotation of atlas ipsilateral to the side to which the neck will neither bend nor rotate. The treatment uses the AAI, applied to the upper cervical spine of the prone patient.

TREATMENT/ADJUSTIVE PROCEDURES

The patient is lowered to the prone position using a Hi-Lo type of table. The primary treatment procedure is the adjustive thrust delivered by the AAI, to spinal, pelvic, and extremity structures. Peters describes an "Activator lift" adjustment for facet syndrome, in which the AAI thrusts into the spinous process some six to eight times, as the patient sits with the spine flexed.[16]

Asked in a 1983 interview, "Do you use adjunctive therapies?" Dr. Fuhr answered "None ... I believe that the only reason a chiropractor goes into physical therapy is because he is at a loss as to how to adjust when he sees an extremely acute patient!"[17] None the less, it seems that AMCT no longer maintains such a purist position on the use of physiotherapy. For example, Frach et al report successful treatment of two cases of Bell's palsy in which AAI adjusting was supplemented with exercise and electrotherapy.[18] Likewise, a case study was presented in which chronic sciatica was treated by AAI adjusting supplemented by a video assisted stretching program.[19]

OUTCOME ASSESSMENT

AMCT claims no originality in assessing clinical outcomes, as compared with other health disciplines. It claims to be part of a growing consensus that variables such as pain, patient satisfaction, global range of motion, and neurophysiological function are the primary factors. AMCT has been actively involved in promoting the widespread use of survey instruments such as the Oswestry questionnaire, the visual analog scale (VAS), and the Neck Disability Index.

On the other hand, it remains quite clear that a successful outcome, at least during a given office visit, would also include the amelioration of certain AMCT-specific clinical findings, such as positive isolation tests and leg checks: "Relative equalization of leg length following manipulation is interpreted as a successful intervention."[20]

Considerable effort has been expended to measure objectively relative leg-length changes using an optoelectric measuring apparatus. One of the particularly interesting findings was that "net changes in position measures were much larger during the active isolation tests than the passive isolation tests, suggesting that voluntary effort must be utilized to induce leg movement."[21]

SAFETY AND RISK FACTORS

We are aware of no contraindictions to care that are specific to AMCT, different from chiropractic care in general. AMCT is at best dubious about the value of side-posture manipulation in cases of low-back disk herniation, and has also questioned the utility, much less the necessity, of achieving an audible "crack" when using spinal manipulative therapy. The percussive AAI is thought to lower the risk of iatrogenic postmanipulative injuries: "The Activator technique, because of its controlled force and displacement, is widely considered to be a safe, non-traumatic method of chiropractic care."[22]

EVIDENCE OF EFFICACY

Due to the relative abundance of Activator-related articles in the literature, we categorize the relevant literature as either diagnostic or treatment-oriented. In addition, we also list a few other studies that bear on AMCT, even though they did not intend to study it per se.

Diagnostic efficacy

Youngquist et al[12] found good interexaminer reliability when two examiners performed an isolation test for C1 subluxation on 72 subjects. They concluded that the isolation test in conjunction with a prone leg check might reliably identify somatic spinal dysfunction. Fuhr and Osterbauer[2] reported "fair" to "good" interexaminer reliability in the determination of relative leg-length inequality in prone subjects. Nguyen et al[23] reported high reliability (kappa = 0.66) between two examiners.

DeWitt et al[24] used optoelectric equipment to measure objectively changes in leg length during isolation testing. The prone subject wore fracture boots to which infrared light-emitting diodes were attached, displacement of which could be recorded by an external apparatus. Cervical extension was shown to produce leg retraction. During the head-up procedure, patients showed more asymmetrical heel motions than did controls, suggesting that isolation testing may be able to discriminate between the two groups. Letters to the editor by Troyanovich[25] and Haas[26] questioning the clinical relevance of the work received an interesting and important response from DeWitt et al,[27] which identifies the primary significance of their work: they have constructed an objective leg position measuring apparatus, which allows determination not only of "absolute net length changes, but trajectories through which each individual foot travels as a result of isolation tests."[27]

Several studies pertaining to the Derifield pelvic leg check (DPLC)[28] have been performed. Researchers have attempted to assess the interexaminer reliability of the DPLC,[2,29-35] but have failed to demonstrate consistent results. Fuhr and Osterbauer did find a measure of reliability,[2] but Haas and Peterson[29] had methodological criticisms of the study. DeBoer et al[33] found good interexaminer reliability in both the knees-extended and knees-flexed positions, but their interpretation of the data was later questioned by Danelius.[31] By comparison, Rhudy and Burk[35] were unable to obtain significant interexaminer reliability in any of four different evaluations of the Thompson leg check system, with Thompson himself participating in part of the study. Shambaugh et al[30] reported good interexaminer reliability for the knees-extended position, but this study has also been criticized for improper statistics.[36,37] Falltrick and Pierson[34] failed to find leg reactivity in response to head rotation, but they were criticized for failing to exert cephalad pressure on the feet during the test.[10] Cooperstein[38] provides a kinesiological interpretation of the DPLC, but this otherwise interesting work is data-free.[39] Venn et al[40] found poor radiographic concordance in prone, supine, and standing radiological leg checks; their statistics were questioned by Osterbauer and Fuhr,[10] who found the study's conclusions insupportable.

Gemmel and Jacobson[41] randomly assigned patients with low-back pain to two groups, one using palpatory pain as a subluxation indicator, and the other a positive finding using a Toftness instrument. Each patient reported less pain after receiving one intervention using an AAI.

Treatment efficacy

Ten patients satisfying very specific criteria for chronic sacroiliac joint dysfunction were culled from a group of 153 consecutive new patients.[42] Each subject was treated for 5 weeks after a 1-week baseline evaluation, three treatments per week, using an AAI. Although no changes could be demonstrated pre- and post-treatment in gait or sway patterns during lateral bending, the patients did show significant reduction in pain and improvement in function (using activities of daily living, or ADL, measures). Five of six respondents reported feeling better in a 1-year follow-up survey.

Yates et al[43] conducted a randomized controlled trial in which hypertensive patients were either activator-adjusted, sham-adjusted, or nontreated. Only the treatment group showed significant short-term reduction in their blood pressure.

Two patients with documented disk herniations and sciatic neuropathy were treated with a variety of methods,[44] including AAI adjusting, pelvic blocking, high-voltage galvanic current, and exercise. Follow-up computed tomographies (CTs) showed complete resolution of the bulge in one case, and reduction in the other. The patients experienced marked reduction in pain and an increase in their functional activities. The research design did not permit attribution of clinical utility to any of the individual components of the regimen, but the authors concluded that the "favorable patient outcomes are somewhat encouraging."[44]

Eleven patients with a history of neck pain following a whiplash injury, nine of whom were acute, were treated in accordance with AMCT protocols,[45] including AAI adjusting (maximum 21 visits). Improvement was noted both on a pain VAS and in cervical range of motion. In addition, the investigators used a "3-D biomechanical analysis system which allows the calculation of finite axis of rotation parameters of the cervical spine during the performance of daily tasks."[45] This apparatus documented objective changes in the subjects that paralleled their clinical improvement.

A case study was presented at the 1992 Seventh Annual Conference on Research and Education,[19] the title of which is quite descriptive: "Treatment of chronic sciatica by mechanical force, manually assisted, short lever adjusting and a video assisted stretching program: a quantitative case report." Ten consecutive new patients who had received a whiplash type of injury to the cervical spine were treated for 6 weeks, using an AAI, while a control group received interferential electrotherapy. Finite helical axis parameters (FHAP) of the cervical spine were obtained before and after treatment. The study is of interest not only because the subjects improved, as manifested by subjective instruments and through range of motion measurements, but also because there were FHAP alterations that mirrored clinical improvement. That is, the FHAP seemed able to discriminate normal from abnormal cervical kinematics.

A 67-year-old geriatric patient with sacroiliac pain was treated with AAI adjusting alone for 2 weeks, following a 3-week baseline period during which no treatment was extended.[46] Following the treatment, the patient manifested improvement in terms of orthopedic testing and in the VAS, and remained improved at a 2-month follow-up.[46] Two cases of Bell's palsy were reported to have been successfully treated, using AAI adjusting, high-voltage galvanic current, and self-administered facial muscle exercise.[18] Activator treatment of a case of coccygodynia was described,[47] as well as a case of postsurgical neck syndrome.[48] A female who had knee pain for several months, and had been diagnosed through magnetic resonance imaging (MRI) as having a medial meniscal tear, markedly improved following adjustments to the knee using an AAI.[49] Although a post-treatment MRI 7 months following the first could not establish a change in the meniscal tear, the patient had become essentially asymptomatic by that time, after receiving 23 treatments over an 11-month period. A female who had experienced shoulder pain for 6 months, and had been diagnosed as suffering from frozen shoulder syndrome (adhesive capsulitis), markedly improved following adjustments delivered primarily to the shoulder and the cervicothoracic spine, with an AAI. The patient was deemed to have fully recovered after 5 months and 35 treatments.[50] A man with a symptomatic lumbar disk herniation improved markedly with Activator adjustive care,[51] as did a woman with multiple cervical disk protrusions.[52]

Gemmell and Jacobson[53] compared the outcome of one treatment, using either a single Meric or AAI, on a group of 30 consecutive patients presenting with acute low-back pain. Although 25 of the 30 subjects reported a decrease in their pain level, there was no difference in the relative improvement experienced by the 16 Meric subjects compared to the 14 Activator subjects. The authors purport this study to be "the first to compare 'name-brand' techniques in chiropractic for the treatment of acute mechanical LBP [low-back pain]."[53]

Phongphua et al[54] provide a short report of the results of using Gonstead, Bioenergetic Synchronization Technique, or Activator Methods Technique on 22 subjects with migraine headaches. Although 5 of the subjects improved, the authors warn not to overinterpret the study, which was quite small, and non-controlled.

Yurkiw and Mior,[55] in a small study, randomly assigned patients with neck pain to either Activator or manipulative treatment. There were no before and after differences in either group in either pain intensity or lateral flexion range of motion. Wood et al[56] performed a similar study, in which neck patients were randomly assigned either to a group receiving AAI adjustments or manual (Diversified) adjustments, with no other treatment modalities used. Both groups showed similar subjective and range of motion improvements, both initially and at 1 month follow-up.

(We have a further comment on this study: see conclusions, below.)

Other relevant studies

Controlled and measured application of the AAI in both "human and dog experiments provided the evidence for vertebral movement in response to a chiropractic thrust."[57] There was simultaneous electromyographic (EMG) activity, but it was not clear whether the vertebral displacement was due directly to the thrust or the associated muscular reaction. A follow-up study by Smith et al[58] measured *relative movements* among nearby vertebrae, as compared with the absolute vertebral movements detected in the previous experiment. This earned heated criticism from Triano[59] and a spirited rejoinder.[60]

Kawchuk and Herzog[61] determined the biomechanical characteristics of five common methods of cervical manipulation, including the AAI. Compared with the lateral break, Gonstead, toggle, and rotation, AAI adjusting featured the smallest mean thrust duration, tied with rotation for the smallest mean peak force generated, and showed an approximately average force/time slope.

Nathan and Keller[62] used an AAI in conjunction with a force–acceleration measurement system to investigate lumbar intervertebral motion patterns in response to a "low force, high frequency posteroanterior" thrust. The results showed that the activator thrust produced exponentially damped oscillations in the lumbar motion segment, with measurable intervertebral axial and shear displacements. Thoracolumbar stiffness was greater in a subject with a severely degenerated disk, and smaller in another with retrolisthesis, compared with a normal subject.

Haas et al[63] assessed the ability of blinded examiners to discriminate sham from real articular pressure testing, as manifested by changes in relative leg length. The investigators concluded that "For the population investigated, leg alignment reactivity to rotatory pressure testing can, in the majority of cases, be attributable to background noise" (i.e., only a small proportion of the reactivity can be associated with the pressure challenge). In a follow-up study,[64] the same investigators assessed the reactivity of leg alignment to an actual activator thrust, or a sham activator adjustment. As in the previous study, there appeared to be no difference in the tendency for the legs to react to either real or sham adjustments. Slosberg[65] did not feel that the investigators had adequately emulated the procedures used by AMCT, in that the "pressure testing" described did not appear to resemble bona fide isolation testing in the thoracic spine. Haas and Peterson, in reply, justified having extended interpretation of their work to Activator Methods protocols. Harman felt that Haas et al had displayed bias against light-force adjusting methods.[66]

Interestingly, an AAI was used at a "nontension setting" to deliver sham adjustments in a controlled clinical trial investigating the effect of osseous thrusting in the management of primary nocturnal enuresis.[67] Harman,[66] on the other hand, claims (without citing references) that at least two experimenters got "good, if not better results, by setting the instruments to zero."[66]

Keller et al have done a number of studies investigating various parameters related to adjusting with an AAI: its value and effectiveness as a mechanical impedance measurement tool,[68] increased paraspinal muscle strength as assessed through use of surface electromyography (sEMG),[69] using an AAI equipped with a load cell and accelerometer to quantify the dynamic stiffness of the thoracolumbar spine,[70] and predicting lumbar segmental and intersegmental motion responses to Activator AAI forces on living subjects.[71] Symons et al[72] used sEMG to detect responses to AAI interventions at multiple locations, and found them more local, that is, both quantitatively and qualitatively different, from those obtained using manual manipulation.

CONCLUSIONS

- Although AMCT, like every other technique system in chiropractic, purports to identify and correct subluxations, AMCT proponents readily admit that "The validity and reliability of the subluxation complex, *per se*, is generally unexplored in AMCT theory, as in other theories of chiropractic care."[10]

- It should be noted that AMCT is the first and perhaps only technique system to have applied the Kaminski model for the validation of chiropractic techniques[73] to itself.[10]
- Despite the fact that AMCT researchers have published a rather impressive quantity of articles in the peer-reviewed literature, this literature is underweighted in the area of clinical outcomes. An Expert Panel that rated the clinical utility of several core treatment methods for the low back did not rate well-published methods more highly than methods about which virtually nothing has been published.[74,75] The publication of this study gave rise to a vigorous exchange of views between the investigators, Fuhr, and Smith.[76-81] In brief, Smith strongly contested the use of Activator methods in clinical situations where more studied techniques had been found to be clinically effective. Fuhr felt that Smith had misinterpreted the original study, the authors of which had warned readers that "lack of evidence is not evidence of lack." Four of the original five investigators, for their part, warned readers not to overinterpret the point that "lack of evidence is not evidence of lack." This intriguing discussion spilled over into *Dynamic Chiropractic*, where a number of columns were published.[82-84]
- We conclude that researchers attempting to validate the clinical value of their favored methods might consider placing more emphasis on outcomes, and less on more peripheral matters such as basic science, and the reliability of diagnostic procedures.
- The use of the AAI is prohibited in the province of Saskatchewan, Canada. Colloca[85] reviews the history of this situation and expresses his opposition to this policy.
- The study by Wood et al,[56] in which neck patients received either an AAI or a manual thrust used an interesting design in which the Activator leg-checking procedure, in addition to other more generic examination methods, was used to determine the side and level of adjustive intervention. Given the results of the study – that the instrument and manually adjusted groups had the same clinical outcome – we cannot rule out that the results might have

been different had the manual adjusters not depended on the Activator analytic protocol for listings. We understand that the study design wanted to standardize everything but the intervention, but we are still left wondering what would have happened had the manual adjustors used examination methods more akin to those used in such a setting.

REFERENCES

1. Cooperstein R 1997 Technique system overview: Activator Methods Technique. Chiropractic Technique 9 (3): 108–114
2. Fuhr A F, Osterbauer P J 1989 Interexaminer reliability of relative leg-length evaluations in the prone, extended position. Chiropractic Technique 1 (1): 13–18
3. Fuhr A 1983 Activator Methods. Today's Chiropractic (Jan/Feb): 16–19
4. Fuhr A W 1986 Activator Methods technique. Today's Chiropractic (May–June): 77–78
5. Lee W C, Fuhr A W 1977 Activator Methods. In: Kfoury P W (ed.). Catalog of chiropractic techniques: an overview of current chiropractic methods by 29 authors, pp. 21–22. Logan College of Chiropractic, St Louis, MO
6. Fuhr A W 1992 Non-specific short and long lever chiropractic adjusting: principles and practice. In: Hansen D (ed.) Proceedings of the 7th Annual Conference on Research and Education, "Focus on health policy and technology assessment in chiropractic", pp. 256–257. Consortium for Chiropractic Research/California Chiropractic Association, Palm Springs, CA
7. Osterbauer P J, Fuhr A W, Hildebrandt R W 1992 Mechanical force, manually assisted short lever chiropractic adjustment. Journal of Manipulative and Physiological Therapeutics 15 (5): 309–317
8. Stephenson R W 1927 Chiropractic textbook. Palmer School of Chiropractic, Davenport, IA
9. Cleveland C S I 1992 The high-velocity thrust adjustment. In: Haldeman S (ed.) Principles and practice of chiropractic, 1st edn, pp. 459–482. Appleton & Lange, Norwalk, CT
10. Osterbauer P J, Fuhr A W 1990 The current status of Activator Methods Chiropractic Technique, theory, and training. Chiropractic Technique 2 (4): 168–175
11. Fuhr A 1990 Activator Methods: basic manual, Activator Methods Chiropractic Technique seminars. Activator Methods, Phoenix, AZ
12. Youngquist M W, Fuhr A W, Osterbauer P J 1989 Interexaminer reliability of an isolation test for the identification of upper cervical subluxation. Journal of Manipulative and Physiological Therapeutics 12 (2): 93–97
13. Slosberg M 1987 Activator Methods isolation tests. Today's Chiropractic 16 (3): 41–43
14. Duell M L 1984 The force of the Activator adjusting intrument. Digest of Chiropractic Economics (Nov/Dec): 17
15. Henningham M 1982 Activator adjusting for acute torticollis. Chiropractic Journal of Australia 2 (1): 13–14
16. Peters R E 1984 Facet syndrome. European Journal of Chiropractic 32: 85–102
17. Fuhr A W 1983 Cornerstone: interview. American Chiropractor (July/August): 24
18. Frach J P, Osterbauer P J, Fuhr A W 1992 Chiropractic treatment of Bell's palsy by activator instrument adjusting and high voltage electrotherapy: a report of two cases. Journal of Manipulative and Physiological Therapeutics 15 (9): 596–598
19. Osterbauer P J, Fuhr A W 1992 Treatment of chronic sciatica by mechanical force, manually assisted, short lever adjusting and a video assisted stretching program: a quantitative case report. In: Hansen D (ed.) Proceedings of the 7th Annual Conference on Research and Education, "Focus on health policy and technology assessment in chiropractic," pp. 256–257. Consortium for Chiropractic Research, Palm Springs, CA
20. Fuhr A, Osterbauer P 1991 Strategies for the detection of neuro-mechanical dysfunction: Activator Method's isolation procedures and prone leg check. In: Hansen D (ed.) Proceedings of the sixth Annual Conference of Research and Education, "Emphasis on consensus," pp. 59–60. Consortium for Chiropractic Research, Monterey, CA
21. DeWitt J K, Osterbauer P J, Stelmach G E, Fuhr A W 1994 Optoelectric measurement of leg length inequalities before, during, and after isolation tests. Arizona State University, Activator Methods, Inc.
22. Slosberg M 1988 Activator Methods: an update and review (parts 1 and 2). Today's Chiropractic 17 (5): 83–85, 88
23. Nguyen H T, Resnick D N, Caldwell S G et al 1999 Interexaminer reliability of activator methods' relative leg-length evaluation in the prone extended position. Journal of Manipulative and Physiological Therapeutics 22 (9): 565–569
24. DeWitt J, Osterbauer P, Fuhr A 1993 Optoelectric measurement of leg length changes during isolation tests. In: Hansen D (ed.) The Proceedings of the Consortium for Chiropractic Research's eighth Annual Conference on Research and Education, pp. 156–157. Consortium for Chiropractic Research, Monterey, CA
25. Troyanovich S 1995 Optoelectric measurement of changes of leg length inequality resulting from isolation tests [letter; comment]. Journal of Manipulative and Physiological Therapeutics 18 (5): 322
26. Haas M 1995 Optoelectric measurement of changes of leg length inequality resulting from isolation tests [letter; comment]. Journal of Manipulative and Physiological Therapeutics 18 (5): 322
27. DeWitt J K, Osterbauer P J, Stelmach G E, Fuhr A W 1995 In reply, to letters to editor concerning: optoelectric measurment of changes in leg length inequality resulting from isolation tests. Journal of Manipulative and Physiological Therapeutics 18 (5): 322–323

28. Thompson C 1984 Thompson technique reference manual. Thompson Educational Workshops, Williams Manufacturing, Elgin, Il

29. Haas M, Peterson D 1989 Interexaminer reliability of relative leg-length evaluations in the prone, extended position [letter, comment]. Chiropractic Technique 1 (4): 150–151

30. Shambaugh P, Scolfani L, Fanselow D 1988 Reliability of the Derifield–Thompson test for leg-length inequality, and use of the test to determine cervical adjusting efficacy. Journal of Manipulative and Physiological Therapeutics 11 (5): 396–399

31. Danelius B D 1987 Letter to the editor: inter- and intra-examiner reliability of leg-length measurement: a preliminary study. Journal of Manipulative and Physiological Therapeutics 10 (3): 132

32. DeBoer F F 1987 In reply: inter- and intra-examiner reliability of leg-length measurement: a preliminary study. Journal of Manipulative and Physiological Therapeutics 10 (3): 133

33. DeBoer K F, Harmon R O, Savoie S, Tuttle C D 1983 Inter- and intra-examiner reliability of the leg-length differential measurement: a preliminary study. Journal of Manipulative and Physiological Therapeutics 10 (3): 61–66

34. Falltrick D R, Pierson D S 1989 Precise measurement of functional leg length inequality and changes due to cervical spine rotation in pain-free subjects. Journal of Manipulative and Physiological Therapeutics 12 (5): 369–373

35. Rhudy T R, Burk J M 1990 Inter-examiner reliability of functional leg-length assessment. American Journal of Chiropractic Medicine 3 (2): 63–66

36. DeBoer F F, Wagnon R J 1989 Letter to the editor. Journal of Manipulative and Physiological Therapeutics 12 (2): 151

37. Haas M, Nyiendo J 1989 Reliability of the Derifield–Thompson test for leg length inequality, and use of the test to demonstrate cervical adjusting efficacy [letter; comment]. Journal of Manipulative and Physiological Therapeutics 12 (4): 316–320

38. Cooperstein R 1991 The Derifield pelvic leg check: a kinesiological interpretation. Chiropractic Technique 3 (2): 60–65

39. Hestbaek L, Leboeuf-Yde C 2000 Are chiropractic tests for the lumbo-pelvic spine reliable and valid? A systematic critical literature review. Journal of Manipulative and Physiological Therapeutics 23 (4): 258–275

40. Venn E K, Wakefield K A, Thompson P 1983 A comparative study of leg-length checks. European Journal of Chiropractic 31: 68–80

41. Gemmell H, Jacobson B 1998 Comparison of two adjustive indicators in patients with acute low back pain. Chiropractic Technique (February): 8–10

42. Osterbauer P J, De Boer K F, Widmaier R et al 1993 Treatment and biomechanical assessment of patients with chronic sacroiliac joint syndrome. Journal of Manipulative and Physiological Therapeutics 16 (2): 82–90

43. Yates R G, Lamping N L, Abram C, Wright C 1988 Effects of chiropractic treatment on blood pressure and anxiety: a randomized controlled trial. Journal of Manipulative and Physiological Therapeutics 11 (6): 484–488

44. Richards G L, Thompson J S, Osterbauer P J, Fuhr A W 1990 Low force chiropractic care of two patients with sciatic neuropathy and lumbar disc herniation. American Journal of Chiropractic Medicine 3 (1): 25–32

45. Osterbauer P J, DeBoer K F, Fuhr A W et al 1991 3-D axis of rotation in whiplash injured patients treated chiropractically. In: Haldeman S (ed.) Proceedings of the Scientific Symposium of the 1991 World Federation of Chiropractic, pp. 57–61. World Federation of Chiropractic, Toronto, Ontario

46. Osterbauer P J, DeVita T, Fuhr A W 1991 Chiropractic treatment of chronic mechanical low back pain in a geriatric population: a practitioner-scientist protocol. In: Wolk S (ed.) Proceedings of the Foundation for Chiropractic Education and Research 3rd Annual International Conference on Spinal Manipulation, pp. 230–231. Foundation for Chiropractic Research and Education, Washington, DC

47. Polkinghorn B S, Colloca C J 1999 Chiropractic treatment of coccygodynia via instrumental adjusting procedures using activator methods chiropractic technique. Journal of Manipulative and Physiological Therapeutics 22 (6): 411–416

48. Polkinghorn B S, Colloca C J 2001 Chiropractic treatment of postsurgical neck syndrome with mechanical force, manually assisted short-lever spinal adjustments. Journal of Manipulative and Physiological Therapeutics 24 (9): 589–595

49. Polkinghorn B S 1994 Conservative treatment of torn medial meniscus via mechanical force, manually assisted short lever chiropractic adjusting procedures. Journal of Manipulative and Physiological Therapeutics 17 (7): 474–483

50. Polkinghorn B S 1995 Chiropractic treatment of frozen shoulder syndrome (adhesive capsulitis) utilizing mechanical force, manually assisted short lever adjusting procedures. Journal of Manipulative and Physiological Therapeutics 18 (2): 105–115

51. Polkinghorn B S, Colloca C J 1998 Treatment of symptomatic lumbar disc herniation using activator methods chiropractic technique. Journal of Manipulative and Physiological Therapeutics 21 (3): 187–196

52. Polkinghorn B S 1998 Treatment of cervical disc protrusions via instrumental chiropractic adjustment. Journal of Manipulative and Physiological Therapeutics 21 (2): 114–121

53. Gemmell H A, Jacobson B H 1995 The immediate effect of Activator vs. Meric adjustment on acute low back pain: a randomized controlled trial. Journal of Manipulative and Physiological Therapeutics 18 (7): 453–456

54. Phongphua C, Hawk C, Long C et al 1995 Feasibility study for a clinical trial of chiropractic care for patients with migraine headaches using different chiropractic techniques. Journal of Chiropractic Education 13 (1): 75

55. Yurkiw D, Mior S 1996 Comparison of Two Chiropractic Techniques on Pain and Lateral Flexion in Neck Pain Patients: A Pilot Study. Chiropractic Technique 8 (4): 155–162

56. Wood T G, Colloca C J, Matthews R 2001 A pilot randomized clinical trial on the relative effect of instrumental (MFMA) versus manual (HVLA) manipulation in the treatment of cervical spine

dysfunction. Journal of Manipulative and Physiological Therapeutics 24 (4): 260–271

57. Fuhr A W, Smith D B 1986 Accuracy of piezoelectric accelerometers measuring displacement of a spinal adjusting instrument. Journal of Manipulative and Physiological Therapeutics 9 (1): 15–21

58. Smith D B, Fuhr A W, Davis B P 1989 Skin accelerometer displacement and relative bone movement of adjacent vertebrae in response to chiropractic percussion thrusts. Journal of Manipulative and Physiological Therapeutics 12 (1): 26–37

59. Triano J 1989 Letter to the editor regarding "Skin accelerometer displacement and relative bone movement of adjacent verterbrae in response to chiropractic percussion thrusts." Journal of Manipulative and Physiological Therapeutics 12 (5): 406–408

60. Smith D B 1989 Rejoinder to Triano's letter to the editor regarding Smith's "Skin accelerometer displacement and relative bone movement of adjacent verterbrae in response to chiropractic percussion thrusts." Journal of Manipulative and Physiological Therapeutics 12 (5): 408–411

61. Kawchuk G N, Herzog W 1993 Biomechanical characterization (fingerprinting) of five novel methods of cervical spine manipulation. Journal of Manipulative and Physiological Therapeutics 16 (9): 573–577

62. Nathan M, Keller T S 1994 Measurement and analysis of the in vivo posteroanterior impulse response of the human thoracolumbar spine: a feasibility study. Journal of Manipulative and Physiological Therapeutics 17 (7): 431–441

63. Haas M, Peterson D, Panzer D et al 1993 Reactivity of leg alignment to articular pressure testing: evaluation of a diagnostic test using a randomized crossover clinical trial approach. Journal of Manipulative and Physiological Therapeutics 16 (4): 220–227

64. Haas M, Peterson D, Rothman E H et al 1993 Responsiveness of leg alignment changes associated with articular pressure testing to spinal manipulation: the use of a randomized clinical trial design to evaluate a diagnostic test with a dichotomous outcome. Journal of Manipulative and Physiological Therapeutics 16 (5): 306–311

65. Slosberg M 1994 Reactivity of leg alignment to articular pressure testing evaluation of a diagnostic test using a randomized crossover clinical trial approach [letter; comment]. Journal of Manipulative and Physiological Therapeutics 17 (7): 496–498

66. Harman R D 1993 Responsiveness of leg alignment changes associated with articular pressure testing to spinal manipulation: the use of a randomized clinical trial design to evaluate a diagnostic test with a dichotomous outcome [letter; comment]. Journal of Manipulative and Physiological Therapeutics 16 (9): 616–617

67. Reed W R, Beavers S, Reddy S K, Kern G 1994 Chiropractic management of primary nocturnal enuresis. Journal of Manipulative and Physiological Therapeutics 17 (9): 596–600

68. Keller T S, Colloca C J, Fuhr A W 1999 Validation of the force and frequency characteristics of the activator adjusting instrument: effectiveness as a mechanical impedance measurement tool. Journal of Manipulative and Physiological Therapeutics 22 (2): 75–86

69. Keller T S, Colloca C J 2000 Mechanical force spinal manipulation increases trunk muscle strength assessed by electromyography: a comparative clinical trial. Journal of Manipulative and Physiological Therapeutics 23 (9): 585–595

70. Keller T S, Colloca C J, Fuhr A W 2000 In vivo transient vibration assessment of the normal human thoracolumbar spine. Journal of Manipulative and Physiological Therapeutics 23 (8): 521–530

71. Keller T S, Colloca C J, Beliveau J G 2002 Force-deformation response of the lumbar spine: a sagittal plane model of posteroanterior manipulation and mobilization. Clinical Biomechanics (Bristol, Avon) 17 (3): 185–196

72. Symons B P, Herzog W, Leonard T, Nguyen H 2000 Reflex responses associated with activator treatment. Journal of Manipulative and Physiological Therapeutics 23 (3): 155–159

73. Kale M 1984 The upper cervical specific. Today's Chiropractic (July/August): 28–29

74. Cooperstein R, Perle S M, Gatterman M I et al 2001 Chiropractic technique procedures for specific low back conditions: characterizing the literature. Journal of Manipulative and Physiological Therapeutics 24 (6): 407–424

75. Gatterman M I, Cooperstein R, Lantz C et al 2001 Rating specific chiropractic technique procedures for common low back conditions. Journal of Manipulative and Physiological Therapeutics 24 (7): 449–456

76. Fuhr A W 2003 Rating specific chiropractic technique procedures for common low back conditions. Journal of Manipulative and Physiological Therapeutics 26 (1): 62–64

77. Perle S M, Robert C, Lantz C, Schneider M J 2003 Rating specific chiropractic technique procedures for common low back conditions. Journal of Manipulative and Physiological Therapeutics 26 (1): 60–61

78. Fuhr A W 2003 Rating specific chiropractic technique procedures for common low back conditions. Journal of Manipulative and Physiological Therapeutics 26 (1): 59–60

79. Smith J 2003 Rating specific chiropractic technique procedures for common low back conditions. Journal of Manipulative and Physiological Therapeutics 26 (1): 57–58

80. Fuhr A W 2002 Rating specific chiropractic technique procedures for common low back conditions. Journal of Manipulative and Physiological Therapeutics 25 (3): 197–198; author reply 198

81. Gatterman M I 2002 Rating specific chiropractic technique procedures for common low back conditions [reply]. Journal of Manipulative and Physiological Therapeutics 25 (3): 198

82. Cooperstein R, Lantz C, Perle S, Schneider M 2002 Growing pains? We don't think so! Dynamic Chiropractic 20 (19): 32–33, 35

83. Mootz R 2002 The next big research thing. http://www.chiroweb.com/columnist/meemoophil/

84. Mootz R 2002 Growing pains. http://www.chiroweb.com/archives/20/15/03.html

85. Colloca C 2001 Activator and other mechanical adjusting devices ruled illegal. X-ray next? http://www.idealspine.com/AJCC_new/April2001/canada.htm

11

Applied Kinesiology (AK)

INTRODUCTION

Cooperstein, before enrolling in chiropractic college, was a chiropractic patient under the care of a Sacro-Occipital Technique (SOT) practitioner. One day, attending as usual for an adjustment, he was greeted by a chiropractor who explained he was substituting that day for the usual doctor. The fact that the substitute doctor used side-posture manipulation, rather than the usual pelvic blocking, was already quite interesting to Cooperstein, but the best was yet to come. The doctor, explaining he had just taken an AK seminar, undertook some muscle-testing procedure, which resulted in Cooperstein being informed he was allergic to gluten and should give it up. Asked "what foods contain gluten?" the doctor said bread, some cereals, and more. "You mean – bread? Give up *bread?*" Needless to say, Cooperstein did not give up bread, and even went on to take several seminars in AK, elements of which are manifested in his practice today … but definitely not muscle testing to determine food allergies.

Gleberzon also has an interesting first encounter with AK. He attended a weekend seminar held in Toronto by a prominent AK chiropractor, on cranial fault corrections for temporomandibular joint dysfunctions. He found the presentation very interesting, although somewhat bizarre in nature. During a break, he found himself in the bathroom with the lecturer. Having taken the customary position with the obligatory empty urinal between them, he asked: "Doc, I really find your presentation very interesting and plan on telling students about it. However, the students in the college where I teach will press me for explanations. They

will want answers in terms of anatomy, physiology, and biochemistry. They will want to know why certain apparently unrelated muscles, joints, organs, and nutritional supplements are all related; how treating the psoas muscle is supposedly related to the third tricuspid tooth or the spleen or whatever. What should I tell them?"

Gleberzon will never forget the answer, as the speaker turned his head sideways (the best he could do under the circumstances, standing in front of urinals): "To be honest, I don't know why certain muscles are associated with certain joints and certain organs. All I can tell you is that those of us using AK methods in the field have found these associations time and time again, and that patients respond very well to this approach, even those patients who have suffered for a long time." Somehow, the simplicity of this answer invigorated Gleberzon. When the presenter did not have the answer, he simply said "I don't know." He did not default to strange invocations of quantum mechanics, previously non-described energies, or alternative physiologies, or pure metaphysics. That was very refreshing.

The AK practitioner is the archetypal example of chiropractic "weird stuff" – and we don't mean that pejoratively … Some of our best friends are AK practitioners, who often revel in making fun of themselves in just that way. As the doctor pokes and prods, or has the patient touch a part of his or her own body, muscles get weak, muscles get strong; and the doctor seems to be some sort of magician. Although reflex techniques tend to be less forceful than other techniques, nothing prevents a *reflex* practitioner from using a highly accelerated thrusting technique, and AK is no exception. AK is one of the two major reflex techniques (the other being SOT) used by chiropractors today. A chiropractic reflex technique purports to examine or treat the patient by means of physiological pathways that tend to lie outside what has been scientifically established.

AK is central enough in chiropractic technique to have spawned a number of other kinesiologies (Ch. 12), the essence of whose methods is well-represented in this current chapter. Most of the spinoff technique advocates are very frank and appreciative in their acknowledgment of Dr. Goodheart, founder of AK, as their inspiration. He is the man without whom their technique would never have existed. We have also seen many allied healthcare practitioners, including medical doctors, nurses, and psychotherapists, absorb large chunks of AK procedures (minus manipulative procedures, we hope!) into their practice. Not surprisingly, this emphasis on kinesiology, the study of the mechanics and anatomy in relation to human movement, has allowed AK practitioners to make big inroads into sports medicine (call it sports chiropractic if you like) as athletic trainers and team physicians. This has greatly added to the burgeoning movement toward introducing chiropractic care into interdisciplinary settings, and added to the credibility of AK procedures despite their occasionally weird character.

OVERVIEW

AK intends to create a unified approach to the identification and treatment of body distortion and dysfunction. It is concerned with functional disturbance in particular, and how it relates to disruption of homeostasis and the causation and maintenance of disease. AK intends that its methods find application in many different health-related fields, and in that sense, it is not a chiropractic methodology exclusively. It aims to restore postural balance, correct gait impairment, and improve range of motion; and considers itself prophylactic of future degenerative changes.

AK uses the body's muscular system as an indirect indicator of the structure and function of its musculoskeletal system, the viscera, and the nervous system. The goal is to normalize neurologic functioning, especially dysfunction related to afferent nervous function. Manual muscle testing both establishes the presence of neuropathology and confirms its removal. In addition, AK practitioners believe there is a functional relationship between specific muscles and glands or other organs, so that their physiological states would be interdependent. AK regards its procedures as essentially diagnostic in nature, so that it could be considered adjunctive to any doctor's pre-existing therapeutic approach. McCord, a diplomate of the International College of Applied Kinesiology (ICAK) since 1978, provides a definition of AK:

The science of applied kinesiology can be defined as a system of diagnosis and therapeutics using information derived from the observation of neuromuscular and musculoskeletal relationships, primarily determined by manual muscle testing. The fundamental objective of the system is the evaluation and correction of bodily dysfunction through the application of natural therapies, thereby aiding in the prevention of disease and the promotion of health.[1]

Table 11.1 lists a few of the sources from which AK, one of the most eclectic of chiropractic techniques,

Table 11.1 Primary sources for Applied Kinesiology procedures

Procedure	Source
Cranial fault correction	William G Sutherland, DO (1929) Nephi Cottam, DC (1929)
Acupuncture meridian therapies	Oriental medicine
Therapy localization, challenging	L L Truscott, DC[2]
Strain–counterstrain	H Jones, DO (1954)
Trigger points, spray and stretch	Janet Travell, MD (1940s)
Foot reflexology	Many sources, ancient and current
Neurolymphatic point treatment	Frank Chapman, DO (1937)
Neurovascular point treatment	Terence Bennett, DC (early 1930s)
Temporal sphenoidal line treatment	M L Rees, DC (early 1940s)
Categories and pelvic blocking (Sacro-Occipital Technique)	Major DeJarnette, DC
Hand reflexes	Vivian Bates, DC[3]

has borrowed its diagnostic and therapeutic armamentarium.

HISTORY

Originator George Goodheart graduated from the National College of Chiropractic in 1939.[4] He claims to have originated AK in 1964, after having observed that postural distortion, in the absence of congenital pathology, is often associated with weak muscles. The seminal case that was described involved winging of the scapula.[5] Following the observation that tender nodules were often palpable in muscles, at their origin and insertion, Goodheart learned to treat the muscle dysfunction through digital mobilization of these areas. Following this, the posture would then improve.[6] Although Goodheart would incorporate into AK theories and procedures derived from many other disciplines (e.g., osteopath Chapman's "neurolymphatic reflexes" and chiropractor Bennett's "neurovascular points"), much of what he developed was original. The ICAK was founded in 1974.[7] The vertebral challenge and therapy localization diagnostic methods were imported from the work of chiropractor LL Truscott.[2,8] Leroy Perry was selected as the team chiropractor by Antigua in the 1976 Olympic games, and Goodheart was the first non-medical doctor to serve as a member of the US Olympic team Sports Medicine Committee in 1980.[9] John Thie, a student of Goodheart, simplified AK procedures for use by the general public, producing a method[10] and manual[11] called *Touch for Health*. The ICAK was founded by a group of doctors who had been teaching AK classes. In the mid-1980s, the organization divided itself into chapters representing Europe, Canada, Australasia, and the USA.

DEFINITION OF TECHNIQUE-SPECIFIC TERMS

- Strong, weak muscles: used by AK practitioners, these terms do not have the same connotation that they have in an orthopedic setting. The so-called weak muscle may be weak on manual muscle testing, and yet found to be normal in strength using an objective measuring device such as a dynamometer. The terms "strong" and "weak" muscles have to do with the ability of the nervous system to mobilize a response to the command to "resist," usually when accompanied by a provocative challenge (below) of some kind, such as therapy localization (below)

- Previously strong indicator muscle (PSIM): during the procedure of manual muscle testing, the PSIM is established as a muscle that is strong in the clear (below), when it is not being tested during a challenge procedure of some kind. The PSIM is thus suitable to be used as an outcome measure following a clinical intervention

- Challenge: a provocative test applied to a patient, such as pushing on a bone in a specific direction, to see how the strength of a PSIM is affected. Challenges can be physical, mental, or chemical[3,6]

- Therapy localization: a testing procedure in which the patient lightly applies a finger to a location of his or her own body, in order to test it for dysfunction, as would be identified by a PSIM weakening (Fig. 11.1)

- In the clear: this term refers to testing a muscle in the absence of any provocative interventions or challenges

- Five factors of the intervertebral foramen: when a muscle tests weak, each of the following etiologic factors are considered, all of which supposedly relate to the intervertebral

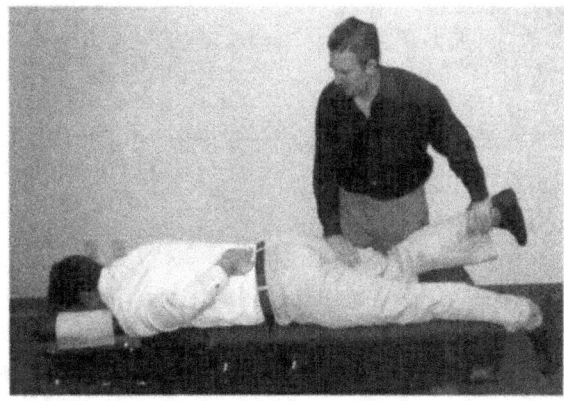

Figure 11.1   Therapy localization.

foramen: the nervous system, the neurolymphatic reflexes of Chapman, the neurovascular reflexes of Bennett, cerebrospinal fluid flow, and acupuncture meridian connectors.[12] Each of these is discussed below under Treatment/adjustive procedures

- Neurologic disorganization: refers to an inability of the nervous system to respond in a coordinated way to stimuli, the "result of afferent receptors sending conflicting information for interpretation by the central nervous system"[13]
- Switching: refers to right/left functional mix-up: the patient furnishes exactly wrong responses to stimuli, due to neural disorganization
- Reactive muscle: a muscle that tests weak only after its related muscle has contracted; that related muscle is termed the primary muscle
- Vertebral challenge: a diagnostic method in which a hypothetical thrust is applied to a putatively subluxated bone, whereby a weakening of a previously strong indicator muscle would indicate the appropriateness of that line of drive
- Eyes into distortion: weakening of a PSIM when the patient gazes in a particular direction
- Temporal tap: a method in which tapping on the temporal bone is used temporarily to disturb sensory filtering mechanisms in the brain; this is accompanied by the administration of some other input (auditory, visual) so as to effect a change in the patient's behavior, or in the results of therapy localization.[3]
- Fixation: lack of normal motion involving three (not the more typical two) vertebrae
- Neurolymphatic reflexes: points on the body originally developed by Chapman, an osteopath, and thought to govern lymphatic drainage of the associated body portion, and digitally treated to strengthen muscles made weak by their involvement
- Neurovascular reflexes: points on the body originally developed by Bennett, a chiropractor, and thought to govern vascular flow in an associated body portion, and digitally treated for such purposes. Although Bennett described these points as occurring everywhere, AK practitioners have only been

able to incorporate the cranial neurovascular points into their treatment regimen

- Temporal sphenoidal line: a line along the temporal sphenoidal suture, discovered by Rees, that purportedly includes points related to muscle and organ function. Walther once stated: "The temporal-sphenoidal line (TS line) is an infallible indicator and valuable diagnostic aid"[14]

PHYSIOLOGICAL MECHANISMS AND RATIONALE

Probably the most basic assumption in AK, the one from which all else follows, is that every myofascial, neuromusculoskeletal, or organ dysfunction is associated with specific muscle weaknesses, from which it follows that a doctor can diagnose and treat diseases and other body problems through muscle testing and balancing. AK doctors consider it very important to understand that most muscle hypertonus or spasm is not primary, but rather results from weakness of the antagonistic muscle;[9,15] thus the goal of care is less to stretch or weaken strong muscles, than to find a way to strengthen weak muscles. Box 11.1 lists the kind of problems that are thought to cause a muscle to be weak on manual muscle testing.[16]

A close relationship has been described for organs and muscles. When a muscle tests weak "in the clear," or in relation to some type of intervention, supposedly it may indicate a problem with an organ or organ system thought to be

---

Box 11.1 Problems detected by manual muscle testing

- Myofascial dysfunction
- Peripheral nerve entrapment
- Spinal segmental dysfunction and deafferentiation (loss of proprioception)
- Neurologic disorganization
- Viscerosomatic phenomena
- Nutritional inadequacy[17]
- Toxic chemical influences
- Disruption of cerebrospinal fluid production or flow
- Adverse mechanical tension in the meninges
- Meridian system imbalance
- Lymphatic vascular impairment

related in a functional way to that muscle. For example, a weakness in the infraspinatus muscle, since that muscle is supposedly related to the thyroid gland, *may* reflect disease of that organ.

Goodheart[12] quotes DD Palmer: "Too much or not enough nerve energy is disease." When it comes to nerve interference, "deafferentiation" is considered particularly significant. When a joint is fixated or subluxated, the aberrant movement causes inappropriate stimulation of local joint and muscle receptors. This in turn supposedly causes inappropriate ascending neurological information, and then inappropriate descending (efferent) commands to both muscles and glands.

Walther believes that, in the case of the vertebral challenge, pushing a bone into a corrective direction stretches hypertonic muscles that have pulled a bone into lesion. This would supposedly cause an increase in muscle hypertonus, which pulls the bone into further lesion, which weakens the previously strong indicator muscle.[14]

It has been hypothesized that the reactive muscle phenomenon results from muscle spindles in the primary muscle of the reactive muscle group being "set too high":[18] "Thus, when there is activation of the primary muscle, the Ia afferent impulses cause an overabundant inhibition of an antagonist muscle through the inhibitory interneuron."[13]

DIAGNOSTIC/ANALYTIC PROCEDURES

Without a doubt, manual muscle testing is the primary diagnostic method. The methods used derived from the work of Kendall et al,[19] and great effort is made to isolate individual muscles during the testing procedure.[20,21] Muscles becoming or remaining weak or strong is the primary examination finding, while the doctor employs a *challenge* of some kind. A challenge is a mental, chemical, or physical provocative (i.e., diagnostic) intervention of some kind, such as applying light pressure, a putative corrective line of drive, a nutritional substance,[17] a heel lift, or even a color.[22] Klein feels it is more efficient to emphasize challenge procedures over therapy localization.[23] The instantaneous effect on the muscle (or lack thereof) provides information as to the

---

Box 11.2 Technique-specific diagnostic methods used in AK

- Vertebral challenge
- Therapy localization
- Temporal sphenoidal line
- Eyes into distortion
- Manual muscle testing as functional neurology
- Vertebral challenge
- Temporal tap

---

indications for the agent that was used to effect the challenge.

Box 11.2 provides a representative list of technique-specific diagnostic methods, all of which are defined and discussed above, that are used in AK. Practitioners point out that, in addition to these, they use other diagnostic methods that are common to chiropractors in general, including range of motion testing, static and motion palpation, posture[15,20,24] and gait analysis, history taking, a standard physical examination, and laboratory testing.[16]

TREATMENT/ADJUSTIVE PROCEDURES

Although the primary effort involves correcting structural imbalance caused by poorly functioning muscles[21] (as already discussed), AK is essentially diagnostic.[25] If there is anything distinctive about AK treatment procedures, it is the vast array of therapeutic and diagnostic procedures and modalities incorporated into AK from other complementary and alternative healthcare disciplines. As an example, Goodheart wrote a two-part article[26,27] explaining when to use the spray and stretch technique of Travell et al,[28] or the strain–counterstrain muscle-shortening technique of osteopath Jones.[29] In addition to these, AK practitioners may utilize any or all of the adjustive and ancillary procedures used by chiropractors in general: high-velocity, low-amplitude (HVLA) manipulation, mobilization techniques, pelvic blocking, and drop-table methods. In addition to generic nutritional advice, such as eating a balanced diet including whole foods, the AK practitioner invariably gets involved in far

---

Box 11.3 Technique-specific treatment procedures used in AK

- Cranial techniques[30]
- Acupuncture meridian therapies[3]
- Myofascial techniques: origin-insertion work, strain–counterstrain treatment, fascial release, spray and stretch, pitch, yaw and roll technique[31]
- Nervous system coordination procedures: cross-crawl, temporal tap, switching correction[3]
- Neurolymphatic point treatment[3]
- Neurovascular point treatment[3]
- Temporal sphenoidal line treatment[3]
- Miscellaneous reflex procedures: stress receptors, hand reflexes, foot reflexology
- Clinical nutrition
- Limbic technique[31]

---

less mainstream nutritional advice. This includes prescribing a myriad of supplements, some quite esoteric and poorly validated. Box 11.3 lists several treatment methods that are typical of AK practitioners.

OUTCOME ASSESSMENT

Manual muscle testing remains the mainstay of outcome assessment, just as it is central to diagnosis in the first place. AK practitioners also use more conventional outcome assessment measures, such as leg checks, patient questionnaires, and laboratory testing.

SAFETY AND RISK FACTORS

Manual muscle testing is contraindicated in some cases due to age, severe disease, acute pain, and local pathology and inflammation.[16] Other than that, since the technique is largely diagnostic, there appear to be no contraindications.

EVIDENCE OF EFFICACY
Diagnostic efficacy

We cover the reliability and validity of manual muscle testing in Chapter 6. As stated there, manual muscle testing has not been found to be very reliable. A pair of review articles[32,33] summarized research on manual muscle testing and its

neurophysiological basis respectively, emphasizing research conducted within the AK milieu. Motyka and Yanuck[32] find the research equivocal, sometimes confirming reliability and validity, other times disconfirming, and often simply irrelevant due to various design flaws. However, some degree of interexaminer reliability was found for manual muscle testing of the pectoralis and piriformis muscles, but not for the hamstrings or the tensor fascia lata muscles.[34] More recently, in two articles,[35,36] Caruso and Leisman investigated the force/displacement characteristics of manual muscle testing, finding that a relatively steep slope – meaning the tested limb moves through a large distance when the force application is large – predicts with 98% accuracy that an experienced manual muscle tester would find this to be a weak muscle. A less experienced muscle tester would get it right, under the assumption that the force/displacement curve is definitive, only 64% of the time. The authors conclude: "The experiment lays the groundwork for studies of the objectivity of muscle-strength assessment in applied kinesiology."[35]

Three studies that investigated the muscle/organ relationship produced equivocal results.[37–39] Another study showed that AK testing could identify thyroid dysfunction.[40] Haas et al found no important link between manual muscle testing and either the vertebral challenge or spinal manipulation.[41] Kenney et al found that AK methods were unable to assess nutrient status.[42] Although Friedman and Weisberg attempted to test certain AK procedures, their study simply listed the data and lacked any statistical analysis,[43] making it difficult to interpret. There are a host of other studies of questionable value, mostly inhouse publications of the ICAK. Rosen and Williams provide an annotated list of research projects pertinent to AK,[44] and Rosen also provides a review of this research[45,46] Klinkoski and LeBoeuf[47] reviewed 50 AK studies published by the ICAK between 1981 and 1987, and found none that satisfied minimal criteria for validity.

Schmitt and Leisman[33] used manual muscle testing to identify 19 subjects as having 21 food allergies, as demonstrated by muscle weakening when the suspected allergen was placed in the mouth. Immunological serum testing, including both a radioallergosorbent test (RAST) and immune complex test for immunoglobulin E (IgE) and IgG, tested positive in 19 of the 21 suspected allergens. According to the investigators, the results of this pilot study warrant further investigation of whether manual muscle testing can provide a means to predict the clinical utility of using nutritional supplements.

Treatment efficacy

We are aware of one study looking at the effect of muscle spindle/Golgi tendon organ technique. Grossi,[48] testing whether this technique would increase the strength of the rectus femoris muscle, found no significant increase in strength whether the subjects received the real treatment or a placebo. However, the investigator did not report on any tests of statistical significance.

In a non-randomized retrospective study in a private chiropractic practice,[49] Froehle found that 46 children aged 5 years and under tended to have fewer symptoms of ear infection when receiving a mixture of pelvic blocking procedures and "the doctor's own modified applied kinesiology." This is obviously difficult to interpret.

CONCLUSIONS

- As practitioners ourselves, we hear patients explain in their own words what they think chiropractic is, what chiropractors do. Although most of them seem to think chiropractors "pop joints" (meaning, perform manipulation), many of them, either through direct experience or word of mouth, think the chiropractor is a specialist in "weird stuff." Some of them wind up in our offices because of that belief, others in spite of it. Reflex techniques often claim undocumented connections between body parts and functions, such as a specific point on the thumb that would relate to cardiac function, or a tender point in the trapezius muscle that would influence uterine function. We should not confuse such reflex techniques with other procedures or examination findings involving the word "reflex," such

as the "deep tendon reflex" or "pathological reflexes."
- Applied Kinesiologists regard their procedures as essentially diagnostic in nature,[1] so they could be considered adjunctive to any doctor's pre-existing therapeutic approach. On the other hand, the reflex treatment procedures that have been developed by AK practitioners are distinct enough, even though related to reflex procedures used in other techniques, for us to consider AK having a therapeutic arm as well.
- Although the correlation between manual muscle testing and objective muscle strength-measuring equipment has been poor, AK practitioners are not overly concerned. They feel that these two ways of measuring muscle strength are like apples and oranges: "they simply do not test or evaluate the same thing on the human body."[25] Recently, supportive evidence has come forth on that point.[35,36]
- Although AK advocates claimed to have published as many as 2000 clinical research papers in 1996,[7] very few have been in the generally accessible peer-reviewed literature, and thus it is difficult to draw any conclusions as to the accuracy or significance of such a comment. As an example, Goodheart wrote about how nutritional absorption affects muscle strength:[17] "A so-called double blind study was also done in which neither the doctor nor the patient knew the nature of the substance that the patient was to chew. The response was appropriate, immediate and highly individualized."[17] What study, published where?
- This type of "study," not subject to peer review or discussion, provides AK practitioners with unjustified confidence in their methods. In a published study, Triano,[38] in conjunction with members of the ICAK, tested whether the strength of the latissimus dorsi muscle would be affected by any of four different nutritional extracts (cardiac, thymic, pancreatic, and testicular glandular products). The expectation was that the pancreatic extract would tend to strengthen the muscle, whereas the other extracts would not. Both the patients and the muscle-testing doctors were blinded. The

experimental hypothesis was invalidated, in that the pancreatic extract did not have a relatively greater impact on the latissimus dorsi muscle. This contradicts the results of Goodheart's uncited double-blind study in the paragraph above.

- AK doctors, although sometimes reasonably self-critical in addressing the oddity of some of their theories and procedures, have also been at times quite self-serving in terms of their interpretations. For example, commenting on Triano's finding[38] that the latissimus dorsi muscle strengthened 25% of the time in response to pancreas extract, Rosen and Williams[46] chose to emphasize that the muscle did indeed respond 25% of the time. They do not deal with the fact that it also responded 25% of the time to three other non-predicted substances, so that the study invalidates the specificity of the latissimus–pancreatic extract relationship.

- AK practitioners seem quite alarmed at how popular diagnostic muscle testing has become, in some cases taken up by lay therapists, and in other cases, performed improperly or out of the multifactorial diagnostic array that AK doctors recommend using.[25,50]

- One of the main AK principles is the muscle–organ relationship. That is, when a muscle tests weak "in the clear," or in relation to some type of intervention, it may indicate a problem with an organ or organ system thought to be related in a functional way to that muscle.

However, no real reason is provided as to why this should be the case. This has been a particularly controversial component of AK. It is one thing to derive subluxation listings from muscle testing, a procedure that may be inaccurate, but perhaps no more so than generally accepted methods of subluxation identification, such as motion palpation. It is quite another thing to tell a patient, perhaps one with no symptoms, that there is "liver congestion" based on a rhomboid muscle weakness. We have seen patients carry this emotional baggage around for years, and even make life-altering decisions based on unproven assertions, even on passing comments, like this.

- It is far from obvious what would cause muscles to weaken and strengthen in response to challenges and other interventions. The ICAK has been quite forthright in admitting that the physiological mechanisms underlying several of the AK diagnostic procedures are not known.[50] We have come across a study in which tactile stimulation of the T2–3 dermatome (overlying the pectoralis major muscle) reduced the strength of the shoulder abductors, as assessed by both Cybex instrumentation and manual muscle testing.[51] (Muscle strength decreased by 8% as measured by Cybex, and by 17% measured by manual testing.)

- Tom and Carole Valentine have written a short book about AK,[52] intended for patients wishing to find out more about it.

REFERENCES

1. McCord K M 1991 Applied Kinesiology: an historical overview. Digest of Chiropractic Economics (September/October): 20, 22, 24, 27
2. Frisbie G K 1976 Truscott system of angular analysis and controlled adjusting. The essence of chiropractic, 3rd edn. Neyenesch, San Diego, CA
3. Walther D S 1981 Applied Kinesiology, vol. I. Systems DC, Pueblo, CO
4. Goodheart G 1989 Applied kinesiology – the beginning. Digest of Chiropractic Economics 31 (6): 15–23
5. Goodheart G J 1989 Applied Kinesiology – the beginning. Digest of Chiropractic Economics (May/June): 15, 17–20, 22–23
6. Goodheart G J 1993 The Applied Kinesiology Technique. Today's Chiropractic 22 (July/August): 56–58

7. Anonymous 1996 An historical overview of Applied Kinesiology. Applied Kinesiology Review 6 (1): 5–6
8. Gin R H, Green B N 1997 George Goodheart Jr, DC, and a history of applied kinesiology. Journal of Manipulative and Physiological Therapeutics 20 (5): 331–337
9. Mladenoff E 1986 Kinesiology corner. Why practice AK? American Chiropractor (February): 61
10. Thie J E, Schmitt W H Jr 1984 The history of applied kinesiology. American Chiropractor (May): 49–50, 52, 54–55
11. Thie J 1994 Touch for health (1st edn 1973). T H Enterprises, Sherman Oaks, CA
12. Goodheart G J 1977 Applied Kinesiology. In: Ktoury P W (ed.) Catalog of chiropractic techniques, pp. 117–119. Logan College of Chiropractic, Chesterfield, MO

13. Walther D S 1988 Applied Kinesiology: synopsis. Systems DC, Pueblo, CO
14. Walther D S 1976 Applied Kinesiology. Systems DC, Pueblo, CO
15. Goodheart G J 1987 Posture: 30 years of observation and some logical chiropractic conclusions part I. Digest of Chiropractic Economics (July/August): 14–16, 119–120
16. Anonymous 1996 Applied Kinesiology status statement. Applied Kinesiology Review 6 (1): 1–3
17. Goodheart G J 1987 Structural imbalance and nutritional absorption. Today's Chiropractic 16 (1): 19, 21–24, 30
18. Perle S M 1995 Technique system overview: Applied Kinesiology (AK). Chiropractic Technique 7 (3): 103–107
19. Kendall H O, Kendall F P, Wadsworth G E 1971 Muscle testing and function, 2nd edn. Williams & Wilkins, Baltimore, MD
20. Goodheart G J 1987 Posture: 30 years of observation and some logical chiropractic conclusions part II. Digest of Chiropractic Economics (September/October): 34, 36–37, 39–41
21. Maffetone P, Durlacher J 1989 Celebrating Applied Kinesiology's gold and silver. Digest of Chiropractic Economics 31 (6): 14–15
22. Walther D S 1983 Muscle testing to evaluate nutrition. Synectics 1 (2): 1,12
23. Klein R 1988 Part two of a series: using the challenge based Applied Kinesiology protocol. Digest of Chiropractic Economics (March/April): 58, 60–61
24. Goodheart G J 1987 Posture: 30 years of observation and some logical chiropractic conclusions part III. Digest of Chiropractic Economics (November/December): 62, 64–65, 67, 128–129
25. Blaich R 1988 Interview: Dr. Robert Blaich, International College of Applied Kinesiology. American Chiropractor (November): 12–15
26. Goodheart G C 1995 Cerebellar strain and counterstrain patterns, part II. Digest of Chiropractic Economics (March/April): 20, 22–26
27. Goodheart G C 1995 Cerebellar strain and counterstrain patterns, part I. Digest of Chiropractic Economics (January/February): 14–16, 18, 20, 23
28. Travell J G, Simons D G 1992 Myofascial pain and dysfunction: the trigger point manual. The lower extremities. Williams & Wilkins, Baltimore, MD
29. Jones L H 1981 Strain and counterstrain. American Academy of Osteopathy, Colorado Springs, CO
30. Walther D S 1981 Applied Kinesiology, vol. II. Systems DC, Pueblo, CO
31. Goodheart G C 1988 The limbic technic. Digest of Chiropractic Economics (Sept/Oct): 22–24, 25–31
32. Motyka T M, Yanuck S F 1999 Expanding the neurological examination using functional neurologic assessment part I: methodological considerations. International Journal of Neuroscience 97 (1–2): 61–76
33. Schmitt W H Jr, Leisman G 1998 Correlation of applied kinesiology muscle testing findings with serum immunoglobulin levels for food allergies. International Journal of Neuroscience 96 (3–4): 237–244
34. Lawson A, Calderon L 1997 Interexaminer agreement for applied kinesiology manual muscle testing. Perceptual and Motor Skills 84 (2): 539–546
35. Caruso W, Leisman G 2000 A force/displacement analysis of muscle testing. Perceptual and Motor Skills 91 (2): 683–692
36. Caruso W, Leisman G 2001 The clinical utility of force/displacement analysis of muscle testing in applied kinesiology. International Journal of Neuroscience 106 (3–4): 147–157
37. Rybeck C H, Swensen R 1980 The effect of oral administration of refined sugar on muscle strength. Journal of Manipulative and Physiological Therapeutics 3: 155–161
38. Triano J J 1982 Muscle strength testing as a diagnostic screen for supplemental nutrition therapy: a blind study. Journal of Manipulative and Physiological Therapeutics 5: 179–182
39. Jacobs G E 1981 Applied kinesiology: an experimental evaluation by double blind methodology. Journal of Manipulative and Physiological Therapeutics 4 (3): 141–145
40. Jacobs G E, Franks T L 1984 Diagnosis of thyroid dysfunction: applied kinesiology compared to clinical observations and laboratory tests. Journal of Manipulative and Physiological Therapeutics 7: 99–104
41. Haas M, Peterson D, Hoyer D, Ross G 1994 Muscle testing response to provocative vertebral challenge and spinal manipulation: a randomized controlled trial of construct validity. Journal of Manipulative and Physiological Therapeutics 17: 141–148
42. Kenney J J, Clemens R, Forsythe K D 1988 Applied kinesiology unreliable for assessing nutrient status. Journal of the American Dietetic Association 88 (6): 698–704
43. Friedman M H, Weisberg J 1981 Applied kinesiology – double-blind pilot study. Journal of Prosthetic Dentistry 45 (3): 321–323
44. Rosen M S, Williams 1991 The research status of Applied Kinesiology, part II: an annotated bibliography. Applied Kinesiology Review 1: 34–37
45. Rosen M S 1994 The research status of Applied Kinesiology, part I. Digest of Chiropractic Economics (September/October): 17–18, 20, 22–23
46. Rosen M S, Williams L 1995 The research status of Applied Kinesiology, part II. Digest of Chiropractic Economics (May/June): 40–41, 43–46, 48–49
47. Klinkoski B, LeBoeuf C 1990 A review of the research papers published by the International College of Applied Kinesiology from 1981–1987. Journal of Manipulative and Physiological Therapeutics 13: 190–194
48. Grossi J A 1981 Effects of an applied kinesiology technique on quadriceps femoris muscle isometric strength. Physical Therapy 61 (7): 1011–1016
49. Froehle R M 1996 Ear infection: a retrospective study examining improvement from chiropractic care and analyzing for influencing factors. Journal of Manipulative and Physiological Therapeutics 19 (3): 169–177
50. Anonymous 1983 Applied Kinesiology – Adopted status statement of the ICAK. Digest of Chiropractic Economics (November/December): 49, 51
51. Nicholas J A, Melvin M, Saraniti A J 1980 Neurophysiologic inhibition of strength following tactile stimulation of the skin. American Journal of Sports Medicine 8 (3): 181–186
52. Valentine T, Valentine C 1985 Applied Kinesiology. Muscle response in diagnosis, therapy, and preventive medicine. Thorsons, New York, NY

12

Applied Kinesiology spin-off techniques

What if the result of the muscle test is unclear?
"Retest, retest, retest!"[1] (p. 24)

INTRODUCTION

George Goodheart and his Applied Kinesiology have been nothing short of seminal in inspiring the development of other technique systems that we may as well call *Kinesiologies*. We did not think it appropriate to provide separate chapters for most of these, because there is not enough distinctive in them to warrant that. In all fairness to the founders of AK spinoff techniques, they sometimes acknowledge that they are not to be understood as standalone techniques, but methods that dovetail with the doctor's other primary technique(s) of choice.

So what, in the end, is a "Kinesiology"? Dr. Michael Rinaldi, a self-described Kinesiologist, says on his web page:[2]

Kinesiology is a bioenergetic feedback system that uses muscle testing to measure changes in electrical resistance of the body. Bioenergetic testing allows the practitioner to quickly and accurately conduct an interview with any of the body's organs or tissue and energetically evaluate their condition. This type of noninvasive testing can determine the body's electrical reaction to many stress producing substances and influences of modern living-form [sic] allergies, heavy metals, drugs and other chemical toxicities to vitamin and mineral deficiencies ... Kinesiology employs a combination of several therapies including: homeopathy, nutrition, Acupressure, Chiropractic, and physical therapy. It is an organized system that allows the practioner [sic] to apply all available knowledge.

When you get right down to it, the therapy localization, challenging, and manual muscle testing performed by a practitioner of Total Body Modification (TBM) Technique or Neuro-Emotional Technique (NET) is about the same as the therapy localization, challenging, and manual muscle testing performed by an Applied Kinesiologist. On the other hand, each of these Kinesiologies adds something – a somewhat different way of challenging, some new way of addressing the mental side of the Triad of Health,[3] or maybe a heavier emphasis on nutritional supplements. Presto, we have what appears to be a new technique system! Sometimes we are amazed at how little it takes to say that new technique x is different from old technique y, but Kinesiologies in no way monopolize this type of technique-spawning behavior, which also typifies Pierce–Stillwagon as it related to the ancestral Thompson Technique, or at least the earlier years of Chiropractic Biophysics Technique as it related to the ancestral Spinal Biomechanics Technique.

What may have accelerated this type of technique system proliferation in the case of the Kinesiologies is the apparent support and even encouragement from the founders. However, we also see warnings emanating from the International College of Applied Kinesiology (ICAK)[4] about inferior AK lookalikes, knock-off techniques that would corrupt the practice methods and wind up being detrimental to patients, and, of course, the reputation of AK itself. As to the temptation to create new Kinesiologies, we assume it must become competitive out there on the seminar circuit. Although we have no complaints to make about the exigencies of product distinction in a capitalist economy, we did not think it appropriate to provide each of these AK spinoffs with its own chapter.

CONTACT REFLEX ANALYSIS (CRA)

CRA was created by Dick A Versendaal, DC, along with a medical doctor, a clinical nutritionist, a dentist, and a hematologist. Like other Kinesiologies, CRA aims to monitor body functions through the study of body reflexes, to identify nutritional deficiencies and other problems, and treat and prevent illness and its symptoms. It draws heavily upon the method of manual muscle testing to identify: (1) structural problems, such as subluxations and "slipped" disks; (2) diseases, such as hormonal deficiencies and virus infections; (3) nutritional deficiencies; and (4) allergies. Despite the claim that "CRA is not a form of treatment or diagnosis, but is simply a method of determining nutritional needs,"[5] CRA most certainly diagnoses diseases and prescribes nutritional support for an immense number of conditions and symptoms.

The name of the technique is derived from *contact reflex points*, which are specific body locations that, when touched by the doctor in a specific manner, cause muscles to "blow out" when manually tested for strength, indicating a problem of some kind. These are, of course, not unrelated to the myriad of reflex points that one finds in AK. From an original total of about 300 reflex points, founder Versendaal has isolated some 75 (many, but not all, of which are acupuncture points) that form the mainstay of the diagnostic system. Among these are nine master reflex points: the right master allergy, left master allergy, metabolic, master heart/blood quality, hemoglobin, coronary, virus, and yeast reflexes. The claim is that in illness, there is an interruption of nerve energy to these reflexes, so that the reflex is "sick" and an indicator muscle will test weak, whereas in health, the reflex is correspondingly "healthy" and the muscle tests strong. Much is made of the body's electrical nature, with the front of the hand supposedly positive, the back of the hand negative, and the fingers neutral in polarity.

Versendaal's rendering of human physiology has little resemblance to anything one might encounter in a physiology textbook, nor what may be called the standard model of how the body works as presented in any medical or chiropractic college. For example: "Research has shown the human body to be a computer, made up of the BRAIN (electrical generator and memory bank) and hundreds of miles of electrical wire called nerves. These nerves connect every organ, gland and tissues of the body. These nerves also connect with fuses or breaker switches called CONTACT REFLEXES."[5]

The CRA practitioner touches the contact reflex points, as defined above, to identify systemic, allergic, and nutritional deficiencies, as evidenced by weakening of test muscles. Muscle testing may also be used to identify vertebral and extremity subluxations. Sometimes the conclusions drawn from minutely different test procedures are wildly disparate. For example, weakness of the arm abducted to 90° with the palm facing up is supposed to identify C5 subluxation, whereas weakness of the abducted arms with the thumbs pointed downward supposedly diagnoses osteoporosis.[5]

The web page of one CRA practitioner provides a succinct description of the primary diagnostic procedure:

To test a reflex, the doctor will use the patient's arm muscle (or any other muscle) as a "circuit" indicator. When the doctor's fingertip comes near or touches a healthy reflex, the arm muscle will remain very strong. Nerve energy is flowing freely. The doctor will not be able to push the patient's arm down without exerting a lot of force. However, if the arm muscle is suddenly weak, and the doctor can easily push the patient's arm down, a "hot circuit breaker" has been located. The nerve energy has been interrupted. Using this reflex information, the doctor will know if the problem is structural, physical, or nutritional.[6]

Since Versendaal's text includes a page for lab values,[5] one may infer that laboratory diagnosis is within the scope of CRA. Likewise, since the book is heavily laden with nutritional prescriptions based on a multitude of common signs and symptoms, and even features a chapter entitled "Differential Diagnosis" (which is not really that at all) it must be said that CRA has some sense of diagnosing illness that may overlap at times with conventional diagnosis.

Although subluxation identification seems to lie within the scope of CRA, no subluxation reduction procedures are described to our knowledge. Therefore, anything that could be called uniquely CRA treatment procedures is limited to nutritional support. A vast array of products are prescribed, most, if not all, of which are supplied by Standard Process Laboratories, whose products are based upon the discoveries of Dr. Royal Lee.[5]

There are allegations of research in CRA, but none is really presented. Versendaal states that CRA "does not easily lend itself to the double-blind studies required of the current medical orthodoxy for scientific validation."[7] Great benefits for patients are claimed, but no documentation is provided. Many case histories and patient testimonials are said to exist and be part of the training program. After castigating Barrett[8] and others for being "concerned primarily with whether a healing art meets their narrow criteria of scientific validity," CRA defender Clecak opines that "the first question is this: Does it *work*? Does it consistently produce outcomes that patients and doctors seek?"[9] On the other hand, Clecak provides no data that CRA does work, although he states that "tens of thousands of individual cases" are available.[10]

Conclusions: CRA

- CRA is the spinoff from Applied Kinesiology that most specializes in the nutrition area. Since there are no uniquely CRA treatments other than nutritional prescriptions, we are not surprised to learn that medical doctors, veterinarians, and dentists are all said to utilize CRA.[9] Where CRA stands in the health sciences may be more a question for nutritional scientists to grapple with, than for the chiropractic profession.
- CRA's strange interpretation of how the body works must give rise to some concern, leading us to wonder if a CRA practitioner (whether chiropractor, dentist, or medical doctor) puts patients at risk. In a recent article, as an example, Versendaal states:[11] "In the gut, each moment means a new beginning. As in tragedy or happiness, pain or joy, the many

varied chemical events are realized by the atoms of good or bad chemistry." As one goes through the writings, one hopes eccentric statements like this simply have a metaphoric intent, but one cannot safely assume that.

- Although Versendaal feels that CRA is not amenable to double-blind study protocols,[7] one is hard-pressed to see why not. Among the many treatment procedures employed by chiropractors, the clinical benefit of prescribing nutritional supplements (unlike manipulation, for example) is relatively easy to test in a double-blinded trial, just as medical pharmaceuticals are routinely tested. Furthermore, it would be straightforward to design an assessment study to see if blinded CRA practitioners can distinguish people with known pathologies from those without them. Such a study design has been used at least twice to study (and refute) iridology.[12,13]
- The safe and effective dosages of the nutritional supplements prescribed by CRA practitioners are essentially unknown, and some are of unknown value altogether. Therefore it is not possible to state whether one would expect health benefits, adverse consequences, or no consequences at all as a result of their use. By prescribing alternative nutritional treatments for virtually any diagnostic entity that exists, intended rather to replace than to complement medical treatments, the practice of CRA may pose a health risk by interfering with the established medical management of cases.
- Although, in theory, manual muscle testing would provide just one diagnostic input among others in prescribing nutritional supplements in a CRA practice setting, it seems that muscle testing is often the only examination procedure performed.

TOTAL BODY MODIFICATION (TBM)

TBM was founded by Dr. Victor L Frank, II, DC, NMD, DO. The TBM practitioner wants to correct the body's functional physiology, to potentiate in a favorable manner the influence of body structure on body function. According to a web page, "TBM (Total Body Modification) is a technique that is used to find the organ or area of the body that is stressed, determine why it is stressed and correct the problem by restoring balance to the nervous system."[14] TBM, like other spinoff Kinesiologies, uses manual muscle testing to identify supposed reflex points and various means of correcting problems identified in this manner.

It is traditional for chiropractors to maintain that they intervene in structure, in order eventually to affect the body's function. TBM claims to address "functional physiology," apparently posited alongside structure as a codeterminant of the individual's health status. One brochure on TBM posted on the web has a paragraph titled "How Does T.B.M. Work?"[14] It explains that "The nervous system is composed of the Central Nervous System, which runs the voluntary function or movements and the Autonomic Nervous System which runs the involuntary functions of the body, such as heart beat, digestion, etc." (We note the peripheral nervous system is not listed as part of the nervous system.) The brochure goes on to explain that under "sufficient stress," the brain fails to respond properly to afferent information, so that efferent control over body function becomes impaired. "This leaves the organ or body part running out of control." The TBM practitioner can find the problem using manual muscle testing.

The TBM practitioner stimulates specific areas of the spine to "stimulate the neurones in the brain to repolarize (fix the fuse) and allow the brain to regain control of the body and guide it back to health."[14] "Everything, whether living or not, has its own vibrational electromagnetic frequency. Each disease also has its own frequency."[14]

TBM practitioners, much impressed with the fact that a well-functioning nervous system "is a major requirement for health," are of the opinion that their technique (since it helps the nervous system) "can have a part to play in almost any problem and uncover and correct the roadblocks to recovery." Indeed, one web page[15] detailed an array "of conditions thought to be helped by TBM":

- Food, contact and inhaled allergies
- Blood sugar imbalances
- Arthritis
- High blood pressure
- Asthma

- Headaches
- Chronic pain and inflammation
- Learning disabilities/hyperactivity/attention deficit
- Chronic digestive disorders
- Sinusitis
- Obesity
- Hypo-/hyperthyroidism
- Menstrual difficulties and infertility.

Conclusions: TBM

- The reviewers are not aware of any references on TBM except for brochures and advertisements available on the worldwide web. Despite various claims to be read on the web that there is research on TBM, we could not locate any. Our review of Applied Kinesiology is applicable to a large extent.
- Dr. Victor F Frank, originator of TBM, who spends most his time teaching, offers a seminar consisting of four modules:[16]
  - Module 1: "thorough functional physiological exam" with corrections, 165 points in all
  - Module 2: "many new techniques"
  - Module 3: "extended body points" and new techniques that have "been effective in at least 500 cases" (!)
  - Module 4: "new material," and "questions and answers".
- While AK often uses different muscle tests for different organs, TBM uses the same indicator muscle but different body points for different organs. TBM, among the various Kinesiologies, appears to have staked its claim for uniqueness on the correction of functional physiology. TBM practitioners maintain an inventory of at least 300 suspected allergens in vials.[17] When these are individually placed in the patient's hand during muscle-testing procedures, a weak muscle supposedly indicates an allergy to the substance in the vial.
- One TBM brochure available on the web[14] decries the importance of research in chiropractic – indeed, castigates it:[14]

  In the early days of Chiropractic, the "old time Chiropractor" was not restricted or confused by "scientific proof" of what they were able to do.

These old masters found a problem and corrected it, thereby, building the reputation of Chiropractic with their main philosophy being that the power that made the body, could correct the body ... By taking the techniques of the old Chiropractic masters and combining them with modern technology, T.B.M. has been able to duplicate the corrections and restoration to health that the old masters were able to do.

- One would expect it to be challenging for patients to maintain conviction in the safety and clinical effectiveness of a chiropractic technique system that explicitly professes its intention not to be "restricted or confused by 'scientific proof.'"

NEURO-EMOTIONAL TECHNIQUE (NET)

NET appears to have emerged from the AK milieu by the late 1980s, although it is surprisingly difficult to discover any historical information on that. Inventor Scott Walker believes his seminal discovery to be the "neuro-emotional complex" (NEC), a "subjective maladaptation syndrome adopted by the human organism in response to a real or perceived threat to any aspect of its survival."[18] He also defines the NEC as "an emotional scar," or "bodily held emotion, the non-resolving affective component of a past trauma, retained as a spinal memory."[19] The "NEC SnapShot" is the memory of the past trauma, capable of evoking in the present the same physiological pattern that existed at the time of the trauma.[20] The "semantic reaction," a closely related term, is the person's "organism-as-a-whole response to a word, a situation, or some other stimulus. Any such response involves 'intellectual,' 'emotional', and physiological factors," what may be called gut-level responses.[19]

NET has explicitly aimed to address the emotional side of what is usually called the Triad of Health, represented as a triangle whose sides are labeled biochemical, emotional, and structural (or equivalent terms). More recently, it has come up with a new symbol, a four-sided structure called the "Home Run Formula," that has three corners labeled like the triangle, but has a fourth corner labeled toxins/homeopathy. In explaining the

metaphor, it is said that "The goal is to: Make sure every patient is 'safe' at each base."[21]

Walker invokes DD Palmer's triad of traumatism, poisons, and autosuggestion as the causes of disease, emphasizing that autosuggestion amounts to "emotional aberrations," the "missing link." Haldeman's discussion of how subluxation can relate to mental disease, and Pert's opinion that emotions are part of the body at large and not confined to the brain, are also cited.[19]

Walker also believes that memory of remote events evokes the visceral and somatic changes that occurred during these events. Memory is unconsciously expressed through motor behavior, and some memory is stored at the cord level, according to a Slosberg citation.[22] Thus, persistent subluxations would in essence be "emotionally disturbed." All trauma supposedly has an emotional or affective component. Those which are not self-resolving leave "emotional scars, or bodily held emotions, as Neuro-Emotional Complexes." These persist as something like irritable foci in the spinal column, affecting the way interneurons there respond to input.

If the patient is engaged in the memory of the emotional component of a subluxation, the pattern of neuropeptides is somehow physiologically engaged, and the nervous system is made better able to respond to an adjustment. All of the therapeutic differences between NET and any other adjustive system accrue to the patient recalling the emotional event during the adjustment. NET uses the semantic reaction to find the key emotional memories and through them the key subluxations. The diagnostic procedure uses muscle testing and other indicators to identify active reflex points. As an example, Walker discusses a patient with severely limited cervical rotation who was shown by (non-described) "testing" to have a gallbladder involvement. Since the gallbladder has been related to resentment by acupuncturists (according to Walker), the key to this patient's recovery was to adjust T4 while he recalled what had made him resentful.[18]

Walker believes that emotional problems may cause subluxations to recur following correction. He quotes Virgil Strang: "A most trying task for a Chiropractor is to attempt to correct the spine of a genuinely distraught individual."[19] Walker offers up headache and backache as archetypical examples of emotionally related somatic problems, and autoimmune disease, brain cell damage, and crime as further examples of emotionally related non-somatic maladies.

The NET subluxation correction, although it explicitly takes into account emotional factors, does not involve counseling or "talk it out" therapy. In correcting the NEC, in Walker's own words, "Having the patient engage a particular emotional event (memory) just prior to and during the adjustment uniquely engages the patient's nervous system."[19] This supposedly provides a similarly unique opportunity for a greater physical–emotional resolution. Therefore, there are no NET adjustive procedures *per se*; their defining characteristic lies not in what the doctor does, but what the patient thinks about, during the adjustive procedure. One NET practitioner posts a description of the treatment procedure on the internet:

The N.E.T doctor uses muscle testing, body reflex points, and semantic reactions (physiological reactions to memories or words) to assist and guide you to recall a specific negative emotions [sic] and when it first occurred. This engages a specific neuro-emotional pattern, much as a computer operator engages a specific program on a computer screen. While you mentally hold the emotional memory, the doctor adjusts the associated spinal subluxations.[23]

The NET adjustment is bilateral, near the vertebral facets. The vertebrae are adjusted in sequences identified by Ridler and Frank (of Total Body Modification Technique), sequences that are supposedly related to specific organs, which would in turn be related by the acupuncturists to specific meridians and emotions.[18] NET practitioners, in addition to adjusting, and like the Applied Kinesiologists, work with meridians, with Bennett's neurovascular points,[24] and facilitated and inhibited muscles.[18]

At some point NET became involved in the homeopathy business, not only administering homeopathy but also marketing a line of homeopathic remedies. The following comment, which eventually concludes it is acceptable that web readers prescribe their own remedy, is taken from Walker's website:

The best way to determine which remedy, if any, is the right one for you is to visit a NET practitioner who has been trained to test these remedies on you. Everyone is unique and, ideally, should be tested for his or her unique needs. In addition, a NET practitioner will likely address other components of the Home Run Formula to insure you have every chance of a successful healing for your presenting condition. If there are no practitioners near you, you can make a selection based purely on your symptoms – it's that effective.[25]

Conclusions: NET

- The formal structure of what uniquely defines NET is rather simple: the NEC is to the autosuggestion side of the triangle of health what the vertebral subluxation is to the traumatism side. Walker feels that NET is not really a standalone technique, but rather an enhancement to other techniques with which it may interface. He notes affinity with DeJarnette (Sacro-Occipital Technique, Ch. 25), Goodheart (Applied Kinesiology, Ch. 11), and Ward (Spinal Stressology, Ch. 28), as to how structural and biochemical aspects impact upon emotions.[18]
- The whole procedure of using the semantic event to identify the subluxation, and adjusting the patient while he or she recalls the emotional component, constitutes an office visit that takes only 3–5 min. Although no evidence is presented, Walker in 1990 stated he had corrected well over 60 000 NECs, and not one had ever recurred. He said that other NET practitioners had the same success.[18]
- The idea that subluxations contain memory patterns that accumulate in the body also shows up in Network Spinal Analysis (Ch. 22)[26,27] and in Neural Organization Technique (below).[28]
- According to Walker, "the emotions that are fixated in the NEC … may or may not be felt, acknowledged or expressed,"[20] meaning that no outcome measures may be needed beyond the doctor's belief that an NEC is present or has been eliminated.

- We may infer from the following citation that NET practitioners fear being seen as excessively metaphysical or esoteric by others:

NET seeks to normalize a neurological imbalance using a structural correction, allowing a change in physiology. NET does not deal with the spiritual realm. It does not exorcise demons or entities. It does not predict the future or deal, in any way, with parapsychology. It does not tell people what their plan of action may, must, or should be.[23]

- As others have noted concerning Spinal Stressology technique,[29] according to Walker, "NET is not psychotherapy. NET is used by psychotherapists and health care practitioners of all disciplines in tandem with their other techniques to quickly enhance their patients' results."[30] Another NET practitioner posted the following on a website: "N.E.T. is not psychotherapy, it is a treatment aimed at maximizing the physiology of the body through the removal of conditioned reflexes."[31]

- We have seen patients cry or experience other strong feelings during adjustive procedures, and have little basis to dispute NET's contention that there are affective components to somatic dysfunction. Given that these responses may spontaneously arise, the question is whether practitioners who receive little or no training in such areas should encourage them.

- The reviewers have had the opportunity to read through a seminar manual that attendees receive at NET seminars. There one can find the NET core ideologies expressed in a somewhat freer form, unlike the more considered and careful expression that typifies NET founder Walker's articles in the trade journals, as herein cited. Perhaps an example from the manual will suffice:

Therapy Localizing with Polarity Enhancing Posturing can often help with a non-electrical muscle testing situation. It appears to cause a greater polarization, thus greater electrical disparity and reactivity between the "touching" and the "touched" portions of the anatomy of the patient and the doctor. The mechanism is not known to, but thought to, utilize the electromagnetic field patterns as manifested in the formation of the micro spiral of the DNA molecule and the macro spiral of the galaxies. If there is a spiral force pervading these two diverse structures, perhaps there is a same or similar force in the human organism.[32]

CLINICAL KINESIOLOGY (CK)

CK is another spinoff from Applied Kinesiology. According to Levy and Lehr, founder Alan Beardall was one of Goodheart's "most brilliant protégés"[1] in the year 1968. Apparently, his breakthrough discovery was that individual muscles did not function as a unit.[1] Later on, Beardall discovered in the mid-1970s that various thumb–finger positions affected muscle strength, and went on to describe hundreds of these "hand modes." Apparently, having the patient curl the hand into various positions can alter the results of manual muscle testing, and help the doctor identify the particular organs that are dysfunctional.

Because it is so central to understanding the only thing that is really unique about CK, that which distinguishes it from generic Applied Kinesiology, we provide a representative description of the hand modes as applied by Beardall:

Hand modes were first rediscovered and used in this therapeutic form in the mid 1970s by the late Alan Beardall, DC. Using kinesiology with a patient one day, Beardall noticed that he got differing responses in muscle testing despite touching the same aberrant vertebra. He then observed that the patient was intermittently and unconsciously placing the fingers of one hand into a particular position. In fact, each time the patient's hand was placed into this position, it altered the muscle test. This extraordinary occurrence prompted Beardall to realize that he was being shown a specific key for a particular consequence. The hand mode read the body, and told him that a vertebra was subluxed – out of position. This was the beginning of the modern day use of hand modes in conjunction with kinesiology. Over the next few years, Beardall added many more hand modes to his work. He related that over a few days the "shape" of a mode would appear to him, until he was able to see it. He would then use it clinically to verify its nature and use.[33]

These hand modes are thought to be identical to or very similar to *mudras* – a mudra is a gesture or position, usually of the hands, that is said to lock and guide energy flow and reflexes to the brain – as they are used in Buddhism and other venues. Thus, these positions of the hands are thought to represent specific energy patterns easily recognized by the nervous system, and correspond to organs, conditions, and treatment options. These are "the keystrokes that a CK doctor uses to navigate through the 'bio-computer.'"[34]

A very succinct overview of CK appears in a book blurb posted at Amazon.com for Levy's patient-oriented book. It reads:[35]

Discovered by chiropractor George Goodheart in 1964 and developed by him and his student and colleague Alan Beardall in the 1970s, clinical kinesiology (CK) tests the body's energetic feedback system and rechannels it for healing. Chiropractor Levy and Lehr, one of her patients, describe it in detail. Although a recent discovery, CK draws heavily on acupuncture and subcontinental Indian medicine and is thereby related to centuries-old traditions. It claims to identify changes in the body before they appear physically, and via both text and diagrams, Levy and Lehr obligingly present the tests used to ascertain such changes. Treatments are designed to reverse or mitigate the changes and consist primarily of improving nutrition, identifying problems arising from food allergies, supporting the immune system, eliminating antibiotics and other powerful drugs, avoiding unnecessary surgery, and staying away from magnetic fields.

Levy and Lehr[36] (pp. 12–14) like Walker in NET (above), add a fourth element to the traditional chiropractic triangle of health, which includes chemical, structural, and emotional components. Whereas Walker added homeopathy, Levy and Lehr add "electromagnetic imbalance, to be addressed using acupuncture, herbal and homeopathic remedies, magnets, laser therapy, Neuro-Emotional Technique, and Bach and other flowers."[36]

The chapter headings from Levy and Lehr's book[36] give us a sense of what CK treatment is like: acupuncture point stimulation, chakra work, Bach flowers, kundalini, alternative nutrition, stress reduction, meditation, avoiding environmental stressors (electromagnetic fields, allergens, etc.) – a veritable catalogue of alternative healing.

Conclusions: CK

- One assumes that a CK practitioner may at times employ some type of chiropractic adjustive procedure, although Levy and Lehr's

patient-oriented book does not feature the words "manipulation" or "adjustment" in the index. Apparently, high-velocity, low-amplitude thrusting is either avoided or at least not emphasized: "Structural treatments involve gentle chiropractic adjustments, muscle work, therapeutic massage, and others."[36] (p. 13)
- Although most self-professed Kinesiologists point out that manual muscle testing is meant to add to, not replace standard diagnostic testing, including laboratory and X-ray, Levy and Lehr feel that manual muscle testing may provide more valuable clinical information than "CAT [computer-assisted tomography] scans, blood tests, MRI [magnetic resonance imagings]," etc. because these latter "do not take into account the energetic patterns."[36] (p. 8)
- According to Levy, the heart is an especially important organ, and a former colleague of CK founder Beardall confirms it originates in the neck and upper thorax:

The heart represents one of the body's most important organs. Burt Epsy, former colleague of Dr. Beardall, confirms that during body development in the womb, the heart originated in the neck and upper thorax. Thus the heart refers energy mainly to the base of the neck, over the shoulders, to the pectoral muscles, down the arms, and directly beneath the sternum.[36] (p. 10)

- CK does not distinguish itself very much from the group of Kinesiologies that have descended from the AK domain. In this review, much emphasis has been placed on a patient-oriented book for want of any published articles on the technique. (Lawrence's book review is, under the circumstances, charitable:[37] "I cannot therefore offer much in the way of judgement except to say this represents the manner in which these authors practice.") Although this may skew the interpretation to some extent, we are confident that anyone who feels comfortable with the theory and practice of AK, regarding which there is much published material, would feel equally at home with CK. On the other hand, anyone who finds AK procedures of dubious validity and reliability is unlikely to have any confidence in CK.

NEURAL ORGANIZATION TECHNIQUE (NOT)

Originator Carl A Ferreri graduated from the Atlantic States Chiropractic Institute in 1956. His seminar notes[38] indicate that some time in 1976 Ferreri came to the realization that "what we were really dealing with was our ability to survive in our environment. Symptoms weren't the important thing, they just got the patient into the office for treatment." This realization raised some questions in his mind, to which NOT is apparently the answer: "What caused the symptoms? What systems were not accommodating the stress of living? Why weren't they?"[38]

In a report to the Panel of Advisors to the American Chiropractic Association Council on Technique,[38] Ferreri indicates that his primary intent is to deal with the neurological basis of chronic subluxations, the real controlling factor, by improving the body's ability to organize all of its neurological subsystems. He comments that "N.O.T can successfully address any problem which can befall the human condition"[28] and "N.O.T is very specifically a way to organize or reorganize the nervous system if damaged or otherwise compromised in some way to restore the proper homeostasis in the body."[28]

NOT is, to a large extent, a synthesis of AK, Sacro-Occipital Technique, and cranial techniques,[38,39] but with an increased emphasis on organizing "the central nervous system by giving us a means of finding and then correcting any neurological deficits found within the innate neurological survival reflex systems …". Ferreri states as follows:[28]

[NOT] works through the recognized primal survival systems known as feeding, fight/flight, reproduction and the immune system activity. All physiological, neurological, vegetative and cognitive activity must function within these survival systems in an organized and integrated manner. These systems must be organized within themselves first and then must be integrated and synchronized with each other.

According to Ferreri, there are four primal survival systems: the feeding, fight/flight, reproduction, and immune systems. All physiological, neurological, vegetative, and cognitive activities depend on these survival systems in order for the body to survive. These systems must be not only internally organized, but integrated and synchronized with each other, mediated by the central nervous system. Various kinds of stress – physical, emotional, chemical, or environmental trauma – interfere with the harmonious and organized function of these reflex systems and ultimately the central nervous system. NOT recognizes and corrects "any of the disorganisations that may be found within the neural programmes of these primal survival systems if damaged or otherwise compromised."[40]

Ferreri believes (like Walker in NET) that trauma can "disrupt the neural programs within these reflex systems which then send inappropriate signals to the body."[28] He also writes: "The body remembers not only how it was born, how it was injured but also the circumstances of all insults to it – be they physical, chemical, environmental or emotional and the combination of all these circumstances."[28] Like kinesiologists in general, Ferreri upholds a Palmeresque triangle of health theory, with emotional, chemical, and physical components to subluxations. He seems to think that electromagnetic fields are profoundly important and dangerous to our health:[28]

The lines of force of the electromagnetic fields which influence all body function and the brain itself are laid down in the connective tissues, particularly in the bones and in the case of the brain in the cranial bones. Any disturbance of this delicate balance can produce disastrous results in relation to brain and neurological function.

NOT practitioners are very involved, as they see it, with addressing dyslexia and other conditions in which the central nervous system shows signs and symptoms of faulty coordination or lack or organization. Ferreri comments that dyslexia results from four cranial faults, three involving the sphenoid bone and one the temporal bones,[41] not only in dyslexia, but in just about every patient, including those who are asymptomatic. Ferreri heavily emphasizes the need to correct cranial faults: "Because we are dealing with neural integration and integrity, the cranial bones and their function must also be taken into consideration."[28] Ferreri claims that most of the problems in dyslexia can be corrected in one office visit,[41] but provides no evidence that this is true.

NOT synthesizes some of the key components of a variety of other reflex techniques, and thus the elements of craniopathy (Ch. 15), as attributed to both osteopath Sutherland and chiropractor DeJarnette (Ch. 25), the category system of analysis as practiced in Sacro-Occipital Technique (Ch. 25), and, of course, Goodheart (Ch. 11). NOT also leans extensively on some of the other Kinesiologies, such as those discussed above: innovations introduced by Frank (TBM), Beardall (CK), and Walker (NET). Unlike most other Kinesiologists, Ferreri endorses "osseous adjustments" when indicated.[39]

At the risk of being somewhat repetitious, and in order to give the reader a genuine flavor for the work, we think it worthwhile providing a detailed description, in its own native language, of NOT testing and corrective procedures:[41]

By using kinesiological modalities to access and activate the known reflex systems which control posture, gait, balance, reactive muscle function, etc. such as the Labyrinthine/Ocular, the Tonic Neck Righting and the Vestibular/Ocular Head Righting Reflex Systems, the Cloacal Pelvic Centering Reflex Systems, the Cerebella Stretch Reflex, the reactive muscle systems, the spindle cell and Golgi tendon reflex systems (feedback mechanisms in the muscles themselves) and other known systems and sub systems and the structural Category systems (I, II, III), we can profoundly affect all body function on purpose. Then using the body memory banks found with the eyes open and/or closed, in the light, in the dark or in half light and other circumstances including "the scene of the accident for example, we can create the proper circumstance to effectively treat almost any condition or deficit which can befall the human condition."

In addition to somatic conditions, NOT claims to treat associated somatovisceral problems, including "digestive system faults, hiatial [sic] hernia, chronic digestive valve problems, scoliosis, learning disabilities, endocrine, circulatory and cardiac stress syndromes."[28] NOT treatment is aimed at restoring homeostasis to the body "by activating combinations of the known reflex systems, acupuncture meridians, muscle spindles, magnetic energy, cranial and spinal bone balances and nutrition which control these systems."[40]

An article in the *British Osteopathic Journal* describes how the IQ scores of the children in a treatment group improved and their learning disabilities lessened, using AK and NOT methods.[42]

Conclusions: NOT

- Like all Kinesiologists, NOT founder Ferreri makes extensive use of muscle testing. He also uses it for his primary outcome measure, writing: "Once correction of these reflex systems is accomplished, specific and immediate outcome can be demonstrated. The immediate return of muscle strength, function and control of body position will indicate that they are indeed corrected."[43] However, his explanation of the mechanism has a distinctly electromagnetic flavor:

  If there is a functional or structural deficit anywhere in the body, there will be a change in the electromagnetic energy in that part or junction. When that part or reflex area is touched by either the examiner or the patient, there is a distraction to the overall energy field as the body tries to compensate for the change. This change is registered in the test muscle, and the muscle momentarily weakens on stress.[28]

- NOT shares the idea that subluxations have an affective component, stored as a memory of a trauma, with Network Spinal Analysis (Ch. 22)[27] and NET (above).[19]

- A quote from an NOT seminar manual[38] confirms both its similarity to and difference from typical AK literature, in that it invokes the same phenomena, but without as much clarity on the interrelationships:

  The activation of the small intestine neuro-lymphatic reflex by rubbing under the rib cage just below the costal cartilage, with the eyes closed, causes a subluxation at the level of the 7D vertebrae [sic]. This subluxation was not there until this activation was instituted. This subluxation was created by the body to establish an irritant to stimulate a reaction somewhere else (a Lovett reaction at the 4D). In this case to activate the gall bladder. This is manifest as a holographic (bone bent on itself) subluxation at the level of the 4D vertebral [sic]

- In his report to the Panel on Technique, Ferreri claims that there is "A research report published in England on Learning Disabilities in the Children's Bureau Quarterly" and a "Research paper published by Drs Bordie and Keil in Perth, Australia and reports from hundreds of chiropractors around the world using N.O.T. protocols."[39] We were not able to retrieve these using standard searching procedures. We did obtain a copy of a book Ferreri coauthored with Richard Wainwright on treating dyslexia and learning disabilities.[44] This book, in addition to providing more detail on the NOT approach to dyslexia, presents 15 brief case reports.

- Given the exceedingly alternative character of the diagnostic methods employed by NOT, those who practice it are charged with the task of making sure that patients with serious pathologies are receiving a quality of care that is at least equal to what they may have received from conventional assessment technologies (such as laboratory testing and physical examination). For example, on its web page, the Ferreri Institute advises prospective patients of the following: "whiplash and closed head injuries – nothing to do with the neck, muscle or soft tissue damage as generally accepted even though the cervical musculature appears to be involved. It is a loss of coordination between the head and neck righting reflex systems caused by a neuro-muscular reaction due to a sudden disturbance in the Cerebella [sic] Stretch Reflex system."[45]

Conclusions: Kinesiologies

- Although there are yet more Kinesiologies which are descendants of the muscle-testing technology pioneered by Goodheart and at the kernel of Applied Kinesiology, we elected to discuss the five we think are most practiced by chiropractors: CK, CRA, NET, NOT, and TBM. Many of the practitioners who practice any of these, as can be judged by visiting their web pages, use several if not all of them. Each of these offshoots is almost like a specialty practice under the Applied Kinesiology umbrella. From that point of view, we find that CK emphasizes Beardall's hand positions, CRA nutrition, NET the NEC, NOT learning disabilities, and

TBM organ balancing and allergies. Having first visited many of these web pages around 1999, we noticed more recently that many of the practitioners had changed their advertised technique specialty, quite seamlessly, since that time.

- Although we did not think there were enough practitioners of Neurovascular Dynamics (NVD) to include it in this chapter, we would be remiss if we did not note it. Developed by chiropractor Terrence Bennett, NVD postulates that anatomic sites on the surface of the body contain "neurovascular reflexes" that reflect the heath of specific internal organs and physiology. Active reflexes can be found by careful palpation for tenderness and pulsations. Furthermore, digital stimulation of the reflexes supposedly causes a reduction in tenderness and a return to normal internal physiology. Light sustained digital pressure is maintained over the active neurovascular reflex. The examiner attempts to discern a pulsation in the range of about 70–74 beats/min, while lightly tugging across the reflex point. The examiner may have to explore several directions of tug in order to determine the direction that maximizes the palpable pulsations and maintains remote thermal reflex activity. This usually takes about 20–30 s, but could take as long as 5 min. Bennett's followers have published anatomic charts indicating the body sites that correspond to certain organs. The practice of NVD has been incorporated into several of the Kinesiologies. William Nelson wrote several case reports involving NVD treatment.[46–48] (We did not find their findings impressive.)

- We would also be remiss if we failed to mention *Touch for Health*,[49] a lay version of Applied Kinesiology. Since it is not a chiropractic technique, Touch for Health is beyond our scope. Suffice it to say that in 1970, John Thie conceived the idea of making available Goodheart's discoveries and methods to the general public. The lecture, seminar, and workshop programs he set up evolved into the Touch for Health Foundation in 1973. At the current time, workshops and instructor-training programs are conducted all over the world, and Touch for

Health methods may be found in use in many settings: physical therapy offices, psychiatric offices, massage practices, and in doctors' offices.

- Some of the kinesiologists are quite frank in saying that diagnosing through muscle testing is not meant to be a substitute for conventional diagnosis (the best example of this is Applied Kinesiology itself), whereas others seem to pay no attention to "allopathic" diagnostic and treatment methods. This may be a matter of concern to some.

- Given that these technique systems often become heavily involved in the mental/emotional side of the chiropractic triangle of health, there is an ever-present danger of spilling over into lay psychotherapy, as practiced by untrained personnel. Walker of NET is very clear on attempting not to get involved in this type of practice, although we do not know to what extent he and other NET practitioners (not to mention those who practice other

Kinesiologies) succeed. This may also be a matter of concern to some.

- Clearly, given the esoteric methods involved, there is much research to be done. The issue is not really that other chiropractic examination and treatment methods are better validated, because many in common use are not. The issue that Kinesiologists must face squarely is that their methods are relatively poor in face validity, in the eyes of many patients and other external observers. In other words, they just don't seem to *make sense*. Confronted with various examination and treatment methods that are not well-studied or clinically validated, most people (one would think) would opt for the one that seems more plausible, more consistent with one's basic attitudes about how the body works. In the interim, although it does try one's patience, perhaps it would be wise not to reject eccentric methods that are largely unstudied in favor of ones that make more sense, are well-studied - and to a large extent found to be *equivocal*.

REFERENCES

1. Levy S L, Lehr C 1996 Your body can talk. Hohm Press, Prescott, AZ
2. Rinaldi M 2002 Kinesiology. http://www.rinaldichiropractic.com/kinesiology.html: M. Rinaldi
3. Walther D S 1981 Applied Kinesiology, vol. I. Systems DC, Pueblo, CO
4. Anonymous 1983 Applied Kinesiology – adopted status statement of the ICAK. Digest of Chiropractic Economics (November/December): 49, 51
5. Versendaal D A 1989 Contact reflex analysis and applied trophology. DA Versendaal, Vista, CA
6. Roth M Procedure of contact reflex analysis. http://members.tripod.com/drrothdc/
7. Versendaal D, Ulan F 1998 Contact reflex analysis and applied clinical nutrition: an effective analytical tool for the alternative health care professional. The American Chiropractor (Mar/Apr): 8–20, 32
8. Barrett S 1998 Contact reflex analysis. http://www.quackwatch.org/01QuackeryRelatedTopics/Tests/cra.html (accessed 16 April 2003)
9. Clecak P 1996 Giving patients reasonable counsel: the case of contact reflex analysis. The American Chiropractor (July/Aug): 18–23, 53
10. Clecak P 1996 Part two: giving patients reasonable counsel: the case of contact reflex analysis (CRA). The American Chiropractor (Sept/Oct): 13, 23, 52–53
11. Versendaal D, Cameron-Cooper C 1999 Exploring the complex wisdom and interactions of the gut and brain chemistry. The American Chiropractor 21 (2): 39–40
12. Knipschild P 1988 Looking for gall bladder disease in the patient's iris. British Medical Journal 297 (6663): 1578–1581
13. Simon A, Worthen D M, Mitas J A 2nd 1979 An evaluation of iridology. Journal of the American Medical Association 242 (13): 1385–1389
14. HealthPyramid 2002 TBM total body modification – your alternative choice for health care! http://www.healthpyramid.com/bio-energetic/tbmbrochure.html: Health Pyramid
15. Rapkin M 1999 What is TBM? http://www.mindspring.com/~drmaxrap/tbmtxt.html: Center for Nonforce Chiropractic
16. Frank V 2002 http://www.tbmseminars.com/Practitioners/products.htm: TBM [sic]
17. Mercola J 2002 TBM total body modification your alternative choice for health care! http://www.mercola.com/article/mind_body/tbm.htm: Health Pyramid
18. Walker S 1990 The triangle of health: once more, with feeling. Digest of Chiropractic Economics (May/June): 16–25
19. Walker S 1996 Disobedient vertebrae: are they (neuro) emotionally disturbed? Chiropractic Products (Oct.): 22–26
20. Walker S 1992 Ivan Pavlov, his dog and chiropractic. Digest of Chiropractic Economics (Mar/Apr): 36–46
21. Netmindbody.com 2002. What heals? http://www.netmindbody.com/what_heals_2.html: Health Pyramid

22. Slosberg M 1990 Spinal learning: central modulation of pain processing and long-term alteration of interneuronal excitability as a result of nociceptive peripheral input. Journal of Manipulative and Physiological Therapeutics 13 (6): 326–336

23. Babcock B H 2002 How does it work? http://babcockclinic.net/n_how.htm: Babcock Clinic

24. Bennett T J 1960 A new clinical basis for the correction of abnormal physiology. Self-published, Burlingame, CA

25. Walker S 2002 NET remedies. http://www.netmindbody.com/remedies_net_remedies.html

26. Herriot E M 1990 Life-changing chiropractic. Yoga Journal (Sept/Oct): 23–25

27. Russo G Network chiropractic: on the leading edge of growth and transformation. (Publication details not available)

28. Ferreri C 1996 Neural Organization Technique international. Chiropractic Products (Oct): 18–19

29. Sehi T, Proetz J F 1986 New answers for old stress problems – part 2. An exclusive interview with Dr. Lowell Ward. Digest of Chiropractic Economics (March/April): 36, 38–39, 41

30. Walker S 2002 NET and psychology. http://www.netmindbody.com/what_is_net.html

31. Janelle L 1999 The balanced body healing through Neuro Emotional Technique. http://www3.sympatico.ca/drlisejanelle/balancedbody.htm: Babcock Clinic

32. Walker S 1996 Neuro-Emotional Technique. NET, Encinitas, CA

33. Cranialrhythm.com. Kinesiology: a historical perspective. http://www.cranialrhythm.com/Faq/Kineshistory.html: Cranialrhythm.com

34. drgustafson.com 2002 Clinical kinesiology. http://www.drgustafson.com/clinical.htm: drgustafson.com

35. Beatty W 1999 Book review, Your body can talk: how to use simple muscle testing to learn what your body knows and needs: the art and application of clinical kinesiology. http://www.amazon.com/exec/obidos/ts/book-reviews/0934252688/qid – 927815277/002-0934553-6969857: Amazon.com

36. Levy S L, Lehr C 1996 Your body can talk. Hohm Press, Prescott, AZ

37. Lawrence D J 1996 Your body can talk: the art and application of clinical kinesiology (book review). Chiropractic Technique 9 (2): 85

38. Ferreri C A 1991 NOT basic procedures. Ferreri Institute, Brooklyn, NY

39. Ferreri C A 1995 NOT technique assessment (unpublished)

40. Ferreri C 2002 Neural Organisation Technique. http://www.positivehealth.com/permit/Articles/Kinesiology/terr50.htm: positivehealth.com

41. Ferreri C 1983 Dyslexia and learning disabilities cured. Digest of Chiropractic Economics 25 (6): 74, 148

42. Mathews M O, Thomas E 1993 A pilot study of applied kinesiology in helping children with learning disabilities. British Osteopathic Journal 12. http://www.icpa4Kids.org/reseach_children_chiropractic_autism.htm (accessed 9/29/2003)

43. Ferreri C A 1992 The centering and righting reflex systems relating to the moving gaits, posture and cranial injury. Transactions of the Consortium for Chiropractic Research (June 7): 305–306

44. Ferreri C A, Wainwright R B 1984 Breakthrough for dyslexia and learning disabilities. Exposition Press of Florida, Pompano, FL

45. Ferreri C 2002 Whiplash and closed head injuries. http://www.notint.com/disorders.htm: Neural Organization Technique International

46. Nelson W A 1994 Chronic low back pain: a case report. Chiropractic Technique 6 (4): 150–152

47. Nelson W A 1990 Rheumatoid arthritis: a case report. Chiropractic Technique 2 (1): 17–19

48. Nelson W A 1989 Diabetes mellitus: two case reports. Chiropractic Technique 1 (2): 37–40

49. Thie J 1994 Touch for health (1st edn 1973). T H Enterprises, Sherman Oaks, CA

13

Bioenergetic Synchronization Technique (BEST)

INTRODUCTION

Birds are the most studied migratory animals. Although they were once thought to navigate by means of stars or landmarks, we now know they have cells in their heads containing iron oxide crystals that align with magnetic north, just like the needle of a compass. Thus, they are able to sense the angle of magnetic field lines and determine directions. Small magnets attached to their heads cause birds to become disoriented, and natural magnetic anomalies, such as deposits of iron ore, also prevent them from navigating. To use magnetic fields for navigation, an animal must be able to detect magnetism, either directly, or by sensing electric currents induced in body fluids.

Magnetite and other kinds of magnetoreception are common among animals. Magnetite biomineralization is ancient, having evolved about 2 billion years ago in magnetotactic bacteria. Some researchers believe this capacity has been incorporated into humans as well. Indeed, the presence of ferromagnetic materials in biological systems provides a hypothetical explanation of the possible adverse health effects of extremely-low-frequency magnetic fields (ELFs). It may even explain the chiropractic technique known as BEST.

Probably the most distinctive feature of BEST is its theoretical and clinical belief that health and disease are strongly related to the influence of magnetic (not to be confused with electromagnetic) fields on the human body. The thinking is that an energy imbalance will divide the body into areas of north and south magnetic energy, whereas a healthy body does not have this "division" of energy. The further claim is made that the chiropractor can eliminate this division by applying his or her own electromagnetic energy to the appropriate points on the body.

OVERVIEW

According to Morter, "BEST takes its name from the Synchronization of the life (BIO) Energy as it pulsates in total communication within and without the body."[1] This is a decidedly vitalistic technique: "Bio-energy, the electro magnetic energy of the Universal Intelligence that creates and sustains all life, flows through the nervous system naturally."[2,3] Since disease supposedly disturbs intercellular communication, and is manifested by abnormal palpable pulsations, the primary goal of BEST chiropractic care is to "improve communication (confirmed by pulsation) and to even leg length and to remove spasticity (confirmed visually and by testing)."[1] The idea is to normalize the sensory system, to effect structural homeostasis, and to reposition the vertebra.[3,4] BEST aims to balance and synchronize the body's total energy, by removing nerve interference, which is especially high in the nervous system.[5]

The analytic procedures are to a large extent descended from Applied Kinesiologists (Ch. 11) and fellow traveling Kinesiologists (Ch. 12), including especially manual muscle testing (Ch. 6). However, founder Morter does introduce the concept of magnetic fields influencing body physiology, and that is built into and makes unique the BEST's analytic and mostly low-force adjustive procedures.

HISTORY

According to Morter, BEST originated on 20 November 1972 while he was attending a convention in Nassau.[6] He reminisces that, while standing in the water, facing the beach, a wave unexpectedly lifted him up and hurled him on to the beach, so that he landed on his neck and back. Since he was at a chiropractic convention, he asked some of the other attendees to adjust him using a variety of techniques, each to no avail. Upon his return home, he sought out other chiropractic care, but refrained from having his neck adjusted. By his account, he practiced with limited range of motion in his right arm and some discomfort for the next year and a half. Then, on 22 June 1974, while attending an Applied Kinesiology seminar on sacral techniques, he felt increased range of motion of his neck after the unsuccessful attempt by the lecturer to correct his sacrum. Learning of the "Lovett brother" concept that the sacrum and atlas are paired in some way, he embarked, as he puts it, on 24 June 1974 on the path of developing BEST, a new approach to non-forceful chiropractic.[6]

DEFINITIONS OF TECHNIQUE-SPECIFIC TERMS

- Survival segmentation: the body's response to illness, in which it organizes itself into magnetic zones of opposite polarity, occurring in either an "anteroposterior (AP)" or "lateral pattern"
- Subluxation: since, according to Morter, subluxation can occur in the cerebellum or between the thalamus and the hypothalamus,[7] his usage of the term is clearly atypical. He states that subluxation is "an interference which shall include, but not be limited to, vertebral disrelationship which alters nerve function."[4] Indeed, Morter credits Ioftness (Ch. 30) with the idea that the primary source of nerve dysfunction is in the brain, rather than the spinal cord or spinal nerves
- Bio: Morter's version of the *life force*
- Sensory dominant subluxation (SDS): "Any recurring vertebral subluxation complex

caused by sensory nerve interference," caused in the "high brain" and induced by stress[8]
- Pulsation synchronization: cellular and organismal pulsations or "beats" which produce waves[9]
- Sensory engrams: a learned motor pattern or memory which, once established, is used as a guide for the body to follow in reproducing the pattern of movement.[6]

PHYSIOLOGICAL MECHANISMS AND RATIONALE

Morter believes that there are three causes of disease: improper timing, toxicity, and thoughts.[6] Interspersed throughout his works, there are references to DD Palmer's definitions of Innate Intelligence, neural tone, and nerve interference; one reads that the body was created by perfect energy (God) and can only respond to stimuli perfectly.[6]

Highly impressed with the thought that there are 10 times as many sensory nerve endings as motor nerve endings ("We are a sensorium, 10 to 1"[10]), Morter believes that adjustments will not hold if the brain is somehow not made aware of them. He also believes that there are clinically relevant magnetic fields in the human body. In normal tissues, adjacent cells would be magnetically attracted to each other, whereas in a sick person, the body segments into variable patterns of south- and north-pole behavior, usually at the major joints. The breakdown in the synchronization of intercellular communication floods the thalamus with uncoordinated impulses, jamming it and maintaining illness until such time as it becomes unjammed. Morter posits the thalamus as a more important locale for nerve interference than the intervertebral foramina, except perhaps when there is trauma. Indeed, he wonders how X-ray-verified intervertebral foraminal encroachment in the lumbar spine could sometimes not be reflected in symptoms such as sciatica, unless there were some other locus for nerve interference. In a word, nerve interference is thought to be "high" in the nervous system.[11]

Displaying his Logan Basic Technique (Ch. 21) roots, Morter claims that once the disease process is underway, structural weakness allows the sacrum to subluxate anteroinferiorly, with compensatory distortion of the vertebra above.[1] Sometimes, however, one finds thoracic subluxation despite a lack of sacral or lumbar distortion, in which case there must be a "segmented energy pattern" in the supradiaphragmatic region. Morter believes that "primary brain interference" affects the motor system in such a way that vertebral subluxations occur and are maintained.[2,11] He also believes that there are two kinds of subluxation, the "traditional chiropractic motor dominant subluxation, or vertebral subluxation complex," and the BEST-discovered "sensory dominant subluxation," or SDS.[8] The SDS is "stress induced, memory retained, and motor expressed."[12]

The contact points for the BEST adjustment are the occiput, sacrum, and abdomen, forming something of a triangle. Morter stressed that the practitioner should "Complete the Triangle" during each office visit.[6]

DIAGNOSTIC/ANALYTIC PROCEDURES

Morter claims that placing one specific pole of a magnet near a strong arm may make it weak, whereas the opposite pole would be expected to make a weak arm strong, as assessed through manual muscle testing.[10] He also claims that these effects can be brought about by using the hands as surrogates for magnets, in that the right palm and digits 3 and 5 constitute a north pole, and the back of the left hand and digits 2 and 4 a south pole. The thumb is neutral. Morter believes he can palpate bodily "pulsations," that would somehow be related to intercellular communication.

BEST incorporates elements of Applied Kinesiology (Ch. 11), such as the *vertebral challenge*, the *switching* phenomenon, and *therapy localization*. In the vertebral challenge, a suspected line of drive is applied to a putatively subluxated bone; a weakening of a previously strong indicator muscle would indicate the appropriateness of that line of drive. Switching refers to a right/left functional mix-up, and exactly wrong responses to stimuli.[13] Therapy localization

(Morter does not actually use the term, but does use the method) refers to a previously strong indicator muscle weakening when the patient applies a light contact to a point of the body under investigation.[13] BEST also incorporates its version of the Derifield leg check[14] (Ch. 4), although the finding of Derifield positive or Derifield negative does not apparently lead to drop-table adjustments. In the end, muscle testing and leg checks are the mainstays of the diagnostic component of BEST.[7] Interestingly, it is the long leg, and not the short leg, that is found to be clinically involved (weak on manual muscle testing). In a successful clinical situation, the legs must remain even after the patient takes a walk around the office.[3]

TREATMENT/ADJUSTIVE PROCEDURES

BEST treatment has been described as "a nonforce sensory nerve adjustment that will cause the brain to respond with a more normal motor impulse permitting improved function in muscles, glands, and all tissues."[11] At least in 1981, when therapeutic magnetism was not as fashionable as it is today, Morter claimed he did not use magnets for therapy, only for diagnostic purposes.[10] The BEST practitioner, given Morter's descent from the Logan technique milieu, is quite *sacrocentric*. Pulsations are apparently palpated on the sacral base, and then synchronized with other pulsations palpated at various spinal levels. Two fingers on each of the chiropractor's hands are thought to be north poles, two south poles, and the thumbs are magnetically neutral. When imbalance is detected, the hands are held for a few seconds at specific contact points on the patient's body until pulsation is felt, at which times the legs should also even.

The Derifield positive finding indicates the patient's "south energy" should be treated, whereas the Derifield negative patient should have the "north energy" treated. The finding of even legs (no Derifield result) indicates the need for a supine adjustment. Treatment in all cases seems to involve the doctor synchronizing pulsations palpated at the most tender point on the sacral base, and a superior point around the atlanto-occipital joint, or even more cephalad at the external occipital protuberance or glabella. The tender points are said to be usually on the side of the body opposite the side of the patient's complaints. They may feel "edemic" [sic] and may become nodular in chronic cases.[15] Therapy localization is used to help identify the appropriate tender points to treat. With synchronization for about 30 s, the legs apparently even. In Morter's words, "A specific neurological adjustment is more effective than a hundred moves that are of lesser quality."[6]

In making manual contacts, Morter suggests that the practitioner use the north energy of the upper half of the body, on the aspect of the body that is facing away from the surface of the earth; this would be the spinal column if the patient is prone. Likewise, he suggests the practitioner should always use the south energy of the body on the aspect that is closest to the surface of the earth.[6] These contacts should be held for at least 20 s. He also claims that it is always more powerful to use the left hand on the abdomen.[6]

Morter maintains that specific adjustments of the vertebral articulations will release fixations while simultaneously stimulating sensory fibers around the articulation, thus allowing the sensory fibers to carry impulses to the brain for position evaluation.[6] However, Morter also suggests that the specific BEST adjustment activates sensory systems to carry a message of vertebral position to the brain. In turn, this permits the spasticity of the paravertebral muscles to relax, allowing the balance of muscle tone around the vertebra.[6]

Morter does not eschew manipulative (high-velocity, low-amplitude) techniques. He simply believes that not all patients can tolerate them, and therefore the chiropractor must have a low-force technique such as BEST available at least for such cases. He also believes that a BEST adjustment delivered before a more traditional vertebral adjustment will help it go better, and after a vertebral adjustment, hold better.[11] He emphasizes how the affective demeanor of the patient must be taken into account to optimize the outcome of care.[2,12,16]

OUTCOME ASSESSMENT

North–south segmentation is thought to have been eliminated[15] when:

- muscle testing the arms shows strength with eyes open or closed
- the legs are even
- there is equal spasticity in the legs
- pulses are synchronized and equal in intensity.

Evening the legs during the office visit, both supine and prone, appears to be central to outcome assessment, although there is some mention of improvement in general health status and pain reduction as goals of care.[11]

SAFETY AND RISK CONSIDERATIONS

Morter says he obtains X-rays on all of his patients, except pregnant women and babies.[4] Therefore, the biohazards of ionizing radiation must be taken into account. Apart from that, given the low-force nature of BEST adjustments, it would have to be considered a relatively safe technique (which is not to say that any other technique systems are dangerous!). One area of concern is whether BEST practitioners might be overly optimistic in their assessment of what type of patient problems are amenable to chiropractic treatment, as evidenced by BEST in a 1980 case report,[17] discussed below.

EVIDENCE OF EFFICACY

There is a case report from 1980,[17] of a man who fractured his pelvis in a motor vehicle accident, and received concurrent care from the hospital and BEST practitioners. Although the man appears to have made a good recovery, there is no obvious way to apportion treatment benefits to the medical and chiropractic providers.

Hawk and Morter[18] used the Medical Outcomes Study Short Form-36 Health Survey, Rand modification 1.0, to assess the impact of BEST care on the general health status of 41 subjects. Each subject attended a 4-day "comprehensive and intensive program of chiropractic care," involving suggestions for lifestyle modification in addition to daily adjustment sessions. Fourteen of the 41 subjects completed a mailed follow-up questionnaire. Subjects' Rand-36 scores ($P < 0.01$) improved in every subscale, and Global Well-Being Scale (GWBS) scores ($P < 0.01$) also improved immediately postintervention. At 8-week follow-up, scores tended to have slipped below the postintervention levels, but were higher than the pretreatment baselines.

Noting the relatively low follow-up rate of Hawk and Morter's study, Blanks and Dobson[19] replicated it in a larger patient sample of 215 patients, who attended one of 10 consecutive 4-day, in-residence health programs (Health Weeks). Unlike the pilot study, in which 62% of the subjects presented with musculoskeletal complaints, the present study (in which the patients were self-selecting) showed a reverse pattern, in which 62% presented with non-neuromusculoskeletal complaints, such as psychologically related problems. The program consisted of 4 days of intensive BEST care, including lifestyle and nutritional education. As in the pilot study, patients received both the Rand-36 health survey and the GWBS just prior to Health Week, then at its conclusion, and again 8 weeks following the conclusion of the program. There were immediate and significant improvements ($P < 0.006$) in six of the eight subscales of the Rand-36, and also significant improvement ($P < 0.006$) in the GWBS, with a 57% response rate. This improvement continued through the 8-week follow-up surveys.

Morter and Schuster[20] studied the effect of the BEST program on salivary pH levels. Under the assumption that pH levels may reflect autonomic imbalance, 24 patients were separated into two gender-and age-matched groups of 12 subjects each, based on clinical indications (as conceived by BEST) of suffering from either predominantly sympathetic (S-group) or parasympathetic imbalance (P-group). Study subjects were tested for fasting salivary pH, and completed the Rand-36 General Health Status survey. Following treatment, pH values increased significantly in the S-group, and decreased significantly in the P-group, and greater pre–post improvement in general health status was observed in the S-group, suggesting a greater overall treatment effect in the S-group compared to the P-group. The investigators concluded: "These preliminary findings support clinical observations suggesting that this approach is associated with restoration of autonomic balance."[20]

Phongphua et al[21] provide a short report of the results of using Gonstead, BEST, or Activator Methods Technique on 22 subjects with migraine headaches. Although 5 of the subjects improved, the authors warn not to overinterpret the study, which was quite small, and non-controlled.

CONCLUSIONS

- Several technique systems in recent years have drawn a distinction between two types of subluxation, one of which is generally seen as post-traumatic or mechanical, and the other of which seems to involve the central nervous system (or the meninges), or is associated with some sort of systemic disease or emotional disturbance. Network Chiropractic (Ch. 22), Spinal Stressology (Ch. 28), and BEST each have some version of this distinction.

- As an example of yet another technique tradition upon which it draws, BEST's descent from the Logan Basic Technique (Ch. 21) family tree is evidenced in Morter's emphasis on the sacrum, as well as his bimanual treatment approach with one hand on the sacrum while the other palpates cephalad structures.

- BEST must be considered a reflex technique, in the sense that it draws its rationale from physiological models that are not mainstream. Morter's belief that patients' body sections bifurcate into north and south magnetic poles, and that the doctor's hand is also so bifurcated, and that there are treatment implications, seems highly speculative. Through it all, Morter also invokes normal physiology (frequently citing Guyton's *Textbook of Medical Physiology*) on behalf of BEST concepts and procedures, with varying degrees of success, as we see it.

- One of the core beliefs in BEST, that spinal problems accrue more to primary sensory distortion than motor dysfunction (i.e., garbage in, garbage out) is reasonable, and not only dates back to the theories of DD Palmer, but would find much support in the modern era. How the BEST treatment approach, on the other hand, directly addresses "sensorium" problems, is an open question.

- Morter seems to believe that patient affective disturbances give rise to sensory disturbance, a belief well in line with modern thinking on psychosocial effects on back pain, somatization, and symptom magnification. On the other hand, BEST practitioners do not describe any particular way of addressing these matters, beyond "synchronizing pulsations."
- There are studies suggesting magnets may influence physiology,[22–29], although none of these sheds direct light on the BEST implementation of magnetic fields.
- The three substantive outcome studies[18–20] on BEST certainly bode well for this treatment approach, although the study designs do not permit ascribing the patient benefit to lifestyle modification, the curative value of the group experience, or some uniquely BEST-like aspect of the adjustive approach.
- As we comment about Network Chiropractic (Ch. 22), reading through some of the BEST writings is not for the faint of heart. What are

we to think upon reading comments like: "However, different regions of like cells (or linked tissues or organs) in one organism can oscillate at slightly different frequencies (heart vs. lung vs. stomach), a special super-impositional pattern emerges when they overlap"?[9] What are we to think upon learning that "biological field energy has been qualitatively demonstrated through Kirlian photography,"[9] supported only by a 1961 reference, when we are aware of the fact that Kirlian photography has long been thoroughly discredited? Finally, what are to make of the following *trans-Newtonian* procedure called *Assessment by Intention*?

Establishing an inter-relationship with the patient's energy field is accomplished with the practitioner assuming a standing position at the foot end of the supine patient. The practitioner, while observing the patient's leg length, mentally envisions a series of questions, anticipating an inaudible yes or no answer from the patient. This yes or no response from the patient, prompted by intention from the doctor, similar in construct to the currently recognized technique of non-contact communication referred to as Therapeutic Touch, is consistently detected through specific changes in leg length and muscle strength. The purpose of the non-contact intention questioning is to access the patient's biofield through which the body responds physically.[9]

REFERENCES

1. Morter M T 1981 Bio Energetic Synchronization Technique part II. American Chiropractor (March/April): 66, 68–69, 71, 78–79
2. Morter M Jr 1989 Subluxations can be just a memory. American Chiropractor (August): 46–51
3. Morter M T 1989 Bio Energetic Synchronization Technique: the sensory specific technique. American Chiropractor (November): 48–49
4. Morter M T 1985 BEST Bioenergetic Synchronization Technique. American Chiropractor (April): 30–36
5. Morter M 1977 Bio Energetic Synchronization Technique. In: Kfoury PW (ed.) Catalog of chiropractic techniques, pp. 65–70. Logan College of Chiropractic, Chesterfield, MO
6. Morter M T, Morter T III, Morter M 1991 Seminar notes, level I (timing/toxicity), level II (timing/toxicity) and level III (thoughts/toxicity) [seminar manual notes]
7. Morter M T 1982 Bio Energetic Synchronization. American Chiropractor (July/August): 46–50

8. Morter M T 1993 The Bio-Energetic Synchronization Technique: a breakthrough in subluxation detection. Today's Chiropractic 22 (5): 68–69
9. Morter T Jr 1998 The theoretical basis and rationale for the clinical application of Bio-Energetic Synchronization. Journal of Vertebral Subluxation Research 2 (1): 23–24 http://www.jvsr.com/1/c32/2198-0040_theoretic.pdf
10. Morter M T 1981 Bio Energetic Synchronization Technique part I. American Chiropractor (January/February): 42–43, 46, 66, 90
11. Morter M T 1986 Bio-Energetic Synchronization Technique. Today's Chiropractic 15 (3): 81–83
12. Morter M T Jr 1995 Chiropractic for the next 100 years. The American Chiropractor 17 (3): 14–16
13. Walther D S 1981 Applied Kinesiology, vol. I. Systems DC, Pueblo, CO
14. Thompson C 1984 Thompson technique reference manual. Thompson Educational Workshops, Williams Manufacturing, Elgin, Ill

15. Morter M T 1981 Bio Energetic Synchronization Technique part III. American Chiropractor (May/June): 22, 25, 61

16. Morter M T Jr 1992 BEST corrects defense physiology. Today's Chiropractic 21 (4): 28–30

17. Morter M T 1980 Bio Energetic Synchronization Technique case study. Digest of Chiropractic Economics (July/August): 76–79

18. Hawk C, Morter M 1995 The use of measures of general health status in chiropractic patients: a pilot study. Palmer Journal of Research 2 (2): 39–44

19. Blanks R H I, Dobson M 1999 A study regarding measures of general health status in patients using the Bio Energetic Synchronization Technique: a follow up study. Journal of Vertebral Subluxation Research 3 (2): 78–85

20. Morter T, Schuster T I. 1998 Changes in salivary pH and general health status following the clinical application of Bio-Energetic Synchronization. Journal of Vertebral Subluxation Research 2 (3): 35–41

21. Phongphua C, Hawk C, Long C et al 1995 Feasibility study for a clinical trial of chiropractic care for patients with migraine headaches using different chiropractic techniques. Journal of Chiropractic Education 13 (1): 75

22. Caselli M A, Clark N, Lazarus S et al 1997 Evaluation of magnetic foil and PPT insoles in the treatment of heel pain. Journal of the American Podiatric Medical Association 87 (1): 11–16

23. Harper D W, Wright E F 1977 Magnets as analgesics [letter]. Lancet 2 (July 2): 47

24. Hong C Z, Lin J C, Bender L F et al 1982 Magnetic necklace: its therapeutic effectiveness on neck and shoulder pain. Archives of Physical Medicine Rehabilitation 63 (10): 462–466

25. Lin J C, Singleton G W, Schaeffer J N et al 1985 Geophysical variables and behavior: XXVII. Magnetic necklace: its therapeutic effectiveness on neck and shoulder pain: 2. Psychological assessment. Psychological Report 56 (2): 639–649

26. Vallbona C, Hazlewood C F, Jurida G 1997. Response of pain to static magnetic fields in postpolio patients: a double-blind pilot study. Archives of Physical Medicine and Rehabilitation 78 (11): 1200–1203

27. Weintraub M 1998 Chronic submaximal magnetic stimulation in peripheral neuropathy: is there a beneficial therapeutic relationship? American Journal of Pain Management 8 (1): 12–16

28. Weintraub M I 1998 Magnetotherapy: a new intervention? [letter; comment]. Archives of Physical Medicine and Rehabilitation 79 (4): 469–470

29. Weintraub M 1999 Magnetic bio-stimulation in painful diabetic peripheral neuropathy: a novel intervention – a randomized, double-placebo crossover study. American Journal of Pain Management 9 (1): 8–17

14

Chiropractic Biophysics® (CBP) Technique

This chapter is partially based on previously published material, and is printed with the permission of the National University of Health Sciences

INTRODUCTION

New chiropractic technique systems rarely come out of the blue – they take root in pre-existing technique systems. Don Harrison states that he parted ways with Pettibon and his Spinal Biomechanics Technique around 1980, due to what Harrison saw as the latter's slowness to effect changes, to found his own Chiropractic Biophysics (CBP) technique.[1] It would take years of divergent evolution, at least as we see it, for these two techniques to become separate and distinct.

At the risk of exaggerating the point, let us stipulate that, for CBP practitioners, posture isn't everything, it is the only thing. The goal of research is to determine the ideal posture, of clinical examination to measure the patient's posture, and of chiropractic care to move patients toward that ideal posture as much as possible. In CBP, the objective is to correct the overall posture (global positioning of the spinal column), rather than individual spinal segments. That puts CBP clearly in the camp of the structural approach to chiropractic, which descends from Carver more than any other individual.[2] The subluxation is postural deviation, and the adjustment is postural correction.

Chiropractic research got off to a slow start, but has increased its quantity and quality dramatically during the last two decades. A large proportion of this research has been conducted in chiropractic colleges, but clinician-scientists have also made a major contribution. In that regard, CBP has contributed to this impressive body of research more than any other of the technique systems, and has been published in venues where chiropractors don't often go. Even those who have looked askance at some elements of this body of research (such as Cooperstein), which has truly been a lightning rod for criticism,[3] must acknowledge the immense effort that it represents, and provide congratulations where congratulations are due. In our Conclusions, we take more issue with some aspects of CBP than we do with virtually any other technique system in this book. That is not because we find more with which to disagree; rather, this reflects our extreme respect for these serious researchers, who thrive on serious critical commentary.

OVERVIEW

CBP technique posits a system of postural analysis and correction based on mechanical engineering principles,[4] with the ultimate goal of reducing nerve interference (Fig. 14.1). It hypothesizes a "normal human posture," mathematically defined in both the frontal and sagittal planes. Heavily invoking the work of Breig,[5] CBP technique practitioners believe that even minor deviation from this normal posture results in adverse mechanical tension in the central nervous system.[6,7] This tension in turn is said to lead to extremely-low-frequency and piezoelectrical electromagnetic effects that would result in neuropathic consequences.[1,8] Posturally oriented spinal care intends to normalize the functioning of the nervous system, and through it the functioning of the entire body.[9] CBP practitioners believe, such is the importance of posture, that "abnormalities of posture (global subluxations) can account for the histopathology,

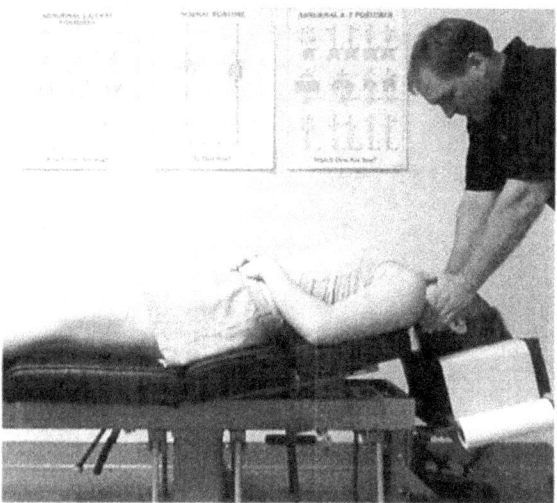

Figure 14.1 The Mirror Image® adjustment for correction of anterior head translation is shown utilizing the Omni drop table. With the patient supine, the thoracic piece must be elevated to cause sufficient posterior head translation. The patient is asked to flex the head forward slightly to eliminate cervical extension. The doctor's contact is the zygomatic bones of the cheek area.

myopathology, neuropathophysiology, and kinesiopathology encountered in patients presenting to the chiropractic professional's office."[10] A theme common to most, if not all, of the moves, and of the patient exercises as well, is the emphasis on "mirror-imaging" the patient,[11,12] which involves prestressing the patient toward postural correction.

CBP is a full-spine, fundamentally osseous technique. For the most part, it does not identify itself with any particular mechanical corrective style, although it does explicitly refer to its manipulative style as "diversified". In this usage, the term "diversified" appears to have more to do with the sense of being eclectic, and has little to do with the proprietary, named technique system called Diversified. Cooperstein addresses this twofold sense of diversified technique in another publication (Appendix 2).[13] CBP practitioners may employ side-posture, prone, and anterior setups; they may use drop tables, hand-held or floor-mounted mechanical percussive devices, and Sacro-Occipital Technique-style wedges to serve as fulcrums to supply mechanical advantage. Ancillary procedures are generally supported, including mirror-image rehabilitative exercise.[11,12] On the other hand, craniopathic procedures, motion palpation, paraspinal heat reading, muscle testing, and what may be termed "reflex technique"[14] phenomena are not supported, with the possible exception of an occasional leg check. Patients are offered symptomatic relief, but encouraged to participate in long-term spinal reconstructive, posturally oriented care.

The patient's three-dimensional posture is correlated with precise radiographic analysis to avoid the confusion inherent in analysis based on X-rays alone, stemming from the vagaries of mapping three dimensions on to a flat plane. Postural deviations are described using an orthogonal nomenclature system adapted from White and Panjabi.[15] The normal (optimal, ideal, etc.) posture is identified as a perfectly straight spine in the frontal plane, featuring sagittal curves in which the segments comprise arcs of circles (or other similar structures), the radii of which would conform to specified boundary conditions. (The factors that would govern the radii of such circles or other structures have shown some interesting changes over the years, and are discussed below.) The full-body posture is then considered as a particular permutation among all the various theoretically possible postures, as mathematically calculated using combinatorial expressions.[16] As a global distortion model, the CBP concept of subluxation explicitly situates itself as exclusive of and alternative to segmentalist chiropractic theories and practice.[17]

HISTORY

CBP technique has its roots in Upper Cervical chiropractic.[18,19] Wernsung had presented a model of the normal spine in the 1930s that influenced both Palmer and Grostic. Later on, Pettibon would develop his "Spinal Bio-Mechanics" technique[20] starting from the upper cervical work of Grostic, Gregory, and others in the Upper Cervical milieu. He enlarged the model to include the sagittal plane, with a significant contribution from the work of Ruth Jackson on the cervical syndrome,[21] and the thoracolumbar spine. All the essential components of CBP technique – the mathematical definition of the normal spine, an emphasis on posture, a mechanical definition of subluxation, an electromagnetic field slant on nerve interference, exacting X-ray technique, specific mirror-imaged rehabilitative exercises, instrument adjusting, and mirror-image prepositioning for adjustments – were in place in the Pettibon milieu, c. 1980.

Donald D Harrison stated that he originated CBP technique in December 1980,[1] because he was "disenchanted with slow changes in the Pettibon procedures,"[22] and also stated his brother Glen Harrison had been a cofounder.[11,12] CBP technique retains the distinct upper cervical flavor of it roots, as reflected, for example, in the practice of attempting to correct the patient's global posture by applying a "light force to the area of the atlas vertebra's transverse process while the patient's abnormal posture is stressed into its mirror image."[23]

Dr. Harrison and his associates have been very prolific over the years, having published many volumes of CBP technique texts, many peer-reviewed articles, and a newsletter c. 1987 that led by February 1991 to a quarterly publication currently called *American Journal of Clinical Chiropractic*. The various CBP technique texts and articles have shown much redundancy of material, frequently reproducing various drafts and other rewrites of articles. Dr. Harrison and his colleagues contributed a few chapters to Sweere's *Chiropractic Family Practice: A Clinical Manual*,[24] which were reviewed in passing (not especially favorably) by McGregor.[25] A two-volume set of CBP textbooks, *Spinal Biomechanics: A Chiropractic Perspective*[26] and *Chiropractic: The Physics of Spinal Correction. CBP Technique*[27] represents the work of Harrison and other contributors in biomechanics, physiology, and chiropractic technique. Drs Donald and Glenn Harrison presented CBP technique to the Seattle Consensus Conference in 1990.[28,29] The most recent book publication is *CBP Structural Rehabilitation of the Cervical Spine*.[30]

DEFINITION OF TECHNIQUE-SPECIFIC TERMS

There is no terminology unique to CBP technique, although there are many terms borrowed from

engineering, mechanics,[31] mathematics,[32] and other chiropractic techniques that may be obscure to some readers. Some examples are provided.

- Catastrophe theory: Thom's mathematical term, applied to sudden changes in spinal equilibrium[1]
- Isoperimetric: a mathematical term that refers to "different possible configurations of the same arc length"[1]
- Prestressing, post-tensioning: mechanical engineering terms, applied to spinal structures[33]
- Lower angle, upper angle, into the angles/kinks: these and other terms are taken from Upper Cervical X-ray line-marking systems
- Mirror-image adjusting: a procedure in which the patient is prepositioned prior to an adjustive thrust, so as to reverse postural deviations
- Mirror-image rehabilitative exercise: patients are taught how to move their "global body parts"[34] into a postural configuration that is the opposite of their postural distortion pattern
- Subluxation: usually regarded by CBP technique to involve "vertebral misalignment ... with some type of nerve interference,"[35] although a distinction is drawn between "relative" (segmental) and "absolute" (global) subluxation.[23] The word is sometimes used in a more general sense as well, for example: "Subluxation is defined as the loss of the mechanical integrity of the spine"[19]
- Adjustment: historically regarded in chiropractic to involve specific contacts and short lever arms,[36] the term "adjustment" is redefined by CBP technique to involve a specific corrective force that would change the "mathematical configuration of the spine toward normal"[23]
- Manipulation: compared with an adjustment, "manipulation" is redefined to involve the utilization of cavitation to increase range of motion[23]
- Torque: CBP claims to use the term "torque" correctly,[26,37] as compared with many, if not most, other chiropractic techniques; Herzog[38] felt that Harrison et al[37] had also misused the term
- Coupling patterns: described in 1987,[39] and more carefully covered in a two-part article by Harrison et al,[40,41] coupling patterns are

said to occur in six degrees of freedom, and not simply in rotation and lateral flexion, the directions they claim are stressed by other technique systems.

PHYSIOLOGICAL MECHANISMS AND RATIONALE

Rosenthal contrasts the "structural" and "segmental" approaches in chiropractic[2] in a manner that leaves little doubt that CBP practitioners must be considered to be strict structuralists. CBP structuralists see postural distortion as the subluxation in and of itself, and offer up a language of listings that describes the linear and angular relationship of entire regions of the spinal–pelvic articulations. A given motion segment may exhibit more signs and symptoms of dysfunction than another, but this would be the consequence rather than the cause of the primary postural distortion. For example, the apical vertebra of a lateral curvature may exhibit tenderness or osteophytosis, but the global subluxation remains the lateral curvature, not what occurs at its apex. From this point of view, since the spine tends to subluxate in a regional manner, it should be adjusted accordingly, possibly using relatively non-specific contacts.

The principal tissues affected by poor posture are the spinal ligaments, the intervertebral disks, the vertebrae, and the nervous tissue. Symmetrically, reduction of postural distortion would entirely explain the benefits that patients experience. "Only chiropractic methods and procedures that correct the patient's posture ... will permanently relieve nerve interference."[42] CBP technique practitioners believe that abnormal posture is the underlying cause for somatoautonomic reflexes resulting in visceral disease, pain, diminished range of motion, articular dysfunction, myofascial lesions, aberrant proprioception, and all other forms of nerve interference. Stress on bone due to unbalanced loads is believed to result in osteophytosis, through the mechanism of Wolf's law, while the low-frequency fields generated from the bone are thought to produce electrical nerve interference.[19] Mirror-image treatment methods, apart from directly correcting the

posture, are "thought to produce a temporary resetting of the proprioceptors."[19]

Central to the physiological rationale for CBP technique is the definition of the "normal" (occasionally "optimal" or "ideal") spine in both the anteroposterior and lateral views. Proponents of CBP technique have focused most of their attention on the lateral view, since they believe the book closed on the frontal plane, where the spine must (in their view) be straight. Various numbers for the normal cervical lordosis have been put forth over the years, ranging from the 60° C1–T1 value supported by Pettibon and Loomis,[43] to the 42° C2–C7 value derived from Delmas, as cited by Kapandji,[44] to the 34° C2–C7 value that emerged from their own normative data on the average pain-free neck: "Two typical geometric configurations of the cervical spine were identified as a normal circular lordotic arc of 34 degrees and an ideal normal of 42 degrees."[45] Work similar to the cervical modeling has now been conducted on the thoracic and lumbar spines, featuring hypotheses on the normal shapes of these spinal regions. There are further comments in the Conclusions below, pertaining to the CBP model of the normal cervical lordosis.

DIAGNOSTIC/ANALYTIC PROCEDURES

CBP technique is an X-ray-intensive technique. The series taken may include some non-standard projections, such as the sitting (Ferguson projection) lumbopelvic view, and the nasium cervical view. The full-spine X-ray is not supported.[46] In conjunction with direct postural evaluation (visualization, plumb-line), postural evaluation through X-ray is the diagnostic cornerstone. Here is a representative summary statement from CBP technique practitioners Gambale and DeGeorge: "In our practice we primarily rely on the patient's posture and corresponding X-ray images. We look at the patient's symptoms, leg length, and heat patterns; restricted motion, taut muscles, and orthopedic/neurologicals as nothing more than presenting symptoms of an underlying spinal structural misalignment (subluxations). That is not to say that the aforementioned are not helpful as indicators; however, they are more useful as a rearview mirror than a means of direction."[47] At one time, some CBP technique practitioners used the Metrecom, a computer-assisted goniometer, developed by Faro technologies,[48] a tool we believe is no longer commonly used, following some negative studies on its accuracy.[49,50]

TREATMENT/ADJUSTIVE PROCEDURES

CBP technique is a full-spine, osseous technique. The patient is "mirror-imaged": that is, prepositioned in a postural configuration opposite the incoming distortion pattern. (The term "mirror-imaging" is somewhat misleading, since there is no way to mirror-image abnormal sagittal curves, such as hypolordosis; the term should be restricted to frontal plane lateral curvatures.) These setups may require props like foam wedges and pillows, and more than one doctor may be needed to prestress the patient toward postural neutrality. The doctor may use drop tables with sections capable of vertical motion, lateral flexion, and even y-axis rotation. The adjustive thrust is generally applied to the prepositioned body area, but may be applied elsewhere. For example, a patient may be prepositioned to reverse an abnormal full spine posture, but receive a thrust applied to the upper cervical area. Some of the drop-table moves are performed with the patient in side-posture, a somewhat unusual position for the patient.

More or less conventional side-posture, prone, and anterior moves are employed, mostly to improve the range of motion. Some CBP doctors may still use the side-posture moves descended from the long-levered moves developed by Pettibon (Ch. 27) – not very descriptively called the "1 move," "2 move," etc. – with contact points on the innominate bone that are well removed from the joints to be moved. Although the moves are generally high-velocity, low-amplitude (HVLA) thrusts, activator-style percussive instruments,[51] either large floor-mounted models or hand-held devices, are often used, especially for the upper cervical area. Some interest has been expressed and experience reported in treating horses chiropractically, adapting the Sharp method to CBP postural procedures.[52]

Ancillary procedures such as physiotherapy, therapeutic exercise, and extremity care are generally supported. Cryotherapy (ice, etc.) may be used to reduce inflammation and pain, and is utilized along with passive motion during the acute phase of care following injuries. Soft-tissue manipulation is also encouraged,[23] including trigger point therapy, transverse friction massage, strain–counterstrain technique, and proprioceptive neuromuscular facilitation technique.[19]

CBP technique has always been very committed to cervical and, more recently, lumbar traction, harking back to its origin in the Pettibon milieu. DeGeorge provides a historical account of how several individuals contributed to the development of CBP traction protocols: "The evolution of chiropractic extension traction has been a result of the efforts and insight of many people."[53] The primary purpose is to stretch the anterior spinal tissues, especially the anterior longitudinal ligament "into the viscous and plastic deformation ranges."[54] Many methods, including a rather novel *extension-compressive* method, are described.[34] Therapeutic exercise (stretching, strengthening) has also been important since the early days of CBP technique. Drs Kim Christensen[55,56] and Michael Schneider (authority on Receptor-Tonus Technique)[57,58] have each been published in the CBP quarterly journal (currently called the *American Journal of Clinical Chiropractic*) in recent years, suggesting an expanded interest in neurologically enhanced muscular and myofascial rehabilitation procedures.[10] Patient education and ergonomic advice are also recommended.[19] Indeed, "Postural chiropractic adjustments, active exercises and stretches, resting spinal blocking procedures, extension traction and ergonomic education are deemed necessary for maximal spinal rehabilitation."[10]

OUTCOME ASSESSMENT

CBP technique is distinctly unimpressed with symptom reduction as a long-term outcome measure, and has found the Mercy Guidelines (Ch. 37) on duration and frequency of care adequate only for the treatment of acute and chronic pain syndromes.[19] In this setting, CBP may utilize standard measurements of subjective complaints, such as the Oswestry questionnaire, and visual analog scales (VAS). When it comes to spinal rehabilitation and a more long-term time frame, postural improvement is paramount, as assessed by X-ray, at one time the Metrecom device, or direct observation.[19] CBP technique is not impressed with range of motion as an outcome measure, frequently mentioning the poor interexaminer reliability studies and citing evidence that range of motion increases are only temporary.[59]

SAFETY AND RISK FACTORS

The usual contraindications to traction are listed: history of stroke, hypertension, etc. Furthermore, the extension-compressive traction method would not be used on a patient exhibiting posterior spurring or stenosis[54] or who has other problems related to spinal extension.[34] Inflammation is sometimes indicated as a special problem, but it is not clear if this contraindicates certain maneuvers. In the absence of a reference to the contrary, it is probably (but not definitely) the case that CBP technique would support the usually listed contraindications to osseous adjusting: osteoporosis, malignancy, recent fracture, etc.

EVIDENCE OF EFFICACY

X-ray line-marking reliability and validity

Several X-ray line-marking reliability studies have been published. To determine the reliability of the closely related Pettibon X-ray line-marking procedures, six practitioners read and reread 30 X-rays, assessing them for atlas laterality.[60] Statistical analysis showed "very good" reliability, both for stability over time and equivalence over experts, although Keating and Boline reanalyzed the data and showed that the measurement errors may have been too large for the method to be clinically useful, in spite of the good interexaminer reliability.[61,62] In another study designed to test the intra- and interexaminer reliability of

CBP technique practitioners in X-ray line-marking, three examiners marked 65 subject films for several pertinent segmental and global parameters. All the reliabilities exceeded 0.70, from which the investigators concluded that "these measurements in CBP technique would be considered accurate enough to provide measurements for future clinical studies."[63] Troyanovich et al[64] showed good CBP lateral lumbar X-ray line-marking procedures to be very reliable (except for marking the arcuate angle). More recently, Troyanovich et al[65,66] demonstrated intraclass correlation coefficients (a measure of agreement) of above 0.7, some very much above 0.7, showing good reliability for a variety of line-marking methods typically used by CBP practitioners to analyze the lumbopelvis and the cervicothoracic spinal regions.

Janik et al[67] showed that a new method for calculating lateral flexion from C3 to T3 from anteroposterior radiographs had high intra- and interexaminer reliability. The same study[67] featured a validity component, which assessed the accuracy of one examiner in using the line-marking method compared with known rotation angles of a plastic C3 vertebra. The average error was only 14% (less than 1°) between -5° and +5°. Harrison's posterior tangent method of X-ray line marking the lateral cervical film, to quantify the degree of lordosis, was found to be more reliable than the Cobb angle method.[68] The posterior tangent and Cobb angle methods were found to be equally reliable ($r > 0.94$) for the thoracic spine lateral view analysis,[69] and a similar conclusion was drawn for the lumbar spine.[70]

As this book went to press, a study was published showing the reproducibility of CBP radiographic patient-positioning procedures.[71]

Clinical effectiveness

A small study[72] found no difference in degree of pain reduction or cervical range of motion increase in two groups of patients, one treated with CBP procedures and the other with the (non-described) "Palmer Package." Both groups improved to some extent, from 5.7 to 7.0 in their Oswestry scores, and about 7° in their cervical range of motion.

DeGeorge and Gambale present a case report involving the reduction of a disk herniation, published in the CBP quarterly publication.[73] Peet reports on the correction of "vertebral subluxations and postural permutations" in a case of cerebral palsy.[74] Pope presents a series of 24 well-documented case reports.[75] All of these reports involve the cervical spine and its lordotic angle, and the results of treatment involving the extensive use of traction. According to Pope, three of the cases demonstrate the reversal of spinal arthritis and marked regeneration of degenerated disks. If these results can be verified, they would amount to a significant breakthrough in the treatment of cervical degenerative joint disease.

A blinded clinical trial was conducted to determine if cervical extension–compression traction, combined with diversified and drop-table adjustments, would alter the cervical spinal configuration.[76] There were two treatment groups, one of which received both the traction and adjustments, while the other received the adjustments only. A control group received no treatment at all. After approximately 60 treatments during a 3-month period, the traction group showed a significant change in all the radiographic parameters that were checked, including: a 13.2° increase in their C2–7 lordotic angle, a 9.8° increase in their C1-horizontal angle, and a 6.8 mm posterior translation of the head. Neither the non-tractioned experimental group nor the control group showed significant radiological changes. The investigators concluded that extension–compression traction, combined with cervical adjusting, did indeed markedly increase cervical lordosis and change other parameters. These results must be considered to be very dramatic, given the general paucity of evidence that chiropractic care measurably alters spinal structural parameters. Plaugher et al, for example, found no such global changes in their study.[77] A critique of the Harrison study[78] and the investigators' response[79] appear in the *Journal of Manipulative and Physiological Therapeutics* of January 1995.

A study published in 2002[80] involving extension traction of the lumbar spine showed that chronic low back patients showed an 11.3° increase in their lordotic lumbar angle, and experienced a significant improvement in the VAS scores. This is all the more important given the previous demonstration[81] that chronic low back pain is correlated with lumbar hypolordosis.

A 2002 study[82] showed that a combination of cervical manipulation and extension traction lowered VAS scores and increased the cervical lobb angle by 12.1°, in addition to effecting improvement in other radiological parameters, compared with a control group in which no changes occurred.

Unlike the previous study,[76] whose outcome measure was radiological, the current study showed a significant pain reduction in the experimental subjects. These results were similar to the 2002 lumbar spine study.[80]

As this book was going to press, an article was published showing, once again, that cervical manipulation plus extension traction can increase the lordotic angle of the cervical spine.[83]

CONCLUSIONS

- Blurring its traditional distinction from what many chiropractors would call an *adjustment*, CBP redefines "manipulation" so as to involve the utilization of cavitation to increase range of motion.[23] This revisionist distinction of adjustment from manipulation clearly leads away from the mechanics of the thrust and toward the mere *goal of the thruster*: "The basic difference between a spinal adjustment and spinal manipulation/mobilization lies in the intent of the practitioner."[23] We are forced to conclude that, in the eyes of CBP practitioners, the only thrust to be considered an "adjustment" is one intended to move the patient's spine toward what the Harrison spinal model defines as "normal."

- CBP investigators have worked hard to establish the reliability (and, to a lesser extent, the validity) of X-ray line-marking procedures, and have also written the most comprehensive review article on the subject.[84] They find good reliability across a broad spectrum of X-ray line-marking procedures in chiropractic including, but not limited to, their own. They have also shown reproducibility of CBP radiographic positioning procedures.

- In our view, the CBP literature is often infused with forced terminology and scientific factoids of unknown significance. For example, we find the term "harmonic," which in classic physics refers to an integral multiple of a fundamental frequency, used to describe the sagittal curves of the spine. As another example, CBP practitioners have stated that the theoretical number of full-body postural configurations is in excess of 128 million,[34] but they seem to believe only one, to the nearest degree, would be normal.

- Harrison appears to believe that the case for a perfectly straight anteroposterior spine is so compelling that contrary views, such as those expressed in *Gray's Anatomy*[85] or by Kendall et al,[86] are not worthy of discussion. He states: "It would appear that debate on an Ideal Normal Static model of the spine should be restricted to the lateral view."[87] This also seems to explain the vehemence of his critiques of Johnston,[88] who wrote an intriguing and utterly benign article in 1966 on how "the compensated, functional spine with least manifestation of symptoms is the form of a tight spiral"[89]; and of Ressel, who mentioned Johnston approvingly in his 1986 article on chiropractic pediatrics.[90] Ressel, in defending himself,[91] argues that Harrison's critique has missed the point by confounding resiliency and strength when discussing the durability of the spine.

- Given how much emphasis has been placed by CBP theorists on defining the normal cervical lordotic angle, it is surprising how frequently different numbers pop up, both over time and within the pages of a single article. For example: "Two typical geometric configurations of the cervical spine were identified as a normal circular lordotic arc of 34 degrees and an ideal normal of 42 degrees."[43] It is also surprising how many different reasons are provided in support of these numbers. Some time around 1996,[92,93] the CBP theorists started paying much more attention to normative data, that is, the importance of symptoms such as neck and back pain (or lack thereof) than they had previously. From that point on, the models they elaborated for the normal spine included not only abstract mathematical parameters, but also elements of clinically relevant, patient-centered findings. We believe this is an important, progressive development.

- Although as we go to press Harrison and his colleagues now favor either a C2-7 34° or 42° figure[92] for the cervical lordosis, depending on how one interprets their comments, at one time Harrison vigorously defended a 45° value, based on Pettibon and Loomis's radius = chord length formula.[93] This formula resulted from the theorem that the normal neck would be a portion of an arc of a circle whose radius equals the vertical length — that is, the chord length — of the neck.[93] Pettibon and Harrison stated in 1981[94] that the radius = chord length arrangement succeeds in "providing the spine with the strongest possible resistance to gravity and the best possible levers for muscle action." These results were explained both geometrically[95] and in terms of the post-tensioning and pre-stressing of radially loaded structures, likening the cervical spine to both arches and dams.[33]

- The Harrison Spinal Model, c. 1981, stuck to the 45° figure, but apparently felt the radius = chord "assumption" needed to be supplemented by the "isoperimetric" solution. This entailed a proposed compromise between the opposing requirements that the cervical spine's bending moment be minimized while its (poorly defined) "inherent lever arm" for movement be maximized.[4] This compromise solution,[96] although a data-free assumption, led to the rather surprisingly strong conclusion that "This 60° arc of a circle is forever established as the 'NORMAL' SPINAL SECONDARY CURVE!!!" (Harrison's own emphasis.)[97] It should be noted that the aforementioned 60° figure is for C1-T1, corresponding to 45° for C2-7.[94] Finally, at about the same time, Harrison provided yet another pathway to a similar cervical lordotic angle, derived from the Delmas index, as cited by Kapandji.[44]

- Indeed, right up to the present, CBP technique has for many years placed enormous weight on Kapandji's single *unreferenced* mention of a certain "Delmas Index: the ratio of the vertical height of the vertebral column to its length as measured along its curves."[44] Following Kapandji, Harrison opines that the ratio for a normal Delmas index must lie between 0.94 and 0.96, with 0.95 considered optimal. This corresponds to sagittal curves that lie between 69° and 56°, a range that contains both the C1–T1 60° lordotic angle favored, according to Harrison, by Pettibon,[97] as well as the 63° lordotic angle favored by Harrison in later formulations.[87] No explanation is provided as to how "this Delmas criteria [sic], together with the assumption that the spinal curves are arcs of circles, can be used to determine an ideal cervical, ideal thoracic, and ideal lumbar curve in the lateral view."[87]

- More recently, the assumptions of the Harrison spinal model have been altered in such a way that the normal or optimal cervical lordosis now features a Delmas index of approximately 0.97.[92] This corresponds to a very significant decrease in the "normal" C2–7 lordotic curve, from the former approximately 42–45° angle to a more plausible 34° angle,[92,93] which is more in line with other typical estimates.[98,99] Patients previously thought to have been hypolordotic would now be seen as falling within normal limits.

- In their definitive 1996 *Spine* article,[92] Harrison et al found that their geometric spinal model predicted the average cervical spine among 400 subjects. Moreover, there was virtually no difference between the lordotic angles found among all 400 subjects, and a subset of 252 subjects without cervicocranial symptoms: each group had lordotic cervical angles of about 34°, with a standard deviation of about 9°.

- It is very important to see what this means. Although the normal cervical lordosis is defined normatively, as the average of pain-free subjects, people in pain were found to have about the same average lordotic angle, suggesting that being "Harrison-normal" did not predict feeling better than Harrison-abnormals. Not only that, but the standard deviation of 9° tells us that 95% of the asymptomatic patients had lordotic angles between 16° and 52°, suggesting that the value of the cervical lordosis is not very clinically important. Nevertheless, Harrison et al suggest in their recent textbook[30] that a patient with a 21°

cervical lordosis (well within that range that contains 95% of asymptomatics) has sustained a 29% loss of lordosis, compared to a putative normal of 29.4°, a figure obtained by producing a weighted average of the results of Harrison et al[92] with those of Gore et al.[100]

- Why isn't this patient reassured that his lordotic angle lies well within the range manifested in 95% of asymptomatic patients (29 ± 18°)? Telling him he has a 29% loss of lordosis is like advising a patient with blood sugar of 100 mg/dl that he needs treatment, because he is above the midpoint of the normal range of 64–126 mg/dl. Hariman, apparently unsuccessfully, tried to make a similar point in his 1995 reply to a letter to the editor penned by DD Harrison.[101] Although Hariman's actual suggestion was that normal values for the cervical lordosis should be reported as *ranges*, not point values, Harrison seemed to think that Hariman was opposed to using the *average* cervical lordosis (however defined) for a normal.

- Although it is interesting that several dozen office visits involving manipulation and extension traction lower pain and increase lordotic values in the cervical and lumbar spines, and that such changes do not occur in control groups, it is misleading to suggest this makes the case for protracted chiropractic care. The 30 subjects entered into the 2003 study[83] were either about 2 standard deviation units or more below the Harrison ideal 34° cervical spine (12.7°), or exhibited segmental regional cervical kyphosis. Since we do not know how typical these patients are in a CBP practice setting, we do not know if the results achieved would be clinically relevent to patients who are not kyphotic or who are more lordotic. It is entirely possible that they may have achieved similar reductions in their VAS values without such protracted care, and more importantly, without changes in their lordotic angles. We must always be careful not to confound association with causation, and keep in mind that many chiropractic adjustive methods not especially concerned with lordotic values have shown their ability to lower pain scores. The increased lordosis seen in this study, given the large range of lordotic angles consistent with being pain-free, may be an incidental finding of little or no clinical significance. There is clearly no point in increasing lordotic angles just because we can.

- When similar curve-fitting methods were applied to the lumbar spine, an interesting and different result was obtained. After having first conducted and reported on normative data,[102] CBP investigators noted[81] that the lumbar spines of both normal subjects and subjects with low back pain could be modeled by an ellipse, but not by the same ellipse. Moreover, among the painful subjects, the spines of the chronic subjects tended to be less lordotic than the normals, whereas the spines of the acute subjects tended to be more lordotic. Therefore, the CBP investigators found that in the lumbar spine, unlike in the cervical spine, there is a relationship between the lordotic angle and the clinical status of the patient.

- Although the case made by CBP practitioners for rehabilitation protocols seems reasonable enough, obviously the degree of treatment deemed necessary greatly depends on the goal of care. If that goal includes convergence upon some spinal structure said to be normal, whereas in fact that goal is not validated, then the degree of rehabilitation that is appropriate and clinically necessary may also be questioned.

- CBP has been so extensively published in recent years that we could not make reference to every article in this chapter. Besides, many of these articles, although written by CBP theorists and/or practitioners, are more about spinal biomechanics than about clinical chiropractic, and therefore were beyond the scope of this chapter. A list of CBP publications is available on the web.[103]

REFERENCES

1. Harrison D D 1981 Chiropractic biophysics phase I. Harrison Chiropractic Seminars, Sunnyvale, CA
2. Rosenthal M J 1981 The structural approach to chiropractic: from Willard Carver to present practice. Chiropractic History 1 (1): 25–29
3. Troyanovich S 2003 The Harrison spinal model: a chiropractic "lightning rod" for criticism. http://www.chiroweb.com/archives/14/25/26.html (accessed 29 June 2003)
4. Kukurin G W 1985 Normal characteristics of the cervical spinal curve. Digest of Chiropractic Economics 28 (2): 12
5. Breig A 1960 Adverse mechanical tension on the nervous system. John Wiley, New York, NY
6. Harrison D D 1992 Deformation of the lumbar spinal ligaments. Journal of Clinical Chiropractic 2 (2): 20–21
7. Garde R E 1992 Deformation of the CNS. In: Harrison D D (ed.) Spinal biomechanics: a chiropractic perspective, pp. 443–482. Harrison CBP Seminars, Evanston, WY
8. Harrison D D, Harrison D L 1992 Subluxation: an electrical phenomenon. In: Harrison D D (ed.) Spinal biomechanics: a chiropractic perspective, pp. 207–228. Harrison CBP Seminars, Evanston, WY
9. Murphy D J 1992 Posture and systemic health. In: Harrison D D (ed.) Spinal biomechanics: a chiropractic perspective, pp. 365–378. Harrison CBP Seminars, Evanston, WY
10. Troyanovich S J, Harrison D E, Harrison D D 1998 Structural rehabilitation of the spine and posture: rationale for treatment beyond the resolution of symptoms. Journal of Manipulative and Physiological Therapeutics 21 (1): 37–50

11. Harrison D D, Harrison G R 1990 Chiropractic biophysics technique: an overview presented at the Consensus Conference in Seattle, Washington. Harrison CBP Seminars, Evanston, WY
12. Harrison D D, Troyanovich S, Payne M R 1993 The Chiropractic Biophysics Technique. Today's Chiropractic (August): 64–67
13. Cooperstein R 1995 Diversified technique: core of chiropractic or "just another technique system"? Journal of Chiropractic Humanities 5 (1): 50–55
14. Cooperstein R 1995 Contemporary approach to understanding chiropractic technique. In: Lawrence D (ed.) Advances in chiropractic, vol. 2, pp. 437–459. Mosby Year Book, Chicago, IL
15. White A A, Panjabi M M 1978 Clinical biomechanics of the spine, 1st edn. J B Lippincott, Philadelphia, PA
16. Harrison D D 1992 Abnormal human posture: permutations of the rotations and translations of the skull, thorax, and pelvis in three dimensions. In: Harrison D D (ed.) Spinal biomechanics: a chiropractic perspective, pp. 43–59. Harrison CBP Seminars, Evanston, WY
17. Pettibon B R, Harrison D D 1980 Spinal biomechanics and the Pettibon spinal model. Today's Chiropractic (November): 14–15, 34, 42–44, 46, 58
18. Harrison D D 1985 History of scientific chiropractic and spinal correction. Digest of Chiropractic Economics (January/February): 20–22
19. Robertson G 1994 Technique outline, CBP, a report presented to the Panel of Advisors to the ACA Council on Technique (unpublished)

20. Pettibon B 1989 Introduction to Spinal Bio-Mechanics. Pettibon Spinal Biomechanics Institute, Tacoma, WA

21. Jackson R 1977 The cervical syndrome. Charles C Thomas, San Francisco, CA

22. Harrison D D 1982 Spinal biomechanics and the Harrison model. Today's Chiropractic (May/June): 25–27, 46–50

23. Troyanovich S J, Robertson G A 1992 Physiological mechanisms of spinal manipulation. In: Harrison DD (ed.) Spinal biomechanics: a chiropractic perspective, pp. 303–363. Harrison CBP Seminars, Evanston, WY

24. Sweere J (ed.) 1992 Chiropractic family practice: a clinical manual. Aspen Publishers, Gaithersburg, Maryland

25. McGregor M 1993 Book review, Chiropractic family practice: a clinical manual. Journal of Manipulative and Physiological Therapeutics 16 (3): 202–206

26. Harrison D D (ed.) 1992 Spinal biomechanics: a chiropractic perspective. Harrison CBP Seminars, Evanston, WY

27. Harrison D D 1994 Chiropractic: the physics of spinal correction. CBP technique. Harrison CBP Seminars, Evanston, WY

28. Sawyer C E 1990 Summary of roundtable II: treatment/therapeutic methods. Chiropractic Technique 2 (3): 155

29. Phillips R B 1990 Summary of roundtable I: analytic/diagnostic methods. Chiropractic Technique 2 (3): 154

30. Harrison D E, Harrison D D, Haas J W 2002 CBP structural rehabilitation of the cervical spine. Harrison Chiropractic Biophysics Seminars, USA

31. Harrison D 1987 Basic mechanics applied to the spine (part one of two). Today's Chiropractic (Nov/Dec): 53, 55, 57, 65

32. Harrison D D, Janik T J, Harrison G R et al 1996 Chiropractic biophysics technique: a linear algebra approach to posture in chiropractic. Journal of Manipulative and Physiological Therapeutics 19 (8): 525–535

33. Harrison D D 1981 Spinal biomechanics and the model, part II. Today's Chiropractic 10 (1): 12–13, 42–47, 58–59

34. Troyanovich S J, Harrison D D 1996 Chiropractic biophysics (CBP) technique. Chiropractic Technique 8 (1): 30–35

35. Harrison D D 1992 Subluxation: a mechanical engineering definition. In: Harrison D (ed.) Spinal biomechanics: a chiropractic perspective, pp. 11–32. Harrison CBP Seminars, Evanston, WY

36. Leach R A 1986 The chiropractic theories, 2nd edn. Williams & Wilkins, Baltimore, MD

37. Harrison D D, Colloca C J, Troyanovich S J, Harrison D E 1996 Torque: an appraisal of misuse of terminology in chiropractic literature and technique. Journal of Manipulative and Physiological Therapeutics 19 (7): 454–462

38. Herzog W 2000 Torque: an appraisal of misuse of terminology in chiropractic literature and technique. Journal of Manipulative and Physiological Therapeutics 23 (4): 298–299

39. Harrison D 1987 Basic mechanics applied to the spine (part three of three). Today's Chiropractic (Nov/Dec): 35–39

40. Harrison D E, Harrison D D, Troyanovich S J 1998 Three-dimensional spinal coupling mechanics: part I. A review of the literature. Journal of Manipulative and Physiological Therapeutics 21 (2): 101–113

41. Harrison D E, Harrison D D, Troyanovich S J 1998 Three-dimensional spinal coupling mechanics: part II. Implications for chiropractic theories and practice. Journal of Manipulative and Physiological Therapeutics 21 (3): 177–186

42. Harrison G 1989 Posture. Chiropractic Biophysics Newsletter 2–3

43. Pettibon B R, Loomis W P 1973 Biomechanical research by Pettibon & Associates #5. Today's Chiropractic (April–May): 12–15

44. Kapandji A 1974 The physiology of the joints, vol. 3. Churchill Livingstone, Edinburgh

45. Harrison D D, Janik T J, Troyanovich S J, Harrison D E, Colloca C J 1997 Evaluation of the assumptions used to derive an ideal normal cervical spine model. Journal of Manipulative and Physiological Therapeutics 20 (4): 246–256

46. Harrison D D, Harrison D E, Troyanovich S 1996 The anterior–posterior full-spine view: the worst radiographic view for determination of the mechanics of the spine. Chiropractic Technique 8 (4): 163–170

47. Gambale A, DeGeorge D 1992 Patch vs. fix. Alabama Journal of Clinical Chiropractic 2 (4): 4

48. Robertson G A 1993 An evaluation of the metrecom chiropractic biophysics program for three dimensional postural analysis. American Journal of Clinical Chiropractic 3 (2): 24–25

49. Walsh M, Breen A C 1995 Reliability and validity of the Metrecom Skeletal Analysis System in the assessment of sagittal plane lumbar angles. Clinical Biomechanics (Bristol, Avon) 10 (4): 222–223

50. Mior S A, Kopansky-Giles D R, Crowther E R, Wright J G 1996 A comparison of radiographic and electrogoniometric angles in adolescent idiopathic scoliosis. Spine 21 (13): 1549–1555

51. Fuhr A 1990 Activator methods: basic manual, Activator Methods chiropractic technique seminars. Activator Methods, Inc., Phoenix, AZ

52. Harrison D D 1988 Dr. Don adjusts two horses using the Sharp method. Chiropractic Biophysics Newsletter 3

53. DeGeorge D 2000 The sum of the parts is greater than the whole. http://www.idealspine.com/AJCC_new/apr2000/traction.htm.Dec. 10

54. Payne M 1991 A brief overview of the CBP traction protocol. Journal of Clinical Chiropractic 1 (2): 2, 31

55. Christensen K 1992 Isotonic "mirror-image" rehabilitation. Journal of Clinical Chiropractic 2 (1): 9–11

56. Christensen K 1993 Isotonic "mirror image" rehabilitation. Journal of Clinical Chiropractic 3 (2): 27

57. Schneider M 1993 Post-isometric muscle relaxation. American Journal of Clinical Chiropractic 3 (2): 32

58. Schneider M 1993 Muscular dysfunction and postural distortion. American Journal of Clinical Chiropractic 3 (1): 21

59. Kuhn K W 1993 A response to the Mercy conference: literature based frequency and duration of care. American Journal of Clinical Chiropractic 3 (2): 1, 6, 8

60. Jackson B L, Barker W, Bentz J, Gambale A 1987 Inter- and intra-examiner reliability of the upper cervical X-ray marking systems: a second look. Journal of Manipulative and Physiological Therapeutics 10 (4): 157–163

61. Keating J C, Boline P D 1988 The precision and reliability of an upper cervical X-ray marking system:

lessons from the literature. Journal of Chiropractic Research, Study and Clinical Investigation 1 (2): 32–42

62. Keating J C Jr, Cooperstein R 1996 Technique system overview: Chiropractic Biophysics technique (CBP) (letters to the editor). Chiropractic Technique 8 (3): 140

63. Jackson B L, Harrison D D, Robertson G A, Barker W F 1993 Chiropractic biophysics lateral cervical film analysis reliability. Journal of Manipulative and Physiological Therapeutics 16 (6): 384–391

64. Troyanovich S J, Robertson G A, Harrison D D, Holland B 1995 Intra- and interexaminer reliability of the chiropractic biophysics lateral lumbar radiographic mensuration procedure. Journal of Manipulative and Physiological Therapeutics 18 (8): 519–524

65. Troyanovich S J, Harrison D, Harrison D D et al 2000 Chiropractic biophysics digitized radiographic mensuration analysis of the anteroposterior cervicothoracic view: a reliability study. Journal of Manipulative and Physiological Therapeutics 23 (7): 476–482

66. Troyanovich S J, Harrison S O, Harrison D D et al 1999 Chiropractic biophysics digitized radiographic mensuration analysis of the anteroposterior lumbopelvic view: a reliability study. Journal of Manipulative and Physiological Therapeutics 22 (5): 309–315

67. Janik T, Harrison D E, Harrison D D et al 2001 Reliability of lateral bending and axial rotation with validity of a new method to determine axial rotation on anteroposterior cervical radiographs. Journal of Manipulative and Physiological Therapeutics 24 (7): 445–448

68. Harrison D E, Harrison D D, Cailliet R et al 2000 Cobb method or Harrison posterior tangent method: which to choose for lateral cervical radiographic analysis. Spine 25 (16): 2072–2078

69. Harrison D E, Cailliet R, Harrison D D et al 2001 Reliability of centroid, Cobb, and Harrison posterior tangent methods: which to choose for analysis of thoracic kyphosis. Spine 26 (11): E227–E234

70. Harrison D E, Harrison D D, Cailliet R et al 2001 Radiographic analysis of lumbar lordosis: centroid, Cobb, TRALL, and Harrison posterior tangent methods. Spine 26 (11): E235–E242

71. Harrison D E, Harrison D D, Colloca C J et al 2003 Repeatability over time of posture, radiograph positioning, and radiograph line drawing: an analysis of six control groups. Journal of Manipulative and Physiological Therapeutics 26 (2): 87–98

72. Zaleski B, Wood J 1992 A comparison of Palmer package and chiropractic biophysics for the treatment of pain. In: Callahan D L (ed.) Proceedings of the International Conference on Spinal Manipulation, pp. 39–40. Foundation for Chiropractic Research and Education, Chicago, IL

73. DeGeorge D, Gambale A 1993 CBP case study. American Journal of Clinical Chiropractic 3 (2): 11

74. Peet J B 1993 Vertebral subluxations with postural permutations at birth in athetoid-ataxic cerebral palsy. American Journal of Clinical Chiropractic 3 (1): 14

75. Pope M J 1994 Applied chiropractic biophysics: case studies. In: Harrison D D (ed.) Chiropractic: the physics of spinal correction, pp. 12-1–12-58. CBP Technique, Evanston, WY

76. Harrison D D, Jackson B L, Troyanovich S et al 1994 The efficacy of cervical extension–compression traction combined with diversified manipulation and drop table adjustments in the rehabilitation of cervical lordosis: a pilot study. Journal of Manipulative and Physiological Therapeutics 17 (7): 454–464

77. Plaugher G, Cremata E E, Phillips R B 1990 A retrospective consecutive case analysis of pretreatment and comparative static radiological parameters following chiropractic adjustments. Journal of Manipulative and Physiological Therapeutics 13 (9): 498–506

78. Hariman D G 1995 Letter to the editor regarding Harrison et al's The efficacy of cervical extension–compression traction combined with diversified manipulation and drop table adjustments in the rehabilitation of cervical lordosis: a pilot study. Journal of Manipulative and Physiological Therapeutics 18 (1): 42

79. Harrison D D, Troyanovich S J, Robertson G A, DeGeorge D J 1995 Letter to the editor in reply to Hariman's critique of The efficacy of cervical extension–compression traction combined with diversified manipulation and drop table adjustments in the rehabilitation of cervical lordosis: a pilot study. Journal of Manipulative and Physiological Therapeutics 18 (1): 42–43

80. Harrison D E, Cailliet R, Harrison D D et al 2002 Changes in sagittal lumbar configuration with a new method of extension traction: nonrandomized clinical controlled trial. Archives of Physical Medicine and Rehabilitation 83 (11): 1585–1591

81. Harrison D D, Cailliet R, Janik T J et al 1998 Elliptical modeling of the sagittal lumbar lordosis and segmental rotation angles as a method to discriminate between normal and low back pain subjects. Journal of Spinal Disorders 11 (5): 430–439

82. Harrison D E, Cailliet R, Harrison D D et al 2002 A new 3-point bending traction method for restoring cervical lordosis and cervical manipulation: a nonrandomized clinical controlled trial. Archives of Physical Medicine and Rehabilitation 83 (4): 447–453

83. Harrison D E, Harrison D D, Betz J J et al 2003 Increasing the cervical lordosis with chiropractic biophysics seated combined extension–compression and transverse load cervical traction with cervical manipulation: nonrandomized clinical control trial. Journal of Manipulative and Physiological Therapeutics 26 (3): 139–151

84. Harrison D E, Harrison D D, Troyanovich S J 1998 Reliability of spinal displacement analysis of plain X-rays: a review of commonly accepted facts and fallacies with implications for chiropractic education and technique. Journal of Manipulative and Physiological Therapeutics 21 (4): 252–266

85. Williams P L, Warwick R (eds) 1980 Gray's anatomy, 36th edn. Churchill Livingstone, Philadelphia, PA

86. Kendall H O, Kendall F P, Wadsworth G E 1971 Muscle testing and function, 2nd edn. Williams & Wilkins, Baltimore, MD

87. Harrison D D 1992 The ideal normal upright static human spine. In: Harrison D D (ed.) Spinal biomechanics: a chiropractic perspective, pp. 33–42. Harrison CBP Seminars, Evanston, WY

88. Harrison D D 1987 Vertical spine in the AP view versus Johnston's c-spine spiral theory. ICA International Review of Chiropractic (January/February): 35–49

89. Johnston L C 1966 The paradox of the functional spine. Journal of the Canadian Chiropractic Association (June–July): 7–10

90. Ressel O J 1986 Chiropractic and children. ICA International Review of Chiropractic (May/June): 44–50

91. Ressel O J 1986 Reply to Harrison regarding Ressel's chiropractic and children: a rationale for care. ICA International Review of Chiropractic (September/October): 73–74

92. Harrison D D, Janik T J, Troyanovich S J, Holland B 1996 Comparisons of lordotic cervical spine curvatures to a theoretical ideal model of the static sagittal cervical spine. Spine 21 (6): 667–675

93. Harrison D D, Troyanovich S J, Harrison D E et al 1996 A normal sagittal spinal configuration: a desirable clinical outcome. Journal of Manipulative and Physiological Therapeutics 19 (6): 398–405

94. Pettibon B, Harrison D 1981 Pettibon Spinal Bio-Mechanics: theory and implications. Pettibon Biomechanics Institute, Vancouver

95. Garde R E 1980 The three-dimensional bio-dynamic congruance [sic] of the spine with gravity. Today's Chiropractic (June): 10–11, 34–35, 46–47, 56–59, 62, 74

96. Harrison D D 1982 The normal spine: a compromise solution of an isoperimetric problem. In: Suh C H, Coyle B A (eds) Thirteenth Annual Biomechanics Conference on the spine, pp. 239a–252. Palmer College of Chiropractic-West, The International Chiropractors Association, and The University of Colorado, Sunnyvale, CA

97. Harrison D D 1988 Chiropractic: physics of spinal correction, vol. 4, p. 49. Harrison CBP Seminars, Evanston, WY

98. MacRae J E 1974 Roentgenometrics in chiropractic. Canadian Memorial Chiropractic College, Toronto, Canada

99. Anderson A 1980 Radiology lecture notes. Western States Chiropractic College, Portland, Oregon

100. Gore D R, Sepic S B, Gardner G M 1986 Roentgenographic findings of the cervical spine in asymptomatic people. Spine 11 (6): 521–524

101. Hariman D G 1995 The efficacy of cervical extension–compression traction combined with diversified manipulation and drop table adjustments in the rehabilitation of cervical lordosis: a pilot study. Journal of Manipulative and Physiological Therapeutics 18 (5): 323–325

102. Troyanovich S J, Cailliet R, Janik T J et al 1997 Radiographic mensuration characteristics of the sagittal lumbar spine from a normal population with a method to synthesize prior studies of lordosis. Journal of Spinal Disorders 10 (5): 380–386

103. CBP research projects as of October 2002. http://www.idealspine.com/index.html: Chiropractic Biophysics On-Line; 2003. Jan. 27

15

Cranial Therapies (CT)
Craniopathy, Craniosacral Therapy (CST)

INTRODUCTION

The skull is composed of six separate bones – the frontal bone, the occipital bone, two parietal bones, and two temporal bones – that are called cranial bones. These bones come together in joints made up of strong, fibrous, elastic tissues, joints called cranial *sutures*. It is still common to find anatomists and others who maintain that such joints, although movable in an infant, are completely fused in adults, devoid of movement. On the other hand, many authorities have long believed that the bones of the cranium are mobile. Attitudes remain fixed, and this area remains contentious.

Although craniopathic procedures may or may not have originated within the chiropractic profession, they find wide use among chiropractors, hence their inclusion in this book. Some chiropractors believe that cranial adjusting is effective as a standalone technique system, just as some find Upper Cervical care a standalone technique system. To continue the analogy, some chiropractors, although they may treat patients using a full-spine approach, believe that spinal adjustments will hold longer if the patient's cranial faults are also addressed. We have seen similar attitudes expressed regarding Upper Cervical care: correct the atlas, and other subluxations will either self-correct or hold their adjustments longer. In reviewing the literature on craniopathy, in some cases we chose to acknowledge works by non-chiropractors (e.g., Upledger), simply due to their impact on chiropractic practitioners. In chiropractic, the major technique systems that deploy craniopathic procedures are Sacro-Occipital Technique (Ch. 25) and the Kinesiologies (Chs 11 and 12).

It is a woeful understatement to declare that the field of CT is vast. CT do not have a standard definition and a review of the approaches comprising this form of healthcare demonstrates a mercurial scope of practice that fluxes with the intent of the practitioner. For our purposes, we have collapsed the different approaches to craniopathy into a broad, generic description, attempting to capture the essence of what makes CT distinct. With this in mind, CT refers to that group of procedures, both diagnostic and therapeutic, that are predicated on the theory that movement restrictions of the cranial sutures of the skull negatively affect purportedly palpable rhythmic impulses produced by cerebrospinal fluid (CSF) which surrounds the central nervous system from cranium to sacrum.[1] One of the more prominent forms of CT, CST, has been defined as a: "systematic approach to evaluating and treating dysfunctions occurring within the articulations of the skull."[2] (p. 95) In a more developed form, it is defined thus:

Craniosacral ... includes a structural diagnostic process that evaluates the mobility of the osseous cranium, the related mobility of the skull and sacrum and the palpation of the CRI (craniosacral rhythm impulse) throughout the body. Craniosacral osteopathic manipulative techniques attempt to restore motion to restrictions within individual sutures of the skull, the skull as a total entity, and the skull in relation to the sacrum, and apply inherent force to the articulations of the vertebral axis, rib cage and extremity.[3] (pp. 182–183)

OVERVIEW

As in chiropractic, the purported aim or therapeutic intent of CT changes depending on the source. While one group of cranial therapists states its intention to be the restoration of functional motion rather than structural change,[4] the more traditional cranial therapists maintain that, since it is structure that governs function, they physically alter the cranial environment, including the alignment of the cranial bones. For example, one internet web page describes the theory underpinning one form of CT as follows: "The interference of structural integrity creates an opportunity for aberrant nerve conduction, neurological summation and irritant reflex arcs that alter the physiological mechanisms of the body, causing different altered functions."[5] Moreover, the procedures used by some craniopaths involve what can only be described as an attempt physically to reposition cranial bones.

Several chiropractic technique systems, notably Applied Kinesiology (Ch. 11) and its spinoffs (Ch. 12), and Sacro-Occipital Technique (Ch. 25), use various forms of craniopathy as a means to manipulate manually the cranial vault, cranial faults, or other related anatomic structures thought to affect subdural and membranous tensions aberrantly.[4] However, unlike other licensed health disciplines, cranial therapy is surprisingly unregulated and we find cranial techniques being offered by chiropractors, osteopaths, dentists, medical physicians, massage therapists, and members of the lay public.

HISTORY

There are historical records from folk medicine in Greek, Chinese, Russian, and Arabic describing healers who use cranial-like methods, although little (if anything) of these approaches seems to have survived into modern times.[4] For example, shiatsu massage relies on the application of pressure and spreading motions along sutural lines in a predetermined way in response to general symptoms.[4] Modern cranial techniques, however, go far beyond this basic mechanical approach and tend to focus on the effects of cranial bone positions and the tension they produce on different membranes within the skull.

William Garner Sutherland is credited as the first investigator into cranial manipulation as a second-year osteopathy student in 1899.[4] While observing a disarticulated skull, Sutherland thought that the surface of the temporal bone was "beveled like the gills of a fish indicating articular mobility for respiratory mechanism."[5] The use of the term "respiratory" was perhaps unfortunate, since this mechanism appears to be separate and distinct from the pulmonary system. Later, Sutherland added the term "primary" to the respiratory mechanism, because he considered its appearance the first sign of life and its disappearance a harbinger of death.[4]

Sutherland posited that the cranial bones were mobile, with the sutures functioning like osseous joints that could potentially be affected by manipulation, thus influencing the vitality of the CSF flow.[4,5,7,8] Sutherland focused on the intracranial ligaments and fascia, believing that they acted as a "reciprocal tension membrane" balancing the motions within the skull.[9] Recognizing that this model fell outside the realm of normal science, Sutherland acknowledged that "the idea of bony movement taking place without muscular action is to say the least unique [and] to a degree difficult to follow."[6] He placed particular emphasis on the sphenoid, and to a lesser extent, the basilar bone, due to their central position in the skull. In essence, Sutherland believed that the hydrokinetic pressure within the cranium as the result of CSF production and flow would constitute a counter force that would alter the meningeal system, the brain environment, and ultimately neuronal function.[8] Fluctuation of the CSF was thought to be transmitted through the falx cerebri and the tentorium cerebelli to cause motions of the cranial bones.[10] Sutherland further theorized that trauma, myofascial tension, and stress could cause disruption to the meningeal/osseous relationship.[8]

In order to test his theories, Sutherland often engaged in self-experimentation. One anecdote tells of Sutherland testing his theories on himself by binding his own skull with straps and monitoring any physiological or emotional changes that ensued. Over time, he began to incorporate palpatory examination of patients' skulls into his experiments. He observed skull mobility in normal asymptomatic individuals as well as abnormal cranial motions in symptomatic patients, attempting to correlate a patient's history with these palpatory findings and to those noticed during his self-experimentation.[4,5,8] Based on these findings, Sutherland introduced craniopathy to the osteopathic profession in the 1930s. However, there was apparently little interest in Sutherland's "cranial osteopathy" until he self-published *The Cranial Bowl*[6] in 1939.[4] In one famous anecdote from that text, Sutherland recounts resuscitating an inebriated man from drowning.[4] He began teaching the principle of CT in the 1940s, and there has been a traceable growing interest in training, experimentation, and literature in the cranial field.

The chiropractor Nephi Cottam was an early pioneer in the field of craniopathy and, according to one source, his observations of the movement of sutures may have predated Sutherland's work by several years.[4] Cottam's technique is verifiable to at least 1928, when he applied for a US patent of his technique, and he published the first text, *The Story of Craniopathy*, in 1936.[7] Cottam believed that cranial bone motion was palpable, but his procedures relied more on the observation of cranial landmarks and asymmetries than palpation, as well as symptoms reported by the patient.[9] Cottam advocated the use of strong direct manual pressure or, in one instance, the use of external pneumatic pressure.[4] In Cottam's work, there is minimal mention of anatomy, neurology, or physiology, nor are there examples of independent research or external literature reviews.

In the early 1930s, Major DeJarnette, a chiropractor and osteopath who developed Sacro-Occipital Technique (Ch. 25), began his investigations of cranial analysis and manipulation.[8] Through his theory of decompartmentalizing the human body, he developed the category system of analysis and treatment, thus further formalizing the field of craniopathy by identifying specific manipulative corrections depending on the category into which the patient falls.[8] In 1952, DeJarnette published his manipulative cranial technique and further integrated craniopathy into the field of chiropractic. In much the same way, Goodheart came to include craniopathy in the protocols of Applied Kinesiology (Ch. 11). Some prominent Applied Kinesiology practitioners concentrate on "cranial faults," described as *dysrelationship* of cranial bones or their internal osseous architecture.

More recently, the osteopath John Upledger further expanded the field of cranial technique. As the story goes, Upledger was assisting during a surgical operation to remove a patient's spinal tumor.[11] Asked to hold the spinal cord for the surgeon, Upledger tells of his embarrassment in finding this to be a much more difficult task than he would have thought, as the cord was rhythmically moving. Seeking answers to this phenomenon, Upledger joined the Department of Biomechanics at Michigan State, teaming up with anatomists, biophysicists, and bioengineers. Upledger eventually identified a continuous nerve plexus in the ventricles and cranial sutures with stretch and pressure mechanoreceptors. In one group of experiments involving monkeys, Upledger reported that he was able to disrupt this rhythm by applying slight pressure to the animal's coccyx. Similarly, Upledger reported he could alter headache pain of patients by moving their coccyx. These findings led Upledger to develop the concept of a craniosacral system. Along with Vredevoogd, Upledger proposed the "Pressurestat model" that theorized that a cranial rhythmic impulse (CRI) was the result of CSF flow, the obverse of Sutherland's "primary respiratory mechanism."[9,12] He established the Upledger Institute in 1985, and the derivative of craniopathy, Craniosacral Therapy (CST), which he trademarked. CST is taught at seminars restricted to healthcare providers throughout Canada and the USA, although this was not always the case, as CST instruction was at one time offered to anyone.

Several textbooks of cranial technique have been written by chiropractors, mostly those practicing Sacro-Occipital Technique (Ch. 25). Some of these are listed in Table 15.1.

Table 15.1 Some craniopathic books in chiropractic

Title of craniopathic book	Author
1979–1980 DeJarnette Cranial Technique Anatomy and Physiology of the Cranium	DeJarnette
Practical Guide to Cranial Adjusting	Getzoff
Cranial Procedures Outline	Unger
Cranial Sutures: Morphology, Analysis, and Manipulative Strategies	Pick
Applied Kinesiology, vol. II. *Head, Neck, and Jaw Pain and Dysfunction – The Stomatognathic System*	Walther
A Study Guide to Cranial Procedures	Miles (ed.)

DEFINITION OF TECHNIQUE-SPECIFIC TERMS

- Cranial rhythm (CR): the pulse wave created by CSF production from the ventricles and pumped under tension through the dura to the sacrum.[3] The ventricles are thought to flex and extend in a motion similar to that of gills, along with associated movements of the sacrum, thus creating the CR. This movement is thought to create a palpable rhythm of 6–12 cycles a minute, distinct and separate from either the respiratory or heart rate
- Cranial rhythmic impulse (CRI): sometimes also referred to as the "Sutherland wave."[9] The CR provides a force that moves the bones of the cranium, called the CRI, palpable at various points of a person's body. The cranial therapist appreciates not merely the rate of the CRI, but also its quality, vitality, and bilateral symmetry. Five separate motions are thought to comprise the CRI (see diagnostic/analytic procedures, below)
- Craniosacral system: a system composed of the cranial structures, neural elements, and sacrum
- Diaphragm: in craniopathy, the body is divided into separate regions or diaphragms, predominantly along the lines of fascia orientation. Collectively, the thoracic outlet, respiratory and urogenital diaphragms are often referred to as the sternal pump[9]
- Entrainment: the integration or harmonization of the different oscillators in the body. McPortland and Mein[9] posited that the CRI is the palpable perception of entrainment, the harmonic frequency that incorporates the rhythms of multiple biological oscillators
- Listening station: a point on the patient's body the therapist contacts in order to assess the CRI
- Pressurestat model: postulated by Upledger, this model purports that the craniosacral system functions as a semiclosed hydraulic system containing CSF
- Primary respiratory mechanism: a system composed of the mutually interdependent brain, CSF, reciprocal tension membranes of the skull, and bones of the skull and sacrum. It does not refer to the pulmonary system, being independent of both cardiac and pulmonary systems, but rather to the motion of the CRI
- Still point: a point on the patient's body that, upon palpation by the examiner, would result in the cessation of the CRI. That is, the craniosacral system becomes still or inactive. This activity is thought to be therapeutic; once released, is it believed that the CRI will resume with better symmetry and vitality. As one source described it: "The still point is somewhat like the eye of a hurricane – a therapeutic place where all the forces that hold us in place or unease become balanced"[13]
- Tissue memory: this concept holds that any tissue of the body has stored memories of emotionally charged events in a person's life that can be liberated during CT. These awakened emotions may indicate unresolved tensions or unconscious memories
- Therapeutic release: a specific technique used by craniopaths to release various tissues, such as the cranial bones, diaphragms, meninges, and so on
- Cranial fault: misalignment or movement restriction of the cranial bones, where they articulate at the sutures.

PHYSIOLOGICAL MECHANISMS AND RATIONALE

The fundamental premise of CT is that the cranial sutures do not close during a person's lifetime, allowing for palpable cranial motions in the sutures and a rhythmic impulse within the cranium.[4] These motions are understandably thought to be subtle: witness Magoun's cautions to a clinician: "Do not look for movements as in other joints of the body. This is merely resiliency – a combination of slight yielding or suppleness in the articulations plus the flexibility of live and pliant bone."[14] In general, craniopaths posit that production of CSF from the choroid plexus of the ventricles produces a palpable wave-like, bilaterally symmetrical cycle transmitted from the cranium to the sacrum. The vitality of this flow can be negatively impacted by several factors, including birth trauma, traumatic brain injury, emotional scarring, or exhaustion caused by pathological diseases such as cancer.[3,4,9]

For some craniotherapists, however, it is consciousness itself that somehow governs the structure of the cranium, and the sum of all earthly forces (called "life forces") that alter the flow of the cranial rhythm.[5] Production of CSF operates as a negative-feedback loop, although the exact form of homeostatic control of the CSF is not known:[4] as the CSF is produced, it causes the dural membrane to expand, thus stretching the sutures of the skull. When the stretching reaches a threshold value, a signal is sent to the plexus to halt further CSF production, causing the cranial sutures to approximate. "The brain involuntarily and rhythmically moves within the skull," wrote Sutherland in 1939, and "This involuntary rhythmical movement involves dilation and contraction of the ventricles during respiratory periods. The ventricle dilation and contraction in turn effects [sic] cerebrospinal fluid circulatory activity: and the circulatory activity effects [sic] movement of the arachnoid and dural membranes; and through the special reciprocal tension membranes ... mobility of the basilar articulations."[6] (pp. 51–52). In general, we notice very little divergence between Sutherland's original theories and the literature of contemporary CT.

Since the dura is attached tightly from the skull to C2 and to S2 (it is relatively mobile between these segments), it is further theorized that there is an association between cranial movements and distinct sacral motions. According to CT practitioners, during sphenobasilar flexion, the cranium widens transversely, the sacral apex moves

anteriorly, while the sacral base counternutates, and the extremities rotate externally.[10,15] Conversely, during the extension phase, the cranium narrows in the transverse dimension, the sacral apex moves posteriorly while the sacral base nutates, and the extremities rotate internally.

In addition to the possibility of cranial bone misalignments, abnormal membranous tension is thought to interfere with the venous sinus within the skull, or perhaps vice versa. Furthermore, increased pressure from venous pressure may contribute to a patient's ill health. Upledger and Vredevoogd[11] have theorized that dural attachments to cranial nerves may compromise nerve fibers and be a source of "noisy" sensory signals, and describe how mechanical restrictions (usually dural sleeve tension) can affect cranial nerves. Cranial therapists believe that mechanical repositioning of cranial bones, by correcting cranial faults, or by reducing subdural and membranous tensions, results in clinical benefits.[4,10]

According to Sutherland's theory of a primary respiratory mechanism, there are five components acting as the driving force behind the CRI, all of which find expression in contemporary CT.[10] These are:

- inherent motility of the brain and spinal cord
- fluctuation of the CSF
- motility of the intracranial and intraspinal membranes
- articular motility of the bones of the cranium
- involuntary mobility of the sacrum between the ilia.

We would be remiss in not mentioning that there are other theories to account for cranial motion. Magoun[16] has suggested that the direct electrical current carried within the brain creates an electrical and magnetic field, causing the neural tube to coil and uncoil cyclically as the field collapses and discharges. Lastly, an oft-cited study posits that the glial cells pulsate in vitro and that the summation of these pulsations translates into the CRI.[17]

It comes as no surprise that the term "subluxation" is not commonly associated with CT, in light of the fact that subluxations are usually confined to the spine and perhaps to the appendicular skeleton. However, in one review article,[9] we see an attempt to describe the "cranial subluxation." Moreover, the use of the term "cranial fault" is widespread, and so we must consider the word "fault" to constitute a subluxation-equivalent. Pederick[7] contends that a cranial subluxation comprises abnormal function (especially motion) of the sutures, abnormal neurological function (usually indicated by changes in muscle tone and sudomotor and vasomotor effects), and possible malposition of the suture within its normal range of motion.[7]

At the extreme, some experts consider craniosacral dysfunction to be the underlying cause of all bodily ills (see examples in Pederick[7]). Alternatively, at the very least, some cranial experts believe that "the mechanical cause of disease is more deeply rooted and of greater, fundamental significance than the chemical,"[14] and that this deep-rooted cause is more often than not craniosacral dysfunction.

Cranial therapists claim to manage successfully a long list of clinical conditions. These appear in Box 15.1, adapted from Pederick.[4] Other conditions purporting to benefit from CST include epilepsy, attention-deficit disorder, dyslexia, dysfunctions of the autonomic nervous system (i.e., Raynaud's phenomenon), acute systemic infection, scoliosis, and cerebral ischemic episodes.[4,9] Upledger also addressed a US Senate Subcommittee investigating the possible link between autism and vaccination, claiming that many cases of autism have been successfully treated by CST. (See further discussion of this point in conclusions, below.)

Box 15.1 Clinical conditions successfully managed by cranial therapy[4]

- Head trauma injuries, either direct (sports-induced) or indirect (whiplash)
- Pressure effects from a prolonged birthing
- Inflammatory reactions affecting cranial structures (otitis, conjunctivitis, sinusitis, pharyngitis, and meningitis)
- Major emotional disturbances, including depression and subtle "cognitive and perceptual issues"
- Disturbances of cranial nerves
- Sleep disorders
- Headache

DIAGNOSTIC/ANALYTIC PROCEDURES

A detailed description of the diagnostic procedures used by cranial therapists is beyond the scope of this textbook, as it fills volumes of osteopathic and chiropractic seminar notes and textbooks. Suffice it to say that the patient is usually instructed to lie in a supine position while the examiner sits at the head of the patient. Gently grasping the patient's skull in a variety of possible positions, the therapist focuses on detecting mobility of the cranial sutures as well as the patient's CRI for both its rate and amplitude.[3,9,10] Although this is hard for us to fathom, the CT practitioner, while palpating the patient, typically visualizes "a state of rapport in the fluid continuity between the physician and the patient by melding the hands with the head"[16] and by "shifting into right-brained thinking."[11]

Greenman et al[10] describe the process of craniosacral analysis in two parts. The first part is the appreciation of mobility of the base of the cranium at the sphenobasilar junction and the associated movement of vault bones. The second component is direct mobility testing of the various sutures that are palpable in the vault, cranial base, and face. Elsewhere, Greenman and McPartland[3] opine that, although each suture contributes a small amount of motion to the overall capacity of the skull to move, and while each movement is itself barely perceptible, the summation of all these motions is none the less sufficient to be measurable by human palpation. The temporal bone is given special attention, as it "has been designated as a troublemaker in the craniosacral literature."[10] (p. 885)

In addition to palpation of cranial or sacral structures, cranial therapists may also use reflexive diagnostic tests adopted from other chiropractic systems, such as Sacro-Occipital Technique or Applied Kinesiology. Manual muscle testing and various other challenges are often used by cranial therapists to determine cranial position. Examples include the "hand modes" or mudras developed in Alan Beardall's Clinical Kinesiology (Ch. 12) which, according to one web-page, are thought to "talk directly to the homunculus of the cerebral cortex," as well as other tests adopted from John Thie's *Touch for Health* (Ch. 12).[5] One group of cranial therapists described the use of a tongue challenge to determine the side of laterality of the occiput on the atlas. For this test, the patient thrusts out his or her tongue and to the corners of the mouth. According to one source, "This activated the lexicon of cranial nerves operating through the tongue; cranial, autonomic supply and cervical plexus and recruits through facilitated segments."[5] Empirical evidence, they claim, indicates that a change in muscle tonus on challenge is indicative of a lateral occiput. This group of CT practitioners sadly reports that "notwithstanding the widespread intercommunication with the vagus, our digestion is often put out due to this lesion pattern."[5]

TREATMENT/ADJUSTIVE PROCEDURES

Not surprisingly, a therapy with so many interpretations and theoretical models has spawned an equally large number of therapeutic approaches. In general, the same supine position used for patient assessment is used for patient treatment. Applications of low levels of force for relatively long durations are preferred, initially in the direction of least resistance of motion.[4] Greenman and McPartland suggest that the two cardinal principles of manual medicine, the barrier concept and activating force, are applicable to CST.[3] In the barrier concept, the clinician identifies a "restrictor" within the available range of movement and a method is used to enhance the motion in the restricted motion. The barrier approach has the therapist generate a motion in the direction of lost motion, analogous to a thrusting procedure on a spinal joint found to be restricted in a particular direction. There is also a description of the "exaggeration" method, in which the therapist generates a movement in the direction opposite the restrictor, providing an activating force in the normal direction. "The indirect method," Greenman and McPartland continue, "finds a point of maximum ease between the restrictive barrier in one direction and the normal barrier in the opposite and maintains that point of maximum ease for a variable period."[3] (p. 187)

Alternatively, the activating forces are classified as extrinsic (activities performed by the therapist), and intrinsic (activities that occur within the patient's inherent system). According to Greenman et al,[10] the extrinsic activity consists of guiding the cranium, particularly the sphenobasilar symphysis, in various directions. The intrinsic activities are those of the primary respiratory mechanism (see definition above).[3] We'll let Greenman et al describe this process, allowing the reader to capture the flavor of this approach: "The most common intrinsic activating forces used are membranous tension and fluid fluctuations. When a load is applied in one direction of the membranous system, the force generated throughout the balanced membranous system results in mobility and symmetry of motion of the cranium."[10] (p. 888)

Among the majority of CT practitioners, during both analysis and treatment, a contact described as 5 g of pressure, which is about equal to the weight of a nickel on a person's eyelid, is used for treatment purposes. The examination room is typically quiet, creating an environment with few possible distractions or background noises.

Pederick has written that the practitioner should progress from the least articulated, most peripheral bones to the more intricately articulated, most central bones.[4] Echoing the comments of Greenman et al,[10] Pederick suggests that some motions are in the direction of ease, while others are into resistance.[4] Pederick also suggests the practitioner starts by minimizing imbalances within the torso and extremities that could affect the operation of the "sternal pump" or that could have direct mechanical influences on the cranial motions.

Still points are palpated and held, allowing for the reinvigoration of the CRI. It should be noted that there are other therapeutic techniques listed throughout the CT literature, including the parietal lift, the sphenobasilar compression–decompression, temporal techniques, and the dural tube rock or glide. In addition to the restoration of cranial suture motion, sacral dysfunctions could also be corrected.

Since the Sacro-Occipital Technique and Applied Kinesiology literature is replete with case studies on the successful resolution of patients' suffering from temporomandibular dysfunction using CT, there are several proposed methods of examining this structure. In one Applied Kinesiology manual describing cranial corrections, there is mention of assessing the patient's mandibular and walking gait along with cranial motions.[18] In that manual, cranial faults are addressed, with particular attention to the cruciate suture (found in the upper part of the hard palate), as it is considered to be the key to unlocking all other cranial faults. Some Applied Kinesiology practitioners associate particular nutritional supports with certain cranial faults, for example, the recommendation of folate supplementation with sphenobasilar correction.[18]

The concept of entrainment is relatively new to healthcare, but we have noticed that it appears more and more frequently in the literature. McPortland and Mein hypothesize that the CRI is the perception of entrainment, the harmonic frequency of biological oscillators, including the cardiac pulse, diaphragmatic excursion, contractile lymphatic vessels, CSF production, pulsating glial cells, electrical fields generated by cortical neurons, cortical oxidative metabolism, and perhaps still other phenomena.[9] They write that this phenomenon was first observed by Christiaan Huygens in 1665 when he noticed that clocks with the same pendulum length begin to swing in synchrony with each other, with the clock with the heaviest pendulum establishing the overall rhythm.[9] They cite other examples of harmonizing oscillators in biological systems, such as the synchronous flashing of fireflies, harmonious chirping of crickets, and women whose menstrual phases cycle together.[9]

OUTCOME MEASURES

Outcome measures are essentially the same as examination findings, showing that treatment does or does not negate the initial findings.

Greenman et al[10] summarized the goals of cranial adjusting (Box 15.2). To quote Pederick, the goal of cranial adjusting "to remove such tensions and restore optimal motion to the cranial bones could enable homeostatic mechanisms to restore balanced membranous tension, enhanced

---

Box 15.2 Goals of cranial care (adapted from Greenman et al[10])

- Improve motion of restricted cranial articulation
- Reduce intracranial membranous tension restrictions
- Improve circulation (via the venous return system in the brain)
- Reduce neural entrapment from exit foramina at the base of the skull
- Reduce pressure effects on cranial nerves within their dural attachments
- Improve the quality and quantity of the craniosacral rhythm impulse

---

venous flow, reduced neural entrapment, with a consequent reduction in associated neurological effects, and allow a normal CRI rate with good quality and amplitude of motion."[4] (pp. 5–6)

SAFETY AND RISK FACTORS

By any definition, CT is a low-force, gentle technique. According to cranial therapists, the primary contraindications for care are acute intracranial hemorrhage, intracranial aneurysm, fracture, herniation of the medulla oblongata, signs of meningeal irritation, and increased CSF pressure.[4]

EVIDENCE OF EFFICACY

We thought it best to examine the question of the efficacy of craniopathic procedures by exploring whether:

- the cranial bones are freely mobile, and if the sutures have anatomic connections to intracranial membranes
- this cranial motion can alter CSF flow, and such flow changes can alter the intracranial environment
- these motions can be detected by palpation, or some other procedure, with an acceptable degree of interexaminer reliability
- gentle pressure on the cranium or other identified points can alter CRI in a measurable way, and be shown to have clinical benefits.

Mobility of the cranial bones

The studies most frequently cited in support of cranial sutures remaining open are by Todd and Lyon from 1924.[19, 20] While they concluded that cranial suture closing was much more delayed than previously thought, there is a selection bias problem in that study.[1] Pederick[4] reviews the literature investigating the closure of cranial sutures, including a review by Retzlaff et al.[21] In addition, Green et al,[1] in a systematic review using a well-designed strategy, found nine studies[19, 20, 22-29] investigating the mobility or fusion of cranial sutures, four of which involved live subjects. In one classic study, Frymann[24] made electronic tracing of cranial bone motions that were then compared to similar tracings of respiratory and pulse rates. In that study, Frymann[24] reported that cranial movements varied between 0.005 and 0.001 in. (0.127 and 0.025 mm). Unfortunately, the study design was poorly described, hampering efforts to assess its quality and observed validity.[1] (Perhaps more problematic was the statement by Greenman and McPortland that the perception threshold was found to be 0.5 mm/s.[3]) In another study, Greenman[23] correlated X-ray with clinical observations. Despite the heterogeneous nature of these often poorly described studies, the preponderance of evidence supports the theory that the adult cranium may not solidly fuse with age and that minute movements between cranial bones is possible.[1] As Upledger put it: "Rather, the microarchitecture demonstrates a general lack of instrasutural [sic] ossification, with the presence of collagen and elastic fibers [sic], a generous supply of vascular structures and nerve plexuses, as well as free nerve endings"[30] (quoted in Pederick[7]). However, no research has demonstrated that these motions can be detected by manual palpation.[1]

The existence of the CRI

Green et al[1] found 10 studies examining the motion of CSF, none of which was undertaken by members of the craniosacral community.[31-41] In general, Green et al reported that the methodological strength of these studies rested on the fact that many of them used measurement tools capable of producing valid and reproducible observations, including intracranial pressure monitoring, magnetic resonance imaging, encephalograms, and myelography.[1] The consistency of the observed phenomenon, coupled with the fact that these studies arose from outside the CT world, support the contention that there is a cranial pulse or rhythm distinct from cardiac or respiratory activity.

Palpating the CRI

We are not surprised to learn that intrarater reliability of CRI palpation exceeds the interrater reliability, as has been the case in similar studies investigating the reliability of motion palpation of spinal joints, leg-checking procedures, and manual muscle testing (Section 2).

Green et al[1] found five studies assessing the interrater reliability of craniosacral dysfunction.[15, 42-45] Most of these studies involved blinded observations, competent observers, and procedural protocols suitable for converting observations into raw data. On the negative side, the studies tended to be small (usually less than 30 patients) and may not have constituted a representative sample of patients.[1] For example, one study by Upledger[42] examined only preschool children, and the study by Wirth-Pattullo and Hayes[44] examined only children with a history of trauma. In that study, Wirth-Pattullo and Hayes concluded that resulting reliability of −0.02 was unacceptable for clinical decision making. Similarly, Hanten et al[15] found poor interexaminer reliability, but excellent intraexaminer reliability (0.78–0.83) in their study of 40 healthy adults being examined by two examiners with 9 months' experience.[15]

Another problem identified by Green et al[1] is that none of the studies used a kappa index of concordance analysis. That is, there was no attempt to determine statistically whether the results obtained were merely the result of chance. Thus, the conclusion by Upledger[42] that there was an aggregate high level of agreement between himself and three other observers (86% ± 0.5) must be interpreted cautiously, especially in light of the fact that these findings have not been replicated in the intervening 25 years. There is a similar problem with the study by Upledger and Karni,[43] reporting that the examiners' subjective impressions of change in craniosacral mechanics correlated well with objective measures including strain gauges and electrocardiographic and electromyographic readings. Again, there were no statistical analyses to support this contention, and, as Green et al point out,[1] the results of this study have not been replicated since it was published in 1979.

As the name implies, CST presupposes reciprocal movements between the cranial bones and the sacrum, an association referred to as "the core-link" hypothesis by some craniotherapists.[46] Zanakis et al,[47] in a study that recorded the movement of surface markers on skin overlaying cranial bones while an experienced practitioner simultaneously palpated apparent sacral motion, reported a 92% level of agreement between the examiners. However, a study by Moran and Gibbons[46] came to a very different conclusion.

In the study by Moran and Gibbons, two registered osteopaths palpated 11 healthy subjects. One examiner was placed at the subject's head and the other at the patient's feet. Each then recorded what they perceived to be the "full flexion" phase of the CRI by activating a silent foot switch. Examiners were blinded to the other's results and could not communicate with each other. The researchers reported that the intraexaminer reliability for palpation of the CRI at the same position ranged from fair to good (+0.52 to +0.73), but the results for a single examiner palpating the CRI at the head and sacrum revealed no concordance. Perhaps not surprisingly, interexaminer reliability for palpation of the CRI ranged from poor to non-existent (−0.09 to +0.05).[46]

We found the study by Hanten et al to be refreshingly honest and well-balanced in reporting that "a single examiner may be able to palpate the rate of CSR consistently, if that is what we truly measured. It is possible that the perception of CSR is illusory. The rate of CSR palpated by two examiners is not consistent ... It appears that a subject's CSR is not related to the heart or respiratory rates of the subject or the examiner."[15]

(p. 213) This left Green et al no choice but to conclude that "the highest quality inter-observer agreement studies have found that assessment of Craniosacral dysfunction by practitioners of Craniosacral therapy is unreliable."[1] (p. 33)

Relationship between aberrant CRI and health

Five studies had the research objective of providing direct evidence of an association between craniosacral dysfunction and poor health outcomes.[48–52] A study by Woods and Woods in the early 1960s[48] measured the CRI rate of 102 psychiatric patients and 62 healthy subjects The CRI of the healthy patients was found to be an average of 12.47 cycles/min. By contrast, the CRI of the psychiatric patients was reported to be on average 6.7 cycles/min. A study by Frymann[49] later that decade explored the possible relationship between symptomatology in newborns and anatomic–physiological disturbances of the craniosacral system. Among the 1250 infants examined, it was found that symptoms, including vomiting, hyperactive peristalsis, tremor, hypertonicity, and irritability, were more prevalent in patients with an increase in the severity of "Craniosacral strain patterns."[49,3] Similarly, Upledger[50] assessed 203 children, attempting to determine a relationship between CRI and developmental problems in grade school. The major problem with these two studies was that health states were subjectively measured, no explicit classification criteria were used to establish content validity, and categories were arbitrary, lacking face validity.[1] Again, Green et al were left to conclude that there is no "significant strength of association, experimental confirmation, specificity of relationship and/or consistency of observed evidence" between craniosacral dysfunction and health.[1] (p. 14)

There have been two case studies published in the chiropractic literature reporting on the benefits of CT among infants. In one case study, Van Loot[53] reported that a 3-month-old child with a history of colic and vomiting responded well to Diversified and Webster pediatric adjusting techniques, in addition to CST. Unfortunately, Van Loot did not describe the method of CT used.

Another article by Hewitt described two infants experiencing problems with breastfeeding who responded well to CST. In one case, Hewitt describes the method she used as a gentle traction to the frontal bone in an anterior direction, and to the temporal and vomer bones in a lateral direction. She describes decompressing the occipital condyles, and applying simultaneous traction to the sacrum to "normalize dural tube mobility."[54] (p. 242) The other child was treated similarly, but also received Diversified-style adjustment to the upper cervical region.

Craniosacral treatment effectiveness

Green et al[1] found seven retrievable studies documenting the purported association between CST and its clinical effectiveness. Study designs were retrospective case control, retrospective case series, before–after, and case reports.[3, 55–60] We discuss two of these studies.

In the first study, Philips and Meyer[58] sought to determine whether the addition of chiropractic care (consisting of Diversified, Thompson, Logan, and/or Webster adjustment techniques) as well as CST in addition to a regimen of standard obstetrical care during pregnancy would result in fewer obstetrical interventions during labor and delivery. The addition of chiropractic care and CST during pregnancy did not result in any observable benefits or detriments with regard to obstetrical interventions during labor and delivery. Green et al suggested that the researchers' interpretation that these results suggest that chiropractic care and CST may be safely employed for pregnancy-associated disorders without complications on labor or delivery is unwarranted.[1] We are forced to disagree with this criticism by Green et al, as Philips and Meyer suggested that "it seems that chiropractic care and Craniosacral therapy may be safely employed for pregnancy-associated disorders, *especially those related to neuromuscular disorders during pregnancy without complication on labor or delivery* [italics added]."[58] (p. 527) That is to say, while chiropractic care and CST may not impact on the obstetrical component of a patient's outcome, if the patient is experiencing low-back pain as the result of her pregnancy

(muscular strain, ligament sprain, facet dysfunction, or subluxation), she can safely seek out this form of therapy without undue concern of a detrimental effect on the delivery of the child. We agree with Green et al's comments that the study may have been too small (63 subjects) to make any conclusions either way.[1]

The second was a before-and-after study by Frymann et al,[56] that examined 186 children, aged 18 months to 12 years, with neurological, structural, or medical problems, over a 3-year period. In addition to the problem of a staggering attrition rate of 46% in this study, as well as possibly invalid comparison groupings, it is difficult to determine the effectiveness of any intervention over so long a period in a group of subjects as rapidly developing as children.

CONCLUSIONS

- We mentioned in our introduction that CT merits inclusion as a chiropractic technique because many chiropractors use it as a stand-alone technique or in order to enhance the results of their spinal adjusting. To go one step further, some see the cranial suture faults as equivalent to spinal subluxations, and use the concept of membranous tension as others use the concept of nerve interference. In craniopathy, we frequently see references to a divine power and the inherent healing abilities of the patient, reminding us of the term "Innate Intelligence."

- Much of the language found in other technique systems is heard in CT. Among the common root terms are "ease" or "dis-ease" (Palmer Hole-In-One, Network Spinal Analysis, Torque Release), nerve tension or interference, entrainment (Network Spinal Analysis), as well as the importance of developing a rapport between the doctor and patient (Bioenergetic Synchronization Technique).

- It is fair to say that the practice of CT meets some of the criteria we might list for face validity, meaning that it just makes sense: there is evidence that the cranial bones remain mobile late into life, and the craniosacral rhythm impulse seems to be a viable and measurable phenomenon, at least in principle detectable by palpation. On the other hand, in reading the work of the craniopaths in and out of chiropractic, we note some exceedingly eccentric language and ideas that may make it more difficult to design and implement studies to improve our knowledge base.

- Pederick[4] is of the opinion that cranial adjusting deserves provisional acceptance, according to the parameters espoused by the Kaminski et al[6] model for the validation of chiropractic technique procedures. He felt CT was well defined and described in the literature, had measurable observations, a plausible science behind it, and had been the subject of experimentation and testing. On the other hand, as we see it, the clinical evidence for CT primarily consists of anecdotal evidence and a few studies with design flaws.

- We have noticed that craniopathy has enjoyed a ground swell of popularity in the media and public domain as of late; so much so that Upledger, a leading figure in the CranioSacral Therapy world, was recently invited to speak before a hearing of the US House of Representatives. The Committee was investigating the apparent rise in the prevalence of autism among children. Upledger described this approach as follows:

  The manual stretching of the restrictive dura mater by the CranioSacral Therapy techniques has provided impressive improvements in autism. The therapy must be continued until the child has reached full growth, because once the dura mater has lost its accommadative [sic] ability, it must be physically stretched by a therapist. CranioSacral Therapy accomplishes this task non-invasively by using the various related bones to which the dura mater attaches as handles to stretch the membranes.[62]

- Oddly enough, we have seen some CT practitioners, when writing about craniopathy, almost pleased to note documented cases of CT resulting in iatrogenic side-effects. Perhaps, in an odd way, this only lends credence to the assertion that something substantive occurs during a cranial treatment, given the skepticism commonly afforded craniopathy. One study reported that 55 patients (5%) treated in the Michigan State University Traumatic Brain Injury program experienced some form of iatrogenic reaction to the treatment. These reactions included a worsening of vertiginous symptoms, increase in psychiatric symptoms (outbursts, paranoia) and a case of total body spastic reaction.[3] Perhaps cranial therapists, just like any practitioner of a specialized technique that requires extra training, want to impress upon others that craniopathy can be dangerous if used inappropriately – that it is best left in the hands of knowledgeable experts. Paradoxically, this belief, were it to be the case, would run counter to the fact that CT instruction has been historically available to any interested person, regardless of level of education or professional credentials. The admission of the lay public to the craniosacral lecture circuit for certification is troubling.

REFERENCES

1. Green C, Martin C W, Bassett K B, Kazanjian A 1999 A systematic review and critical appraisal of the scientific evidence on craniosacral therapy. British Columbia Office of Health Technology Assessment, Centre for Health Services and Policy Research, University of British Columbia
2. Rogers J S, Witt P L 1997 The controversy of cranial bone motion. Journal of Orthopedic and Sports Physical Therapy 26 (2): 95–102
3. Greenman P E, McPartland J M 1995 Cranial findings and iatrogenesis from craniosacral manipulation in patients with traumatic brain syndrome. Journal of the American Orthopathic Association 95 (3): 182–188
4. Pederick F O 1997 A Kaminski-type evaluation of cranial adjusting. Chiropractic Technique 9 (1): 1–15
5. Cranialrhythm.com Kinesiology: a historical perspective. www.cranialrhythm.com/Faq/CFDintro.html
6. Sutherland W G 1939 The cranial bowl. Free Press, Mankato, MN
7. Pederick F O 1993 Cranial adjusting – an overview. Chiropractic Journal of Australia 23 (3): 106–112
8. Pick M G 1994 A preliminary single case magnetic resonance imaging investigation into maxillary frontal-parietal manipulation and its short-term effect upon the intercranial structures of an adult human

brain. Journal of Manipulative and Physiological Therapeutics 17 (3): 168–173

9. McPortland J M, Mein E A 1997 Entrainment and the cranial rhythmic impulse. Alternative Therapy 3 (1): 40–45

10. Greenman P E, Mein E A, Andary M 1996 Craniosacral manipulation. Manual Medicine 7 (4): 877–895

11. Upledger J E, Vredevoogd J D 1983 Craniosacral therapy, pp. 2–25. Eastland Press, Seattle, WA

12. Upledger J E 1995 Research and observations support the existence of a craniosacral system, pp. 1–17. Upledger Institute Enterprises

13. Hollenbery S, Dennis M 1994 An introduction of craniosacral therapy. Physiotherapy 80 (8): 528–532

14. Magoun H J Sr 1951 Osteopathy in the cranial field, 3rd edn, p. 94. Journal Printing Company, Kirksville, MO

15. Hanten W P, Dawson D D, Iwata M et al 1998 Craniosacral rhythm: reliability and relationships with cardiac and respiratory rates. Journal of Orthopaedic and Sports Physical Therapy 27 (3): 213–218

16. Magoun H I 1976 Osteopathy in the cranial field, 3rd edn. Journal Printing Company, Kirksville, MO

17. Lumsden C E, Pomerat C M 1951 Normal oligodendrocytes in tissue culture. Experimental Cell Research 2: 103–114

18. Leaf D W 1995 Seminar notes on cranial fault corrections for TMJ dysfunctions. Self-published, Plymouth, MA

19. Todd T W, Lyon D W Jr 1924 Endocranial suture closure: its progress and age relationship. Part I: adult males of white stock. American Journal of Physical Anthropology VII (3): 325–384

20. Todd T W, Lyon D W Jr 1925 Cranial suture closure: its progress and age relationship. Part II: ectocranial closure in adults males of white stock. American Journal of Physical Anthropology VIII (1): 23–25

21. Retzlaff E, Upledger J, Mitchell F L Jr, Walsh J 1968 Ageing of cranial sutures in humans. Anatomy Record 193: 663

22. Baker E G 1971 Alteration in width of maxillary arch and its relation to sutural movement of cranial bones. Journal of American Osteopath Association 70 (7): 559–564

23. Greenman P E 1971 Roentgen findings in the craniosacral mechanism. Journal of the American Osteopath Association 70 (9): 928–945

24. Frymann V M 1971 A study of the rhythmic motions of the living cranium. Journal of the American Osteopath Association 70 (9): 928–945

25. Hubbard R P, Melvin J W, Barodawala I T 1971 Flexure of cranial sutures. Journal of Biomechanics 4 (6): 491–496

26. Kokich V G 1976 Age changes in the human frontozygomatic suture from 20 to 95 years. American Journal of Orthodontics 69 (4): 411–430

27. Heifetz M D, Weiss M 1981 Detection of skull expansion with increased intracranial pressure. Journal of Neurosurgery 55 (5): 811–812

28. Pitlyk P J, Piantanida T P, Ploeger D W 1985 Noninvasive intracranial pressure monitoring. Neurosurgery 17 (4): 581–584

29. Kostopoulos D C, Keramidas G 1992 Changes in elongation of falx cerebri during craniosacral therapy techniques applied on the skull of an embalmed cadaver. Cranio 10 (1): 9–12

30. Upledger J E 1984 Craniosacral system: clinical applications and research. In: Greenman P E (ed.) Concepts and mechanisms of neuromuscular functions, pp. 66–69. Springer Verlag, Berlin

31. O'Connell J E 1943 The vascular factor in intracranial pressure and the maintenance of the cerebrospinal fluid circulation. Brain 66: 204–228

32. Du Boulay G, O'Connell J E, Currie J et al 1972 Further investigations on pulsatile movements in the cerebrospinal fluid pathways. Acta Radiologica [diagn] (Stockholm) 13: 496–523

33. Cardoso E R, Rowan J O, Galbraith S 1983 Analysis of the cerebrospinal fluid pulse wave in intracranial pressure. Journal of Neurosurgery 59 (5): 817–821

34. Takizawa H, Sugiura K, Baba M et al 1983 Spectral analysis of cerebrospinal fluid pulse wave [English abstract]. No To Khinkwi 35 (12): 1227

35. Avezaat C J, van Eijndhoven J H 1986 Clinical observations on the relationship between cerebrospinal fluid pulse pressure and intracranial pressure. Acta Neurochirurgica (Wien) 79 (1): 13–29

36. Enzmann D R, Rubin J B, DeLaPaz R, Wright A 1986 Cerebrospinal fluid pulsation: benefits and pitfalls in MR imaging. Radiology 161 (3): 773–778

37. Feinberg D A, Mark A S 1987 Human brain motion and cerebrospinal fluid circulation demonstrated with MR velocity imaging. Radiology 163 (3): 793–799

38. Ursino M 1988 A mathematical study of human intraspinal hydrodynamics, part 1: the cerebrospinal fluid pulse pressure. Annals of Biomedical Engineering 16 (4): 379–401

39. Ursino M 1988 A mathematical study of human intracranial hydrodynamics, part 2: stimulation of clinical tests. Annals of Biomedical Engineering 16 (4): 403–416

40. Zabolotny W, Czosnyka M, Walencik A 1995 Cerebrospinal fluid pulse pressure waveform analysis in hydrocephalic children. Childs Nervous System 11 (7): 397–399

41. Li J, He W, Yao J, Wen H 1996 Possibility of observing the changes of cerebrospinal fluid pulse waves as a substitute for volume pressure test. Clinical Medical Journal (English) 109 (5): 411–413

42. Upledger J E 1977 The reproducibility of craniosacral examination findings: a statistical analysis. Journal of the American Osteopath Association 76 (12): 890–899

43. Upledger J E, Karni Z 1979 Mechano-electric patterns during craniosacral osteopathic diagnosis and treatment. Journal of the American Osteopath Association 78 (11): 782–791

44. Wirth-Pattullo V, Hayes K W 1994 Interrater reliability of craniosacral rate measurements and their relationship with subjects' and examiners' heart and respiratory rate measurements. Physical Therapy 74 (10): 908–920

45. Rogers J S, Witt P L, Gross M T et al 1998 Simultaneous palpation of the craniosacral rate at the head and feet: intrarater and interrater reliability and rate comparisons. Physical Therapy 78 (11): 1175–1185

46. Moran R W, Gibbons P 2001 Intraexaminer and interexaminer reliability for palpation of the cranial rhythmic impulse at the head and sacrum. Journal of Manipulative and Physiological Therapeutics 24 (3): 183–190

47. Zanakis M F, DiMeo J, Madonna B F A et al 1996 Objective measurement of the CRI with manipulation

and palpation of the sacrum (abstract). Journal of the American Osteopath Association 96: 551

48. Woods J M, Woods R H 1961 A physical finding related to psychiatric disorders. Journal of the American Osteopath Association 60: 988–993

49. Frymann V 1966 Relation of disturbances of craniosacral mechanisms to symptomatology of the newborn: study of 1250 infants. Journal of the American Osteopath Association 65 (10): 1059–1075

50. Upledger J E 1978 The relationship of craniosacral examination findings in grade school children with developmental problems. Journal of the American Osteopath Association 77 (10): 760–776

51. White W K, White J E, Baldt G 1985 The relation of the craniofacial bones to specific somatic dysfunctions: a clinical study of the effects of manipulation. Journal of the American Osteopath Association 85 (9): 603–604

52. Baker E G 1971 Alteration in width and maxillary arch and its relation to sutural movements of cranial bones. Journal of the American Osteopath Association 70: 559–564

53. Van Loot M 1998 Colic with projectile vomiting: a case study. Journal of Clinical and Chiropractic Pediatrics 3 (1): 207–210

54. Hewitt E G 1999 Chiropractic care for infants with dysfunctional nursing: a case series. Journal of Clinical and Chiropractic Pediatrics 4 (1): 241–244

55. Blood S D 1986 The craniosacral mechanism and the temporomandibular joint. Journal of the American Osteopath Association 86 (8): 512–519

56. Frymann V M, Carney R E, Springall P 1992 Effect of osteopathic medical management on neurologic development in children. Journal of the American Osteopath Association 92 (6): 729–744

57. Greenman P E, McPartland J M 1995 Cranial findings and iatrogenesis from craniosacral manipulation in patients with traumatic brain syndrome. Journal of the American Osteopath Association 95 (3): 182–188

58. Philips C J, Meyer J J 1995 Chiropractic care, including craniosacral therapy, during pregnancy: a static-group comparison of obstetric during labor and delivery. Journal of Manipulative and Physiological Therapeutics 18 (8): 525–529

59. Joyce P, Clark C 1996 The use of craniosacral therapy to treat gastroesophageal reflux in infants. Infants and Young Children 9 (2): 51–58

60. Thom S 2003 Pregnancy, birth, and post partum applications of cranial fluid dynamics. http://adhumanitas.com/pages/ArticlesPostPartum: Ad Humanitas

61. Kaminski M, Boal R, Gillette R G et al 1987 A model for the evaluation of chiropractic methods. Journal of Manipulative and Physiological Therapeutics 10 (2): 61–64

62. Upledger J E 2000 Autism: present challenges, future needs – why the increased rates? Hearing before the Committee on Government Reform. 106th Congress, House of Representatives. Serial no. 106–180: 430–443

16

Distraction Manipulation (Cox: CDM) Technique
Flexion–Distraction Technique

INTRODUCTION

In the early 1980s, there was a chiropractic college that kept a so-called Cox table upright in a closet in one of its outpatient clinics. Everyone, including all the interns, knew it was there. Every now and then, one of them would bring in an obvious disk herniation case, and judiciously ask permission to use the Cox table. This permission was never granted. The clinic director would explain that the president of the college did not consider flexion–distraction to be a *chiropractic* technique. That college, incidentally, now offers CDM through its continuing education program.

The question squarely posed by CDM, more than by any other technique system covered in this book, is *what is a chiropractic technique?* Although founder James Cox is not reticent in explaining that his methods constitute a blend of chiropractic and osteopathic principles, even that is not the crux of the matter. Motorized and non-motorized traction and mobilization methods can be found inside and outside chiropractic, there is nothing proprietary about that. Unlike any of the other technique systems we describe, the *only* distinctive feature of CDM is the use of a piece of *equipment*, the proprietary Chiro-Manis® and/or Zenith®-Cox® flexion–distraction, or other tables with similar capabilities.

This question of CDM's credentials as a (narrowly defined) chiropractic technique system came up again in 1995–1996 when Cooperstein and four other investigators convened an expert panel to formulate procedure-specific, condition-specific ratings for the treatment of common low-back conditions.[1,2] In selecting treatment procedures to include in the study, they knew from the outset that Cox's distraction methods would be included, but it took a while to figure out how to rationalize that. After all, the literature is full of examples of traction methods that are utilized by medical and other healthcare providers. So what, therefore, qualifies CDM as a chiropractic adjustive method? The investigators eventually decided that there were two distinctive attributes of CDM that justified inclusion in the study: since the doctor places one hand on the segment that is being treated, this traction method, unlike most others is first, manually assisted and second, segmentally specific. The investigators discussed, but did not feel the need to resolve the question, whether CDM should be correctly classified as a *manipulation* method. We comment further on this matter in the conclusions below.

OVERVIEW

The treatment principle is squarely contained within the descriptive nature of the name of the technique: flexion plus distraction. CDM requires specialized treatment tables that allow the operator to apply these coupled vectors. These tables include a section underlying the lower part of the body from the pelvis down that the clinician can lower by means of a tiller, thus flexing the lumbopelvis on the trunk, and exerting traction to the lumbar spine. Although CDM is usually thought of as a treatment for herniated lumbar disk, it is also used for most other commonly seen lumbopelvic conditions. Moreover, practitioners have been actively extending its treatment principle to the cervical spine and cervical conditions, so that it is no longer, if it ever was, designated for the low back only. Although the CDM table and the distraction method it facilitates are clearly the defining aspects of CDM, the practitioner engages the patient on several more expansive levels, including but not limited to physical therapy, exercise, rehabilitation, vocational training, nutritional counseling, and lifestyle modification.

HISTORY

Founder James Cox graduated from the National Chiropractic College in 1963. In 1964, as the result of an unsuccessful experience in attempting to treat a herniated disk case using traditional side-posture manipulation, he began his study and deployment of osteopathic traction therapy using a specially equipped McManis table. Floyd Blackmore, DC, DO, was instrumental in exposing him to these treatment principles. After some 9 more years of continued development of his methods and equipment, including the development of the Chiro-Manis table, Cox coined the term "flexion–distraction manipulation" to refer to his distractive treatment method. The table itself had evolved into the Zenith-Cox table by 1984, when Williams Manufacturing Company took over its fabrication.

Apart from Cox's experience with patient care, it was his own experience *as a patient* that really cemented his interest in flexion–distraction methods. After some 10 years of chronic low-back pain, he seriously exacerbated his low-back condition in 1981 during a fence-building project. After 3 weeks of unsuccessful treatment for a herniated lumbar disk and excruciating leg pain, treatment that included flexion–distraction, Cox's problem had progressed to cauda equina syndrome, replete with the bladder and bowel deficits that beg immediate surgical decompression. The microdiscectomy that followed, in a word, worked. Following that very personal experience, Cox devoted himself not only to teaching flexion–distraction, as a conservative alternative before the need for surgical intervention has become clear, but also to teaching patients to take care of themselves so as to avoid winding up in surgical situations, as he had.

By 1990 a certification program for educating chiropractors in flexion–distraction was in place at the National Chiropractic College. A cervical component has been developed for the table that permits the doctor to do for herniated cervical disk what the caudal section of the table permits for herniated lumbar disk. Several editions of Cox's textbook, *Low Back Pain: Mechanism, Diagnosis, Treatment*,[3] have been published, in addition to many research articles having to do not only with clinical outcomes but with the basic science of how flexion–distraction affects the intervertebral disks. The National Chiropractic College (now called National Health Sciences University) and Loyola University Medical School have conducted federally funded collaborative research on the flexion–distraction procedure.

DEFINITION OF TECHNIQUE-SPECIFIC TERMS

- Flexion–distraction: the term "flexion–distraction," although seeming to be generic in one sense, is virtually synonymous with Cox's concept and clinical application, as described throughout this chapter, and thus warrants being considered a technique-specific term.

PHYSIOLOGICAL MECHANISMS AND RATIONALE

Since the intervertebral disks do not have an ample blood supply, they depend on vertebral movements both to obtain metabolites and to rid themselves of the waste products of metabolism. During lateral flexion movements, for example, fluid and solutes are expressed from the disk on the side to which bending takes place, and imbibed on the side away from the direction of bend.

In addition to the nutritive value of introducing movement into restricted lumbopelvic joints, the immediate effect of lumbar traction is the reduction of intradiscal pressure. Cox believes this pressure drop effectively "sucks back" the herniated nuclear material. As a companion factor, the tension upon the posterior and anterior longitudinal ligaments that is created by traction is thought to push the disk back into the space between the vertebral bodies.

By these two factors, the pressure drop and ligamentous centripetal force, CDM is designed to have a directly structural impact on the intervertebral disk, by increasing disk height, and reducing annular fiber and nucleus pulposus distortion. This in turn is thought to restore more normal movement patterns and posture to the locomotor system. Either the herniated disk is repositioned, or the adjacent vertebral bodies are realigned. Restoration of a more normal nucleus structure may in turn reduce irritation of pain-sensitive nerve fibers in the annulus.

Summarizing, flexion–distraction is thought to improve vertebral motion and positional relationships, free up longitudinal adhesions, relieve nerve root pressure, separate the facet joints, improve circulation in and around the intervertebral foramina, improve metabolite transport into the disks, and reduce hydrostatic pressure in the disks.[3] (p. 274)

DIAGNOSTIC/ANALYTIC PROCEDURES

There are no unique or specific CDM diagnostic procedures. A patient presenting at a CDM clinic provides a detailed history, and then receives a thorough physical examination. This examination includes a particularly comprehensive battery of orthopedic and neurological tests, including tests for symptom magnification and/or malingering. Patients who have been involved in trauma, or have a history of systemic disease, or who have signs of cauda equina syndrome or spinal cord compression, necessarily receive imaging procedures (possibly including computed tomography or magnetic resonance imaging) and specialized neurologic tests such as electromyogram (EMG). Other patients may receive a trial round of care without having received this level of diagnostic testing. However, if they have not improved by 50% within about a month, unless there is a suggestion of patient non-compliance, they are considered eligible for these elective diagnostic procedures.

TREATMENT/ADJUSTIVE PROCEDURES

Flexion–distraction starts by first having the patient lie prone on the table, which often requires the doctor's assistance. The table itself is designed to flex the pelvis on the trunk, simultaneously generating traction, by means of a tiller bar (handle) at the foot of the table, that allows depression of the table's caudal piece. There are straps available to secure the patient's ankles, to increase the distractive force. Once the patient is prone, tolerance testing is performed to make sure the patient experiences diminished intensity of pain and/or centralization of symptoms (i.e., fewer distal symptoms). The doctor places his or her hand on the segment above the level of disk herniation, while the other hand applies downward pressure to the tiller bar to effect flexion and distraction of the patient's legs and lumbopelvis below the stabilized segment. The table moves about 2 in. (5 cm) maximum, less for a shorter person.

Once patient tolerance is demonstrated, the treatment can begin. Three sets of treatments are applied, each set consisting of five 4-s flexion procedures, or 20 s apiece. At least 10 s are allowed between sets, so that the entire procedure can take under 2 min. The patient's legs may be left free, unsecured by the ankle straps, so that gravity alone provides the distractive force; or the doctor may add some distractive force by pressing upon the patient's ankles; or, finally, the straps may be used to secure the patient's ankles, to provide a maximum of distractive force. All is done according to patient tolerance.

It must be understood that, although the archetypal patient seen in a flexion–distraction has discogenic symptoms, patients with facet syndrome, sacroiliac problems, scoliosis, and spondylolisthesis receive condition-specific "specialized" Cox distraction procedures, the details of which are beyond our scope to describe. The reader is advised to review Cox's textbook[3] for such details.

Flexion–distraction is supplemented by a variety of ancillary procedures. These include not only physical therapy modalities, such as hot/cold therapy and galvanic currents, but also soft-tissue methods like trigger point work. Bracing is provided to the patient as needed; the patient is also instructed in exercises and attends a back wellness school.

OUTCOME ASSESSMENT

The orthopedic tests that served as diagnostic indicators also serve as outcome measures. These are supplemented by survey instruments, including the Oswestry Pain Index, the Roland–Morris Pain Questionnaire, and pain drawings. Re-examinations are conducted every 2–3 weeks.

Patients with severe pain and/or sciatica are seen daily, whereas patients who have less severe and/or non-sciatic pain may be seen less frequently, perhaps two to three times per week. Obtaining a 50% reduction in symptoms in about a month would be considered a favorable treatment outcome. Cox provides three algorithms for the management of the low-back patient: one for general screening, another for radicular low-back cases, and a third for non-radicular low-back cases. The clinician's choice of treatment approach, visit frequency, concurrent care options, and so forth depend on the nuances of the particular cases. These are beyond our scope to describe in this chapter, but the reader may refer to Cox's textbook[3] for a full presentation.

SAFETY AND RISK FACTORS

Cox feels it must first be established that the patient is able to tolerate the distraction procedures. The main factor involved in non-tolerance is excessive pain during the first 1–3 days after an injury, during which time analgesic modalities such as ice and galvanism are indicated to reduce the amount and impact of acute inflammation. Apart from patient tolerance, there are also specific, named conditions, the presence of which would exclude a patient from consideration for flexion–distraction treatment. These include cauda equina syndrome, fracture, dislocation, cancer, infection, diabetes, arthritides, vascular and systemic diseases, and hard and/or progressive neurologic signs.[3] (p. 288)

EVIDENCE OF EFFICACY
Basic science research

From a basic science point of view, it has been found that medial and posterolateral herniated nuclear material responds to distraction methods better than laterally herniated material. It has also been found in a cadaveric radiographic study[3] (p. 262) that vertebral motions occur during flexion–distraction, with L5 flexing 6° on S1 while the posterior disk height increased by 3 mm (3.5° and 1.7 mm at L4–5). (Although in retrospect, one wonders how results like this could *not* have been obtained, it was still necessary to obtain the measurements.) In another study on live subjects, it was found that the average intervertebral flexion going from the intermediate table position to the extreme flexed position increased by 3.2°. In a surface EMG study, patients under treatment sustained a one to five times increase in electrical activity compared to their pretreatment activity. (Nevertheless, this may not be as significant as it seems, given that the resulting EMG signal was still only 2–12% the level they achieved when asked to exert maximal muscle contraction.) Traction on a cadaveric specimen showed a reduction in intradiscal pressure, in accordance with Cox's theory, and the decrease tended to be larger to the extent the pre-treatment disk pressure was higher – the more abnormal the patient, the greater the reduction in intradiscal pressure that would be expected to occur. All of these points are documented by Cox.[3]

CLINICAL EFFECTIVENESS RESEARCH

Although there are many case reports and some case series involving several patients, there would be no point in reviewing any of them given that we have what amounts to a case series involving no fewer than 1000 patients.[4] This study, combining data collected in two previous studies, involved 30 chiropractors, all using the same paperwork and treatment protocols, each collecting data on at least 20 consecutive low-back cases entering their practices. Although patients may have received modalities such as electrical stimulation, massage, hot/cold therapy, trigger point therapy, and bracing, flexion–distraction was the primary treatment method used in 92% of the cases.

Patients' responses to care, not surprisingly, depended on their diagnosis – the condition being treated. About 83% of patients with lumbar sprain or strain at L4 and L5 had a good to excellent response to care. Disk herniations at L4 and L5 had 61% and 66% good to excellent responses, respectively. The treatment of spondylolisthesis came in somewhat lower, with 59% of responses judged good to excellent.

Looking across the multiple conditions treated in this large case series, it must be noted that only 8.7% of the patients progressed to chronicity, defined as symptom persistence after 12 weeks of treatment. This is probably less than the 10–20% of untreated patients who progress to chronicity, but how much less depends on whether that number is closer to 10% or 20%. The mean number of days required to obtain maximal improvement was 29 days, with maximal improvement defined as 3 months of conservative care, re-establishment of the pre-injury state, or 100% relief of pain.

Apart from the impact on spinal pain, there is some evidence that flexion–distraction is safe and effective for some types of organic dysfunction, such as chronic pelvic pain in women.[5]

CONCLUSIONS

- In our introduction we questioned whether a piece of equipment could uniquely define a chiropractic technique system. In closing, we would question the appropriateness of classifying flexion–distraction as a method of *manipulation*. We examined this term in Chapter 2, where we made the point that usage varies, from essentially "treatment by hand" in some (mostly extrachiropractic) contexts, to high-velocity, low-amplitude manual thrusting in other contexts, including chiropractic. Therefore, how helpful is it to consider flexion–distraction a manipulative technique?
- Of course, the same problem is posed by instrument adjusting, where the forces are applied by a hand-assisted machine. Some instrument

adjustors eschew the term "manipulation" anyway, which they consider medicalized, so there are no issues posed for them in defining instrument adjusting as manipulation technique. Other instrument adjustors, such as Activator practitioners, are wont to use the term "manipulation," no doubt for some reason shared with flexion–distraction practitioners.

- There is no doubt about it, flexion–distraction really is a one-size-fits-all type of treatment. Without wishing to overinterpret, we must none the less heed Cox's own declaration: "Along the lines of McManis and Stoddard, I treat all low back conditions with axial distraction treatments ... not just intervertebral disc herniation."[3] (p. 275)
- Since the flexion–distraction approach is predicated upon having a structural impact on the herniated disk, whereby it attempts to suck the disk back in or use tension in spinal ligaments to force it centripetally, one is hard pressed to understand why Cox simply notes, without comment, that symptoms are unrelated to the size of the disk herniation.[3] (p. 284) If that is the case, why bother trying to reduce the size of the herniation? How can we reconcile the comment that symptoms and size of disk correlation are unrelated, with the further comment that a "2-mm difference in canal size is all that is needed to determine whether a person will have low back pain ... [such as can be caused by] disc protrusion"?[3] (p. 285)
- It is impossible to conclude this chapter without noting that Cox's flexion–distraction technique is not the only conservative method expressly designed to treat disk and sciatic conditions conservatively. Robin McKenzie developed his very different approach as a physical therapist, so his extension methods remain beyond the scope of a book limited in scope to chiropractic techniques. On the other hand, we might mention that: (1) his target patients are the same as those who commonly receive flexion–distraction; (2) he usually, but not always, treats his patients in *extension*; and (3) it is not entirely clear how a clinician might decide to choose between Cox's flexion or McKenzie's mostly extension-based methods.

- McKenzie believes we should treat the patient using vectors that "centralize" symptoms like pain and paresthesia, i.e., treat so as to make symptoms less distal, even if that increases local back symptoms. Usually this involves extending the spine (e.g., by having the patient perform prone press-ups) but sometimes it may involve flexing the spine.
- Cox leaves little doubt about how he feels about applying extension–distraction for herniated disk. Among the undesirable consequences, he lists decrease in posterior disk height, disk protrusion with canal stenosis, buckling of the ligamentum flavum into the canal with further stenosis and possible compression of the cauda equinum, closure of the vertebral canal by 2 mm, closure of the facet joints, increased discal pressure, posterior movement of the nucleus pulposus, and intervertebral foraminal encroachment and resulting nerve root pressure.[3] (pp. 275–276) Given all these negative comments, one surmises that Cox does not support spinal extension therapy. However, assuming this to be true, one is hard-pressed to explain the demonstrated clinical value of McKenzie procedures.[6,8]
- On another front, the rehabilitative methods of Pettibon,[9] Harrison and Troyanovich,[10] and Troyanovich[11] all employ extension traction. These practitioners, although they present precious little clinical data on outcomes that would be relevant to a patient (e.g., pain reduction), do suggest these procedures may change the sagittal curves to some extent.[12]
- The expert panel convened by Gatterman et al,[1] as well as two other publications spawned from this project,[2,13] all find strong clinical support for the safety and clinical effectiveness of flexion–distraction procedures. After all, one cannot dismiss reportage on 1000 consecutive cases.[4] On the other hand, 1000 case reports are just that, 1000 case reports. In the absence of a randomized and controlled clinical trial, we cannot be entirely certain that the 50% improvement in about a month's time that Cox considers treatment success is a superior clinical outcome to alternative treatments, including no treatment.

REFERENCES

1. Gatterman M L, Cooperstein R, Lantz C et al 2001 Rating specific chiropractic technique procedures for common low back conditions. Journal of Manipulative and Physiological Therapeutics 24 (7): 449–456
2. Cooperstein R, Perle S M, Gatterman M L et al 2001 Chiropractic technique procedures for specific low back conditions: characterizing the literature. Journal of Manipulative and Physiological Therapeutics 24 (6): 407–424
3. Cox J M 1999 Low back pain: mechanism, diagnosis and treatment, 6th edn. Williams & Wilkins, Baltimore, MD
4. Cox J M, Feller J, Cox-Cid J 1996 Distraction chiropractic adjusting: clinical application and outcomes of 1000 cases. Topics in Clinical Chiropractic 3 (3): 45–57
5. Hawk C, Azad A, Phongphua C, Long C R 1999 Preliminary study of the effects of a placebo chiropractic treatment with sham adjustments. Journal of Manipulative and Physiological Therapeutics 22 (7): 436–443.
6. Faas A 1996 Exercises: which ones are worth trying, for which patients, and when? Spine 21 (24): 2874–2878; discussion 2878–2879.
7. Donelson R, McKenzie R 1992 Effects of spinal flexion and extension exercises on low-back pain and spinal mobility in chronic mechanical low-back pain patients. Spine 17 (10): 1267–1268.
8. Taylor D N 1993 Treatment of disc herniation and fragmentation by spinal extension distraction. Chiropractic Technique 5 (3): 111–118
9. Pettibon B R 1989 Pettibon Spinal Bio-Mechanics. Pettibon Bio-Mechanics Institute, Tacoma, WA
10. Harrison D D, Troyanovich S 1996 Chiropractic Biophysics Technique. In: Lawrence D (ed.) Advances in chiropractic, vol. 4, pp. 321–348. Mosby Year Book, Chicago, IL
11. Troyanovich S J 2001 Structural rehabilitation of the spine and posture: a practical approach. MPAmedia, Huntington Beach, CA
12. Harrison D D, Jackson B L, Troyanovich S et al 1994. The efficacy of cervical extension-compression traction combined with diversified manipulation and drop table adjustments in the rehabilitation of cervical lordosis: a pilot study. Journal of Manipulative and Physiological Therapeutics 17 (7): 454–464
13. Cooperstein R, Perle S M 2002 Condition-specific indications for low back chiropractic adjustive procedures for the low back: literature and clinical effectiveness ratings of an expert panel. Topics in Clinical Chiropractic 9 (3): 19–29

17

Diversified Technique (DT)[1]

INTRODUCTION

Around 1995, Cooperstein began writing a string of articles on technique systems in chiropractic, using a template that had been devised by the Panel of Advisors to the American Chiropractic Association Council on Technique: Sacro-Occipital Technique,[2] Activator,[3] Chiropractic Biophysics,[4] and Thompson:[5] all done without a hitch, published in the journal *Chiropractic Technique*. (Some of the other members of the Technique Panel also contributed articles.) However, turning to DT, Cooperstein sadly informed the Panel, much to its surprise – and perhaps horror – that it simply could not be done. Instead, he wrote an article on the history of DT that was published in the *Journal of Chiropractic Humanities*,[1] summarized in Appendix 2.

The problem with the term "diversified" begins with the fact that it has been subject to diverse interpretations in the chiropractic milieu, to the point that it is not even clear whether or not the word should be capitalized. For some individuals, "diversified" is an adjective, in the sense of "eclectic," whereas for others, "Diversified" is a noun, representing the name of a specific chiropractic technique system. The issue cannot be explained away as mere semantics, in that the differences in usage underscore divergent historical legacies. The usage of the term "diversified" has ranged from an expansive descriptor of the core of things chiropractic, all the way to a restrictive label for just another named chiropractic technique. As the core of chiropractic, DT is too global to describe succinctly, whereas as a named technique, it is too eclectic to describe distinctly. Maybe that is why

Kfoury, who edited a catalog of chiropractic techniques in 1977[6] that included such notable entries as "Perianal Postural Reflex," and the "Von Fox Combination Technique," did not include DT.

Diversified chiropractic technique is like a close friend with a somewhat fuzzy past, whose true identity must remain unknown until that past is known. Cooperstein,[1] as well as Green and Johnson,[7] have tried to uncover that history. In the meantime, against our better judgment, since by all accounts DT (whatever it is) is the most widely practiced technique system in chiropractic,[8] we are going to do a round-peg-in-a-square-hole job on DT. We will bravely attempt to confine it to the same template we have used for the other technique systems, thus pretending it actually is some kind of technique system; this in spite of the fact that there is precious little in DT that can be considered proprietary. There are no unique terms, no distinctive physiological rationale, no examination procedures unlike any that would be performed in any chiropractic office in the world. It's when we turn to the *adjustive procedures* that we have our first glimpse of a somewhat unique Diversified style, as we describe below.

OVERVIEW

Diversified is the most generic of all technique systems. It starts from the broadest of philosophical tenets: chiropractors adjust subluxations (sometimes, avoiding the term, they correct subluxation-equivalents, as discussed in App. 2), to prevent nerve interference, so the body can heal itself. Diversified practitioners identify subluxations through patient history, palpation, X-ray, thermography, leg checks, and a variety of reflex procedures. They are full-spine chiropractors and usually, but not always, treat the extremities. They perform both high- and low-velocity adjustive procedures (manipulation and mobilization, respectively), sometimes use specialized tables (usually drop or flexion–distraction tables) or other equipment (such as padded wedges), and may use adjusting instruments as an alternative to manual interventions. Adjunctive procedures might include physical therapy modalities, soft-tissue and myofascial work, reflex methods, heel lifts, orthotic devices, nutritional advice and supplements, exercise instruction, rehabilitation procedures, and activities of daily living (ADL) counseling.

HISTORY

The roots of the Diversified approach to chiropractic technique lie within a broad-scope, less personalized reaction to the Palmeresque fundamentalism that emanated from the "Fountainhead" during chiropractic's first several decades.[1] Indeed, the philosophies and methodologies of the loyal opposition – primarily Carver, Langworthy, Smith, Forster, Howard, and "the Big Four" (Firth et al) – amount to a sort of "proto-diversified" technique, even though the methods associated with these individuals remained either deliberately or accidentally proprietary, not yet truly eclectic and depersonalized. Proto-diversified technique eluded BJ Palmer's attempt to dominate the burgeoning chiropractic profession, many of whose leading individuals did not accept his autocratic position. Green and Johnson develop the thesis that Metzinger and his colleagues were important proponents of early DT.[7]

In addition to the substantive differences between their methods and those of the Palmer milieu, the loyal opposition conformed to a more mainstream method of accumulating knowledge. Compared to the essentially antiestablishment position struck by BJ Palmer, they stuck closer to, and for the most part declared allegiance to, the existing body of scientific knowledge, which they intended to improve (but not necessarily replace) through the accretion of chiropractic knowledge.

Here then, are the roots of DT – not merely a body of clinical practice, but an approach to sustained chiropractic development. BJ Palmer greatly accelerated the development of competitive schools of chiropractic by demanding in 1924 that all chiropractors adopt the neurocalometer,[9,10] and in the early 1930s that they abandon vertebral adjusting below the level of C2.[11]

It is safe to say that DT took shape in substance before assuming the appellation "diversified," the origin of which remains appropriately obscure.[12] Nevertheless, the classic expression of DT can be either probably[13] or unequivocally[12] attributed to Joe Janse, DC. There is no doubt that his 1947 *Chiropractic Principles and Technic*[14] remains DT's crowning achievement. Although the book assumes some fairly revisionist, antifundamentalist ideological positions – e.g., "To say that subluxation is the one and only cause of disease is wrong"[14] – what really qualifies Janse as the mentor of DT is the tremendous scope of clinical chiropractic procedures he describes. Moreover, of particular importance is the way he describes them: Janse was able to present chiropractic diagnostic and therapeutic methods in a generic, non-proprietary manner. In Janse's hands, chiropractic is no longer an alternative to medical science, but rather a complementary science (even though he did discount the existence of communicable diseases, therefore rejecting the practice of vaccination).

In Janse's book,[14] according to Grice and Vernon,[15] "more than 117 procedures were presented including spinal adjustments, peripheral joint adjustments, and sinus and organ techniques. These techniques, with only slight modifications, continue to be used by the majority of chiropractors and often are referred to as 'diversified techniques'." That Janse himself most likely endorsed the term "Diversified" may be inferred from his introduction to States' 1967 illustrated chiropractic technique manual: "Roentgen studies reveal that no two spines, and their relating lumbosacral and sacroiliac mechanisms, are totally alike. There are variances in the composite and mechanical dispositions, as well as in the symmetry and architecture, of the articular motor beds. These factors alone make *diversification* [emphasis added] of adjusting procedures imperative."[16]

DEFINITION OF TECHNIQUE-SPECIFIC TERMS

There quite simply are none. A Diversified practitioner who uses terms like "subluxation" and "adjustment" does so in an entirely generic manner. Although such a practitioner may employ a term that takes origin within the narrow confines of a technique system, say, "therapy localization," there are no proprietary Diversified terms. Subluxations tend to be named according to how the vertebral body has misaligned, unlike Gonstead listings that use the spinous process as a reference point. Some Diversified practitioners seem to eschew the use of the term "subluxation," because in their view it is misleading: stripped of meaning as a result of being used as a default option for whatever is wrong with the patient, or because it means too many different things to different chiropractors and technique systems.

PHYSIOLOGICAL MECHANISMS AND RATIONALE

Diversified practitioners believe the concept of subluxation/spinal dysfunction includes both misalignment and movement restriction: "crooked bones and sticky joints." Although there is very little information on which, if any, specific directions of restriction result from specific misalignments, Diversified takes under its wing a composite world-view in which statics (alignment) and dynamics (movement) share center stage. Some Diversified practitioners prefer the term "vertebral subluxation complex (VSC)" to the simple unadorned "subluxation," a more narrow term, but that is a mere detail: in a DT setting, any old subluxation-equivalent will do,[17] or even none at all. The subluxation is thought either to cause nerve interference directly by compressing or irritating nerve roots, or results in visceral and/or somatic dysfunction through more complex mechanisms that involve reflexes (such as facilitated states) and vicious cycles (like the pain–spasm–pain cycle).

The effects of subluxation are thought to affect both afferent (sensory, proprioceptive) and efferent (muscles, glands, and other organs) function, and indeed, many Diversified practitioners support a

---

Box 17.1   Proposed mechanisms of spinal manipulation (adapted from Meeker & Haldeman[18] and Meeker et al[19])

- Alleviation of entrapped facet joint tissue (i.e., meniscoid)
- Repositioning of posterior annular material from intervertebral disk
- Alleviation of stiffness derived from fibrotic tissue caused by injury, trauma, or degenerative changes
- Inhibition of excessive reflex activity in intrinsic spinal musculature or limbs and/or facilitation of inhibited muscle activity
- Reduction of compressive or irritative insults to neural tissue

---

GIGO model – garbage in, garbage out – of nervous system dysfunction and adverse health consequences. However, we are also aware of some Diversified practitioners who are not nearly as tied to any obligatory nerve interference; that is, the benefits derived from the chiropractic adjustment (or manipulation) are more mechanical in nature than neurological. Box 17.1 summarizes the mechanisms that DT practitioners believe are involved in spinal adjusting and manipulation.

DIAGNOSTIC/ANALYTIC PROCEDURES

Diversified practitioners use any or all of the following to identify subluxations/spinal dysfunctions: patient history, static and motion palpation, postural assessment, gait analysis, X-ray line marking, thermography, leg checks, and a variety of reflex procedures (including manual muscle testing, challenges, and therapy localization).

Probably the most agreed-upon examination procedure for DT practitioners is palpation, despite continuing debate on its reproducibility and clinical utility. We find the PARTS acronym (Box 17.2) a useful summary of what may be considered a generic DT examination protocol.

TREATMENT/ADJUSTIVE PROCEDURES

DT practitioners are full-spine chiropractors, and also tend to treat the extremities. By full spine, we

Box 17.2 The PARTS acronym[20]

P Pain
A Asymmetry or alignment
R Range of motion (segmental or region)
T Temperature, texture, tone
S Special tests (leg checks, thermography, and so on)

mean they do not restrict their focus to any one region of the body such as the atlas (upper cervical spine, Chs 32 and 33) or the sacrum (as in Logan Basic Technique, Ch. 21). They perform both high- and low-velocity adjustive procedures (manipulation and mobilization, respectively), sometimes use specialized tables (usually drop or flexion–distraction tables), and may use adjusting instruments as an alternative to manual interventions. In spite of all this adjustive diversity, we usually think of the "osseous thrust" as the hallmark of DT: a high-velocity, low-amplitude thrust accompanied by audible release, or cavitation. Adjunctive procedures might include physical therapy modalities, soft-tissue and myofascial work, reflex methods, heel lifts, orthotic devices, nutritional advice and supplements, exercise instruction, rehabilitation procedures, and ADL counseling. Good[21] describes the biomechanics of various adjustments he classifies as Diversified, emphasizing resisted vs assisted approaches – which joints are affected by different types of thrusting procedures.

We are finally able to identify one characteristic of DT that may be proprietary, at least in the eyes of some. Diversified high-velocity, low-amplitude thrusts sometimes deploy rotation in either the setup (the preadjustive tension phase) or the thrust itself, especially in the cervical and lumbar spines. This is only an issue for those who eschew rotation vectors, at least anything beyond a minimum, such as Gonstead practitioners. Most of the rotated cervical moves, such as the modified rotary break, are done with the patient in the supine position, although there is also a prone cervical break and a sitting rotary break. Although few would support side-posture "million dollar roll" procedures for adjusting the low back (for a limited defense, see Cooperstein[22]), in

which there is extreme counterrotation of the pelvic and shoulder girdles, Diversified practitioners are not reluctant to use some degree of rotation in their low-back setups and thrusting procedures. Given how widespread the practice of Diversified is, and the lack of a founding figure type as authoritative as, say, Goodheart in the case of Applied Kinesiology, or DeJarnette in Sacro-Occipital Technique, we are not surprised to find that the corpus of moves that may be called "Diversified" extensive is highly variable.

OUTCOME ASSESSMENT

Diversified outcome measures are more or less the same as the examination procedures, as is the case with most technique systems: reverse the positive examination finding, confirm the correction of the subluxation.

SAFETY AND RISK FACTORS

Given the diversity of Diversified adjustive and adjunctive procedures, we cannot draw any conclusions about their safety beyond a few isolated remarks that apply to virtually all things chiropractic. The incidence of major adverse consequences, like stroke following cervical manipulation[23] or cauda equina syndrome following lumbopelvic manipulation,[24] is extremely small. The incidence of minor adverse consequences is as much as one in two[25,26] but these are self-resolving and within a few weeks of care the majority of patients are improved compared with their precare baseline conditions.

Much inquiry and debate has surrounded the safety of cervical manipulation, especially Diversified-like maneuvers that employ a rotational vector. As discussed in Chapter 38, the current best evidence indicates that not only are the serious adverse consequences rare, unpredictable, and idiosyncratic occurrences, but there is very little, if any, irrefutable evidence to support the contention that one form of cervical manipulation carries more risk of injury than any other form of cervical manipulation.

EVIDENCE OF EFFICACY

The broadness of DT precludes us from commenting on its efficacy, as if that were different from the effectiveness of mainstream chiropractic methods in general. The effectiveness of spinal manipulative therapy is established by high-quality evidence for low-back pain, cervical pain, and headache. We provide a few representative citations, which themselves are review articles rather than primary research.[27-30] There are also pragmatic studies[31] looking at chiropractic vs alternative (usually medical) treatment, and studies, sometimes controversial, assessing its cost-effectiveness, such as the Manga report.[32] The results for visceral conditions are much more equivocal, and we decline the temptation to review that sketchy, confusing, and controversial body of evidence.

Sometimes an investigator or author simply states that "Diversified" was used, usually meaning purely manual high-velocity, low-amplitude thrusting. Sometimes it may mean more than that. For example, Hsieh et al[33] tell us they used "the 'Diversified' technique," but in their context this includes drop-table moves and sitting moves that would usually not be taught in courses called "Diversified." We read:

Each patient received therapy three times per week for 3 weeks. Experienced licensed chiropractors with a 5-year minimum of clinical experience delivered joint manipulation at both sites. The joint manipulations, consisting of high velocity and short-amplitude specific thrusting manipulations (the "Diversified" technique), were performed in the lumbar and/or sacroiliac regions (i.e., the tender locations indicated by the examiner on the Assessment Recommendations form or other levels clinically deemed by chiropractor to need therapy). Side or sitting posture was allowed. Drop table techniques also were allowed. All treatments were given on Leander Model 900 EZ Tables (Leander Health Technologies, Port Orchard, WA). No flexion distraction or mobilization was allowed.[33]

CONCLUSIONS

- Ironically, as the years went by, DT, which originated as a liberating, eclecticizing response to the myriad of narrowly defined and often cultistic technique systems of the day, found itself more than just occasionally arranged alongside, rather than alternative to them – as yet another technique system. However paradoxically, it appears that modern DT is chiefly distinguished from all of the others by its poor distinction from any one of them.

- The allure of brand-name techniques shows surprising resilience, in that many contemporary practitioners seem to prefer the cookbook-ishness of a technique system to the clinical freedom of generic technique,[34] or at least an uneasy mingling of the two.[35] How an individual practitioner regards DT may directly reflect how he or she feels about chiropractic technique in general. Someone who prefers eclectic practice may well endorse the descriptor "diversified," small d, and resist any attempt to have his or her methods characterized from a technique systems point of view. Conversely, the type of practitioner who professes to practice "Diversified" with a capital D may believe it best to specialize in a particular technique system, and object to having his or her technique defined away into the essence of all things chiropractic.

- Some contemporary chiropractors and authors regard DT as a named technique system, parallel to all the others, largely but certainly not exclusively identified historically with the former National Chiropractic College (now called National University of Health Sciences). From this point of view, DT is sometimes seen as a corpus of moves, lacking a distinct philosophical, ideological, or mechanical foundation as compared with other technique systems. Other contemporaries consider DT to be immense and generic, comprising the totality of chiropractic therapeutic and diagnostic procedures that, by virtue of overwhelming acceptance, have come to comprise the core of chiropractic technique itself. In a way, the two positions are opposite sides of the same coin: as a named technique, DT is too eclectic to describe distinctly, whereas as the core of chiropractic, it is too global to describe conveniently. The great majority (95.9%) of chiropractors themselves claim to use "Diversified," and 73.5% of their patients received DT.[8]

- Several of the chiropractic colleges teach courses in their core curricula that are called "Diversifed," but there are huge differences in the mix of moves supported. Hinz, in his article on DT methods, the Northwestern College, and John B Wolf,[36] seems to intend by the usage of the term "Diversified" all of the following: emphasis on the basic sciences, educational excellence, avoidance of dogmatic debates over technique and scope of practice. According to Hinz, "the system advocated an analysis of the patient, using the knowledge obtained through previous courses and experience, in order to utilize the technique or adjuncts which would fit the particular patient's need. This type of teaching was liberal in the sense that the school did not strictly adhere to any one technique, but studied many techniques and utilized the ones that were deemed most beneficial through deduction from the basic sciences and personal clinical experience."[36]

- The opposition one encounters to the DT use of rotation in adjustive setups and thrusting is not evidence-based, since there are no data supporting the view that rotational vectors are more hazardous than other vectors,[22] and thus by definition reflects simple bias and prejudice.

- We have seen some comments to the effect that Diversified adjustments are non-specific, intended to increase range of motion, rather than correct subluxations and associated nerve interference through specific contacts and vectors. We are at a loss to understand how anyone could conceive this denigrating thought, and strongly oppose it.

NOTE

The dual nature of DT as simultaneously technique system and technique umbrella was heavily manifested in our struggle to collaborate on this chapter. Cooperstein as a student studied Diversified at Life West, where it is taught as a technique system, whereas Gleberzon attended Canadian Memorial Chiropractic College, the technique curriculum of which heavily emphasizes Diversified in the sense of an umbrella term for many things chiropractic. In working on this chapter we came to realize that the Canadian Diversified umbrella differs in some ways from the American Diversified umbrella. The Canadian Diversified practitioner, granted the umbrella connotation, (1) is less likely to be comfortable with the "subluxation" term; (2) emphasizes nerve interference less; (3) is more reliant on standard orthopedic tests; and (4) is more heavily dependent on palpation as opposed to other classic chiropractic examination procedures (leg checking, X-ray line marking, thermography). The Canadians often substitute for "subluxation" any number of synonyms they believe more clinically informative: joint dysfunction, spinal irritation, facet dysfunction, and the like. Likewise, they can happily exist without the conceptual anchors of "nerve interference" or "spinal adjustment," focusing instead on a patient's symptoms and the intervention with "spinal manipulative therapy."

REFERENCES

1. Cooperstein R 1995 Diversified technique: core of chiropractic or "just another technique system"? Journal of Chiropractic Humanities 5 (1): 50–55
2. Cooperstein R 1996 Technique system overview: Sacro Occipital Technique. Chiropractic Technique 8 (3): 125–131
3. Cooperstein R 1997 Technique system overview: Activator Methods Technique. Chiropractic Technique 9 (3): 108–114
4. Cooperstein R 1995 Technique system overview: Chiropractic Biophysics Technique (CBP). Chiropractic Technique 7 (4): 141–146
5. Cooperstein R 1995 Technique system overview: Thompson Technique. Chiropractic Technique 7 (2): 60–63
6. Kfoury P W (ed.) 1977 Catalog of chiropractic techniques. Logan College of Chiropractic, St Louis, MO
7. Green B N, Johnson C D 1995 Unveiling an enigma: the origins and development of Diversified chiropractic technique. In: Cleveland III C, Gibbons R (eds) Conference proceedings of the Chiropractic Centennial Foundation, p. 34. Chiropractic Centennial Foundation, Davenport, IA
8. Christensen M G 2000 Job analysis of chiropractic. A project report, survey analysis and summary of the

practice of chiropractic within the United States.
National Board of Chiropractic Examiners, Greeley, CO

9. Gibbons R W 1992 Medical and social protest as part of hidden American history. In: Haldeman S (ed.) Principles and practice of chiropractic, 2nd edn, pp. 15–28. Appleton & Lange, East Norwalk, CT

10. Keating J C 1991 Introducing the neurocalometer: a view from the fountainhead. Journal of the Canadian Chiropractic Association 35 (3): 165–178

11. Montgomery P D, Nelson M J 1985 Evolution of chiropractic theories of practice and spinal adjustment, 1900–1950. Chiropractic History 5: 71–77

12. Gitelman R, Fligg B 1992 Diversified technique. In: Haldeman S (ed.) Principles and practice of chiropractic, 2nd edn, pp. 483–501. Appleton-Century-Crofts, New York, NY

13. Peterson D 1987 Diversified technique and short lever specific contact procedures. In: Coyle B, Mootz R D, Menon M K (eds) Second Annual Conference on Research and Education. Pacific Consortium for Chiropractic Research, Belmont, CA

14. Janse J, Houser R 1947 Chiropractic principles and technic. National College of Chiropractic, Lombard, IL

15. Grice A, Vernon H 1992 Basic principles in the performance of chiropractic adjusting: historical review, classification, and objectives. In: Haldeman S (ed.) Principles and practice of chiropractic, pp. 442–458. Appleton & Lange, Norwalk, CT

16. States A Z 1967 Spinal and pelvic techniques. National College of Chiropractic, Lombard, IL

17. Cooperstein R, Gleberzon B J 2001 Toward a taxonomy of subluxation-equivalents. Topics in Clinical Chiropractic 8 (1): 49–60

18. Meeker W C, Haldeman S 2002 Chiropractic: a profession at the crossroads of mainstream and alternative medicine. Annals of Internal Medicine 136 (3): 216–227

19. Meeker W C, Mootz R D, Haldeman S 2002 The state of chiropractic research. Topics in Clinical Chiropractic 9 (1): 1–13

20. Bergmann T 1993 PARTS joint assessment procedure. Chiropractic Technique 5 (3): 135–136

21. Good C J 1992 An analysis of diversified (lege artis) type adjustments based upon the assisted-resisted model of intervertebral motion unit prestress. Chiropractic Technique 4 (4): 117–123

22. Cooperstein R 1997 The reverse double whammy leg check. Dynamic Chiropractic 15 (16): 35–38

23. Haldeman S, Carey P, Townsend M, Papadopoulos C 2001 Arterial dissections following cervical manipulation: the chiropractic experience. Canadian Medical Association Journal 165 (7): 905–906

24. Shekelle P, Adams A H, Chassin M R et al 1992 Spinal manipulation for low back pain. Annals of Internal Medicine (117): 7

25. Senstad O, Leboeuf-Yde C, Borchgrevink C 1996 Predictors of side effects to spinal manipulative therapy. Journal of Manipulative and Physiological Therapeutics 19 (7): 441–445

26. Leboeuf-Yde C, Hennius B, Rudberg E et al 1997 Side effects of chiropractic treatment: a prospective study. Journal of Manipulative and Physiological Therapeutics 20 (8): 511–515

27. Shekelle P, Adams A H, Chassin M R et al 1992 The appropriateness of spinal manipulation for low back pain: indications and ratings by an all-chiropractic expert panel. RAND, Santa Monica, CA

28. Shekelle P, Adams A H, Chassin M R et al 1991 The appropriateness of spinal manipulation for low back pain: indications and ratings by a multidisciplinary expert panel. RAND, Santa Monica, CA

29. Hurwitz E L, Aker P D, Adams A H et al 1996 Manipulation and mobilization of the cervical spine. A systematic review of the literature. Spine 21 (15): 1746–1759; discussion 1759–1760

30. Bronfort G, Assendelft W J, Evans R et al 2001 Efficacy of spinal manipulation for chronic headache: a systematic review. Journal of Manipulative and Physiological Therapeutics 24 (7): 457–466

31. Meade T W, Dyer S, Browne W et al 1990 Low back pain of mechanical origin: randomized comparison of chiropractic and hospital outpatient treatment. British Medical Journal 300: 1431–1437

32. Manga P 1993 The effectiveness and cost-effectiveness of chiropractic management of low-back pain. Kenilworth, Richmond Hill, Ontario, Canada

33. Hsieh C Y, Adams A H, Tobis J et al 2002 Effectiveness of four conservative treatments for subacute low back pain: a randomized clinical trial. Spine 27 (11): 1142–1148

34. Cooperstein R 1990 Brand name techniques and the confidence gap. Journal of Chiropractic Education 4 (3): 89–93

35. Gleberzon B J 2000 Name techniques in Canada. Current trends in utilization rates and recommendations for their inclusion at the Canadian Memorial Chiropractic College. Journal of the Canadian Chiropractic Association 44 (3): 157–167

36. Hinz D G 1987 Diversified chiropractic: Northwestern College and John B Wolf, 1941–1984. Chiropractic History 7 (1): 35–41

18

Directional Non-Force Technique (DNFT)

INTRODUCTION

It was probably a bad idea for DNFT originator Van Rumpt to use the word "non-force" to describe his technique, because it gave people some funny ideas about what DNFT practitioners do. Obviously, it takes force to accomplish work, such as moving a bone through a distance (unless Newton had it all wrong). DNFT practitioners know there is a problem here: witness John's comment: "The term 'non-force' is slightly inaccurate … It is, rather, light-force or low-force in nature."[1]

Unfortunately, this does not solve the problem, because "non-force" is not slightly inaccurate, it is *completely* inaccurate. DNFT myofascial work, often involving goading the skin with a wood dowel, can be extremely forceful; and Van Rumpt himself attributed his clinical success to "heavy palpation." Van Rumpt may not have originated the concept of the functional short leg, and he himself attributes some version of the Derifield leg check to the osteopathic profession, but he certainly had a lot to do with promulgating the concept. His "reactive leg reflex" was an important impetus to the development of reflex techniques in general, and it is no coincidence that Van Rumpt collaborated with DeJarnette (Ch. 25). Fuhr also acknowledges the impact of Van Rumpt on Activator Methods Chiropractic Technique (Ch. 10). Although we have reason to believe that there may not be many DNFT practitioners, and although DNFT advocate Christopher John complains "There has been more discrimination against DNFT chiropractic than you can imagine,"[1] we are of the opinion that Van Rumpt's influence casts a long shadow over the world of contemporary chiropractic technique.

OVERVIEW

The primary goal of DNFT is the removal of nerve interference. An advertisement for DNFT states: "DNFT BASIC PREMISE: In the tradition of DD Palmer, find the subluxation, fix it, and leave it alone. No subluxation – no adjustment."[1]

Central to DNFT is a leg-check procedure for detecting the presence and exact location of subluxation, and a unique, low-force thumb thrust for correcting subluxations.[2] The technique is not so much full-spine as full-body, in that it addresses vertebrae, ribs, muscles, disks, cranial bones, soft tissues, extremities, ligaments, and organs. DNFT practitioners pride themselves in being able to correct subluxations in a relatively small number of visits, provided the subluxation diagnosis is correct and the thrusts are correctly delivered.

HISTORY

Richard Van Rumpt, the founder of DNFT, provided his first interview at the age of 82 in 1987,[3] and to our knowledge never published anything about his technique except a contribution to a catalog of chiropractic techniques in 1977.[4] In the 1987 interview (which was actually compiled over many years by the interviewer) he describes how he first began developing what became known as DNFT while still a chiropractic student at the National College, from which he graduated in 1923. A patient whom he had simply palpated, albeit "heavily," came in the next day (believing she had been adjusted) markedly improved. At about the same time, Van Rumpt read in a Rosicrucian magazine that the fingers on the hand are alternately either positive or negative, which led him to wonder if that could be turned into a principle of treatment. Early on he developed the "reactive leg reflex" concept, perhaps the first concept in chiropractic of the functional short leg, and he also claimed originality for being the first to use the thumb to adjust the body.[3] Van Rumpt began teaching DNFT in New York around 1940, and at one point was "De Jarnette's first and only so-called Director of the Sacro Occipital Research Society."[3] He died on 23 September 1987, after having appointed Christopher John and Phillip Convertino to carry on his work, teaching seminars and conducting research.[3] There are currently about 100 fully certified practitioners worldwide.[5]

DEFINITION OF TECHNIQUE-SPECIFIC TERMS

- Adjustment, subluxation: used generically, with no elements proprietary to DNFT[3]
- Thumb toggle thrust: refers to the type of contact used by the doctor, in which the overlapped thumbs are used to apply a highly accelerated but very light force to the patient, in an overall style that resembles the toggle-recoil thrust minus the recoil[3]
- Reactive leg reflex: refers to Van Rumpt's leg-check procedure, in which a "challenge" into tissue results in the leg pulling up if there is subluxation[2,3]
- Distortions: adaptations or compensations for subluxation, that should not be adjusted
- Thrust vs adjustment: a thrust only becomes an adjustment when it "succeeds 100% in correcting the subluxation and removing the nerve interference."[6] An adjustment, by comparison, does succeed in removing the subluxation and all the nerve interference
- Misalignment: does not exist except as part of a subluxation, and the subluxation necessarily involves nerve interference.

PHYSIOLOGICAL MECHANISMS AND RATIONALE

Van Rumpt believed that Innate Intelligence could be contacted by "visualization – thought projection – thought materialization – projection of mental energy or mind power" to arrive at a chiropractic subluxation analysis or listing.[4] He felt that Innate Intelligence could also be used to remove nerve interference, and that fixation was not so much a primary problem as a protective response to nerve insult. Specific correction of all the components of the subluxation removes the body's need to maintain hypomobility.[1] Likewise, such correction can result in the amelioration of regional distortions like scoliosis.

DNFT practitioners believe that subluxations are not corrected a little bit at a time, but rather all at once with a single thrust. This requires that both the listing and the thrust are perfect. Indeed, DNFT takes great pride in correcting subluxations in very few visits, ideally two to six.[2] Articular noises (audibles) are of no significance to a DNFT practitioner, since the noise does not establish realignment; i.e., the concepts of misalignment and realignment are of central significance. DNFT practitioners believe that it does not take much force to correct a subluxation if the doctor has the right listing and uses the right thrust.[7]

DIAGNOSTIC/ANALYTIC PROCEDURES

The primary, proprietary discovery of Van Rumpt is the "reactive leg reflex."[4] It is used to analyze the entire body for evidence of nerve interference. This procedure is said to identify where the nerve interference is, the direction of subluxation, how to correct it, and how to confirm correction. The procedure involves placing a "positive or a negative" finger over a misalignment, while turning the patient's feet outward.[5] If there is a subluxation present, one leg – the reactive leg – temporarily appears shorter than the other. Following an effective adjustment, this reflex is abolished. The procedure uses light challenges in potential directions of misalignment, which result in characteristic reactions in the leg positions that rule in or out the different possibilities. DNFT believes the leg check provides a direct window into the workings of Innate Intelligence.[6] According to John, if the leg check is performed within 3s of the challenge, and a subluxation is indeed present, then "there is a pull-up of the 'reactive leg,'" a shortening that "is dramatic and is generally ½-inch to one full inch [1.25–2.5 cm]."[1]

X-ray is not supported to determine subluxations or to generate listings, and never provides evidence of nerve interference.[2] However, X-rays are supported to rule out contraindications, determine pathology, for medicolegal reasons, and to "help sell the chiropractic principle and make clear to the patient the need for chiropractic service."[4]

TREATMENT/ADJUSTIVE PROCEDURES

The term "non-force" in DNFT is clearly a misnomer: "The term 'non-force' is slightly inaccurate … It is, rather, light-force or low-force in nature."[1] John provides a clear statement of DNFT's disavowal of manipulative (i.e., high-velocity, low-amplitude) treatment methods:[6] "DNFT is the original innate non-force technique in Chiropractic. There are no cervical rotaries, lumbar rolls, bone popping thrusts, or in Palmer's words, 'playing piano on the spine.'"

Unique to DNFT, the thumb toggle thrust is used to correct subluxations. DNFT practitioners pride themselves on being able to correct subluxations in a small number of visits. This requires getting the perfect listing, and applying the perfect thrust.[7] There is a claim for a direct correction of a bulging or even herniated disk, including some unusual types of disk herniations (anterolateral cervical disks) and unusual locations (thoracic disks).[6,8] Sometimes, particularly in treating an intervertebral disk, a modified dowel is applied between the transverse processes of the vertebrae.

DNFT includes regimens for soft-tissue adjustments, craniopathy, extremity adjustments, the eyes, and in fact "all articulations or tissues of the body that can be reached." There are special procedures for many visceral conditions, such as hiatal hernias and appendicitis.

It is very important in DNFT, so they say, to steer clear of "distortions," which are adaptations or compensations for subluxation. Since they are supposedly self-correcting when the primary subluxations are corrected, distortions should not be treated.

OUTCOME ASSESSMENT

The same leg-check procedure that identifies subluxations and how they might be corrected is also used to confirm correction. Indeed, the doctor is to apply the exact same pretest as posttest, to prove success in having completely corrected the subluxation and removed the nerve interference.

SAFETY AND RISK FACTORS

DNFT manifests an extreme distaste for high-velocity, low-amplitude thrusting, which it regards as "unpleasant force," and dangerous to the patient. Although Van Rumpt states that X-ray could be useful to identify contraindications for adjustments, he also states that "there is never a contra indication for giving a DNFT adjustment!"[4] The light forces that DNFT practitioners claim to generate *may be* relatively safer than high-velocity, low-amplitude manipulations.

EVIDENCE OF EFFICACY

We are aware of no published studies on the efficacy of specific DNFT treatment procedures. On the other hand, the similarity of the thumb thrust to other widely used procedures, about whose clinical effectiveness a little more is known (e.g., instrument-assisted thrusting, toggle-recoil adjusting), suggests there may be some clinical utility. Likewise, the clinical effect of using a dowel to goad paraspinal soft tissues may resemble that of the more well-known and validated trigger point work as done in medicine, physical therapy, and chiropractic (i.e., Nimmo Receptor-Tonus technique, Ch. 24).

CONCLUSIONS

- The world-view of DNFT, apart from the fact that it eschews forceful thrusting, is otherwise very traditional and mainstream. The definitions of subluxation, adjustment, and misalignment, and the central therapeutic intent to remove misalignment and nerve interference are at the center of almost all of the chiropractic theories.
- Van Rumpt leaves little doubt what he considers to be his central innovation:

  Regarding our very special leg reflex – this reflex has very little or nothing to do with an actual traumatic or congenital short leg. Our leg check is in no way related to any other type of leg check now or heretofore ever used by any other D.C. or person now or ever alive. It is a 100% Van Rumpt discovery, based on 53 years of research. This reflex, plus innate, tells us all we need to know to make a perfect subluxation analysis, adjustment, and post test to prove correction of subluxation and removal of nerve interference.[4]

- John clarifies that the leg check is entirely different from the Derifield, Activator, National Upper Cervical Chiropractic Association, or any other leg-measuring systems in chiropractic.[1] The Activator Methods leg check, their use of the term "leg reactivity," and the practices of "isolation testing" and "pressure testing" are inspired by DNFT, which Fuhr and Osterbauer name as an antecedent.[9]

- Van Rumpt's "visualization" procedure, a "thought projection" process by which he arrived at a subluxation listing,[4] so much resembles the "Assessment by Intention" procedure later to be used by Morter[10] in Bioenergetic Synchronization Technique (Ch. 13) that we must presume a connection.
- The unfortunate use of the term "non-force" may have created some unnecessary confusion about what DNFT hopes to achieve and how it hopes to achieve it. Virtually every diagnostic and therapeutic procedure described by DNFT authors occurs in some related form in other techniques (e.g., Activator Methods, Thompson, Full-Spine Specific), where their use has been less controversial.
- According to John,[1,11] a subluxation can be corrected in two to six visits, and maintenance care in a DNFT setting involves one visit in 1–4 months. Van Rumpt himself said his average patient was seen and made subluxation-free in four visits.[3]
- Sadly, near the end of his life, Van Rumpt stated: "There is a move to limit field research but I really believe chiropractic would have died long ago if it were not for the field researchers who eliminated much of the rough, knock 'em down, drag 'em out chiropractic."[3] We presume Van Rumpt mistook calls for more rigor in research for an effort to limit research by clinician-scientists, as field researchers have been described.

REFERENCES

1. John C 1994 The Directional Non-Force Technique. Today's Chiropractic 23 (4): 30–32
2. John C 1992 The Directional Non-Force Technique of chiropractic. American Chiropractor (July/August): 15–16
3. Author unknown 1987 Van – the innate man [Interview with Van Rumpt]. American Chiropractor (September): 4–7
4. Van Rumpt R 1977 Directional Non-Force Technique. In: Ktoury P W (ed.) Catalog of chiropractic techniques, pp. 13–16. Logan College of Chiropractic, St Louis, MO
5. Rapkin M 2002 Directional Non-Force Technique. chiropractor-doctors.com
6. John C (undated) Directional Non-Force Technique seminars. Christopher E. John, Beverly Hills, CA
7. Gensler R 1987 In memory of Van – the 'Innate' man. Chiropractic Journal (November): 13
8. John C 1989 The Directional Non-Force Technique of chiropractic. American Chiropractor (July): 14–15
9. Fuhr A E, Osterbauer P J 1989 Interexaminer reliability of relative leg-length evaluations in the prone, extended position. Chiropractic Technique 1 (1): 13–18
10. Morter T Jr 1998 The theoretical basis and rationale for the clinical application of Bio-Energetic Synchronization. Journal of Vertebral Subluxation Research 2(1): 23–24
11. John C 1989 The Directional Non-Force Technique. American Chiropractor (July): 14–15

19

Full-Spine Specific (FSS) Technique

Meric Technique, Meric Recoil Technique[1,2]

INTRODUCTION

Some years ago, one of us (Cooperstein) found himself sitting next to CS Cleveland, Jr at a dinner featuring members of the Panel of Advisors to the American Chiropractic Association Council on Technique. We spent most of the evening discussing the innovative animal research he had conducted three decades earlier, in which a mechanical splint was used to create vertebral subluxations in rabbits, while monitoring their systemic consequences. That research was very consistent with the theory and practice of FSS Technique, which from its inception in the early years of chiropractic to the present time has always stressed how segmental subluxations affect visceral function. Whereas others both before and after his time frequently enjoined debate on the somatovisceral question in a data-free zone, CS Cleveland, Jr quietly conducted his own research on the matter. (Yes, his rabbits developed kidney disease.)

To tell the truth, we could have easily merged our comments on FSS Technique into our chapter on Diversified Technique (Ch. 17). After all, the goals of care, terminology, examination procedures, adjustive procedures, and outcome measures are similar to those that could be found in any Diversified practice setting in the world. On the other hand, there were some considerations in favor of a separate chapter: (1) the uniqueness of applying the toggle-recoil adjustive procedure to the full spine, rather than limiting it to atlas; and (2) the retention of this technique tradition through four generations of Clevelands and the two Cleveland colleges (Kansas City, Los Angeles).

The National Board of Chiropractic Examiners reported in 2000[3] that 19.9% of chiropractors used "Meric" and that 6.5% of their patients received "Meric" care. Now, maybe that is accurate as stated, but it is not obvious what survey respondents understood by the term "Meric": the Meric System of BJ Palmer, the Meric Technique, or even Mears Upper Cervical Technique. How many of these respondents use Meric adjustive methods in a mechanical sense, how many depend on Meric spinal level/visceral problem relationships in their clinical thinking, and how many use and depend on both? In any case, its distinctive mechanical style and staunch emphasis on somatovisceral phenomena continue to define the FSS approach to traditional chiropractic technique. At the same time, the commitment of four generations of Clevelands to chiropractic education continues to impress all those who make themselves aware of this proud history.

OVERVIEW

The primary goal is the elimination of vertebral *positional subluxation*, in order to remove nerve interference.[2] A secondary goal is to reduce immobilization or aberrant intervertebral motion, caused by the subluxation. Meric technique is a very traditional manual, specific, short-lever technique, featuring high-velocity, low-amplitude (HVLA) thrusting. The thrust is delivered to any of the vertebrae of the prone patient, featuring a recoil mechanism that resembles the well-known toggle-recoil adjustment of the atlas.[1]

HISTORY

FSS, formerly known as Meric Technique,[1] is as old as chiropractic itself. In fact, among those techniques in common use today, it more closely resembles the technique of the Palmers (prior to BJ Palmer's adoption of Upper Cervical technique in 1930) than any other technique. FSS represents the core of the technique program at the two Cleveland Chiropractic Colleges, in Los Angeles and Kansas City. Three generations of Carl Clevelands have served as the president of Cleveland Colleges. At this time, at least at the Cleveland Colleges, the term "Full-Spine Specific" is preferred to Meric Technique for a number of reasons: (1) to underscore that it has to with a particular mechanical adjusting style, with an emphasis on specificity; (2) to indicate that it is not identical to the Meric analytic (symptom-specific); and (3) to make clear that the entire spine, not simply the upper cervical spine, is assessed and adjusted.

The recoil adjustment used in FSS directly descends from the original mechanical style of the Palmers and Stephenson.[2] The Meric System was worked out by BJ Palmer and Palmer School of Chiropractic faculty member James C Wishart, around 1910.[4-6] By the term "meres," BJ Palmer referred to specific segmentally related areas of the body. In the Meric System, the doctor would first identify all the subluxations, and then decide, based on which were "hot boxes" and on the results of "nerve tracings," which segments were to be adjusted. The Meric System eventually took on the connotation of adjusting the segments neurologically related to a diseased viscus, whereas the FSS today has more to do with a mechanical style of adjusting segments that have been determined to be misaligned and/or fixated.

Dr. CS Cleveland, Jr conducted a series of innovative pilot animal studies that were described in a 1965 publication.[7] Splints were devised that could subluxate the middle vertebra among three in a domestic rabbit, while the physiological and structural consequences were monitored over a period of time. In his report, Cleveland reported that, after several weeks of having T12 iatrogenically subluxated, each of the two rabbits developed kidney disease, although different diseases.

DEFINITION OF TECHNIQUE-SPECIFIC TERMS

- Meric: refers to the "vertemeres" of the spine, the segments of the vertebral column, so that the term "Meric Technique" has to do with segmental specificity[6]
- Toggle-recoil adjustment: has a dual sense, involving the recoil of the doctor's contact hand away from the patient after the thrust, and also the transmission of the force through the patient following the impact
- Meric chiropractic arch: refers to the doctor's hand position, with the wrist fully extended with ulnar deviation and flexion of the metacarpophalangeal joints to 90°
- Nerve tracing: we can do no better than cite the founder, DD Palmer himself: "The chiropractor should trace sensitive, swollen, longitudinally contracted nerves, for the purpose of locating their impingement and tension ... There is no better way to locate the cause of disease, or demonstrate to a prospective patient how bones and nerves are related to each other and why such relationship accounts for health and disease, than by palpation and nerve-tracing"[8] (p. 102)
- Hot boxes: locations of elevated temperature along the spine, detected either with the back of the fingers or with the neurocalagraph, and thought to indicate subluxated vertebrae.[9]

PHYSIOLOGICAL MECHANISMS AND RATIONALE

Since the nervous system governs the entire body, Meric Technique, however local its application, is thought to determine the health of the entire body and all of its organ systems.[2] The nervous system governs the health of the body, and interference with the nervous system resulting from vertebral subluxation results in disease, owing to the inability of the organism to maintain its adaptation to environmental variables.

We provide a representative statement[10] from Dr. CS Cleveland, Sr:

THE PURPOSE OF AN ADJUSTMENT is NOT to depress or NOT to stimulate! BUT to remove interferences with transmission, or pressures, from the affected nerve thus restoring normal nerve supply, THEN innate intelligence, or nature, with her exact knowledge, decreases or increases activities in the various organs or parts, as she finds necessary. With our limited conscious knowledge, we can not educationally substitute such limited conscious knowledge and control on the outside, for innate intelligence's unlimited knowledge and control on the inside.

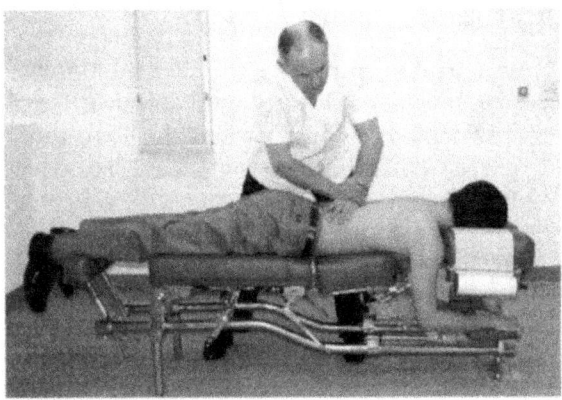

Figure 19.1 Full-spine specific.

DIAGNOSTIC/ANALYTIC PROCEDURES

In the sense that "Meric" refers to the Meric System, then the identification of a diseased viscus or organ system forms part of the diagnostic input in determining the level to be adjusted. Although Meric Technique evolved within a static listing paradigm, in which segments are identified as misaligned, contemporary practitioners are just as likely to apply these methods to the correction of vertebral fixations. The two Cleveland Colleges of today (Los Angeles and Kansas City) teach a full program of diagnostic procedures, proceeding from the history to the physical examination and then on to the more narrowly defined "chiropractic procedures." Although the anteroposterior full-spine X-ray remains important to FSS practitioners, at the current time they use history and palpatory findings as their main tools, followed by X-ray to confirm the findings. The X-ray generates the specific subluxation listings that determine where and how the adjustments are to be performed, whether to use a spinous or lamina contact (based on which was more misaligned).

TREATMENT/ADJUSTIVE PROCEDURES

The Meric Technique employs an HVLA maneuver, virtually always on prone patients (Fig. 19.1). Originally, the technique was performed on prone patients whose abdomens were suspended

across a gap in the table, a precursor to today's Hi-Lo tables with breakaway chest and/or abdominal pieces. The suspension of the abdomen across a breakaway section of the table permits an "open wedge" at the anterior margin of the disk space, a setup that is thought to reduce the resistance to a posteroanterior thrust. The thrust itself is applied perpendicular to the spine. The segmental contact point is either the spinous process or lamina, using the nailpoint one and nailpoint two contacts on the doctor. The patient's face is turned toward the side of laterality of the subluxation, if there is a lateral component to the listing, or to the side of restriction, if that is the listing, and is kept neutral if there is not.

OUTCOME ASSESSMENT

The outcomes are not distinguished from the diagnostic criteria. Thus, X-ray demonstration of vertebral realignment is considered of prime significance, as would be palpatory demonstration of improved motion.

SAFETY AND RISK FACTORS

The only contraindications to care are those that are germane to HVLA manipulative techniques in general, e.g., fractures, dislocations, tumors.[2] Meric Technique is always applied to a prone patient, and rotational and side-posture adjustments are avoided.

EVIDENCE OF EFFICACY

There are many published and often high-quality studies that demonstrate the clinical and cost-effectiveness of HVLA thrusting. In all likelihood it would be fair to expect that the Meric Technique, as an HVLA technique, would share in this beneficial outcome.

An interesting blinded, randomized trial was conducted by Cleveland and several colleagues,[11] apparently within the Cleveland Chiropractic College system, and thus almost certainly emphasizing, if not exclusively using, Meric Technique methods. In this study, experimental subjects showed improved two-point discrimination and force estimation tasks following adjustments, and to a lesser extent followed coarser manipulations than a non-treated control group.

No difference was found between the results of a single office visit using the Meric Technique as compared with the Activator Methods technique, although both groups showed reduced low-back pain as measured using a visual analog pain scale.[12] A patient with cervical spondylotic radiculotherapy responded well to Meric treatment methods in eight visits over a 26-day period, and remained pain-free, without neurological deficits, at a 4-month follow-up.[13]

CONCLUSIONS

- In view of the fact that the Meric System of analysis, having to do with visceral concomitants of segmental subluxation, is historically related to Meric Recoil Technique (or FSS), an HVLA specific adjusting method, it can be challenging to tease the two apart.
- Carpenter et al studied the relationship of organ irritation and spinal mobility, in an investigation having to do with the Meric analytic system.[14] CS Cleveland, Jr, in his animal research report,[7] quoted heavily from the infamous Winsor report,[15] which related visceral disease seen on autopsy with spinal curvatures.
- The Cleveland study,[11] which found enhanced peripheral nervous system sensory function in adjusted subjects compared to controls, was a well-done study conducted in what may as well be considered the prehistory of chiropractic research, and deserves to be acknowledged for that; so must be the animal research of CS Cleveland, Jr.[7]
- The Meric system of analysis has become increasingly controversial over the years (see, for example, Nansel and Szlazak,[16] but the Meric system of vertebral adjusting remains as mainstream and well-regarded as ever.

REFERENCES

1. Thomas R 1991 Full Spine Specific (Meric) Technic. In: Hansen D (ed.) Transactions of the Consortium for Chiropractic Research, pp. 295–302. Consortium for Chiropractic Research, Monterey, CA
2. Claus C 1995 Technique assessment outline: Meric Technique. In: Report to the Panel of Advisors to the ACA Council on Technique, p. 7 (unpublished)
3. Christensen M G 2000 Job analysis of chiropractic. A project report, survey analysis and summary of the practice of chiropractic within the United States. National Board of Chiropractic Examiners, Greeley, CO
4. Dye A A 1969 The evolution of chiropractic – its discovery and development. Reprint of 1939 edition published by author. Richmond Hill, NY
5. Leach R A 1986 The chiropractic theories, 2nd edn. Williams & Wilkins, Baltimore, MD
6. Cleveland C S I 1992 The high-velocity thrust adjustment. In: Haldeman S (ed.) Principles and practice of chiropractic, 1st edn. pp. 459–482. Appleton & Lange, Norwalk, CT
7. Cleveland C S, Jr 1965 Researching the subluxation on the domestic rabbit. Science Review of Chiropractic 1 (4): 5–28
8. Palmer D D 1914 The chiropractor. Press of Beacon Light, Los Angeles, CA
9. Burcon M 2002 BJ's $50000 Timpograph still captures our imagination after more than fifty years. Digest of Chiropractic Economics 38 (3): 54–55
10. Cleveland C S Sr 1951 Chiropractic practic and principles – outline. C S Cleveland Sr, Kansas City, MO
11. Cleveland III C 1982 Spinal correction effects on motor and sensory functions. In: Mazzarelli J P (ed.) Chiropractic interprofessional research, pp. 21–31. Offset Olona, Milano, Italy
12. Gemmell H A, Jacobson B H 1995 The immediate effect of Activator vs. Meric adjustment on acute low back pain: a randomized controlled trial. Journal of Manipulative and Physiological Therapeutics 18 (7): 453–456

13. Gemmell H A 1994 Cervical spondylotic radiculopathy treated with the Meric technique: a case report. Chiropractic Technique 6 (1): 14–16
14. Carpenter S, Hoffman J, Mendel R 1979 An investigation into the effect of organ irritation on muscle strength and spinal mobility. Journal of Clinical Chiropractic 3 (1): 42–60
15. Winsor H K 1921 Sympathetic segmental disturbances – II. The Medical Times (November): 267–271
16. Nansel D, Szlazak M 1995 Somatic dysfunction and the phenomenon of visceral disease simulation: a probable explanation for the apparent effectiveness of somatic therapy in patients presumed to be suffering from true visceral disease. Journal of Manipulative and Physiological Therapeutics 18 (6): 379–397

20

Gonstead Chiropractic Technique (GCT)

This chapter is partially based on previously published material, and is printed with the permission of the National University of Health Sciences

INTRODUCTION

GCT was less well-known in the Canada of the mid-1980s, when Gleberzon was a student at the Canadian Memorial Chiropractic College, than it is now. And so it was, that with great enthusiasm, he took advantage of a rare opportunity to attend a seminar put on by Gonstead doctors straight from Mount Horeb, where Clarence Gonstead himself had practiced and taught his seminars. There were hundreds of chiropractors and chiropractic students in attendance. The first 2 h were filled with venerable old-time Gonstead practitioners recounting tales of what can only be described as miraculous cures, as though there were a divine power at play. (Were these doctors from Mount Horeb, as they claimed, or Mount Sinai?) Gleberzon could not help but be impressed.

At the break, the speakers offered to adjust any members of the audience who thought they needed an adjustment. When it was Gleberzon's turn, the Gonstead doctor sat him down and proceeded to palpate his neck, finding several of the kind of unhappy joints that often lurk in the necks of first-year chiropractic students. Then, without taking a history, or performing any other physical examination procedures, he asked permission to adjust his neck. Gleberzon, figuring he had come this far and may as well let it go all the way, nodded assent. Now, he had only been adjusted by a few chiropractors up until then, and has been adjusted by many since, but Gleberzon can honestly say at the current time that this Gonstead adjustment was the hardest

he has ever received; not hard in the sense of painful, but hard in the sense of *powerful*.

Gonstead is a very widely practiced technique system. According to the National Board of Chiropractic Examiners survey,[1] some 59% of the respondents say they use it, although not exclusively, and 29% of their patients receive Gonstead care. Vear[2] thinks its analytic and adjustive methods are so typical of the mainstream of chiropractic, so generic, that GCT should hardly be considered a technique system – but we disagree. One need simply ask the next Gonstead practitioner who walks by: "Hey, is Gonstead a technique system, or an umbrella for all things chiropractic?" There can be no doubt what the answer would be. Although flattered by the suggestion that their technique includes so much that is considered mainstream and essential to chiropractic, we would find our Gonstead friends (affectionately called *Gondroids* by some) most willing to point out how their methods differ from so many of the other technique systems. GCT is big enough to have what may be called Gonstead tendencies, adherents who espouse somewhat different types of Gonstead-inspired practices of chiropractic. As we have seen in the case of other technique systems, such as Sacro-Occipital Technique (Ch. 25), the passing of the founder eventually led to a splintering, and some acrimony as to which individuals would be the legitimate heirs. We know in advance we will not be able to impress all of the Gonstead adherents equally with the accuracy of our work, and yet we hope they will all think we have captured the spirit of the methods of Clarence Gonstead.

OVERVIEW

In a phrase, the Gonstead practitioner seeks to "Give the Right Adjustment at the Right Place and at the Right Time."[3, 4] The "right adjustment" is a specific high-velocity, low-amplitude (HVLA) thrust that corrects a subluxation, and with it, the associated nerve interference. Firczak quotes Dr. Gonstead as having said: "it only takes three adjustments on the wrong vertebra to make it a subluxation."[5]

The GCT fosters a multifactorial examination procedure directed at identifying the various components of the vertebral subluxation complex, which is congruently regarded as a multidimensional entity. The evaluation procedures include history taking, visual inspection, general physical examination, static and motion palpation, static and dynamic (stress) radiography, and instrumentation (primarily thermography). The adjusting strategy itself emphasizes specificity, HVLA thrusting with audible release, lines of drive that favor posteroanterior and eschew rotational vectors, and avoiding thrusts directed against hypermobile compensations.

HISTORY

Dr. Clarence Gonstead saw his engineering education interrupted by World War I, at which time he was drafted into the military. After serving as an aviation technician, he rejoined civilian life to take a BS degree. While a university student, he became disabled with rheumatic fever. Although medical doctors were unable to help him, a chiropractor enabled him to resume his studies within a month. Following this personally impressive experience with chiropractic, Gonstead completed a chiropractic education and began practice in the year 1923.[6,7] The neurocalometer, developed at the Palmer College during his term there, formed an important element of his practice from the beginning. His practice grew to be so immense that by 1964 he had to construct an inn to lodge the many patients who flocked to his new and very large clinic in Mount Horeb, Wisconsin. A licensed pilot, he would fly his own plane from his personal airstrip to the laboratory of the Lincoln College of Chiropractic, where he would dissect and study cadaver spines. This led to an elaborate model of spinal derangement, with special emphasis on discopathy. He typically worked 6½ days per week, from 7.00 a.m. until late at night, while somehow being able to pursue a very active teaching and lecturing schedule as well. His personal rapport with patients was legendary.

During his long and distinguished career, Gonstead pioneered the use of many instruments for the detection of "nerve pressure." He also perfected multispeed X-ray screens, developed the use of the knee–chest table, refined the Zenith Hi-Lo table, and worked out many new concepts for the chiropractic profession. Among these, perhaps his "disk concept" of the mid-1930s, discussed below, has left the most indelible mark on the profession.

Two Palmer graduates, brothers Alex Cox (1964) and Douglas Cox (1967), joined the Gonstead Clinic staff to help Dr. Gonstead with documenting his work.[8] In 1974, Gonstead sold his chiropractic holdings, including the Mount Horeb facility, the Gonstead Seminar of Chiropractic, Gonstead Management Services, and a motor hotel, to the Cox brothers.[3,8] Dr. Gonstead passed away in 1978, leaving his entire estate to the chiropractic profession as "student chiropractor scholarships" and "teaching chairs" for the chiropractic colleges.[8]

DEFINITION OF TECHNIQUE-SPECIFIC TERMS

There is not much jargon utterly unique to the Gonstead system, but there are a number of phrases that take on such importance, and are used so characteristically, that it is worthwhile listing and briefly discussing a few.

- Subluxation: "A vertebral misalignment that results in nerve interference;"[9] "The disrelationship of the facets is the result of, and secondary to, the misalignment at the ... intervertebral disc"[10]
- Compensation: "A misalignment in the spine created as a result of the body trying to offset

or overcome the imbalances created by a subluxation"[7]

- Level foundation: the sacrum is considered the base of the spine:[10] vertebrae that begin lateral inclinations of the spine in relationship to the sacral level base are considered possible *subluxations*, whereas those vertebrae that terminate these lateral inclinations by regaining a parallel relationship to the sacral base would be termed *compensations*

- Lateral wedge, open wedge, "high side of the rainbow": all of these expressions refer to the convex side of a lateral flexion malposition, thought to result from ipsilateral shifting of the nucleus pulposus

- "Through the plane line of the disc": Gonstead practitioners are adamant about adjusting vertebrae posterior to anterior, with a thrust parallel to the disk plane. Herbst goes so far as to suggest that contrary strategies "may have altered the course of our profession by convincing thousands of chiropractors that 'adjusting' a vertebra cannot change its position, does not get people well, and is painful to the patient"[10] (p. 81)

- Posteriority: Gonstead practitioners believe that, with the exception of atlas, a vertebra must subluxate posteriorly in relationship to the segment below (for opposing views, see Harrison[11])

- Intersegmental range of motion (IROM) motion palpation: a type of motion palpation, intended to identify segmental loss of full ROM in any of the six degrees of freedom; it is to be contrasted with the other main type of motion palpation, end-feel or end-play joint assessment.[12]

- Sympathetic and parasympathetic nervous systems: Dr. Gonstead believed that the spinal range C5–occiput and below L5 governed the parasympathetic nervous system, and C6–L5 the sympathetic nervous system.[13] (p. 357)

PHYSIOLOGICAL MECHANISMS AND RATIONALE

Subluxation is thought to result from trauma to the spine, which initiates damage to the intervertebral disk and initiates a sequence of events that culminates in nerve interference. According to Cremata et al,[14] Gonstead theorized that subluxation developed in stages, starting with fixation, progressing to misalignment and cumulative damage to the disk, and finally to nerve interference. Contemporary practitioners strongly believe that "the most important part of spinal misalignment is posteriority…the least important of spinal misalignments is rotation."[15] The goal is always to move the vertebral body into a more normal position relative to the disk.

Some GCT practitioners state that *subluxation* refers to misalignment of the disk, especially the nucleus pulposus. "The disc, as always, is the key."[5] According to a 1973 newsletter,[16] Gonstead formulated his disk concept in the mid-1930s after doing a number of dissections: "I wanted to see how it was that the nerve pressure was produced. I found that the vertebra slipped on the disc dislodging the nucleus which protruded into various parts of the disc producing the pressure on the nerves. I found that the most common area for this occurrence was at the intervertebral foramen. The technique of adjusting I developed consisted of moving the segments onto the disc repositioning the nucleus. Therein lies the uniqueness of my work."[16]

It has been suggested that an adjustment directed *below* the level of involvement usually fails to improve the patient, whereas an adjustment directed *above* the fixated segment will worsen the patient and increase the pain. The explanation is that fixations are generally accompanied by compensatory hypermobility in superior segments, with ligamentous instability and a tendency toward neurological dysfunction.

Gonstead practitioners tend to be suspicious of pain as a diagnostic indicator, and certainly address non-painful areas of the spine with as much attention as painful areas. They believe that asymptomatic subluxations in a given area may interfere with improvement in a symptomatic, treated area.[7]

DIAGNOSTIC/ANALYTIC PROCEDURES

Cremata et al,[14] after describing vertebral subluxation as a multivariate complex, recommend that the diagnostic regimen feature multiple components. Although they recognize that for the most part there is nothing uniquely Gonstead in any one of their procedures, they nevertheless claim originality for at least one point: "the concept of using most, if not all, of these examination procedures routinely to assist in the identification of subluxated motion segments and the weighing of the relative value of each test based on the magnitude of the deviation from normal, rather than solely the variable the test is assessing."[14]

In order of importance, Alex Cox lists the following diagnostic procedures for identifying the "Right Place" to adjust: "instrumentation, digital palpation, motion palpation, visual analysis, and finally, X-ray."[3] On the role of X-ray, Cox attributes the following remark to Clarence Gonstead: "It is very important to find the subluxation on the patient, and then take the x-ray to verify the findings."[3] Indeed, "x-ray examination of the patient is absolutely necessary whenever possible."[7] Plaugher has described the difference between medical and chiropractic usage of diagnostic radiology, especially in terms of establishing in specific cases the safety of HVLA adjusting.[17]

The preferred spinographic procedure involves a 14×36 in. (35×90 cm) anteroposterior (AP) full-spine view, and a unique lateral view involving two 14×18 in. (35×45 cm) exposures taken in a single 14×36 in. (35×90 cm) film (a "split-screen" exposure). The lateral view is said to provide most of the information, given the primacy GCT affords to the disk. The AP view has been stated to provide information primarily about the pelvis.[18] Some contemporary Gonstead practitioners have stressed the value of functional radiographic analysis, primarily stress plain films taken in lateral flexion and flexion/extension.[14] There has also been some recent experimentation and experience with videofluoroscopy.[19]

The fundamental importance of instrumentation (primarily thermography) is thought to be that it establishes the "Right Time": that is, when the adjustment is most likely to benefit the patient. Gonstead clinicians subscribe to the classic conception that, while other examination procedures may pertain to vertebral misalignment and movement abnormalities, it is instrumentation that confirms nerve interference. According to Alex Cox, "If there is no pressure on the nerve, adjusting is not necessary."[18] Cremata et al further explain that "bilateral temperature differential instrumentation and galvanic skin response testing are used to identify areas that may be suggestive of local autonomic disturbances or local changes due to inflammation and the subsequent production of heat."[14]

The classic Gonstead vertebral subluxation listings generally include three components: P for posteriority, R or L for the side of spinous process deviation, and S (superior) or I (inferior) for lateral flexion malpositioning. Although his idea does not appear to have been taken up, Troxell proposed adding a quantitative component to the Gonstead listings (e.g., $P_{18}L_5S_{10}$).[20] Other contemporary practitioners favor the use of an orthogonal system which considers all six degrees of freedom.[13,14]

Gonstead used a "nerve tracer,"[5] now known as an electrical conductor scanner (ECS) or galvanic skin response (GSR) instrument. This is consistent with the Gonstead conception that subluxation is always accompanied by nerve interference, which will inevitably result in autonomic nervous system dysfunction. Following negative research findings,[21,22] this tool appears to have been abandoned.

TREATMENT/ADJUSTIVE PROCEDURES

The GCT is fundamentally a full-spine, osseous technique, emphasizing specific HVLA thrusts. The GCT's staunch support for HVLA-style treatment is confirmed by Cox's rejection of non-force and soft-tissue techniques: "Chiropractic was founded, designed, and built on osseous spinal adjusting procedures ... the most sound approach in chiropractic today."[3] "All corrections should be audible ... a single, solid sound is much more representative of a good vertebral correction than the typical 'rattle' heard in general manipulation."[7] The intent of the thrust is to move the vertebral body toward a more normal weight-bearing position on the disk. This is best effected by a posterior to anterior thrust, with little or no rotation.

Unlike some adjusting styles, the doctor releases from the thrust slowly,[7,14] avoiding the rebound that is typical of toggle-recoil type of adjustments.

The criteria for the "Right Adjustment" include the doctor's contact point, the contact on the patient, the line of drive, the depth of the thrust, and the table used.[3] Gonstead doctors often praise the great care Upper Cervical practitioners devote to analyzing and adjusting the atlas, and Cremata et al add that the GCT extends this same specificity and precision to the other vertebrae and the sacroiliac joints. "The most important tool in the reduction of the vertebral subluxation complex is the specific vertebral adjustment."[14] Plaugher also emphasizes this specificity in his heavily Gonstead-influenced chiropractic book, *Textbook of Clinical Chiropractic: A Specific Biomechanical Approach*[13] and in a book chapter.[12] Although as a general rule the thrust is directed so as exactly to reverse the specific subluxation listing, some Gonstead practitioners will also take into account global motion asymmetries,[14] which may play even a dominant role in determining side-specificity. Some GCT practitioners emphasize the importance of not adjusting the sympathetic and parasympathetic nervous systems (although these are characterized somewhat unconventionally) on the same office visit, at least in the case of an acute patient. In a representative statement, GCT practitioner Firczak states: "Never mix the systems when dealing with any visceral problem."[5]

There are a few treatment procedures and pieces of equipment which, although not unique to the GCT, find their greatest application within it. The knee–chest table,[23,24] originally invented for the purpose of cervical adjusting, is said to improve mechanical advantage in adjusting, especially in the case of obese, pregnant, or very large patients. The cervical chair permits adjusting the articulations cephalad to T3 with the patient in a seated position. According to Cox," Its effectiveness comes from the ability to use a posterior to anterior and inferior line of drive ... [this] allows a deep adjustment to the disc while taking into consideration the flat cervical facets."[7]

Gonstead clinicians almost always use the "cervical chair" for sitting cervical adjustments.[25]

It is a chair with an adjustable hinged back, used in conjunction with a strap that fixes the patient's torso when the thrust is delivered. The "lift and set" motion[25] is thought to explain how the clinician can thrust through the plane line of the disk without jamming the cervical facets, which are quite oblique to the disks. In an unusual endorsement of muscle spasm, one Gonstead clinician theorizes that the cervical chair move causes "a splinting reaction by the muscles which serve this joint ... [and] is necessary so that the patient doesn't lose too much of the correction between visits."[25]

Unlike most other chiropractic practitioners (or so it would seem), a few Gonstead authorities are not in general averse to treating certain fractures, such as compression fractures of the mid thoracic/lumbar area.[5,13,26] There is also a case report describing the adjustive care of a patient with a lamina fracture of C6, although thrusting procedures were not applied to that segment specifically.[27] Plaugher et al acknowledge the clinical need to identify fractures prior to initiating chiropractic adjusting, in a case report.[28]

There are a large number of Gonstead technique provisos, a few representative examples of which may be worth mentioning in passing:

- A segment must go posterior first in order to subluxate.
- The most posterior segment must be adjusted.[19]
- With the exception of C1, all vertebral adjustments must be directed through the plane line of the disk.[7]
- "Starting from the bottom, adjust the lowest subluxation three to five times before moving up."[5]
- Nerve interference occurs on the open side (i.e., divergent disk angle side) of the wedge.
- Adjust through the "plane line of the disc," on the "high side of the rainbow."
- List the innominate on the side to which the body of L5 has rotated.
- The segment cephalad to a hypomobile subluxation is usually a hypermobile compensation.

- Gonstead procedures must not be mixed with other technique procedures, lest this "reduce the quality of its application."[15]

ANCILLARY PROCEDURES

At the time of a 1984 interview,[29] Cox claimed that the Mount Horeb clinic, in order to comply with the scope of chiropractic practice laws of the state of Wisconsin, confined its procedures to hands-only adjustment, some advice on nutritional supplements, and general advice on nutrition and exercise. Many, if not most, Gonstead practitioners are quite content, in whatever state they practice, to limit their ancillary practice to these procedures. Cremata et al state: "As a rule, Gonstead practitioners tend to be full spine adjusters who use minimal adjunctive services. Adjunctive therapies are commonly used only as they assist in the reduction of the vertebral subluxation complex."[14] Physical therapy is therefore unimportant at best, and better avoided: "If the patient requires therapy we would like to refer him to people who are in that business specifically" (Alex Cox, quoted by Blaurock-Busch.[15] Thus, physical therapy is by and large not supported.

OUTCOME ASSESSMENT

There is no effective distinction between the Gonstead diagnostic procedures and outcome measures. The goal of care is the reduction or elimination of the signs and symptoms of the vertebral subluxation complex, although it may be asymptomatic in some cases. Pain is seen as something of a "great deceiver," just as likely, if not more likely, to manifest a hypermobile compensation as a true hypomobile subluxation.

SAFETY AND RISK FACTORS

GCT practitioners generally acknowledge the same contraindications to HVLA thrusting as other osseous practitioners. None the less, in some cases they have de-emphasized commonly listed contraindications (e.g., managing and even adjusting some types of fractures.[26])

Gonstead clinicians typically enjoin a tremendous opposition to rotational adjustment/ manipulation, as manifested in the following representative statement: "The most dangerous technique in spinal manipulation is excessive rotation of the spinal column." This has led to rather harsh judgments of non-Gonstead manipulative procedures: "We wouldn't want to be associated with a doctor who lumbar-rolls a patient both sides, or does his cervical adjustments supine" (Alex Cox); "There is nothing specific about the osteopath's approach. They just move a bone without any feeling or concern" (Doug Cox).[18]

The prohibition of rotational manipulation owes some of its militancy to the alleged relationship of vascular accidents to rotatory cervical adjustments. GCT practitioners believe that "the use of Gonstead cervical adjustments will minimize the risk of vascular accidents."[5] Likewise, the elimination of flexion and rotation in the adjusting line of drive is thought to reduce the potential for damage to the lumbar disks.[14]

Plaugher and Lopes[24] describe a few contraindications specific to the knee–chest table, including "fractures of the lamina, severe osteolytic activity and any segment exhibiting normal or hypermobility." Severe lumbar hypolordosis presents a special problem, as does severe hyperlordosis of both the lumbar and cervical spines, which is unlikely to benefit from a thrust which increases extension. A patient who has trouble relaxing is unlikely to be treated effectively on a knee–chest table. WA Cox lists each of the following as contraindications to knee–chest adjusting: pain on lumbar extension, lumbar kyphosis, lower-spine spondylolisthesis, and advanced low-back spondylosis, osteoporosis, or osteoarthritis.[7,14] Cox also lists some rather obvious contraindications for side-posture lumbar adjustments, including osteoporosis, hip prosthesis, and inability to bend the knees.[7]

EVIDENCE OF EFFICACY
Diagnostic efficacy

There have been a number of studies concerning the reliability of Gonstead X-ray line-marking procedures. Phillips[30] compared pelvic X-ray line-marking systems developed by Gonstead, Hildebrandt, and Winterstein. The numerous discrepancies that arose indicated the need for continued research on the reliability and validity of these procedures. Plaugher and Hendricks found "substantial" intra- and interexaminer reliability in using the GCT X-ray line-marking procedures, and in every case the intraexaminer test–retest reliability was greater.[31] On the other hand, Burk et al,[32] in their study of Gonstead X-ray line marking, could not obtain better than "slight" to "fair" interexaminer and "fair" to "moderate" intraexaminer reliability. In a review article, Harrison et al[33] concluded that the Gonstead line-marking procedures are highly reproducible. Another study did at least validate the reproducibility of patient positioning for pelvic radiography, as measured by the Gonstead X-ray line-marking procedures, at 1 h and at 18-day intervals.[34]

There is precious little information available on the *validity* of the Gonstead X-ray line-marking procedures. Nevertheless, Specht and De Boer used them as the analytic engine in their study of the relationship of anatomical leg-length inequality and abnormal spine curves and curvatures.[35] Schram et al[36] X-rayed a dry articulated pelvis in a variety of tilted and rotated positions, and then used Gonstead line marking rules to analyze the films. They found that, although small amounts of rotations did not affect posterior-inferior/anterior-superior (PI/AS) listings, they did dramatically affect internal/external (IN/EX) listings: each degree of rotation produced 1.87 mm change in IN/EX listings. Pelvic tilt had minimal effect on both PI/AS and IN/EX calls. These data suggest that the Gonstead pelvic X-ray marking procedures are likely to generate bogus listings as the result of even minimal patient *y*-axis rotational positioning errors. Both Hildebrandt[37] and Harrison[38] came to similar conclusions.

Jeffery,[39] in a doctoral dissertation performed at the Anglo-European College of Chiropractic, characterized three general methods of radiometry for pelvic torsion. Adapted versions of these methods were then used to calculate innominate tilting of a dry specimen tilted to varying known degrees and radiographed. Since Jeffery did not actually produce pelvic torsion in the dry specimen,

having merely rotated the entire pelvis in the sagittal plane and applied the line-marking rules to one hemipelvis, the work is not entirely satisfactory. That stated, Jeffery found the Gonstead method neither reliable nor sensitive for detecting AS/PI relationships compared with the other two methods, which were both adequate.

Cooperstein[40,41] investigated the effects of pelvic torsion on bilateral innominate measurements through a computer simulation. He concluded that the Gonstead line-marking system for innominate torsion could be potentially validated provided a number of stringent conditions are satisfied: there is a relatively large amount of pelvic torsion, in a patient with a steep sagittal plane sacral base angle, who receives full-spine radiography. The analytic system would not be useful for patients with normal or flattened sacral base angles, nor for small degrees of pelvic torsion, nor in sectional radiography.

Zengel and Davis, having devised a mathematical system for determining X-ray projectional distortion,[42] applied this methodology to calculate the effects of induced vertical and horizontal vertebral body off-centering[43] and of induced lateral flexion malposition.[44] They found that "in every instance, off-centering produced no measurable effect on the position of the constructed Gonstead lines" drawn parallel to the vertebral endplates in an AP X-ray. Therefore, these lines would be interpretable "as is," there being no need to correct for projectional distortion.

It has already been noted that Gonstead and some later GCT practitioners formerly used a GSR instrument. It was thought to identify both spinal subluxations and extremity misalignments,[14,23] according to the belief that articular dysfunction would be manifested by alterations in electrical conductance. However, Nansel and Jansen[45] found very poor test–retest reliability in using the ECS, and furthermore, that the instrument seemed to *create* the lowered electrical resistance it was designed to detect. Another interexaminer reliability test also generated only modest levels of interexaminer concordance, leading the investigators to conclude that the use of the ECS in examining asymptomatic subjects was not presently supported.[22]

Plaugher, in a review of the literature regarding spinal thermography, concluded that the handheld thermocouple devices popular among Gonstead practitioners (which descend directly from the neurocalometer), seem to manifest less interexaminer reliability than infrared devices.[17] His own study of the Nervo-Scope generated at best equivocal results,[46] but with an interesting tendency for intraclass correlations to be higher for a second series of observations: "The authors speculated that as the instrument was used in a repeat sequence, positive findings became more stable and frivolous temperature fluctuations were 'erased.'"[17]

According to Plaugher,[12] there have been no clinical trials aimed at evaluating the value of Gonstead-style intersegmental range of motion assessment (motion palpation). He cautions against coming to any premature conclusions concerning it, pro or con.

Treatment efficacy

From a basic science point of view, Kawchuk and Herzog[47] showed that Gonstead-style thrusts generate forces similar to those generated by similar HVLA styles, and considerably higher than, for example, the force generated by a handheld percussive instrument.

In a study designed to determine if HVLA adjustments could alter static radiological parameters such as retrolisthesis, the extent of the lordotic curves, and Cobb's angle, Plaugher et al[48] measured a statistically significant but very small reduction in retrolisthesis, the only intersegmental subluxation parameter assessed in their study. There was a high degree of interexaminer reliability in measuring some, but apparently not all, of the parameters. There were letters to the editor and rejoinders.

Nansel et al[49] found that a Gonstead cervical chair move, delivered to the lower cervical spine on the side found to be most restricted in lateral flexion by goniometric examination, would dramatically reduce the motion asymmetry. Another follow-up study[50] demonstrated that this amelioration of asymmetry would prove stable for at least 48 h in subjects lacking a previous history of neck trauma, whereas the asymmetry in passive

end-range would tend to return among the subjects who had experienced previous trauma. In yet another follow-up study, again using cervical chair adjusting methods, Nansel et al[51] were able to demonstrate that Gonstead upper cervical adjustments were relatively more effective than lower cervical adjustments at ameliorating cervical rotational asymmetry, whereas lower cervical adjustments were relatively more effective than upper cervical adjustments at ameliorating lateral flexion asymmetry.

There is a case report of successful treatment of a meniscal tear,[52] and another describes resolution of symptoms in a man who had received a clinically unsuccessful discectomy of C6.[53] Lantz and Chen[54] investigated whether HVLA adjustive care (including Gonstead adjustive procedures) would influence the course of adolescent idiopathic scoliosis in curves less than 20°. Since not only Gonstead but Diversified procedures were used, and heel lifts and lifestyle counseling were also available to the patients, we must exercise caution in concluding that Gonstead procedures were ineffective, despite the finding that chiropractic care was not effective in reducing the severity of scoliotic curves.

There are a few case reports and series, and one randomized trial, on the somatovisceral effects of Gonstead-style adjustments. Both Hood[55] (uncontrolled case series) and Plaugher and Bachman[56] (one case report) reported success in controlling hypertension in treatment programs including Gonstead-style specific, short-lever HVLA thrusts. Nansel et al,[57] in examining the effects of similar adjustments on asymptomatic subjects, found no changes in blood pressure, heart rate, or plasma catecholamine levels. There are case reports suggesting that there were adjustive benefits in a case of epilepsy,[52] a reduction of headache-related symptoms in a case of temporomandibular disorder,[58] and improvement in a case of myasthenia gravis.[59] Most recently, Plaugher et al[60] conducted a practice-based randomized controlled-comparison clinical trial of Gonstead adjustments vs massage in patients with essential hypertension. The control group showed the most improvement in their hypertensive state, followed by the adjustive care group; the massage group improved the least.

CONCLUSIONS

- Vear, after distinguishing between what he calls "general adjustive technique" and technique "system approaches," says that the GCT "comes closest to having met his criteria for its acceptance as a non-technique system."[2] It is not obvious that what Dr. Vear meant as a compliment would be taken as such by all Gonstead practitioners, who may prefer being regarded as distinct from other technique systems.

- Gonstead believed C5–occiput and below L5 governed the parasympathetic nervous system, and C6–L5 the sympathetic nervous system.[13] (p. 357) The obvious discrepancy compared with mainstream descriptions of the anatomy of the nervous system warrants further consideration.

- It is common for GCT to recommend palpating for edema and other signs of acute inflammation. For example, Cremata et al state that GCT examination procedures are directed at identifying "swelling, heat, altered function, redness, and pain."[14] Since chronic inflammation is a clinical entity very different from acute inflammation, essentially lacking the cardinal signs such as swelling and redness, it is not obvious why one would expect a chronic patient to display such signs.

- Among the various thermography technologies, Gonstead practitioners usually use dual-probed devices such as the Nervo-Scope, rather than infrared devices that do not touch the skin. As can be seen in obvious reddening of the skin of patients examined using tools like the Nervo-Scope, we cannot rule out that it produces acute inflammation during the examination process.[61,62] Thus, it may *produce* the asymmetry it purports to detect.

- GCT practitioners follow a multivariate approach to subluxation identification, rather than rely on any one or very few examination findings.[14] Given the multiplicity of diagnostic procedures claimed by GCT advocates, and given the claim that it is the concordance of several such procedures rather than any one finding in particular that confirms the subluxation complex, it would be useful to note if indeed clinicians using such a multivariate system would achieve an acceptable degree of concordance. This is especially important given the many negative studies on the interexaminer agreement of *individual tests*.

- Rhudy et al,[63] hypothesizing that better results may accrue when "the findings of several different procedures are interrelated," examined the interexaminer concordance of three trained clinicians when they employed a multifactorial examination procedure consisting of Gonstead-style AP full-spine radiography, motion palpation, and dual-probe thermography. The levels of agreement turned out to be quite low, on the basis of which the investigators concluded "clinical judgements are probably based more on other subjective impressions on the part of the chiropractor than the information derived from the procedures themselves."[63] Jansen and Nansel came to a similar conclusion from a more theoretical point of view by performing a Monte Carlo experiment (a methodology that involves generating random numbers to simulate experimental findings) that determined chance concordance rates in a multiple diagnostic test scenario.[64]

- The Gonstead emphasis on disk pathology, and their discocentric view of the subluxation entity, seem quite consistent with contemporary views on the high rate of occurrence of discogenic back pain.[65]

- The Gonstead advocacy of the AP full-spine radiological view finds support in a review by Taylor,[66] who concludes "full-spine radiography is an effective diagnostic and analytic procedure with an acceptable risk/benefit ratio."

REFERENCES

1. Christensen M G 2000 Job analysis of chiropractic. A project report, survey analysis and summary of the practice of chiropractic within the United States. National Board of Chiropractic Examiners, Greeley, CO

2. Vear H J 1981 Introduction to chiropractic science. Western States Chiropractic College, Portland, OR

3. Cox A W 1992 The Gonstead system. American Chiropractor (November/December): 38

4. Cox W A 1982 The Gonstead system. American Chiropractor (July/August): 68

5. Firczak S W 1988 The Gonstead technique: a review. Today's Chiropractic (July/August): 25–26

6. Butler M 1973 Gonstead: 50 years. Today's Chiropractic (August/September): 24–26

7. Cox W A 1982 Overview of the Gonstead technique. In: Mazzarelli J P (ed.) Chiropractic interprofessional research, pp. 41–46. Offset Olona, Milano, Italy

8. Fernandez P G 1987 The miracle man. Chiropractic Achievers (Fall): 41–44

9. Cox W A 1986 The Gonstead technique. Today's Chiropractic (May/June): 75

10. Herbst A 1980 Gonstead chiropractic science and art: the chiropractic methodology of Clarence S Gonstead. Schichi Publications Mount Horeb, WI

11. Harrison D D 1992 Subluxation: a mechanical engineering definition. In: Harrison D (ed.) Spinal biomechanics: a chiropractic perspective, pp. 11–32. Harrison PBC Seminars, Evaston, WY

12. Plaugher G 1994 Specific-contact, short-lever-arm articular procedures: advances in the Gonstead technique. In: Lawrence DJ, Cassidy D, McGregor M, et al (eds) Advances in chiropractic. Mosby-Year Book, St Louis, MO

13. Plaugher G (ed.) 1993 Textbook of clinical chiropractic: a specific biomechanical approach. Williams & Wilkins, Baltimore, MD

14. Cremata E E, Plaugher G, Cox W A 1991 Technique system application: the Gonstead approach. Chiropractic Technique 3 (1): 19–25

15. Cox W A 1984 Interview [with W Alex Cox]. American Chiropractor (May): 15–20

16. Author unknown 1973 Three expansions: Dr C S Gonstead celebrates 50 years in chiropractic. Today's Chiropractic (August/September): 5

17. Plaugher G 1992 Skin temperature assessment for neuromusculoskeletal abnormalities of the spinal column. Journal of Manipulative and Physiological Therapeutics 15 (6): 365–381

18. Blaurock-Busch E 1984 What's new at Gonstead? An exclusive interview with Drs Alex and Doug Cox, Mt Horeb, WI and Dr. Juan Ferry, South Weymouth, MA. Digest of Chiropractic Economics (May/June): 69

19. Firczak S W 1987 A review of the Gonstead technique. Today's Chiropractic (August): 57–59

20. Troxell J L 1984 An expansion to the Gonstead listing system. Digest of Chiropractic Economics (March/April): 130

21. Nansel D D, Jansen R D 1988 Concordance between galvanic skin response and spinal palpation findings in pain-free males. Journal of Manipulative and Physiological Therapeutics 11 (4): 267–272

22. Plaugher G, Haas M, Doble R W Jr et al 1993 The interexaminer reliability of a galvanic skin response instrument. Journal of Manipulative and Physiological Therapeutics 16 (7): 453–459

23. Firczak S W 1990 Innovations in the Gonstead technique. Today's Chiropractic (July/August): 46–49

24. Plaugher G, Lopes M A 1990 The knee–chest table: indications and contraindications. Chiropractic Technique 2 (4): 163–167

25. Clemen M 1989 The advantages of the cervical chair technique. Today's Chiropractic (July/August): 74–77

26. Plaugher G, Alcantara J, Hart C R 1996 Management of the patient with a chance fracture of the lumbar spine and concomitant subluxation. Journal of Manipulative and Physiological Therapeutics 19 (8): 539

27. Alcantara J, Plaugher G, Abblett D E 1997 Management of a patient with a lamina fracture of the sixth cervical vertebra and concomitant subluxation. Journal of Manipulative and Physiological Therapeutics 20 (2): 113–123

28. Plaugher G, Alcantara J, Doble R W 1996 Missed sacral fracture prior to adjustment. Journal of Manipulative and Physiological Therapeutics 19 (7): 480

29. Cox W A 1984 Interview, W Alex Cox. American Chiropractor (May): 15–20

30. Phillips R B 1975 An evaluation of the graphic analysis of the pelvis on the A-P full spine radiograph. ACA Journal of Chiropractic 9 (December): s139–s148

31. Plaugher G, Hendricks A H 1991 The inter- and intraexaminer reliability of the Gonstead pelvic marking system. Journal of Manipulative and Physiological Therapeutics 14 (9): 503–508

32. Burk J M, Rhudy T R, Ratliff C R 1990 Inter- and intraexaminer agreement using Gonstead line marking methods. American Journal of Chiropractic Medicine 3 (3): 114–117

33. Harrison D E, Harrison D D, Troyanovich S J 1998 Reliability of spinal displacement analysis of plain X-rays: a review of commonly accepted facts and fallacies with implications for chiropractic education and technique. Journal of Manipulative and Physiological Therapeutics 21 (4): 252–266

34. Plaugher G, Hendricks A H, Doble R W Jr et al 1993 The reliability of patient positioning for evaluating static radiologic parameters of the human pelvis. Journal of Manipulative and Physiological Therapeutics 16 (8): 517–522

35. Specht D L, De Boer K F 1991 Anatomical leg length inequality, scoliosis and lordotic curve in unselected clinic patients. Journal of Manipulative and Physiological Therapeutics 14 (6): 368–375

36. Schram S B, Hosek R S, Silverman H L 1981 Spinographic positioning errors in Gonstead pelvic X-ray analysis. Journal of Manipulative and Physiological Therapeutics 4 (4): 179–181

37. Hildebrandt R W 1985 Chiropractic spinography. 2nd edn. Williams & Wilkins, Baltimore, MD

38. Harrison D 1993 The pelvic listings of EX-IN, AS-IN, and PI-EX are figments of your "projected" imagination. American Journal of Clinical Chiropractic 3 (2): 18

39. Jeffery K R 1981 X-ray analysis of differential leg length and pelvic distortion. Anglo-European College of Chiropractic dissertation, Bournemouth, UK

40. Cooperstein R 1992 Roentgenometric assessment of innominate vertical length differentials. In: Hansen D (ed.) Proceedings of the 7th Annual Conference on Research and Education, pp. 273–277. Consortium for Chiropractic Research, Palm Springs, CA

41. Cooperstein R 1990 Innominate vertical length differentials as a function of pelvic torsion and pelvic carrying angle. In: Jansen R D (ed.) Proceedings of the 5th Annual Conference on Research and Education,

pp. 1–14. Consortium for Chiropractic Research, Sacramento, CA

42. Zengel F, Davis B P 1988 Biomechanical analysis by chiropractic radiography: part I. A simple method for determining X-ray projectional distortion. Journal of Manipulative and Physiological Therapeutics 11 (4): 273–280

43. Zengel F, Davis B P 1988 Biomechanical analysis by chiropractic radiography: part II. Effects of X-ray projectional distortion on apparent vertebral rotation. Journal of Manipulative and Physiological Therapeutics 11 (5): 469–473

44. Zengel F, Davis B P 1988 Biomechanical analysis by chiropractic radiography: part III. Lack of effect of projectional distortion on Gonstead vertebral endplate lines. Journal of Manipulative and Physiological Therapeutics 11 (6): 469–473

45. Nansel D D, Jansen R D 1988 Concordance between galvanic skin response and spinal palpation findings in pain-free males. Journal of Manipulative and Physiological Therapeutics 11 (4): 267–272

46. Plaugher G, Lopes M A, Melch P E, Cremata E E 1991 The inter- and intraexaminer reliability of a paraspinal skin temperature differential instrument. Journal of Manipulative and Physiological Therapeutics 14 (6): 361–367

47. Kawchuk G N, Herzog W 1993 Biomechanical characterization (fingerprinting) of five novel methods of cervical spine manipulation. Journal of Manipulative and Physiological Therapeutics 16 (9): 573–577

48. Plaugher G, Cremata E E, Phillips R B 1990 A retrospective consecutive case analysis of pretreatment and comparative static radiological parameters following chiropractic adjustments. Journal of Manipulative and Physiological Therapeutics 13 (9): 498–506

49. Nansel D, Cremata E, Carlson J, Szlazak M 1989 Effect of unilateral adjustments on goniometrically-assessed cervical lateral-flexion end-range asymmetries in otherwise asymptomatic subjects. Journal of Manipulative and Physiological Therapeutics 12 (6): 419–427

50. Nansel D, Peneff A, Cremata E, Carlson J 1990 Time course considerations for the effects of unilateral lower cervical adjustments with respect to the amelioration of cervical lateral-flexion passive end-range asymmetry. Journal of Manipulative and Physiological Therapeutics 13 (6): 297–304

51. Nansel D, Peneff A, Quitoriano J 1992 Effectiveness of upper versus lower cervical adjustments with respect to the amelioration of passive rotational versus lateral-flexion end-range asymmetries in otherwise asymptomatic subjects. Journal of Manipulative and Physiological Therapeutics 15 (2): 99–105

52. Alcantara J, Heschong R, Plaugher G 1998 Chiropractic management of a patient with subluxations, low back pain and epileptic seizures. Journal of Manipulative and Physiological Therapeutics 21 (6): 410–418

53. Alcantara J, Plaugher G, Thornton R E, Salem C 2001 Chiropractic care of a patient with vertebral subluxations and unsuccessful surgery of the cervical spine. Journal of Manipulative and Physiological Therapeutics 24 (7): 477–482

54. Lantz C A, Chen J 2001 Effect of chiropractic intervention on small scoliotic curves in younger subjects: a time-series cohort design. Journal of Manipulative and Physiological Therapeutics 24 (6): 385–393

55. Hood R P 1974 Blood pressure: results in 75 abnormal cases. Digest of Chiropractic Economics (May/June): 36–38

56. Plaugher G, Bachman T R 1993 Chiropractic management of a hypertensive patient. Journal of Manipulative and Physiological Therapeutics 16 (8): 544–549

57. Nansel D, Jansen R, Cremata E et al 1991 Effects of cervical adjustments on lateral-flexion end-range asymmetry and on blood pressure, heart rate and plasma catecholamine levels. Journal of Manipulative and Physiological Therapeutics 14 (8): 450–456

58. Alcantara J, Plaugher G, Klemp D D, Salem C 2002 Chiropractic care of a patient with temporomandibular disorder and atlas subluxation. Journal of Manipulative and Physiological Therapeutics 25 (1): 63–70

59. Alcantara J, Steiner D M, Plaugher G 1999 Chiropractic management of a patient with myasthenia gravis and vertebral subluxations. Journal of Manipulative and Physiological Therapeutics 22 (5): 333–340

60. Plaugher G, Long C R, Alcantara J et al 2002 Practice-based randomized controlled-comparison clinical trial of chiropractic adjustments and brief massage treatment at sites of subluxation in subjects with essential hypertension: pilot study. Journal of Manipulative and Physiological Therapeutics 25 (4): 221–239

61. Cooperstein R 2002 Dual probe thermography: constructive test par excellence. Journal of the American Chiropractic Association 39 (9): 32–34

62. Amalu W C, Tiscareno L H 1994 The evolution of modern paraspinal thermography. Today's Chiropractic 23 (3): 38–41

63. Rhudy T, Sandefur R M, Burk J M 1988 Interexaminer/intertechnique reliability in spinal subluxation assessment: a multifactorial approach. American Journal of Chiropractic Medicine 1 (3): 111–114

64. Jansen R D, Nansel D D 1988 Diagnostic illusions: the reliability of random chance. Journal of Manipulative and Physiological Therapeutics 11 (5): 355–365

65. Bogduk N 1995 The anatomical basis for spinal pain syndromes. Journal of Manipulative and Physiological Therapeutics 18 (9): 603–605

66. Taylor J A 1993 Full-spine radiography: a review. Journal of Manipulative and Physiological Therapeutics 16 (7): 460–474.

21

Logan Basic Technique (LBT)
Logan Basic Methods[1]

INTRODUCTION

Hugh Logan did not invent monosegmentalism in chiropractic. Apparently DD Palmer, the Founder himself, was of the opinion that the most significant subluxations occurred somewhere around the lumbothoracic transitional area. None the less, Logan was certainly one of the earliest chiropractors, if not the first, to erect an entire technique system around the primacy of one bone – in his case, the sacrum. This occurred during the mid-1920s. BJ Palmer, by comparison, announced Upper Cervical Technique to the world in the 1930s. In terms of disease etiology, monosegmentalism claims for itself the same relationship to all of chiropractic as chiropractic does for all of pathology. LBT invokes the supreme importance of sacral subluxation among all possible subluxations, just as subluxation theory invokes subluxation as the most important among all causes of disease.

Logan followed in the footsteps of Willard Carver, chiropractic's first important structuralist,[2] in emphasizing full-spine postural distortions as the basic target of chiropractic care. The structuralist approach, after having sustained a long period of dwindling interest, has experienced something of a renaissance in recent years, with the advent of technique systems like Spinal Biomechanics (Ch. 27) and Chiropractic Biophysics (Ch. 14). Another impetus to chiropractic structuralism has been provided by renewed interest in functional restoration and rehabilitative approaches, and their leading advocates (Hammer, Liebenson, Janda, Lewit). So far, we have not witnessed this contemporary and growing interest in chiropractic structuralism lead to increased interest or practice

of LBT, but we would not surprised if that were to happen, if for no other reason than the rapidly growing multidisciplinary interest in the sacroiliac joint.

Logan was into the sacrum when the sacrum wasn't cool. Indeed, Logan's focus on sacral subluxation in the 1920s preceded the seminal work of Janse and Illi on sacral biomechanics and the gait mechanism by a couple of decades, while medical anatomists largely continued to regard the sacroiliac joint as immobile until perhaps a decade ago, some 70 years after Logan began promulgating his lumbopelvic model.

As you will see, the Logan adjustive approach tends to use extraordinarily light contacts, as little as 2–10 oz (56–280 g) of pressure.[3] Not all chiropractors are comfortable with applying such light forces, and some would castigate such an approach as a reflex technique to be shunned. However, dismissing LBT for that reason would mark a tremendous folly, not only because the clinical utility of the technique is largely unstudied and potentially ample, but because the Logan mechanical model is very accomplished. It is entirely separable from the adjustive procedures, just like Internet Explorer in relation to the Windows operating system (Microsoft's protestations notwithstanding). Nothing prevents a high-velocity thruster from wedding high-velocity, low-amplitude methods to Logan analysis. Not everyone will want to tug on the sacrotuberous ligament for several minutes to correct an anterior-inferior sacrum, as Logan described; and some will prefer thrusting on the contralateral sacral apex with the patient lying in side-posture (similar to Pettibon's not-very-descriptively-named #2 move) or on a drop table (as Thompson described, for sacral apex subluxations).

Logan's legacy lives on, having had a substantial impact on contemporary chiropractic analysis, beyond the 17% of chiropractors who claim to use it, on 7% of their patients.[4] We are aware of two comprehensive textbooks on Logan Basic Technique,[5,6] and of course, the Logan College of Chiropractic is thriving, at 68 years old.

OVERVIEW

The primary intention of Logan Basic is to reduce body distortion and thereby promote health, through elimination of nerve interference and facilitation of homeostatic self-regulation of the body. Logan's most well-known statement, "As the sacrum goes, so goes the spine"[7] indicates the essence of LBT. This means that if the sacrum is not subluxated, then any other subluxations that occur would be self-correcting. Lower-extremity "deficiencies or distortion" are also taken into account, as Hutti explains,[1] in that they may precipitate sacral base inferiority. The sacral subluxation is corrected by a light tugging pressure on the sacrotuberous ligament, as described below.

HISTORY

Hugh B Logan, graduate of the Universal Chiropractic College in 1915, was the founder of the college which still bears his name and originator of one of the oldest techniques in use today. Gabel claimed that the first principles of Basic Technique were formulated as early as 1919.[8] Logan's chiropractic college became the surviving institution of the Carver colleges.[9] (p. 20) The seminal experience was a case of sciatica in which the patient, Logan himself, having been analyzed in the prone position (as was customary at this time, the early 1920s) had not improved following a variety of different treatments. When the patient was examined in the weight-bearing position, the different findings he obtained informed a new treatment approach that eventually resulted in the LBT.[7] According to Schneider et al.[10] (p. 204) LBT is taken from Hurley and Sanders' *The Aquarian Age Healing* (see Further reading).

By about 1930, Logan had pieced together the elements of a standing postural examination, in which he could relate patient symptoms to patterns of spinal distortion and segmental lesions as well. A major piece of the puzzle was to realize the significance of the foundation of the spine: the lower limbs, sacrum, pelvis, and lower lumbar vertebrae. Adjusting techniques were developed that acknowledged the role of muscle guarding in the paraspinal muscles, and that would reduce their need to be dysfunctional by effecting structural improvement in the spine.

According to BJ Palmer, quoted by Dye in 1939, "Basic Technique was a modification of Straight Chiropractic, and I still believe it might be so properly classified."[11] Gabel writes that the first chiropractor to use the sacral apex contact was Francis Dillon,[8] and the piriformis contact has been attributed to Coggins.[12] The first full-spine X-ray was taken by Warren Sausser, for use in conjunction with LBT. Dr. Vinton Logan (the founder's son) gathered the technique together as a posthumous textbook,[6] published in 1950. The Logan College, still going strong, was founded in the 1930s,[13] and the college's own website lists 1935 for the year.

DEFINITION OF TECHNIQUE-SPECIFIC TERMS

There are few terms used in Logan that are unique or used in a non-standard way. At some point Logan said that the word "basic" referred not, as one would suppose, to the *fundamental* nature of his technique, but rather to the *base of the sacrum*. The segmental contacts, or patient contact points, for the application of the procedures are somewhat unique.

- Apex contact: sacrotuberous ligament, opposite side of sacral apex deviation, using 3–6 oz (84–168 g) of pressure;[13] halfway between the ischial tuberosity and the sacrococcygeal joint[13]
- Notch contact: gluteal muscles, inferior sacrum side

- Ulnar contact: near the apex contact, but using more force in severely fixated cases
- Piriformis contact: a posteriorward pressure applied at the insertion of the piriformis muscle at its insertion on the greater trochanter[12]
- Auxiliary contacts: taken as aids in application of the other contacts, in accordance with the lines of muscle pull.

PHYSIOLOGICAL MECHANISMS AND RATIONALE

Logan's key observation was that the sacrum and the pelvis are the foundation of the spine,[1] and the cornerstone of his analysis was that the original subluxation, the one without which all other subluxations in the body would be self-correcting, is that of the sacrum. He felt that forces applied to the sacrum (Fig. 21.1) would be "magnified and reflected" to the rest of the body, while forces applied to the rest of the body (Fig. 21.2) would be "concentrated and reflected to the sacrum."[14] According to Logan, the sacrum drops anterior-inferior with respect to the ilium ("low and anterior") as Thompson would eventually phrase the point.[15] The ilium, with respect to the sacrum, then falls into an "eccentric rotation," in a posterior direction, and will become more so as the condition becomes chronic. The pelvis is carried anteriorly on the side of the low sacrum in order to align the body's center of gravity and the gravity line.

(The anterior pelvis refers to y-axis rotation and should not be confused with an anterior-superior innominate listing.) "The body of the lowest freely movable vertebrae always rotates toward the low side of the sacrum or the foundation upon which it rests and rotates toward the high iliac crest when that crest is high as a result of sacral subluxation."[6,13,16] This gives rise to "a complex, opposed, rotational" lumbar scoliosis, as Logan's forebear Carver would have put it,[17] or "a rotary scoliosis"[6] in Logan's parlance, or a "rotatory scoliosis," as it is typically termed in today's chiropractic terminology. Logan described a series of full-body distortions, in both the frontal and sagittal planes, and carefully illustrated them in his writings.

Although Logan himself considered the mode of correction of his light contact to be purely mechanical, this was in opposition to critics at the time who opined that the basic contact exerted its effects via a neurological reflex, by influencing the ganglion of impar, where the right and left autonomic chains unite near the tip of the coccyx.[18] The assumption is that there is a muscular response to sacral base unleveling, reflecting the body's effort to correct its own subluxations.

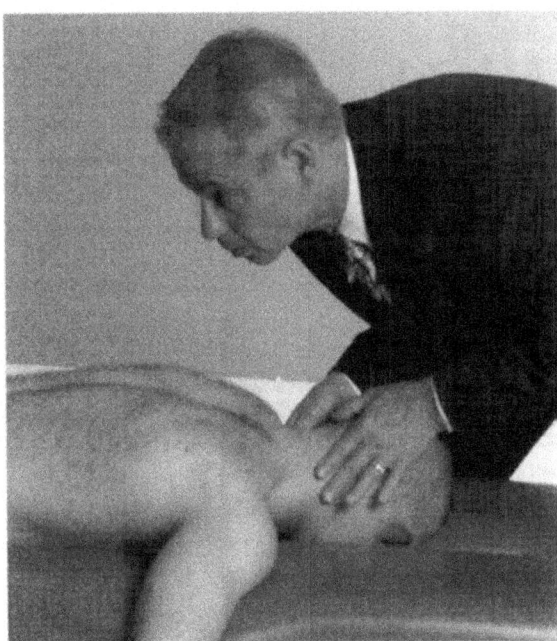

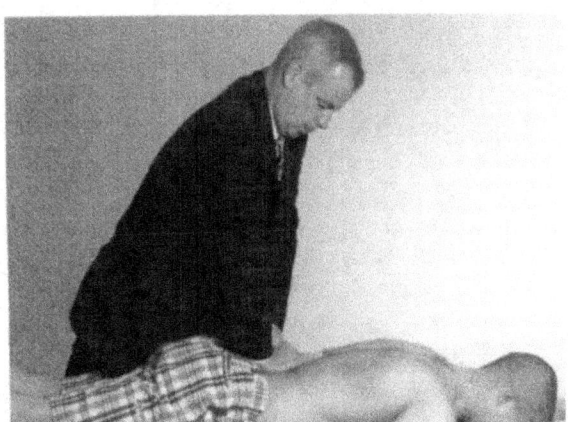

Figure 21.1 Logan Basic Technique applied to low back.

Figure 21.2 Logan cervical technique.

The role of the various contacts, especially on the sacral apex, is to assist that musculature in effecting balance.

DIAGNOSTIC/ANALYTIC PROCEDURES

Logan himself considered the upright, weight-bearing examination of the entire patient to be his primary diagnostic innovation, from which follows the importance of the standing full-spine X-ray. Prominent Logan practitioner Mawhiney also emphasizes the radiological examination: "X-ray interpretation is of prime importance, as it will impart the information necessary to plan the correction procedure."[19] He and possibly other Logan practitioners use a hanging X-ray in addition to the routine anteroposterior and lateral radiographs, used to determine the lowest freely movable vertebra, and to establish a prognosis for scoliosis reduction.[20]

LBT features an exacting X-ray analysis, the main purpose of which is to calculate the amount of heel lift that is required. It takes into account and tries to correct for X-ray distortions, such as that produced by "off-centering" of the patient,[13] as well as the impact of biomechanical factors. Zengel and Davis provide a very articulate account of the Logan line-marking system, emphasizing how it corrects for off-centering and other positional artifacts.[21] From these X-rays and in conjunction with postural evaluation, Logan derived 10 typical distortion patterns of the spine, some having to do with the sagittal and others the frontal planes.

The gluteal crease test[22] involves pressing on the gluteal tissue of a prone patient with the doctor's palms. The gluteal crease is thought to deviate toward the side of an inferior sacral base.

Logan practitioners may use bilateral scales, two scales that independently underlie each foot, recording the body's weight as passed through each of the legs.[14] Mawhiney states that, according to Logan, more weight will be borne on the side of the higher sacral base.[20] Jagusch explores this matter further, and how heel lifts influence bilateral weight distribution.[23]

In addition to the full-spine X-ray, the evaluation of the patient includes postural analysis, static and dynamic spinal palpation, identification of tender points, and sometimes the use of other instrumentation.[7] At the Logan College today, the chiropractic students are taught that the work-up of the new patient involves a case history, physical examination, laboratory, and possibly special studies if the patient presentation so warrants. At this point, the doctor goes on to perform more specifically chiropractic diagnostic procedures. Generally, after having localized a presenting complaint to a segmental lesion, the doctor then performs a full-spine structural analysis, to determine how the base of support of the spine has allowed this subluxation.

TREATMENT/ADJUSTIVE PROCEDURES

LBT is a low-force technique.[1] The primary segmental contact is at the sacral apex, although the doctor may also utilize a notch, ulnar, or auxiliary contact.[13] The apex contact is halfway between the sacrum and the coccyx, and the line of drive for the light pressure applied is lateral and superior. The adjustment to the sacral apex involves very light pressure on the sacrotuberous ligament for a sustained period of time, which may be quite lengthy but rarely exceeds 20 min.[3] Meanwhile, the doctor's other hand monitors the relaxation response of the paraspinal musculature, changes in respiration, and "a pulsation on the end of your thumb."[13] The force is applied on the side opposite the side of sacral apex deviation. A typical time period is 1–3 min,[13] although more time may be required. Hutti explains[1] that, while one hand applies corrective pressure against the sacral apex, the other hand attempts to correct slight displacements of vertebrae that may be causing pain or irritating nerves throughout the spine. Key to success of the sacral apex contact is the following: maximal relaxation of the erector spinae, patient comfort, and corrective support of lumbar hyperlordosis or hypolordosis, if present.[3,14]

Apart from the sacral apex contact, there are also contacts called notch, ulnar, and auxiliary (see definitions above). Pioneered by Coggins, the piriformis muscle may require a light contact at its attachment to the greater trochanter. In addition to these contacts, shoe and ischial lifts, usually temporary, are thought to maintain the adjustments applied to the various contacts; these are considered to play an important role in the Logan technique system. Heel and ischial lifts are used to balance the spine.[13] Although this usually means that the lifts are applied to the anatomic or functional short-leg side, if a lift happens to balance a spine by being applied to the long-leg side, then that is where it should be applied. Logan practitioners recommend patient postural re-education, and the use of orthopedic devices (lumbar cushions, cervical pillows), as well as posturally oriented exercises.[7]

OUTCOME ASSESSMENT

Pre and post X-rays are considered important to establish that the sacral subluxation and the associated spinal distortion have been reduced. In addition, the amelioration or worsening of the original signs and symptoms is also monitored.

SAFETY AND RISK FACTORS

"Logan's program has no contraindications," according to Filson and Johnson.[7] One assumes that this is because there are usually no high-velocity, low-amplitude thrusts in LBT: "Logan uses no impulse, high velocity, high force adjusting in its pure form."[7] According to Lawson, "As a minimal force procedure however, it is particularly indicated for the acutely ill, and the patient in the extreme age groups, ranging from newborn to the very aged."[3]

EVIDENCE OF EFFICACY

Partial support for the validity of Logan–Coggins X-ray marking methods is supplied in a series of papers by Zengel and Davis.[21,24–26] Mannello found fair to moderate interexaminer reliability in assessing radiographs for the side of the basic contact.[27]

Evidence in support of an antihypertensive effect for the apex contact has been presented by Dulgar et al.[16] Subjects receiving a real piriformis contact had a statistically significant reduction in blood pressure compared to both a group receiving a sham basic contact, and a group of controls receiving no intervention whatsoever. Lawson and Sanders,[28] investigating the effects of Logan, Activator, and Diversified techniques, did not find that any of them changed soft-tissue compliance, at least as measured by the somewhat suspect tissue compliance meter.

Logan practitioner Mawhiney describes how to apply Logan methods in cases of tortipelvis, as described by Barge,[29] but provides no data as to its clinical effectiveness. Elsewhere, he reports on the successful application of Logan methods to a case of compression fracture in the lumbar spine,[30] and in another case of mild scoliosis.[31] Mawhiney, although he must be considered a Logan practitioner, also applies extra-Logan methods in conjunction with the sacral apex work, such as thrusting methods and the use of the Leander table. (This piece of specialized equipment allows motorized intermittent traction and the application of belts aimed at reducing lateral curvature in a prone patient.) That stated, he used a combination of methods in treating three cases of scoliosis in a family of young females, each of whom received LBT, Leander tractioning and bracing, hanging exercises, and heel lifts.[32] Although the author claimed improvement in two of the three cases, there are so many inconsistencies and vagaries in the article that we are not comfortable in accepting the author's conclusions.

CONCLUSIONS

- The exacting Logan X-ray analysis leads toward identifying the side to which the sacral apex contact must be applied, and also the prescription of the exactly appropriate size of heel or shoe lift. Logan line-marking methods, including the distortion–correction modules that are so important to its uniqueness, are the lower-body analogs of the Upper Cervical analysis that leads to optimal atlas adjustment (Chs 32 and 33).

- We have already commented that Logan was one of the first important monosegmentalists, emphasizing the importance of one segment above all others. Unlike strict Upper Cervical chiropractors, who argue that *only* atlas and/or axis can subluxate, Logan took a less extreme position on sacral subluxation: if the sacrum was not subluxated, then any other subluxations would be self-correcting.

- Hugh Logan was a model builder, in that he described body distortion as a series of interconnected kinetic chains. Although he recognized that segmental faults occurred, he saw them as consequences of the entire body's faulty posture and biomechanics. He was one of the first chiropractors to identify the relation of lower-extremity findings to those of the axial skeleton. Although we are not in a position to comment on the correctness of his findings, some of which remain unclear at this time, he typically found the lower extremity on the side of sacral inferiority to reflect a flat arch, knee flexion, and decreased joint spaces (ankle, hip, knee). He also described how the pelvis rotated anteriorly around the vertical axis of the body (not to be confused with an anterior-superior ilium) on the side of a low sacrum; this finding was confirmed by the non-chiropractic investigator Friberg,[33] who almost certainly had never heard of Logan.

- Logan was clearly in the spine-straightening business, and thus anticipates the development of modern structuralists such as Pettibon and Harrison (Chs 27 and 14, respectively), although his analysis could hardly be considered purely structuralist in itself, given the heavy emphasis on the sacrum, both etiologically and therapeutically. Filson and Johnson[7] confirm our sense of Logan's bent towards structuralism:

Standing postural examinations were developed, patterns of spinal distortions were categorized, relationships of spinal distortions and segmental subluxations were identified, and clinical trials were tested. Primary reductions of postural faults were followed by secondary reductions in segmental subluxation and reductions in signs and symptoms. This was a major breakthrough in the early chiropractic doctrine by reversing the roles of the primary reduction of the segmental subluxation and secondary improvement in postural attitude. This is not to suggest either to be totally right or wrong, but rather to suggest both to be significant in spinal analysis and treatment.

- Logan wrote: "The body of the lowest freely movable vertebrae always rotates toward the low side of the sacrum ... and rotates toward the high iliac crest when that crest is high as a result of sacral subluxation."[6] In other words, he believed that sacral base inferiority was associated with iliac crest *superiority*, and his various drawings of the basic distortion are consistent with that belief. However, most X-ray studies of the lumbopelvis do *not* find the sacral base and iliac crest moving in opposite directions.[34] Cooperstein discusses the wherewithal for Logan's belief and argues that he is in error.[35,36]

- RB Mawhiney, a Logan practitioner, makes a curious defense of taking a lumbar X-ray *after* lumbar muscle spasm has been corrected, to see what the underlying problem was -- after the fact.[22] We do not believe this unusual use of ionizing radiation constitutes a typical LBT method.

- Mannello[14] provides references[18,37-43] for basic science research that in her opinion supports some of the precepts of LBT. It is beyond our scope to review this body of literature, but any comprehensive attempt to research the putative mechanism of the Logan piriformis contact not only on pain reduction but on visceral function should consult these references.

- It is not entirely clear whether LBT, despite its emphasis on very light contacts, should be considered a "reflex technique" or not. Logan certainly did not consider it to be, and contemporary Logan theorists attempt to explain how the light contacts impact upon somatic and visceral structures using neurophysiological models that can be found in any mainstream medical or chiropractic textbook. This is very different from the invocation of alternative physiologies that one finds among bona fide reflex technique systems.

REFERENCES

1. Hutti L J 1998 Logan Basic Technique: purpose and application. Today's Chiropractic 27 (6): 54–55
2. Montgomery P D, Nelson M J 1985 Evolution of chiropractic theories of practice and spinal adjustment, 1900–1950. Chiropractic History 5: 71–77
3. Lawson D 1991 Logan Basic Technique: short and long lever, mechanically assisted. In: Hansen D (ed.) Sixth Annual Conference on Research and Education, pp. 336–339. Consortium for Chiropractic Research, Monterey, CA
4. Christensen M G 2000 Job analysis of chiropractic. A project report, survey analysis and summary of the practice of chiropractic within the United States. National Board of Chiropractic Examiners, Greeley, CO
5. Coggins W N 1975 Basic Technique – a system of body mechanics. Elco, Willowdale, Ontario, Canada
6. Logan H B 1950 Textbook of Logan basic methods. Logan Chiropractic College, Chesterfield, MO
7. Filson R M, Johnson G 1994 Technique system overview: Logan system of body mechanics assessment. Chiropractic Technique 6 (3): 98–103
8. Gabel R A 1977 Basic Technique. In: Kfoury P W (ed.) Catalog of chiropractic techniques, pp. 7–11. Logan College of Chiropractic, Chesterfield, MO
9. Gibbons R W 1980 The evolution of chiropractic: medical and social protest in America. In: Modern developments in the principles and practice of chiropractic, 1st edn, pp. 3–24. Appleton-Century-Crofts, New York, NY
10. Schneider M, Cohen J, Laws S (eds) 2001 The collected writings of Nimmo and Vannerson: pioneers of Chiropractic Trigger Point Therapy. Self-published, Pittsburgh, PA
11. Dye A A 1939 The evolution of chiropractic – its discovery and development. Reprint of 1969, Richmond Hill, Richmond Hill, NY
12. Moses D E 1991 Studies on Logan Basic piriformis contact. ACA Journal of Chiropractic (December): 35–37
13. Webster L L 1987 An overview of the Logan Basic Technique. Today's Chiropractic (July/August): 71, 111
14. Mannello D 1992 Logan Basic Technique short and long lever technique. In: Hansen D (ed.) Proceedings of the 8th Annual Conference on Research and Education, pp. 158–159, 249–253. Consortium for Chiropractic Research, Palm Springs, CA
15. Thompson C 1974 Thompson technique reference manual, 1st edn. Thompson Educational Workshops, Williams Manufacturing, Elgin, IL
16. Dulgar G, Hill D, Sirucek A, Davis B P 1980 Evidence for possible anti-hypertensive effect of Basic Technique apex contact adjusting. ACA Journal of Chiropractic 14 (September): S97–S102
17. Carver W 1921 Carver's chiropractic analysis of chiropractic principles as applied to pathology, relatology, symptomology and diagnosis, 1st edn. Dunn, Oklahoma City, OK
18. Sparandeo J J, Kadel R E 1982 A neurological model for Basic Technique. Digest of Chiropractic Economics (July/August): 36–38, 140

19. Mawhiney R B 1984 Scoliosis: procedures for case acceptance and treatment. The American Chiropractor (May): 10–11, 13
20. Mawhiney R B 1981 Scoliosis. The American Chiropractor (May/June): 78–81
21. Zengel F, Davis B P 1988 The Logan and modified Logan systems for marking and analyzing spinal radiographs. Digest of Chiropractic Economics (November/December): 36, 38, 40, 43–46, 48, 50
22. Mawhiney R B 1986 Lumbar muscle spasm (tortipelvis) correction using Logan Basic Technique. The American Chiropractor (April): 29, 31, 33–34
23. Jagusch J R 1991 How to use heel lifts in a chiropractic office. Digest of Chiropractic Economics (March/April): 52–55
24. Zengel F, Davis B P 1988 Biomechanical analysis by chiropractic radiography: part II. Effects of x-ray projectional distortion on apparent vertebral rotation. Journal of Manipulative and Physiological Therapeutics 11 (5): 469–473
25. Zengel F, Davis B P 1988 Biomechanical analysis by chiropractic radiography: part I. A simple method for determining X-ray projectional distortion. Journal of Manipulative and Physiological Therapeutics 11 (4): 273–280
26. Zengel F, Davis B P 1988 Biomechanical analysis by chiropractic radiography: part III. Lack of effect of projectional distortion on Gonstead vertebral endplate lines. Journal of Manipulative and Physiological Therapeutics 11 (6): 469–473
27. Mannello D 1993 Inter-rater agreement of Basic Technique radiographic analysis. In: Hansen D (ed.) Proceedings of the 8th Annual Conference on Research and Education, pp. 158–159. Consortium for Chiropractic Research, Monterey, CA
28. Lawson D, Sanders G 1992 Changes in soft tissue compliance in response to spinal manipulation using Activator, Logan Basic, and Diversified Technique. In: Callahan D L (ed.) Proceedings of the International Conference on Spinal Manipulation, p. 137. FCER, Arlington, VA
29. Barge F 1982 Chiropractic technic: tortipelvis. Bawden, Davenport, IA
30. Mawhiney R B 1991 Case study: chiropractic treatment of compression fracture and costovertebral displacement due to trauma. The American Chiropractor 13 (7): 18–21
31. Mawhiney R B 1989 Reduction of minor lumbar scoliosis in a 57 year old female. Journal of Chiropractic Research 2: 48–51
32. Mawhiney R B 1999 Accelerated treatment protocols of the International Scoliosis Research Center on three cases of scoliosis under chiropractic care: case reports. Chiropractic Technique 11 (3): 125–132
33. Friberg O 1987 Leg length inequality and low back pain. Clinical Biomechanics 2: 211–219
34. Vernon H, Bureau J 1983 A radiographic study of the incidence of low sacral base and lumbar lateral curvature related to the presence of an apparent short leg. Journal of the Canadian Chiropractic Association 27 (1): 11–15

35. Cooperstein R 1990 Innominate vertical length differentials as a function of pelvic torsion and pelvic carrying angle. In: Jansen R D (ed.) Proceedings of the 5th Annual Conference on Research and Education, pp. 1–14. Consortium for Chiropractic Research, Sacramento, CA

36. Cooperstein R 1992 Roentgenometric assessment of innominate vertical length differentials. In: Hansen D (ed.) Proceedings of the 7th annual Conference on Research and Education, pp. 273–277. Consortium for Chiropractic Research, Palm Springs, CA

37. Shambaugh P 1987 Acupuncture as a mechanism of chiropractic sacral apex adjustment. American Journal of Acupuncture 15: 349–354

38. Slosberg M 1988 Effects of altered afferent articular input on sensation, proprioception, muscle tone and sympathetic reflex responses. Journal of Manipulative and Physiological Therapeutics 11 (5): 400–408

39. Skoglund C R 1989 Neurophysiological aspects of the pathological erector spinae reflex in cases of mechanical pelvic dysfunction. Journal of Manual Medicine 4: 29–30

40. Simons D G, Hong C Z 1989 The pathological erector spinae reflex: a local twitch response? (letter to the editor). Journal of Manual Medicine 4: 69

41. Silverstolpe L 1989 A pathological erector spinae reflex – a new sign of mechanical pelvic dysfunction (brief communication). Journal of Manual Medicine 4: 28

42. Vleeming A, Van Wingerden J P, Snijders C J et al 1989 Load application to the sacrotuberous ligament: influences on sacroiliac joint mechanics. Clinical Biomechanics 4: 204–209

43. Vleeming A, Stoeckart R, Snijders C J 1989 The sacrotuberous ligament: a conceptual approach to its dynamic role in stabilizing the sacroiliac joint. Clinical Biomechanics 4: 201–203

FURTHER READING

Hurley J, Sanders H 1932 The Aquarian age healing for you, vol I. Haynes, Los Angeles, CA

Hurley J, Sanders H 1933 The Aquarian age healing, vol II. Haynes, Los Angeles, CA

22

Network Chiropractic Technique (NCT) and Network Spinal Analysis (NSA)

INTRODUCTION

One of us (Cooperstein) began reading and writing about Network Chiropractic Technique (NCT) in 1995, but did not at that time write anything intended for publication. Years later, when the idea for this book arose, not surprisingly, we decided to dust off and reuse what had already been written. During production, it became clear that NCT had developed into a related but different healing method that founder Donald Epstein now called Network Spinal Analysis (NSA), beginning around 1994. Not only that, but NSA itself had a tendency to redefine central concepts from time to time, so that it became increasingly difficult to characterize Network Care.

Since, as we describe below, NSA (unlike NCT) must be considered complementary to chiropractic care, rather than a chiropractic technique system *per se*, at some point we began to question the appropriateness of even including it within this book, which is by definition a compendium of *chiropractic* technique systems. From that point of view, although aware of its evolution into NSA, we originally decided to emphasize NCT; it is, or at least was, clearly chiropractic, and we presumed it still claims many practitioners. Therefore, we wrote a chapter on NCT that included short discussions of how NSA differed.

This writing strategy did not work. We eventually realized that it was taking more time than it saved to graft discussion of NSA on to a basic presentation of NCT, especially since new material kept emerging that needed to be acknowledged, even as we were going to press. Therefore, we decided to rework the material so that NSA became more the primary focus, although we thought it best to retain our material on NCT, since it remains of historical interest and continues to inform elements of NSA (Fig. 22.1). NSA, although not a chiropractic technique as such, needs to be described in our book because, as this book goes to press, it is taught only to chiropractors and chiropractic students, who we felt might be very interested in the information and analysis in this chapter.

In this chapter, sometimes we simply use the term "Network," when a point in our opinion seems to refer equally well to both NCT and NSA. From time to time, especially in the terminology section, we will tackle some of the newer jargon and concepts that mark the transition. References older than 1995 may be safely assumed as pertinent to NCT, and from 1995 on, to NSA. In writing about NCT, we usually use the past tense, to

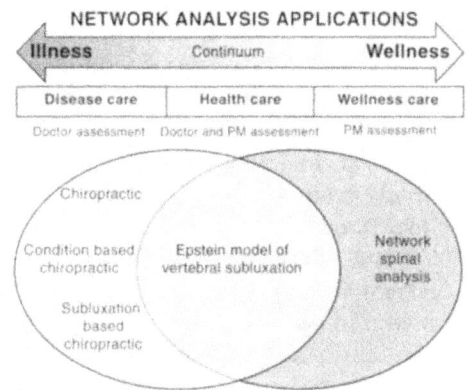

Figure 22.1 Overlap between Network Chiropractic Technique and Network Spinal Analysis.

convey the notion that NSA no longer views some of the procedures that were routinely used in NCT as automatically intrinsic to NSA. This by no means suggests that a contemporary practitioner of NSA eschews such procedures, but only that if he or she does so, that is outside the carefully defined scope of NSA.

OVERVIEW

On a traditional level, the primary purpose of NCT was to detect, classify, and adjust vertebral subluxations, which impair the physiological, emotional, and mental options for growth and development, ultimately resulting in sickness and disease. Subluxations were classified as either Class A structural, or Class B meningeal/facilitated. A good outcome depended on addressing each class with the appropriate type of adjustment and in the right order. The adjustment was prophylactic and therapeutic in addressing subluxation. NCT claimed less to be a distinct technique, than a means of "networking" – that is, sequencing other chiropractic techniques so that the timing is enhanced in terms of when particular adjustments are given. "We now know when, where and how to apply adjustive forces to consistently get exciting results."[1] Network of any kind is unabashedly vitalistic.[2,3]

By comparison, NSA applies gentle forces, often called entrainments, to *spinal gateways*, which are spinal areas having vertebral–dural attachments, in order to shift the mind–body from stress physiology to greater adaptative self-assessment and organization. These light forces bring about two healing waves, in which the patient/practice member undergoes a spontaneous rocking pattern, that ultimately release spinal tension and allow resolution of vertebral subluxations in the standard sense of the term. These waves are called the respiratory wave (generally achieved in Level One care) and the somatopsychic wave (generally achieved in Level Two care), and are presumed to correct vertebral subluxations, and often effect emotional release. The primary goals of NSA care are to promote practice member self-awareness of the spinal structure, initiate the healing waves, detect spinal gateways, detect adverse mechanical spinal cord

tension, administer entrainments, and conduct outcomes research.[4]

HISTORY

Chiropractic has always been a mind–body healing discipline, going back to D D Palmer's triangle of health, which had sides representing autosuggestion, traumatism, and toxins, or, using more contemporary terminology, mind, body, and chemicals. The mind–body concept went mainstream during the 1960s and 1970s, as it became central to the counterculture, the melting pot from which much of what we now call CAM – complementary and alternative medicine – emerged. Donald Epstein originated Network Chiropractic around 1970 as a blend of traditional chiropractic and New Age thinking. Contemporary reinterpretations of Einstein's quantum mechanics and theory of relativity (e.g., *The Tao of Physics*, and *The Dancing Wu Li Masters*, see Further reading) apparently did not escape notice by Epstein and his Network colleagues, who brought the New Physics, as some called it, to the center stage of chiropractic philosophy.

More recently, Epstein has reformulated the technique formerly known as NCT into a method he now calls NSA,[5] an approach to wellness deemed distinct from chiropractic. NSA is only taught to doctors of chiropractic, but Epstein positions NSA as distinct from chiropractic. The relationship of the two is developed in the following passage:

… NSA may also be applied as a form of wellness education, without any representation of diagnosing, treating, attending to, remedying, correcting, preventing or advising in relationship to any condition, including subluxation, malady or symptom. In order for an individual to practice NSA within the context described, it will require at least 3½ years of post-graduate study including a distance learning certificate … These individuals will not be taught to identify or adjust subluxations, nor will practice chiropractic or any health restorative or maintenance discipline.[4]

Donald Epstein, originator of Network, graduated from New York Chiropractic College in 1977 (Fig. 22.2). His first interest was in Upper Cervical specific technique (Ch. 32), relying upon

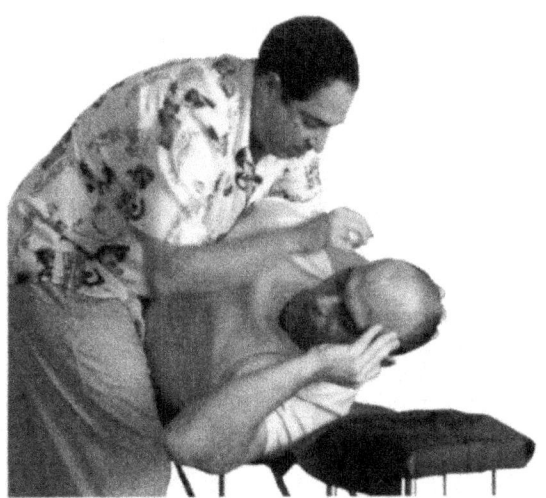

Figure 22.2   Donald Epstein, originator of Network.

thermography, leg checks, and spinography for listings. Although he drew upon Logan Basic Technique (Ch. 21) on the sacrum, Thompson work (Ch. 29) on positive iliums, Pierce's work (Ch. 23) on the fifth cervical, and Pierce–Stillwagon (Ch. 23) pelvic work, Epstein did not like to address the thoracolumbar spine in these years, for fear that it would worsen what he believed to be the primary upper cervical subluxation. Network Chiropractic took shape between the years 1979 and 1984, following the observation that the classic Upper Cervical theory could not explain a number of clinical observations. Overall, Epstein claims substantial influence from the Palmers, Gonstead, Van Rumpt, Fuhr, Harrison, Pettibon, Ward, DeJarnette, Grostic, Walker, and Toftness, among others. Epstein began conducting seminars in Network Chiropractic in 1984.

The term "Network" appears to have been adopted in 1982 when Epstein began "networking" multiple chiropractic techniques. The Network concept of subluxation was also developed in 1982, to which a clinical phasing system was added in 1985, which in turn was organized into three specific levels of care by 1994. It is the introduction of these levels of care that, according to Epstein, distinguishes NCT from NSA.[5] A fourth level of care was added in 2001.[6] By 1999, the term "entrainment" had replaced the term "adjustment," as it became clear to Epstein that both the

cortical and subcortical areas of the brain respond to these low-force contacts. Also in 1999, Epstein hypothesized that vertebral subluxations were symptoms (or adaptations) to another process, involving spinal cord tension patterns, amenable to correction through healing waves. The purpose of the entrainment was then seen as allowing the brain to normalize the conditions that allowed and maintained subluxation, which in turn was no longer the direct target of Network care.

Epstein and NCT/NSA have received a lot of publicity in the national media, including high-circulation magazines and newspapers, and Epstein has made many television appearances. Based on the observation that each person's healing experience has certain attributes characteristic of different stages of consciousness, Epstein has written a best-selling book, *The 12 Stages of Healing* (see Further reading). Another book on NSA is being prepared for publication.

DEFINITION OF TECHNIQUE-SPECIFIC TERMS

As stated above, references older than 1995 may be safely assumed as more pertinent to NCT, and from 1995 on, to NSA. There is considerable continuity and overlap, in as much as NCT terms tend to remain alive and well within the NSA kernel, augmented more than abandoned or fundamentally altered. Exceptions to this generalization are noted.

- Network: in one sense Network has to do with community, in which "a 'family' of chiropractors and practice members share a dedication to the growth, development, health, and well-being of the individual and the planet."[7] In another sense, Network has to do with sequencing moves drawn from other chiropractic techniques so that the adjustments will be more efficient and lasting. Finally, Epstein is said to believe that the body is "a functional network in which everything is linked to everything else."[8]
- Class A subluxation: structural in nature,[5,9] with elements of fixation, misalignment, and nerve interference, it is the classic chiropractic

subluxation, treatable with high-velocity, low-amplitude (HVLA) thrusting

- Class B meningeal subluxation: essentially neurological (facilitated) in nature,[5,9] located within the brain or spinal cord, it involves a "multisegmental facilitation of the paraspinal musculature due to adverse cord–brain tension and interference in the cord, brain, and/or dural sleeves."[10] Furthermore, it is a "concussion of forces" on an emotional or chemical level that overloads the central nervous system. The vertebra displaces secondarily, as an adaptative feature
- Facilitated subluxation: Epstein began to prefer this term to meningeal subluxation,[9] although we can discern no difference between the two terms as they are used[11]
- AMCT: Adverse Mechanical Cord Tension. The term is taken from Breig,[12] redefined by Epstein to include NSA ideology
- Phasing system:[1] consists of five phases of AMCT (Table 22.1), each of which has distinctive palpatory and biomechanical findings and implications for the vertebral level and type of care to be rendered. Once subluxation is determined to exist, the phasing system is then used to determine what levels are to be adjusted
- Levels of care: specifically defines the transition from NCT to NSA.[5] Each of the three levels

(described below) corresponds to a desired outcome of care: basic, intermediate, and advanced care.[1] A fourth level is under development. Each of the five phases within the phasing system occurs within each of the levels of care (Table 22.2)

- Spinal set point: related to the fight or flight posture that represents a "loss of recovery from a specific postural state";[10] an adaptation to adrenal exhaustion, in an attitude of flexion that increases meningeal and spinal cord tension
- SMFU: the spinal meningeal functional unit, associated with increased adrenal stress and an impending "set point positive"[10]
- Meningeal critical: a clinical entity in which the patient is approaching an impending collapse of the nervous system (e.g., disk herniation),[9] and even death
- Practice member: the person formerly known as "the patient"
- Clear-out: the adjustment process in NCT[8]
- Recovery: in the context of NCT, Epstein preferred the term "recovery" to "healing," describing it as a process in which innate intelligence accepts the adjustment[10]
- Respiratory and somatopsychic waves: the spontaneous writhing in which NCT/NSA patients/practice participants typically engage. The respiratory wave is a smooth, rhythmic muscular movement, synchronized with breathing. The somatopsychic wave is a coordinated wave motion of the major muscle groups, gently rocking restricted spinal segments
- Non-linear: this refers to the phenomenon that a relatively small neurological input, or

Table 22.1 Phases of care

Phase one	Sacrum and/or occiput
Phase two	C1 and/or C5
Phase three	Lateral pelvic or sacral sway
Phase four	C2 and/or C3
Phase five	C2 and sacrum, C5 with coccyx

Table 22.2 Levels of care

Level	Target	Comments
Level one (basic care)	New patients/reinitiated care	Mostly reduces Class B subluxations; respiratory wave, 18–51 visits
Level two (intermediate care)	Continuing care	Class A subluxations added; gentle rocking-type spontaneous writhing; about 26–52 visits
Level three (advanced care)	Practice members	Aimed at overall health, not symptom reduction; fully developed spontaneous writhing; 4 months minimum, 34 visits
Level four (unity care)	Adds clavicles and trochanters	Under development[4]

even light corrective adjustment, may result in a much larger response or reaction in the body

- Entrainment: the NSA low-force adjustment-equivalent, given that the term "adjustment" is no longer used in NSA to describe its light force application. Epstein states that "the entrainment contact or impulse is applied to a segmental region of high, free energy in the vicinity of the attachment of the spinal cord … It is not a form of spinal manipulation, nor is it specifically developed to correct fixation, pain, misalignment or subluxation."[13] The term is also used in cranial therapy, to refer to the effect of one pendulum on another, so that they begin to swing in synchrony. Thus, entrainment may refer to the harmonizing oscillations of biological systems
- Point of critical tension: the NSA segmental contact-equivalent; that segmental spinal region which appears to give rise to a specific area of meningeal and/or cord tension.[6,13] According to Epstein, this point varies automatically on a given segment, depending on the directional vectors of the tension. It is often located at the occiput, sacrococcygeal, and lower cervical regions (points where the dura attaches)
- Spinal gateway: we feel compelled to quote Epstein: "access point for auto-assessment … a focal area of free or unbound energy … sensitive to entrained biological fields and to non-local intelligence."[13] The spinal gateway is "an interface between dimensions of tissue,

energy and consciousness" and/or "a nexus for interaction between the passive, active, neural control and the emotional subsystems, contributing to spinal and neural integrity."[13] The points of critical tension apparently identify a spinal gateway for the practitioner to use in order to foster respiratory or somatopsychic waves.[13]

It can be seen that many word and concept substitutions mark the transition from NCT to NSA. Table 22.3 provides some examples.

PHYSIOLOGICAL MECHANISMS AND RATIONALE

NCT invoked a fairly classic triad of health model, after D D Palmer: there are physical, chemical, and emotional causes of subluxation.[10] The chiropractor is to help the patient recover from all these types of stress.[14] NCT also entertained a fairly traditional, D D Palmeresque model of the subluxation: vertebral misalignment, intervertebral foramen narrowing, pressure on the nerve root, and nerve interference.[1] Subluxation bifurcates, as described above, into the Class A structural and Class B meningeal (facilitated) categories.[2]

Like Neuro-Emotional Technique (Ch. 12),[15] NCT proposed that past emotional experiences become bound up with the musculoskeletal system. Furthermore: "The neurological system acts as a conduit for the organization and control of your genetic potentials by the physical personification of your resident (Innate) Intelligence."[16] The vertebral subluxation was thought to initiate, perpetuate, and sustain impaired ability to adapt to the "information in environmental forces."[10] The meningeal subluxations were said to be associated with adrenal exhaustion, as described by Selye (see Epstein[10]). Epstein also invoked the osteopathic theory of facilitation (attributed to Korr), as a further explanation of how subluxation can cause abnormal muscle tone.[10] Citing Speransky, Epstein stated that once the nervous system has been irritated, removal of the irritant may suffice to quiet the process.[10] This is very consistent with the more contemporary NSA view that entrainment can resolve the spinal problem

Table 22.3 Two types of Network

Network Chiropractic Technique term	Network Spinal Analysis equivalent term
Adjustment	Spinal low-force applications; entrainment contact
Subluxation	Spinal and somatic tension patterns; facilitated focus
Subluxation correction	Enhancing spinal and neural integrity
Segmental contact point	Spinal gateways at the point of critical tension
Nervous system	Neural subsystem
Vertebrae, disks, ligaments	Active subsystem
Muscles, tendons	Passive subsystem

that gives rise to vertebral subluxation, a defensive, adaptative process.

In the context of NCT, subluxations were corrected, according to Epstein, so that the patient became more aware of the healing process both in the office and at home. The concept that the patient (or practice participant) is to be directly involved in self-assessment of spinal and neural integrity becomes especially prominent in NSA.[17] In NCT, Class A and B subluxations were treated differently and sequentially (first B, then A), because of their different etiologies. Although the physiological character of the Class A subluxation is easily understood, in that it lies well within the classic description of the chiropractic subluxation, the Class B subluxation is less straightforward. It involves tension in, and even constriction of, the meningeal sleeves. Some of the fine distinctions that follow from this otherwise clear categorization are not especially straightforward to a non-Network practitioner. For example, a posterior atlas transverse subluxation would be classified as a Class A subluxation, whereas an anterior atlas transverse subluxation would be classified as a Class B subluxation. As another example, C3 subluxations were said to be meningeal, whereas C4 subluxations are only rarely meningeal.[18]

Epstein believes that the individual dominated by meningeal subluxations adopts a typical "fight-or-flight" demeanor, with adrenal hyperactivity, increased muscle tone, reduced digestive function, and more.[14] NCT proposed that the order in which subluxations are corrected in the various spinal regions would be critical to the success of the treatment.

Having focused on NCT, we now turn to the physiological mechanisms related to NSA. The differences have far less to do with any changes in the view of how the body works, in health and in disease, and more with how the NSA practitioner might best promote healing. In essence, light force applications to points of critical tension cue the brain to take on new wellness strategies. These are manifested by the respiratory and somatopsychic waves, which "are associated with spontaneous reorganization, redistribution, and release of spinal tension."[4] NSA care is thought to promote greater self-awareness, including that of the relationships of body, mind, emotion, and expression. In a significant reinterpretation of the traditional subluxation model, the vertebral subluxation is no longer seen as the single cause of ill health, but rather as an integral element in a mind–body disconnect, a result of defense physiology and postural distortion. A practice member who becomes more aware of this process, through NSA spinal contacts, is enabled to normalize the process that led to the subluxations and prevent recurrence.[4]

DIAGNOSTIC/ANALYTIC PROCEDURES

To the usual questions that must be answered by any chiropractor (Is there subluxation? Where is it? What is its direction? What direction of force must be applied?) NCT added two more questions: (1) What should be the sequence of adjustments? and (2) What type of force should be applied? It should be noted that at one time Epstein believed that "Symptoms, in no way, play a role in the evaluation utilized within Network Analysis."[19] Epstein stated in 1983, although things have changed somewhat, that his analysis used the following diagnostic means:[19]

- thermocouple instruments (nervoscope, neurocalometer, neurocalograph)
- infrared thermometer (diathermy with graph)
- digital temperature differential instrument (digital readout of temperature)
- microwave radiation detector (a gadget related to the Toftness instrument)
- microwave palpation (placing the hand a few inches (5–10 cm) above the practice member's body, looking for unusual sensations, such as heat, cold, or "emptiness" (akin to non-contact therapeutic touch? Magnetic healing?)
- vertebral challenge, presumably as described in Applied Kinesiology, Ch. 11
- prone leg check – we think this is a Derifield-like procedure (Ch. 4)
- palpation – for bone landmarks, muscles, and energy radiation
- observation for visible distortions, presumably postural evaluation.

The Class A subluxations are identified using classic chiropractic tools, principally leg checks and palpation, but the Class B subluxations may require less classic means of identification. At one time Epstein endorsed the Toftness radiation detector (Ch. 30),[19] but we are not certain what he would say today about that controversial tool. Palpation of the paraspinal musculature is critical in order to make the distinction between the Class A and B subluxations, using very light touch to reveal multisegmental bands of muscle.[20] Palpation identifies not only standard entities, such as bones, but less orthodox identities, such as energies and radiations. "Palpation of the paraspinal musculature … may serve as a critical tool in the clinical practice of vitalistic chiropractic."[20] "Norlyk writes: 'Usually chiropractic treatment is based on what is found in the first visit through X-rays and other means of diagnosing,' says Epstein. 'However, the key factor in Network Chiropractic analysis is the dynamics of how the body accepts the forces. Once you start to reduce some meningeal tension in the spinal cord, most of the structural distortions change vastly.' "[21]

NCT/NSA does not really ask the chiropractor to give up whatever methods he or she is already using, but rather add to them from the Network armamentarium, consisting chiefly in its proprietary diagnostic methods of performing leg checks, palpating, and using instrumentation. In NCT, the use of X-ray was supported, if the doctor was already in the habit of taking them for the purpose of subluxation identification. In NSA, X-rays are not routinely taken, although they may be indicated if examination findings are non-conclusive, the practitioner suspects an anomaly or loss of structural integrity, or a particular force to be used requires radiographic analysis.[6]

As recently as 1996 an NSA practitioner would have included static and motion palpation, muscle palpation, phase indicators, and any of a number of instrumentation procedures (electrocardiogram, X-ray, thermography, muscle testing, etc.) as part of a thorough subluxation identification examination. More recently, it seems that the phase indicators, the items in Table 22.4, which are said to identify adverse spinal cord tension, are the only remaining obligatory NSA examination elements.[6]

Table 22.4 NSA phase indicators

Indicator assessed	Segment level
Leg length	Cord, cervical
Cervical syndrome test	Cervical
Leg crossover	Lumbosacral, lumbopelvic
Ankle eversion stress	Hip, spinal rotation
Heel tension	Hip, lower extremity, spinal flexion/extension
Bilateral adduction stress	Second and third cervicals
Unilateral adduction	Second and third cervicals
Stress Z-flick	Second and third cervicals
Abduction stress (flexion–extension)	Fifth cervical and coccyx
Palpation (motion, static, muscular)	All vertebral segments
Sacrotuberous ligament tension	Lateral bending sacrum
Postural analysis	All vertebral segments
Flexibility (range of motion)	All vertebral segments

TREATMENT/ADJUSTIVE PROCEDURES

NCT was based on classifying subluxations into two categories, and then prioritizing their correction in a way that requires the minimum force. The most severe subluxations, the Class B subluxations that cause the most spinal cord distortion and spinal structural distortion, were treated first and with the least amount of force. Intersegmental Class A subluxations were addressed second. Emotional expression by the patient was common and desirable: "The patient's spontaneous expression of the release of tension and interference is a natural occurrence. In fact, when individuals express their deepest stresses they heal more deeply and more completely."[1]

The Class B (facilitated) subluxations, because they would be located within the neurological system, were treated differently from the Class A subluxations. If a doctor were to adjust a Class B subluxation using a thrusting technique, the patient would tend to be very anxious and resist the adjustment. At this point, the doctor would be counseled just to "hold" that spinal region, while talking to the patient. Examples of Class B corrections included the light-force Logan Basic sacral apex contact (Ch. 21), and a gentle contact on the occiput on the side of the short leg, in order to reduce caudad subluxations.[17]

Class B/meningeal/facilitated subluxations were adjusted with low-force sustained contacts or light, rapid, toggle-recoil actions. Epstein wrote that no patient should receive osseous thrusts "until meningeal tension is released."[10]

The Class A (structural) subluxations amount to the "classical type" of subluxations that chiropractors identify and adjust, with audible release using a thrusting technique. On the web, Epstein states: "A mild structural force may be used to set the restricted segment into motion in order to free the nerve (at the intervertebral foramen)."[22] It is recommended that the doctor use considerable prestress to minimize the force that need be applied to effect the adjustment. NCT is rather indifferent as to which particular mechanical methods are used: rotary break, Carver thrust, thumb move, etc. In that regard, NCT could be said to advocate the use of Diversified methods for adjusting these Class A subluxations. (In 1996, Epstein wrote that NSA uses "hands on, low-force adjustments,"[5] from which we gather that some NSA practitioners might eschew traditional thrusting procedures and joint cavitation.

The NSA corrective procedure does not seem to resemble a conventional chiropractic adjustment, low-force or otherwise. Consider the following description[13] of an NSA force applied to a patient in intermediate care:

It is applied in a fashion similar to a threading a needle. The flexion/extension contact is made just inferior to the spot desired and then an upward scoop allows for the contact point on the finder to provide an anterior to posterior and inferior to superior "lift of the connective tissue" in the appropriate area. The lateral bending contact is made just lateral to the desired Gateway. The force is applied in an anterior to posterior and a lateral to medial direction. The finger contact terminates at the center of the Gateway.

The patient's expression of strong, spontaneous emotions is said to be so common during Network visits, and is so strongly encouraged by the doctor, that it might be fair to regard the encouraging of emoting as an ancillary procedure. Indeed, Epstein remarks: "These somato-emotional releases are not chiropractic any more than a bowel movement is chiropractic. They are processes associated with life itself."[1]

Although more often than not, Network practitioners shy away from making claims about treating specific diseases or conditions, preferring to take the traditional chiropractic position that they treat subluxations, not "medical diseases," an *East West* columnist once claimed that NSA can treat "ulcers, cancer, learning disabilities, alcoholism, cystic fibrosis, dyslexia, paralysis, and more,"[21] and one does routinely see such testimonials posted on Network-related websites.

NSA no longer intrinsically includes subluxation identification and correction, although NSA practitioners are likely to engage in such procedures to some extent as within their chiropractic scope of practice. What is considered uniquely NSA is the application of light force contacts to effect respiratory and somatopsychic waves, which enable the body to cope effectively with subluxations. We have already described how light contacts applied to points of critical tension entrain the body, through spinal gateways, to become more aware of what is required for wellness.

OUTCOME ASSESSMENT

The methods that are used to identify health problems are the same as the ones used to confirm improvement. Although pain reduction itself was not a valid outcome measure in NCT, patient questionnaires used to monitor the course of care are virtually devoid of questions regarding pain.[6,22] Intangibles such as the personal development of the "practice member" are considered critical. The "wave phenomenon" (also known as the respiratory wave or the somatopsychic wave) is considered of paramount importance, and constitutes an important outcome measure in that regard.[5]

Inspection of the patient questionnaires that are reprinted in the NSA literature shows there are many questions about spinal "awareness" and the like, and virtually no questions about pain: its presence, absence, intensity, location, time course, quality, and ameliorating/aggravating aspects.

Network doctors have put numerous testimonials on the internet. The following samples[23] – although we do not think that patient testimonials document outcomes of care – provide a flavor for what Network patients define as good outcomes:

"Having had 'traditional' care previously, I am pleased at a) the effectiveness, b) gentleness, c) overwhelming calm, during my visits" (Steve). "For me, Network Chiropractic has helped me to deepen my meditation practice, by focusing on my body in a very detailed, attentive way. My body begins to reveal to me emotional information that is beyond my mind. I also appreciate the fact that with this type of work, I am being guided towards healing myself as opposed to being healed by someone else" (Nadia). "Physically, after 3 to 4 sessions, the sinus problems I was experiencing for over 1 year, were healed and I recovered the sense of smell too. That was close to a miracle! Three months later, I breathe normally, my neck moves freely with hardly any pain and spiritually there is constant joy in my Self. I experience life differently in that, when problems arise, solutions follow easily and I return to being centred, balanced and happy" (Marie-Chantal).

SAFETY AND RISK FACTORS

Epstein expressed a strong aversion to using some of the standard tests for nerve root tension: Kernig's, Lasegue's straight-leg raise, and Brudzinski's sign.[16] At that time, in 1984, he felt it would be better to identify the meningeal subluxation by less invasive methods, and avoid increasing tension of the cord and meninges for diagnostic purposes. He took the unusual position that only rarely is the real problem (i.e., the meningeal subluxation) even anatomically near the spinal level identified by the orthopedic tests, adding: "It is the contention of Network Chiropractic that what is commonly known as a disc syndrome and spondylolisthesis, are just two of the more common means that the resident intelligence may use to reduce neurological damage in the meningeal critical complex."[16] This is very consistent with the contemporary view of NSA that subluxation is adaptive, a strategic although defensive choice.

The patient is asked not to wear neck jewelry, or any "crystals," because they might "resonate with the 'subluxated' you." Other advice includes not wearing leather, and not eating or drinking alcohol before a visit.

EVIDENCE OF EFFICACY

A large-scale study claims that practice participants under NSA care obtain health benefits.[24] In this retrospective study, data were collected from 156 Network offices on the health status of 2818 patients. The study used a novel survey instrument, which asked the study participants to rate four health domains (physical state, mental/emotional state, stress evaluation, life enjoyment) and overall quality of life at the present time compared with "before Network." The investigators stated there was evidence of improved health in all four health domains, as well as their "health coefficient." The longer the duration of care, the more substantial the health benefits that were assessed by the study participants (We have comments on this study below, in the Conclusions.).

Miller and Redmond[25] reported that patients receiving Network care showed no changes in their skin temperature or electromyogram (EMG) findings, but did show diminished electrodermal activity (i.e., skin electrical conductance, mostly a measure of sweating). By comparison, the only change showed by the control group members, who did not receive any type of sham or placebo treatment, was higher EMG values. The investigators concluded that Network care must have calmed the experimental group while the control group was made anxious during the recording period. (Other interpretations are, of course, possible.) Another study[26] found that the somatopsychic waveform was associated with non-linear data, although it is hard for us to say what that would mean. There is a case report showing a dramatic improvement in psoriasis in a patient under Network care.[27] There is a testimonial about a child with learning deficits, thought to be related to a traumatic birth process, who improved with Network Care.[8]

CONCLUSIONS

- Reading through the NCT/NSA writings is not for those who lack a sense of adventure. One reads that "atoms oscillate and, consequently, vertebrae oscillate," that the short-leg indicator denotes unilateral cord tension, and

NSA employs certain principles of quantum mechanics.[5]

- Confirming NSA's view of its distinctness from chiropractic, Epstein's preamble to a recent seminar manual states: "The resolution of spinal subluxation, whether it be structural or facilitated by nature, may be one of the benefits of enhanced spinal and neural integrity achieved through the application of Network Spinal Analysis, but it is no longer one of its objectives."[13]

- Interest in correcting spinal subluxation in the traditional sense has yielded to: (1) promoting the practice member's self-awareness of spinal structures; (2) the ability to initiate spontaneous, self-generated somatopsychic responses; (3) detecting and enhancing the availability of spinal gateways; (4) detecting the presence of adverse mechanical spinal cord tension; (5) wanting to "enhance precognitive and cognitive self-awareness"; and (6) evaluating the efficacy of the practice member's wellness and quality of life.[6]

- Although NSA "is currently taught exclusively to chiropractors and chiropractic students,"[17] there are reasons to suppose this could change. For example, one also reads: "NSA, as a stand-alone discipline, is positioned as having application for various health practitioners using other approaches to practice member care, including Chiropractors who adhere to correction of vertebral subluxation."[6] Thus, NSA hints at extending its approach to practitioners outside the chiropractic profession, while being very careful to not leave its chiropractic roots behind altogether. Ironically, while chiropractic as a CAM profession undergoes some serious soul-searching, trying to decide if it should emphasize being complementary or alternative, NSA has taken another path: it positions itself as complementary and perhaps even alternative to *chiropractic*.

- The Blanks et al study[24] claiming to show improved health status compared with "before Network," uses a retrospective design, a very unusual methodological approach in using subjective survey instruments. Normally, studies using patient self-assessment surveys determine

a baseline, against which values are compared during the course of care and at regular follow-up intervals. This means that the patients at any moment in time are rating their present health status, a self-evaluation which is likely to be more reliable than their recollections of some past status. Since memories of the past are always colored by the experience of the present, data gathered from self-evaluations based on memory of the past are likely to be less reliable than data gathered in the present about the present. Moreover, any patients who have dropped out of Network care are not part of the survey, so that it would appear to be weighted in favor of those satisfied with their care. Patients who do not feel better in the present compared with pre-Network, who may have discontinued Network care for that reason, are simply not there to be counted, accounting for selection bias. When a significant proportion of the subjects who should be in a survey are not interviewed, selection bias may be introduced whereby those included are systematically different from those who are not included in the survey. Selection bias reduces the generalizability of the results to the reference population of all Network patients. It is worth noting that patients receiving Network care feel better in some ways than before having received their care. However, virtually any study ever done that asked patients if they were satisfied with their chiropractic care found that they were, no matter what technique was used.

Gleberzon was involved in a contentious exchange with Blanks et al concerning their retrospective study.[28,29] Specifically, Blanks et al questioned the motivation behind an article by Gleberzon that detailed, among other things, that the data generated by retrospective studies such as the one cited in the NSA literature must be interpreted cautiously, as the patients in the study may suffer from recall bias (they may wish to substantiate their perceived benefits while under NSA care, especially since that care may be very expensive and time-consuming). Although Blanks et al emphasized that all research studies have methodological limitations, Gleberzon noted that none of these potential limitations had been described at any time in the body of the published retrospective study and disagreed with their position that only NSA follows a rigorous research paradigm.

- Some NSA practitioners entertain a theory of symptom interpretation that certainly raises some red flags, as evidenced by an unsigned patient handout that found its way into our hands. Entitled *Now that you've had your first Network Chiropractic clear out*, it suggests that following Network care the body may develop new symptoms, such as fever, as it recovers from illness.

As you recover, your body will retrace the memory patterns of much of what you have experienced. This means that your physical body may "dream" of old injuries, symptoms or ailments, as it unlearns old, non-constructive subluxation patterns ... you may experience [old] symptoms, although this will be only so long as your body needs to "hold you there" until it grows past the old pattern ... Common recovery changes include change in breathing patterns, elimination, digestion, sensory changes such as tingling, warmth, itchiness, change in blood pressure, hormonal changes, fever, or symptoms associated with your body "cleaning house."

The patient handout continues by warning against the assumption that it may be desirable to have symptoms of organic disease: "The presence, or severity of these symptoms does not necessarily mean that you are better, they can have many meanings." The patient handout does not clarify under what circumstances a doctor, let alone a patient, might find the signs and symptoms of organic disease a favorable finding. Elsewhere, along the same lines, we read: "It is the contention of Network Chiropractic that what is commonly known as a disc syndrome and spondylolisthesis, are just two of the more common means that the resident intelligence may use to reduce neurological damage in the meningeal critical complex."[18]

- Network care involves numerous patient visits. Let us look at NSA visit frequency guidelines according to its levels of care model,[6] which describes basic, intermediate, and advanced care, with a fourth level on the way. Basic care, for new patients or recently reinjured patients that primarily addresses the Class B subluxations, requires 6 weeks to 4 months, 3 visits/week = 18–51 office visits. This is followed by intermediate care, in which primarily Class A subluxations are addressed, requiring 3–6 months, at least 2 visits/week = 26–52 office visits. Finally, the patient graduates to advanced care, requiring at least 4 months, at least 2 visits/week = 34 visits. Therefore, the levels of care model predicts that a new patient will be seen at least 78–137 times in about 1 year of care. At any moment the level 3 patient can sink back to level 1 or 2, and start all over again going through the levels.

- Emotional release on the part of the practice member is one of the recurring themes in descriptions of the NSA experience. The authors, as chiropractic clinicians, have seen patients begin crying or experience other strong feelings during adjustive procedures, and have little basis to dispute Network's contention that there are affective components to somatic dysfunction. Given that these responses may arise spontaneously, the authors' question is whether practitioners who may not be trained as mental health specialists should deliberately aim to evoke them, as seems common in an NSA practice environment.

- We have done our best to describe Network care, despite its ever-changing character, as NSA first weaned itself from NCT, and later went through significant evolutionary changes. The reader is urged to consult the internet to obtain the most recent self-characterizations of Network care, which are very easy to locate by simply searching under the term Network Spinal Analysis (e.g., InnateIntelligence.com, and AssociationForNetworkCare.com).

Just as this book was going to press, Network practitioners found themselves involved in a situation in the Canadian province of Manitoba, wherein the governing board declared Network Spinal Analysis was not a chiropractic technique. Having reviewed some of the same documents we had, it appears they had come a conclusion similar to the one we expressed in our introduction: NSA appears to have evolved into a technique more complementary to than included within chiropractic. Epstein, on the other hand, disputed this view and in a letter to the Manitoba board, advised he was in the process to revising statements at www.associationfornetworkcare.com that may have contributed to misunderstandings.

REFERENCES

1. Epstein D 1995 A revealing interview with Donald Epstein, DC, developer of Network Spinal Analysis. American Chiropractor (September/October): 6–7, 32, 38

2. Epstein D 1993 Network chiropractic: alignment for growth. Innate Intelligence 1 (4): 4

3. Epstein D 1987 The vitalistic practitioner. Digest of Chiropractic Economics (September/October): 64–65

4. Epstein D 2003 The tenets of Network Spinal Analysis and an overview of the Epstein models. Today's Chiropractic 32 (3): 20, 22–27

5. Epstein D 1996 Network Spinal Analysis: a system of health care delivery within the subluxation-based chiropractic model. Journal of Vertebral Subluxation Research 1 (1): 51–59

6. Epstein D M 2001 Theoretical basis and clinical application of Network Spinal Analysis (NSA) ® and evidence based document, XI revision. Innate Intelligence

7. Epstein D 1990 Network chiropractic: alignment for growth 1 (2): 4

8. Herriot E M 1990 Life-changing chiropractic. http://www.at-easewellness.com/reading_articles_litechanging.htm; (Accessed 29 May 2003)

9. Epstein D M 1984 Network Chiropractic explores the meningeal critical. Part I: anatomy and physiology of the meningeal functional unit. Digest of Chiropractic Economics (January/February): 78–80, 82

10. Epstein D 1987 The stress connection: gauging the role of the nervous system. Today's Chiropractic 15 (6): 15–17

11. Epstein D 1992 Network chiropractic: a unified application of chiropractic principles. Innate Intelligence

12. Breig A 1960 Biomechanics of the central nervous system. Almqvist & Wisekll International, Stockholm, Sweden

13. Epstein D 2001 Network Spinal Analysis seminars. Advanced level intensive. Seminar notes

14. Epstein D M 1986 The spinal meningeal functional unit tension and stress adaptation. Digest of Chiropractic Economics (November/December): 58, 60–61

15. Walker S 1996 Disobedient vertebrae: are they (neuro) emotionally disturbed? Chiropractic Products (October): 22–26

16. Epstein D M 1984 Network Chiropractic explores the meningeal critical. Part 2: "the disc syndrome" and the ultimate release. Digest of Chiropractic Economics (March/April): 89, 144–146

17. Epstein D 2003 Wellness and Network Spinal Analysis newly positioned. Chiropractic Journal (in press)

18. Epstein D M 1983 Network Analysis part 2. Digest of Chiropractic Economics (July/August): 18, 20, 21, 23

19. Epstein D M 1983 Network Analysis part 1. Digest of Chiropractic Economics (March/April): 57–58, 138–140

20. Epstein D 1989 Palpation as a critical tool to detect, classify, and understand central nervous system pathological dominance, and the correlation of these findings to various models of the vertebral subluxation. Presented to the research group ARCS

21. Norlyk E M 1989 Beyond bones. A new chiropractic system strives to align body and soul. East West (December): 26–30

22. Epstein D M 1996 Theoretical basis and clinical application of Network Spinal Analysis (NSA), 6th revision. Innate Intelligence

23. Patient testimonials 2003 http://www.trytel.com/~tucker/network/testimonials.html (accessed 29 May 2003)

24. Blanks R H I, Schuster T L, Dobson M 1997 A retrospective assessment of Network Care using a survey of self-rated health, wellness and quality of life. Journal of Vertebral Subluxation Research 1 (4): 15–31 http://www.jvsr.com/1/c32/1497_0041_retrospe.pdf

25. Miller E B, Redmond P D 1998 Changes in digital skin temperature, surface electromyography, and electrodermal activity in subjects receiving Network Spinal Analysis care. Journal of Vertebral Subluxation Research 2 (3): 87–95

26. Bohacek S, Jonckheere E 1998 Chaotic modeling in Network Spinal Analysis: nonlinear canonical correlation with alternating conditional expectation (ACE): a preliminary report. Journal of Vertebral Subluxation Research 2 (4) http://www.jvsr.com/1/c32/2498_0022_chaotic.pdf

27. Behrendt M 1998 Reduction of psoriasis in a patient under Network Spinal Analysis care: a case report. Journal of Vertebral Subluxation Research 2 (4) http://www.jvsr.com/access/abstracts.asp?catalogid=96

28. Gleberzon B J 2001 Letter to the editor. Journal of the Canadian Chiropractic Association 45 (1): 62–64

29. Blanks R H I et al 2001 To the editor in reply. Journal of the Canadian Chiropractic Association 45 (1): 64–65

FURTHER READING

Epstein D M 1994 The 12 stages of healing: a network approach to wholeness. Amber-Allen, San Rafael, CA

Fritjof C 2000 The Tao of physics: an exploration of the parallels between modern physics and Eastern mysticism, 4th edn. Shambhala, Boston

Zukar G 2001 The dancing Wu Li masters: an overview of the new physics. Perennial Classics, New York, NY

23

Pierce–Stillwagon Technique (PST)

INTRODUCTION

In 1991, Walter V Pierce was a featured speaker at a chiropractic research conference. In a concluding session near the end of the conference, a series of professional researchers struck a fairly consistent theme, to the effect that we had a long way to go in the area of researching chiropractic technique procedures. Pierce, following them, and quite oblivious to the somewhat gloomy tone that had been struck, took the microphone with great authority and confidence. He described in the simplest terms possible how he analyzed and corrected subluxations, how he typically restored the cervical lordosis in those who had lost it in one or two visits (a half-dozen in more challenging cases). Unlike the preceding speakers, who had portrayed the road ahead as fraught with potholes, Pierce charged the chiropractors and chiropractic students in the audience to address the future with great alacrity, to take renewed pride in their chosen profession. The electricity in the room was startlingly tangible, as audience members approached the microphone to thank Pierce for his stirring remarks, for having turned the negative mood around and ended the session on a high note.

Of course, Pierce's unbridled optimism was no more justified than the professional researchers' gloominess. He was right to emphasize that, through it all, chiropractic procedures work rather well, but they were right to bring out how poorly we understood how they work, and how that lack of understanding could hinder improving the state of the art. Since that day in 1991, researchers have tended to show more respect for traditional technique procedures, while technique people have acknowledged the need for their methods to be validated, and not simply declared to get great results.

Although PST combines the work of two men, Walter V Pierce and Glenn Stillwagon, the result so clearly resembles the technique of a third man, J Clay Thompson, that we are left with the following question: how similar can two chiropractic technique systems be, and still be considered separate and distinct? We could have written one chapter on drop-table adjusting, with a title like "Integrated Drop-Table Technique," but we chose to afford both PST and the Thompson Technique (Ch. 29) their own chapters. Each of these technique systems claims large numbers of adherents who presumably find them different enough to warrant distinct appellations.

Here are the differences: PST adds two new listings (double posterior-inferior (PI) and double anterior-superior (AS)) to the Thompson system, adds thermography to the analytic work-up, changes the terminology a little bit, customizes a few of the drop-table moves, and leaves out a few of the Thompson listings. Does that make a new technique? In all fairness to Drs Pierce and Stillwagon, they are fully aware of their debt to Thompson, stating in the introduction to their technique manual: "The Thompson Terminal Point Table, as well as his special method of adjusting, has given us the impetus to develop the technique herein described."[1] So be it.

OVERVIEW

PST follows in the tradition of Thompson technique (Ch. 29), and therefore retains much of its flavor: the importance of a Derifield-derived leg-check procedure, the emphasis on the cervical and pelvic areas, and heavy reliance on drop tables.[2,3] It is a full-spine, high-velocity, low-amplitude, drop-assisted technique. Much attention is paid to the postural substrate, even though subluxations are regarded as segmental lesions to which postural aberration is secondary. To the Thompson analysis are added two important pelvic listings (double PI and double AS) and one important cervical listing (the fifth cervical). There is much greater emphasis on the role of X-ray and thermography, both as part of the examination procedure and as outcome assessment.[4] There is considerable scope for incorporating other chiropractic techniques into the scope of PST, including Logan Basic (Ch. 21), Upper Cervical technique (Chs 32 and 33), and Reaver's Fifth Cervical technique.[5-7] When all is said and done, the primary focus of the technique is correction of the vertebral subluxation complex (VSC).[8]

HISTORY

Although Pierce started out as an upper cervical chiropractor, he eventually began study with J Clay Thompson, learning from him the indications for and the usage of a full-spine drop-table technique. He went on to develop his own table in conjunction with Williams Manufacturing, the Model 220 Terminal Point Hy-Lo table. Stillwagon, a 1956 graduate of the Palmer College,[9] heavily relied on thermographic analysis from the beginning, starting out his career with the dual-probed neurocalograph, which closely resembled the original neurocalometer, adding to it a recording capability. Around 1963 Pierce arrived at a new concept for thermographic instrumentation, by which a single-probe infrared device could replace the dual-probe predecessor devices. Pierce, Stillwagon, and Thompson went on jointly to develop what was to become the Derma-Therm-O-Graph,[10] which in turn had evolved into the Visi-Therm by 1983.[10]

Kevin Stillwagon, son of Glenn Stillwagon and a 1980 graduate of the Palmer College, later joined the development team, resulting in much work and many articles on thermography technology and clinical implementation.[2,4,10-22] It seems that Pierce (who passed away in 1993) may have been more involved in table development,[7] videofluoroscopic examination,[23] and image interpretation.[6,11,24] Not long before he died, Pierce associated himself professionally with Dr. Burl Pettibon, who shared many of his ideas concerning the definition of the normal cervical spinal lordosis.[25] The Pierce–Stillwagon Technique lives on, practiced by 17.1% of chiropractors on 6.5% of their patients.[26]

DEFINITION OF TECHNIQUE-SPECIFIC TERMS

- Spine-in-motion study: PST jargon for the Derifield leg check (see Ch. 4, on leg checking), which generates the listings positive ilium, negative ilium, and positive cervical rotation test
- Cervical rotation test: changes in relative leg length as the head is turned from side to side by a prone patient, signifying cervical subluxation
- Positive ilium: Derifield leg-check listing in which the knees-extended short leg crosses over to become the knees-flexed long leg, leading to the prone adjustment of the posterior-inferior iliac spine
- Negative ilium: Derifield leg-check listing in which the knees-extended short leg remains short when the knees are flexed, leading to any number of possible adjustments, depending primarily on X-ray findings and the possible presence of tender points
- PI ilium: a rotational misalignment of the ilium, in which the posterior superior iliac spine (PSIS) moves inferiorward and the symphysis pubis moves superiorly
- Double AS, double PI ilium: these listings are not to be understood as bilateral sacroiliac lesions, but rather as descriptors of the position of the PSISs "in space;" that is, either an anterior or posterior tilting of the entire pelvis, relative to its normal position, accompanied by lumbar adaptation[27]
- Lorphosis: a cervical spine that has a kyphotic region, either in the upper or lower cervical spine[28]

- Approximate normal potential rule: the arc that is traced out by the anterior bodies of the normal cervical lordosis;[24] the gold standard against which hyperlordotic, hypolordotic, and lorphotic cervical curves are rated
- Acu-arc: drafting tool that enables calculation of the radius of curvature of an arc. PST uses this tool to measure the curviness of the spinal regions in the sagittal plane
- Derma-Therm-O-Graph (DTG), Visi-Therm: thermography devices used in PST. The DTG, developed early on, was a dual-probed thermocouple device that was later replaced by the Visi-Therm, an infrared device capable of measuring absolute (as opposed to simply relative) temperatures (and thus cold points; Ch. 8).

PHYSIOLOGICAL MECHANISMS AND RATIONALE

PST practitioners believe that the normal spine in the frontal plane should be straight with the center of the head directly over the symphysis pubis. They further believe that the sagittal plane should manifest four curves: two anterior curves in the cervical and lumbar spines, and two posterior curves in the dorsal and sacral areas. The weakest areas of the spine would be the pelvic and cervical areas, which, when subluxated, give rise to compensations in the lumbar and thoracic spines. The adjustments consist in techniques for the upper cervicals (C1–2), the fifth cervical, the pelvis, and the sacrum.

The Stillwagons are fond of saying that thermography measures "physiology," whereas the other common indicators – leg checks, X-ray, muscle checks – reflect anatomy.[12,14] Their idea is that subluxation reduction normalizes autonomic function, allowing restoration of symmetric blood flow through body tissues, eliminating abnormal thermographic findings. PST is a very "osseous" technique, in that it takes at face value the contention that crooked bones are worth aligning, to normalize nerve function – and that's about it. One does not read of elaborate neural mediations, not even at the relatively simple level one finds in Thompson's writings.

DIAGNOSTIC/ANALYTIC PROCEDURES

A Derifield leg check is performed (Ch. 4), not unlike the Thompson procedure, except that there appears to be no analog for the X-Derifield Thompson listing, and a few other Thompson odds and ends (Ch. 29). Historically, this has been an X-ray-intensive technique, which means that the doctor ultimately takes listings off the film: double or unilateral PI or AS, internal (IN), external (EX), combinations thereof, and cervical listings (Table 23.1). Hinwood and Hinwood reported on the listings frequencies observed in a group of 633 patients.[29]

X-ray examination also forms a vital part of the examination, the analysis of which is not unlike the well-known parameters of the Gonstead analysis. The acu-arc standard of normalcy for the cervical lordosis is sometimes listed as 17 cm[6,30] and sometimes as 17–30 cm.[28] Deviations from this range are considered necessary to correct. Pierce went on to develop videofluoroscopic examination procedures of the cervical spine.[31]

In more recent years, the Stillwagons (in the absence of Pierce, who died in 1993) have to some degree de-emphasized the use of imaging techniques to identify the VSC, as compared with using thermography to get at it from a narrowly defined physiological point of view: "The loss of juxtaposition is such a small range of motion involving the three degrees of movement that we have been unable to see it on anatomical studies or palpate it. We certainly can't see juxtaposition on a flat X-ray ... It is obvious we cannot determine function on anatomical studies or palpation. However, advanced technology using thermal imaging enables us to do this."[32]

Thus, thermographic analysis occupies a central place in subluxation determination.[14] The

Table 23.1 Typical pelvic subluxation listings, as used in PST

Listing	Definition
PI	posterior-inferior
AS	anterior-superior
IN	internal (i.e., medial)
EX	external (i.e., lateral)

importance is well-rendered by the following representative quotation: "Adjust or not to adjust, that is the question. How do you determine the need? B.J. used instrumentation, but then, did he know what he was doing?"[33] Many articles have been written recommending the routine use of thermographic examination. As a special application, they claim thermography to be especially useful in examining geriatric patients, because of a relatively high rate of occurrence of reflex sympathetic dystrophy (RSD).[34]

Finally, the Stillwagons have more recently been advocating the use of scanning electromyography (EMG), which uses surface electrodes as compared to conventional needle EMG.[5,34]

TREATMENT/ADJUSTIVE PROCEDURES

Although PST is a full-spine, drop-table technique, the PST seminar manual[1] only concerns the adjustment of the pelvic area. The pelvic moves are performed either supine or prone, on a drop table (Fig. 23.1). Pierce's *Results*[35] adds the fifth

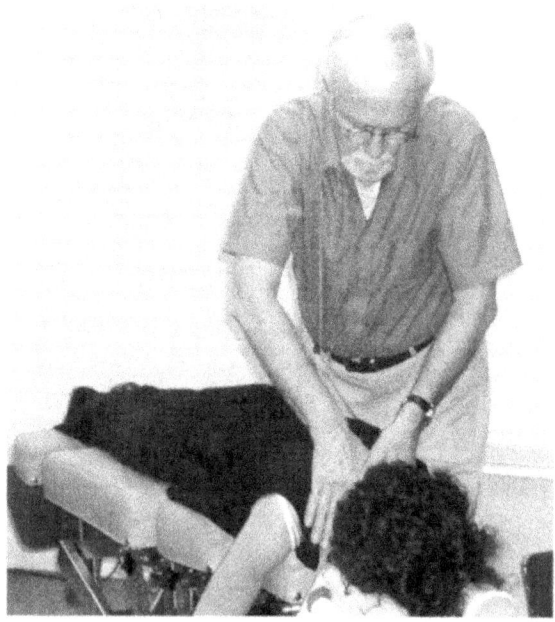

Figure 23.1   Dr. WH Zemelka, drop-table authority, performing the C5 Drop as pioneered by Vernon Pierce.

cervical, toggle, and sacral basic moves; one also finds a typical upper cervical analysis and a toggle-type move described.[6] Pierce's upper cervical roots are manifested in the fact that no thoracolumbar or lower cervical moves are described. In *Results*,[35] Pierce describes using his version of the "none-force" Logan Basic contact (Ch. 21) for treating acute disorders. The Fifth Cervical move amounts to a vigorous drop on C5, intended to restore lordosis rather abruptly to a hypolordotic or even lorphotic neck.

OUTCOME ASSESSMENT

Since the spine-in-motion study (i.e., Derifield leg check) is central to the overall patient examination procedure, not surprisingly, the abolition of a leg-check finding suggestive of vertebral subluxation is central to judging there to have been a good clinical outcome.

One of the principal goals of PST is to ensure adequate cervical lordosis, which is thought to exist when the neck forms an arc of a circle of 17–30 cm radius. PST practitioners certainly are not opposed to reducing symptoms, but their emphasis is strongly on normalizing physiology, as measured using thermography,[22] and realignment, as measured by X-ray.

Restoration of thermographic symmetry is critical to PST outcome assessment: "Using thermography is such a simple solution to this problem. It can give you an immediate indication of how the body is reacting to an adjustment, favorable or unfavorable."[10] The Visi-Therm device is capable of emulating both dual-probed results, by measuring left/right heat asymmetry, and segmental temperature irregularities, by comparing one vertebral level with the levels above and below. The data are colorized for easy viewing using a personal computer and monitor.

Usually, PST practitioners claim that cold spots signify pathology: "Most theories at that time [said] we were reading 'hot' nerves, but we found that this wasn't true. We found that we were actually reading cold areas of the blood vascular system, caused by subluxations. In 1967, we patented the Derma-Therm-O-Graph, a heat measurement device that permits us to spot these cold areas ...."[7]

None the less, Stillwagon and Stillwagon do indicate that acute subluxations would be expected to manifest as hot spots, that would yield to coldness as the stage of chronicity is attained.[13] PST also stresses the importance of X-ray-discernible changes, including restoration not only of normal pelvic and upper cervical alignment, but also of cervical lordosis.

SAFETY AND RISK FACTORS

We are aware of no contraindications to PST different from the contraindications to spinal manipulation in general.

EVIDENCE OF EFFICACY

Stump[36] found that "out of 975 cases treated for sacroiliac syndrome under the PST method of analysis and correction, 23 patients had to be referred for medical care. All other patients responded favorably with the length of treatment ranging from one month to one year at the time of the study." Kesten[37] investigated whether PST could reduce pelvic unleveling. His small group of 5 patients did not show statistically significant amelioration of pelvic unleveling, as measured by a Metrecom goniometric system, but the subjects did report a reduction in their pain levels. The forces generated in drop-table adjusting have been measured and found to be substantial.[38,39] The comprehensive studies by Cooperstein et al and Gatterman et al[40,41] found virtually no clinical trials using drop-table methods.

CONCLUSIONS

- The Stillwagons, confronted with the difficulty of using imaging techniques to demonstrate the presence of the VSC, have recommended placing comparatively more emphasis on demonstrating its physiological components, as identified by thermal imaging (thermography). Here is the problem with X-ray, as they see it:

Have you ever taken an X-ray of a patient which shows that the cervical spine is kyphotic and you tell the patient this is why he is experiencing headaches, or why the hands are numb? Then you tell the patient his neck should be curving the other way and the symptoms will go away. Later, after care, a post X-ray is taken and the cervical spine has only minimal change, and yet the symptoms are gone. What do you tell the patient? Embarrassing, isn't it?[42]

Thus, the Stillwagons recommend using thermographic procedures rather than radiological procedures to identify vertebral subluxation. However, thermography is no less controversial than radiography in identifying spinal pathological states. The Stillwagons acknowledge the possibility of thermal asymmetry in asymptomatic subjects, but do not seem to think this means the diagnostic procedure results in frequent false-positives: "It is not uncommon to find asymptomatic patients with abnormal scans. These patients are shown the abnormality, and tend to follow our recommendations better, because they can "see" the problem."[10] This belief in the importance of the finding of thermal asymmetry, in the absence of correspondence with patient symptoms or other examination findings, is at minimum problematic. We are at a loss to understand why the Stillwagons feel that "Thermography can not meet, nor will it ever be able to meet a basic criterion of a medical diagnostic test: The blinded study."[21] On the contrary, thermography is quite amenable to being studied in a rigorous manner, and has been.[43]

- It took us a while in reading through the PST technique manual to grasp that there are two types of "PI" ilium listings, the posterior-inferior ilium and the positive ilium, and that they are not the same listing. The positive ilium is a sacroiliac listing in which the PSIS *translates* (i.e., moves linearly) posteriorly and inferiorly, relative to the sacrum. The posterior ilium, as discussed in PST, is a different type of sacroiliac listing, in which the innominate bone *rotates* around some (non-discussed) intrapelvic axis of rotation.

- Very little is known on the biomechanics of drop-table adjusting, in terms of how it affects patients differently from non-drop-table methods of intervention. The relatively small distance through which the table drops when actuated, as compared with how far the patient's low back may be moved through space while lying in side-posture, *may* suggest that drop-table low-back interventions are relatively safer than side-posture manipulations. However, even if this were true, it certainly would not mean that side-posture manipulation has ever been shown to be unsafe for the great majority of patients. Apart from patient considerations, it seems reasonable to suggest that drop-table methods may be kinder and gentler to the doctor's own spine, especially if there has already been an injury, compared with side-posture manipulation techniques.

- Although for many years Walter V Pierce and Glenn Stillwagon combined their technique in most ways, Pierce did emphasize more heavily

the status of the cervical lordosis, as well as a few other matters, worthy of some attention. According to Painter, his later work may as well be called the Pierce Results System,[44] a practice style somewhat different from what he had espoused during his years of managing PST with the Stillwagons. He had incorporated stress X-rays (flexion, extension, and/or lateral bending views) and also videofluoroscopy into his work. He was also employing handheld adjusting devices, like those used by Pettibon, Fuhr, and others, as well as a computer-assisted adjusting instrument.[45] Near the end of his life, Pierce combined his work with Pettibon,[25] who, like Pierce had done, continues to emphasize heavily the importance of the cervical lordosis.

REFERENCES

1. Pierce W V, Stillwagon G 1976 Pierce–Stillwagon seminar manual. Pierce-Stillwagon Seminars, Monongahela, PN
2. Stillwagon G, Stillwagon K 1998 The Pierce–Stillwagon technique: procedures and analysis. Part I of II. Today's Chiropractic 27 (3): 34–48
3. Stillwagon G, Stillwagon K 1998 The Pierce–Stillwagon technique: procedures and analysis. Part I of II. Today's Chiropractic 27 (2): 34–39
4. Stillwagon G, Stillwagon K 1998 Vertebral subluxation correction and its affect on thermographic readings: a description of the advent of the Visi-Therm as applied to chiropractic patient assessment. Journal of Vertebral Subluxation Research 2 (3): 1–4 http://www.jvsr.com/1/c32/2398-0030_vertibral.pdf
5. Reaver C 1977 The fifth cervical key. Chirp, Dravosburg, PA
6. Pierce W V 1981 Results. Chirp, Dravosburg, PA
7. Scroggins R I 1982 Successful chiropractic practice built on repeatable patient results. Digest of Chiropractic Economics (March/April): 51
8. Stillwagon G, Stillwagon K L 1995 Chiropractic must stake its claim on the vertebral subluxation complex. Today's Chiropractic 24 (3): 34–38
9. Stillwagon B S, Stillwagon G 1997 There's no CPT code for philosophy! Today's Chiropractic 26 (2): 76–79
10. Stillwagon G, Stillwagon B Chiropractic thermography – visual evidence. http://www.stillwagon.com/articles/Artvisul.htm
11. Pierce W V 1982 Instrumentation. Digest of Chiropractic Economics (September/October): 41–44
12. Stillwagon G 1985 Visi-Therm: non-contact computerized infrared thermography. American Chiropractor (May): 63–67
13. Stillwagon G, Stillwagon K 1985 Early observations of the Visi-Therm. Today's Chiropractic 14 (5): 38–40
14. Stillwagon G, Stillwagon K L 1986 Adjust or not to adjust. Digest of Chiropractic Economics 28 (5): 49
15. Stillwagon G, Stillwagon K L 1986 Thermography: an evaluation tool. Today's Chiropractic 15 (3): 59
16. Stillwagon G 1989 Thermography: is chiropractic ready for it? American Chiropractor (April): 28–31
17. Stillwagon G, Stillwagon K L, Stillwagon B S, Dalesio D L 1992 Chiropractic thermography. ICA International Review of Chiropractic 48 (1): 8–13
18. Stillwagon G, Stillwagon K L 1993 Objective chiropractic model for research. American Chiropractor 15 (5): 20–24
19. Sawyer C E, Meeker W C, Phillips R B 1992 Module summaries from consensus conference 2. Chiropractic Technique 4 (2): 37–45
20. Stillwagon G, Delesio D 1998 Chiropractic thermography for outcomes measurement of the vertebral subluxation complex. Today's Chiropractic (May/June): 96–102
21. Stillwagon G, Stillwagon K L Thermography at the crossroads. http://www.stillwagon.com/articles/Artherm2.htm
22. Dalesio D, Stillwagon G 1998 Chiropractic thermography for outcomes measurement of the vertebral subluxation complex. Today's Chiropractic 27 (3): 96–102
23. Wallace H L, Pierce W V, Wagnon R J 1992 Cervical flexion and extension analysis using digitized videofluoroscopy. Journal of Chiropractic Research and Clinical Investigation 7 (4): 94–97
24. Pierce W V 1979 Curves and curvatures. Chirp, Dravosburg, PA
25. Hochman J I 1992 Pierce and Pettibon combine their systems. ICA Review (January): 84–86
26. Christensen M G 2000 Job analysis of chiropractic. A project report, survey analysis and summary of the

practice of chiropractic within the United States. National Board of Chiropractic Examiners, Greeley, CO

27. Clemen M J 1983 Understanding and adjusting bilateral pelvic unit subluxations. Today's Chiropractic (March/April): 22

28. Stillwagon G, Stillwagon K L 1983 The Pierce–Stillwagon technique. American Chiropractor (July/August): 20–23, 28–31, 65

29. Hinwood J A, Hinwood J A 1983 Sacroiliac biomechanics. Digest of Chiropractic Economics (January/February): 79

30. Pierce W V 1987 Research of the cervical spine. Digest of Chiropractic Economics (September/October): 14–18

31. Wallace H, Wallace J, Resh R 1993 Advances in paraspinal thermographic analysis. Chiropractic Research Journal 2 (3): 39–52

32. Stillwagon G Loss of juxtaposition ... the elusive part of vertebral subluxation complex. http://www.stillwagon.com/articles/Artjuxta.htm

33. Stillwagon G, Stillwagon B Did B J know what he was doing? http://www.stillwagon.com/articles/ArtBJ.htm

34. Stillwagon G, Stillwagon K L 1994 Geriatrics – where does chiropractic fit in? ICA Review (September/October): 49–51

35. Pierce W V 1986 Results. X-Celent Ray, Dravosburg, PA

36. Stump J L 1979 Efficacy of the Pierce–Stillwagon chiropractic technique in clinical application of the sacroiliac syndrome. ICA International Review of Chiropractic 33: 42–44

37. Kesten B S 1991 Multiple case study of five patients with pelvic unleveling. Chiropractic Research Journal 2 (1): 51–56

38. Adams A A, Wood J 1984 Forces used in selected chiropractic adjustments of the low back: a preliminary study. Research Forum 1 (1): 5–9

39. Hessell B W, Herzog W, Conway P J, McEwen M C 1990 Experimental measurement of the force exerted during spinal manipulation using the Thompson technique. Journal of Manipulative and Physiological Therapeutics 13 (8): 448–453

40. Cooperstein R, Perle S M, Gatterman M I et al 2001 Chiropractic technique procedures for specific low back conditions: characterizing the literature. Journal of Manipulative and Physiological Therapeutics 24 (6): 407–424

41. Gatterman M I, Cooperstein R, Lantz C et al 2001 Rating specific chiropractic technique procedures for common low back conditions. Journal of Manipulative and Physiological Therapeutics 24 (7): 449–456

42. Stillwagon G, Stillwagon K L What are we trying to change? http://www.stillwagon.com/articles/Artchang.htm

43. Hoffman R M, Kent D L, Deyo R A 1991 Diagnostic accuracy and clinical utility of thermography for lumbar radiculopathy. A meta-analysis. Spine 16 (6): 623–628

44. Painter F Pierce results system. http://www.chiro.org/LINKS/pierce.shtml

45. Evans J M 2002 The history of computerized fixation imaging. http://www.pulstarfras.com/About_SENSE_TECHNOLOGY.html

24

Receptor-Tonus Technique
(Receptor-Tonus Control Method (RTCM), Nimmo Technique)

INTRODUCTION

Once upon a time, Cooperstein, during a trip to New York to visit with his brother and family, accompanied his sister-in-law to her chiropractor's office. That chiropractor, demonstrating his treatment approach, at one point said "I usually throw in a little Nimmo work." He began randomly rubbing away in the interscapular area, making little circles in the soft tissue that no doubt felt good, and maybe even did some good – however accidentally, as Nimmo would have explained. It is now clear to Cooperstein that what he was doing had nothing to do with actual Nimmo work. It was, for better or worse, the first time Cooperstein had seen a clinical intervention alleged to be Receptor-Tonus Technique.

Raymond Nimmo understood well how and why, given growing interest in "soft-tissue work," a chiropractor might feign skill in Receptor-Tonus Technique, simply by gimping around in muscles without having taken the trouble first to identify actual trigger points; and beyond that, without having taken the trouble to acquire the skill to identify trigger points.

Dr. Raymond L Nimmo was brilliant, heretical and courageous. He introduced what is now called trigger point work into chiropractic at a time when trigger point work was not cool. We are very lucky that M Schneider, J Cohen and S Laws have published an anthology of his writings,[2] about half of which is articles originally published in the *Digest of Chiropractic Economics* and the other half taken from Nimmo's own publication, *The Receptor*. This incredible resource really simplified the task of producing this technique review, and we thank the producers. (Rather than cite the original sources in our own book chapter, we elected to cite the anthology.)

The identification of Nimmo with trigger point work is so total, such a ready-made, that it takes extra effort to get past that solitary fact and appreciate Nimmo the man. Although he was seen by some as antichiropractic (for severely taking to task the bone-out-of-place, nerve-pressure theory), and by others as unchiropractic (because of his emphasis on treating muscles, not bones), the critique he formulated was not of chiropractic per se, but of the chiropractic delivery vehicle. How sad it was, as he saw it, that chiropractors had become anti-intellectual and rigid in their thought processes, ethically challenged in their unbridled pursuit of patients, and hateful in their attitudes about the role and contributions of other healthcare professions. As a largely self-trained clinician/scientist, Nimmo came to understand that the purpose of chiropractic research was not to prove one's ideas, but to seek out the truth; that research was not an end in itself, but intended ultimately to improve patient care.

OVERVIEW

The starting point of Receptor-Tonus Technique is that dysfunctional muscle results in joint restriction and/or misalignment, as well as abnormal visceral function. These problems are often self-perpetuating, and require external intervention to disrupt the reflex arcs. Receptor-Tonus Technique identifies and treats these myofascial trigger points, so as to normalize neurological function, and reduce or eliminate both direct and referred pain. Normalizing receptor function also normalizes effector regulation of muscle and gland function, freeing a muscle or group of muscles from hypertonus, and improving the patient's posture and overall bodily function.

HISTORY

Raymond L Nimmo graduated from the Palmer College in 1926. Early in his career he followed BJ Palmer in practicing the Hole-In-One (HIO) upper cervical technique, but remained perplexed about a couple of personal observations about the neuromuscular system. First, some people (like himself) had nice posture but were racked with pain, whereas others had poor postures and never hurt. Second, it was not clear how and why some people exhibited tight muscles, despite not having voluntarily contracted them. In 1935, Nimmo took up Logan Basic Technique[2] (p. 203–204) (Ch. 21), which, according to Nimmo, was appropriated from Hurley and Sanders' *Aquarian Age Healing* (see Further reading). (Logan attended Hurley's

first class.) Although Nimmo saw that Logan's very light sacral specific work got good clinical results, it was not obvious to him how such light contacts could provide benefit to a 200 lb (90 kg) man lifting a 100 lb (45 kg) weight, throwing his full weight on to each side of the sacrum with each step. He next took up Chromaffin Synapse Therapy, an intrarectal technique thought at the time to affect the sacral ganglia, but which Nimmo thought in retrospect worked on muscles such as the piriformis and coccygeus. Nimmo then became involved in the McIntosh system of Fascia Release, although he eventually understood that the technique actually released tensed musculature.

Apparently, Nimmo's own methods got their start during the 1940s, and he began working exclusively on them in 1954.[2] (p. 17) In a 1977 publication,[3] Nimmo wrote that his seminal discovery, that manual pressure could normalize muscle function, had occurred 25 years previously, suggesting a date in the late 1940s. His treatment methods eventually led him to coin the term "noxious generative points" (Fig. 24.1), which he later concluded

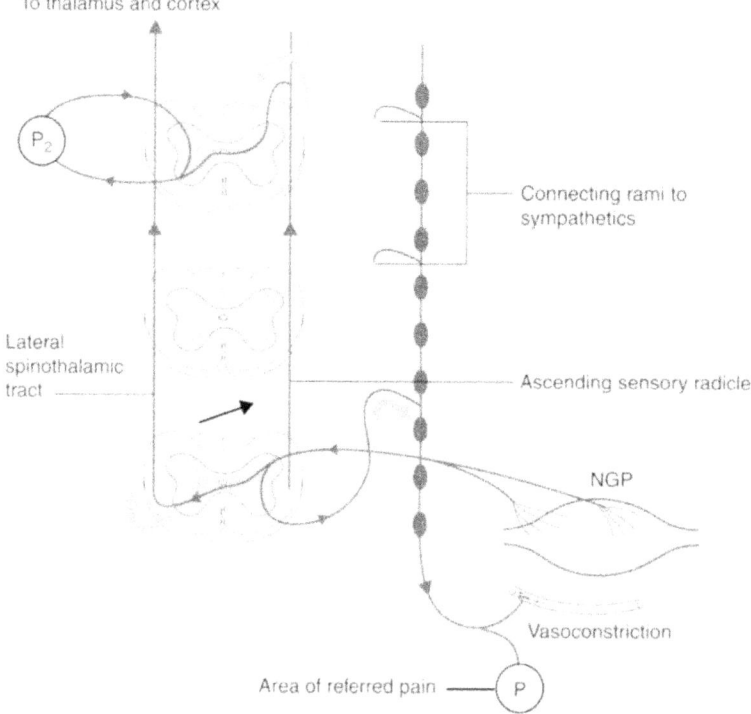

Figure 24.1 Neural routes taken by stimuli from a noxious generative point (NGP).

were identical to the trigger points described by medical practitioner Janet Travell, whose work he had come upon in 1952. In an undated issue of *The Receptor*, which appears to be from 1958, he speaks of the "first year" of RCTM.[2] (p. 25) Travell herself, and thus through her this type of manual therapy, achieved notoriety when she became personal physician to the pain-racked President John F Kennedy. She and coauthor Simons later produced two thorough volumes describing their methods.[4,5] As for Nimmo, he published his first article in the November 1957 issue of the *National Chiropractic Association Journal*.[1] He was later joined by collaborator and coauthor James Vannerson, who, like Nimmo, passed away in the 1980s.

DEFINITION OF TECHNIQUE-SPECIFIC TERMS

Nimmo coined several phrases that are hardly, if ever, used today. He himself was delighted to jettison atypical terms and jargon whenever a more popular phrase existed that meant the same thing. That stated, we will list a few obscure terms that show up in his writings.

- Trigger point, tonoplast, noxious generative point, painful nerve mechanism: a nerve arrangement, myofascial or ligamentous, that generates noxious impulses that bombard the central nervous system, upsetting its balance[2] (p. 19)
- Receptor-Tonus Control Method (RTCM): the treatment of trigger points using ischemic compression
- Aberrative foci: Nimmo's "subluxation-equivalent," as discussed by Cooperstein and Gleberzon[6]
- Hypermyotonia: muscle hypertonus.[7]

PHYSIOLOGICAL MECHANISMS AND RATIONALE

Michael Schneider, a principal proponent of Nimmo's methods today, identified two major premises of Receptor-Tonus Technique:[1] (1) muscle dysfunction often precedes joint dysfunction, so that hypertonic muscles cause fixation and

osseous misalignment; (2) trigger points can provide noxious stimuli to the central nervous system, resulting in referred pain, peripheral nerve entrapment, facilitation of spinal cord interneurons, and somatovisceral/somatosomatic reflexes.

Nimmo was not much impressed by the thought that vertebral misalignment is some sort of primary problem. His starting point was that "bones are where muscles and ligaments put them."[2] (p. 2) In other words, bones don't just decide to misalign, an absurdly simplistic view he derisively termed the "osseous limitation." Therefore, the chiropractor must understand that the trouble is not with bones, but with the nervous system that controls the muscles that control the bones. He argued that the reticular activating system (RAS) controls muscle tone, and thus posture, but that the RAS itself was governed by proprioceptors, or specialized receptors. In opposition to those chiropractors who would attempt to reverse postural distortions via purely mechanical means, efforts which he felt were doomed to failure, Nimmo wrote: "Find the original condition which forced the RAS to distort the body, correct it, and you will see immediate change."[2] (p. 41)

Like DD Palmer, and in opposition to simplistic interpretations of the nerve impingement model, Nimmo believed that the patient's problem arose from too much aberrant input, not excessive output from the nervous system. This was an early application of the GIGO metaphor of the computer age: garbage in, garbage out. Indeed, writing in the 1950s, Nimmo was well aware of "electronic brains," and discussed the confounding impact that would likely result from attaching a high-voltage battery to the innards of the system.[2] He went on to declare: "Perverted reception means perverted action."[2] (p. 20)

The "original condition" identified by Nimmo was the *noxious generative point*, now commonly identifed by its more common and entirely equivalent term, *trigger point*. The trigger point is associated with pain in a characteristic cutaneous distribution, which may not even contain the trigger point. These hypersensitive pain points may precipitate abnormal reflex arcs, resulting in both somatovisceral and somatosomatic reflexes: abnormal visceral and abnormal musculoskeletal function, respectively. Some insult to a muscle – such as overuse or frank injury, a cold draft, or even emotional problems – causes an abnormal increase in afferent input to the spinal cord, which in turn may cause an abnormal stream of efferent impulses back to the muscle, resulting in hyper-myotonia (hypertonus). This mechanism, sometimes called the pain–spasm–pain cycle, becomes a vicious cycle. These abnormal reflex arcs have tremendous staying power, and often require external intervention to break the loop. In addition to the reflex hypertonus of the muscle related to the trigger point, there may be satellite or secondary trigger points, and visceral dysfunction in the organs innervated by the internuncial neuronal pool stimulated by the trigger point.

Among the physiological explanations, Schneider,[8] following Nimmo, invokes two laws:

- Hilton's law: the nerve which supplies a joint also supplies the skin overlying that joint, and the muscles which move that joint. Therefore, when any of the above structures becomes inflamed or painful, it triggers reflex spasm in muscles associated with that joint.
- Davis' law: Any muscle which remains hypertonic or in spasm for a period of time is prone to develop myofascial trigger points. As a muscle shortens, the pull of tonus is increased, and the muscle shortens further. Nature allows no slack in the muscular system.

Figure 24.1 summarizes Nimmo's subluxation pathology, although he would have preferred the term "noxious generative point" to our use of the word "subluxation." The noxious generative point fires impulses into the cord in the afferent loop. The efferent connection produces vasoconstriction and referred pain at location P through connection with the sympathetic nervous system; an ipsilateral somatosomatic reflex; and contralateral symptoms at location P_2. Nimmo and Vannerson go on to explain:

With these brief statements in mind it may readily be seen that any increase in afferent (sensory) stimuli, induced by stress or injury by which receptors in somatic areas are over-stimulated, will also increase motor stimuli passing through the anterior root, which will heighten muscle tonus, evoke vascular

tensions, and perhaps alter visceral functions. It is the constancy of such hypertonus, with the reciprocal action of hypotonus on the opposite muscles, which eventually misaligns spinal segments and produces other distortions of the skeletal frame. There is no other way physiologically possible.[3] (p. 49)

The treatment strategy immediately follows: treat the receptors (i.e., trigger points), to normalize muscles, skeletal structures and visceral function. Nimmo did not argue that other technique methods, such as the sacral methods of Logan Basic Technique or Upper Cervical Technique, did *not* work, but only that they worked by more or less *accidentally* impacting upon receptor-effector mechanisms, and through them muscles, other connective tissues, and organs. Nimmo thought that the results achieved by these other adjustive methods were more transient than those that came about through the deliberate treatment of trigger points.

Although exactly what is effected by ischemic compression is largely unknown, some possibilities suggested by Schneider[1] include: (1) local vasodilation, increasing the drainage of the waste products of metabolism; (2) endorphin release and consequent analgesia; (3) reflex inhibition of muscle hypertonus; (4) and specific stretching of the local contracted muscle fibers. Normalizing muscle function is thought to allow normalization of bone position (posture), joint mechanics and visceral function, and would reduce primary and referred pain complaints.

DIAGNOSTIC/ANALYTIC PROCEDURES

Obviously, what is unique and distinctive in Receptor-Tonus Technique is the identification of trigger points, both primary and secondary. That stated, we note that Receptor-Tonus practitioners also practice standard history taking and physical examination procedures.[1] As Schneider describes it,[1] the trigger point scan involves using moderate finger pressure to locate strands of contracted muscle fibers known as *taut bands*, which may contain localized *knots* or *nodules*. Having identified such structures, the doctor then attempts to elicit referred pain and/or autonomic phenomena, perhaps to reproduce the patient's presenting complaints. Some practitioners use a soft-tissue algometer to objectify their findings.

TREATMENT/ADJUSTIVE PROCEDURES

Although Receptor-Tonus practitioners are likely to use an assortment of clinical interventions, emphasizing but not limited to trigger point work, we need not dwell upon how they implement exercises, counseling on the activities of daily life, and so forth. The medical treatment of trigger points often involves injection techniques, outside the scope of chiropractic, and sometimes the application of ultrasound. Some of both medical and chiropractic providers treat trigger points using a method known as "spray and stretch," which involves cooling down the muscle to be treated (the muscle related to the trigger point, which need not actually be in the muscle at all!) while stretching it. The cooling is achieved either by using a vapocoolant spray, or through ice massage. Nimmo's original trigger point method, still used by many chiropractors and others, even when they acquired their training in a medical milieu, utilizes *ischemic compression* (Travell's term), a strictly manual method.[9]

Schneider advocates applying pressure to the trigger point for 7–10 s,[1] although we have also seen that he and coauthor Cohen recommend as little as 5–7 s (Fig. 24.2).[9] (By comparison, Travell recommended as much as 2 min of compression, as forcefully applied as the patient can tolerate it.[9]) Nimmo sometimes used a slow, gliding pressure applied to larger sensitized areas in a muscle.[10] An office visit may involve three or four applications, and the force level varies from patient to patient. Daily treatments are discouraged, as being too stressful for the patient.[9] Although Nimmo himself relied solely on ischemic compression, some contemporary practitioners add physical therapy modalities as ancillary procedures, and many deploy general muscle stretching and exercises.

OUTCOME ASSESSMENT

Not surprisingly, given the pre-eminence of the trigger point, the patient's improvement is suggested by reduction or elimination of the degree of tenderness to scanning palpation or algometry. On the other hand, given how frequently patients enter a Receptor-Tonus practice setting for a pain complaint, the reduction of that pain is an outcome measure of primary importance. Nimmo, without any doubt, saw himself in the pain reduction business.

SAFETY AND RISK FACTORS

The contraindications to ischemic compression listed by Schneider[1] are all relatively infrequent, suggesting that the method is well-tolerated by most patients without adverse reactions. The listed contraindications are: (1) deep-vein thrombosis or tendency to thromboembolism, especially involving the posterior calf muscles; (2) taking corticosteroid or anticoagulant medications that increase the risk of bleeding; (3) application directly over a bruised or otherwise directly injured muscle location; (4) extremely low pain thresholds; and (5) significant post-treatment bruising. No osseous thrusting is involved, so we need not note its contraindications.

EVIDENCE OF EFFICACY

There is an extensive medical literature on the clinical efficacy of trigger point injections and the

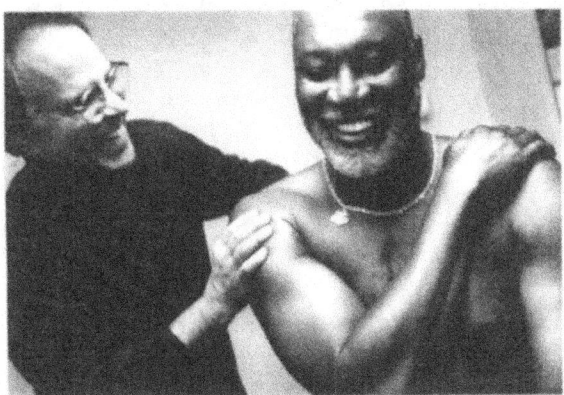

Figure 24.2 Dr. J Cohen performs Nimmo Receptor-Tonus Technique on former Pittsburgh Steeler great LC Greenwood.

spray and stretch techniques, which is certainly relevant to the evaluation of Receptor-Tonus Technique. As Schneider notes, many, if not most, of the studies involve other treatment modalities as well, such as manipulation and physical therapy devices, confounding our ability to ascribe treatment benefits with certainty to the trigger point component. There are examples of studies supporting both visceral consequences of manual trigger point treatment, such as a randomized clinical trial by Delaney et al[11] that showed a reduction in blood pressure and in heart rate; and also examples underscoring pain reduction, such as a trial conducted by Hou et al.[12]

Schneider provides a case report[13] involving a 32-year-old male marathon runner presenting with a painful snapping hip and knee pain. Manually treating myofascial trigger points in the ipsilateral tensor fascia lata and gluteus medius/minimus muscles, and providing home stretching exercises, led to the patient becoming asymptomatic in six office visits.

CONCLUSIONS

- As we read through the Nimmo and Vannerson anthology,[2] we came across too many quotable quotes not to afford these men a posthumous opportunity to speak for their iconoclastic selves.

On the nerve pressure theory, citing Tarsey

Where nerve pressure exists, there is always 'paralysis, paresis, pain' ... No wonder when a chiropractor talks about nerve pressure with the connotation and intent he always means by such, the medic knows he is either an ignoramus or is trying to push his wares.[2] (p. 11)

On traditional chiropractic philosophy:

The customer is always right, and he wants health, not a metaphysical concept of what is wrong. We need to go to work. The patient does not give a hoot about our principle and our philosophy. We need to quit preaching and go to work. You convert a man when you make him well again.[2] (p. 13)

On somatovisceral reflexes:

Crooked spines do not usually cause human disease, except to the degree that such distortion places organs at a mechanical disadvantage.[2] (p. 13)

On X-ray, part I:

When studying an X-ray the doctor should keep in mind there are many things it will not reveal. Function, for example. Too many times X-ray becomes a tyrant and is a complete dictator of procedure. Probably in 9 cases out of 10 the chiropractor could proceed just as successfully without it. If you do not think so, try it. You might find that you will bring to life a talent long buried – the ability to detect the state of tissue by feel, for example.[2] (p. 14)

On X-ray, part II:

It is an established fact that patients become well of conditions with no discernible change whatsoever in vertebral relationships, as proven by precision pre and post X-ray studies.[2] (p. 55)

On correcting postural distortion:

Wiggling machines, stretching machines, and all sorts of mechanical gadgets will not straighten a body. It takes human intelligence, understanding and application.[2] (p. 41)

- In a welcome departure from the professional chauvinism that often impels technique proprietors to coin and utilize atypical and often obfuscating terminology, Nimmo actually preferred terms coined by others that he thought would be more familiar to readers and listeners to his own creations. That is why he abandoned the "noxious generative point" in favor of the term "trigger point."
- As should be abundantly clear by now, Nimmo and Vannerson did not support the traditional subluxation theory, in the sense of bone-out-of-place as some sort of primary problem. On the other hand, like chiropractors in general, at the center of their technique one finds a *subluxation-equivalent*, as we have defined it: "any word or phrase used by a technique partisan that renders that same reductionist thought and serves the same function as the mere word 'Subluxation.'"[6] As the editors of the Nimmo and Vannerson anthology[2] point out, the following quotation is definitive: "Chiropractic is a healing science and art which is concerned with locating and eliminating aberrant foci in the human body which interfere with the normal functional integrity of the nervous system."[2] (p. 56) So there it is: chiropractic is about correcting *aberrant foci*.

- Nimmo well understood that diagnosing and treating trigger points would temporarily increase the patient's pain. He felt that chiropractors who ran "slap-happy" practices, who were only concerned with immediately making the patient feel better, were derelict in their duties as chiropractors. A doctor who knows how to reproduce the patient's complaint is well on the way to being able to vanquish it.

- In Figure 24.1, locations P and P_2, according to Nimmo, can be almost anywhere in the body. This reminds us of fellow Texan William D Harper's proposition that, when it comes to the nervous system, *Anything Can Cause Anything.*[14] (We guess.) Nimmo thought this model adequately explained how D D Palmer would have restored hearing in the first chiropractic patient:[2] (p. 34)

  I think there are certain essentials necessary in order for us to escape from the mossy-fingered grip of orthodoxy and improve when a superior method is evident.

  First, one must have a free and open mind and not fear change. One should cultivate an attitude of gladness when he finds himself in error, realizing that now he is free to correct it. One should feel elated and not depressed and fearful when he finds a hitherto cherished idea to be baseless.

  Two, for honest research one must keep his practice free from economic pressure. Research cannot be valid if influenced by economics. He must hold his practice to a modest level where he can know, study and follow each case. Clinical advances do not come from those with huge practices, only managerial skills.[2]

- Chiropractors have always had to struggle with the concept that so many disparate techniques, ranging from methods that emphasized the atlas, the sacrum, or anything inbetween, using light or vigorous thrusting, seem to get parallel results. Nimmo dealt more squarely with this paradox than any other chiropractor whose work we read in writing this book. He points out that, although we blame misaligned vertebrae for patients' problems, pre and post X-rays do not usually differ, even though the patients improve. He cites the case of the Upper Cervical practitioner, who asserts that there can be no impingement below the neck, despite the fact that many patients whose necks are never touched are restored to health. He also cites the case of the pelvic man, who, opining that the foundation of the spine must be addressed first, is left with no explanation for the success of the Upper Cervical practitioner. Nimmo believed that the success of varying treatment methods ultimately accrued, however unintentionally, to their having had an impact upon receptor-tonus points.

- Poole,[10] citing Vannerson,[15] describes how emotional stress and tension may elicit trigger points and through them somatic pain and hyperactive autonomic function. We think this is a very important point.

- Although Cohen and Schneider state[9] that Receptor-Tonus Technique was one of the first reflex techniques in chiropractic, we are not certain that we agree. Elsewhere in this text, we comment that reflex techniques in chiropractic usually claim to work by means of poorly understood body mechanisms, not described in mainstream works of anatomy and physiology. The reflex arcs that provide the theoretical underpinning of Nimmo's methods, by comparison, are so well-described and plausible that we are not inclined to consider Receptor-Tonus Technique a reflex technique.

- Is there any temptation to classify Receptor-Tonus as a reflex technique simply because it is a low-force technique? In another place,[7] Cohen and Gibbons point out that Nimmo was one of the earliest low-force practitioners, although preceded by Leo Loban and Leo Spears; and Nimmo himself described how he was influenced by Logan's light-force Basic Technique. In our opinion, using light forces does not make a technique a reflex technique. Despite the reflex-like character of his work, in the sense that manual stimulation of various body loci produces or reduces pain in body locations that can be quite far away, Nimmo himself vigorously opposed the notion that his was a reflex technique. "It is not a reflex system, but a direct approach, clearing out entirely all so called 'reflexes.'"[2] (p. 17)

REFERENCES

1. Schneider M 1994 Receptor-Tonus Technique assessment. Chiropractic Technique 6 (4): 156–159
2. Schneider M, Cohen J, Laws S (eds) 2001 The collected writings of Nimmo and Vannerson: pioneers of Chiropractic Trigger Point Therapy. Self-published, Pittsburgh, PA
3. Nimmo R L 1977 Receptor-Tonus Technique. In: Kfoury P W (ed.) Catalog of chiropractic techniques, pp. 63–64, Logan College of Chiropractic, Chesterfield, MI
4. Travell J G, Simons D G 1983 Myofascial pain and dysfunction: the trigger point manual, vol. 1. Williams & Wilkins, Baltimore, MD
5. Travell J G, Simons D G 1992 Myofascial pain and dysfunction: the trigger point manual, vol. 2. Williams & Wilkins, Baltimore, MD
6. Cooperstein R, Gleberzon B J 2001 Toward a taxonomy of subluxation-equivalents. Topics in Clinical Chiropractic 8 (1): 49–60
7. Cohen J H, Gibbons R W 1998 Raymond L Nimmo and the evolution of trigger point therapy, 1929–1986. Journal of Manipulative and Physiological Therapeutics 21 (3): 167–172
8. Schneider M J 1992 Nimmo Receptor-Tonus Technique: advanced. Self-published, Pittsburgh, PA
9. Cohen J H, Schneider M 1990 Receptor-Tonus technique: an overview. Chiropractic Technique 2 (1): 13–16
10. Poole P B 1990 Myofascial therapy: neurophysiological basis of the Nimmo Technique. D C Tracts 2 (4): 199–205
11. Delaney J P, Leong K S, Watkins A, Brodie D 2002 The short-term effects of myofascial trigger point massage therapy on cardiac autonomic tone in healthy subjects. Journal of Advanced Nursing 37 (4): 364–371
12. Hou C R, Tsai L C, Cheng K F et al 2002 Immediate effects of various physical therapeutic modalities on cervical myofascial pain and trigger-point sensitivity. Archives of Physical Medicine and Rehabilitation 83 (10): 1406–1414
13. Schneider M J 1990 Snapping hip syndrome in a marathon runner: treatment by manual trigger point therapy – a case study. Chiropractic Sports Medicine 4 (2): 54–58
14. Harper W D 1974 Anything can cause anything, 3rd edn. Self-published, Seabrook, TX
15. Vannerson J F 1997 Sympathetic vascular malfunctions in disease: part II. Digest of Chiropractic Economics (Sept/Oct): 60–70

FURTHER READING

Hurley J, Sanders H 1932 The Aquarian age healing for you, Vol I. Haynes, Los Angeles, CA

Hurley J, Sanders H 1933 The Aquarian age healing, Vol II. Haynes, Los Angeles, CA

25

Sacro-Occipital Technique (SOT)[1]

This chapter is partially based on previously published material, and is printed with the permission of the National University of Health Sciences

INTRODUCTION

One day about 15 years ago, one of us (Cooperstein), just scrounging around in the medical books section of a used bookstore, stumbled upon a copy of DeJarnette's 1934 book *Reflex Pain*,[2] which appears to be one of his first books. The term "Sacro-Occipital Technique" is already in it, as are the fundamental concepts and reflex methodology that will eventually lead to SOT, chiropractic's first great reflex technique. Applied Kinesiology (Ch. 11) may be larger, in the sense that it leans on more sources and features more nooks and crannies, having imported the bigness of SOT in one key stroke by hitting enter on the chiropractic technique pull-down menu. On the other hand, SOT must be regarded as the historical methodological source of virtually all that is reflex technique today. This is not to say that SOT itself did not have antecedents, as we comment in the History section below.

Those chiropractors, patients, and others who find alternative physiologies central to the appeal of complementary and alternative medicine (CAM) procedures very much appreciate SOT and its fellow travelers, whereas those who turn to CAM in spite of its unorthodox procedures might see SOT and other reflex techniques as simply too much over the line. SOT practitioners, unlike some other reflex folk we know, seem quite aware of their eccentric image, and most willing to disabuse detractors in a non-defensive manner through endless explanation and good-natured exchange of views.

Incidentally, Cooperstein managed to get that 1934 DeJarnette text autographed by him about

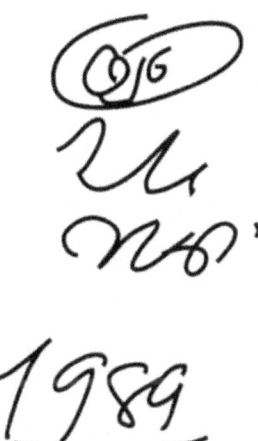

Figure 25.1 DeJarnette's autograph.

3 years before he died in 1992, and here is that "signature" (Fig. 25.1).

OVERVIEW

"Reflex Pain therapy offers you no panacea."[2] The therapeutic intent of SOT is three-pronged, consisting of the specific structural, neurological, and somatovisceral correction of subluxation-related problems.[3] The goal is to "maximize the function of the Primary Cranial Sacral Respiratory Mechanism, to restore weight bearing postural dynamics of the body, and specifically to treat lumbar vertebral, disc, and sciatic nerve problems."[4]

The category system serves as the lynch-pin of structural correction, while Chiropractic Manipulative Reflex Technique (CMRT) represents the mainstay of somatovisceral intervention. From a diagnostic point of view, the ascription of patients to one of three possible categories is central. Category I, "the first level of subluxation to develop" according to Saxon,[5] involves failed coordination between the sacroiliac and cranial-sacral respiratory mechanisms, normally connected by the dural membranes and the flow of cerebrospinal fluid. Category II, following on the heels of an unresolved Category I subluxation, is essentially a post-traumatic clinical entity. It is said to involve the "weight-bearing" function of the sacroiliac joint and "affect the connective tissue of the cranial sutures and spine, the iliofemoral ligaments, the extremities, and the psoas muscle."[4] An unresolved Category II may progress to a Category III, which Unger characterizes as an insult to the lumbosacral cartilaginous system.[6] Saxon adds that it is accompanied by nerve root compression or stretch syndrome,[5] and Getzoff that there is injury to "disc tissue, the surrounding muscles, the sciatic nerve and the pyriformis muscles."[4]

Since the dural ligament connects the cranial vault and the sacrum, category failure, although sometimes narrowly defined in relationship to lumbosacral structures, typically relates to concomitant cranial failure. The importance of the craniopathic component of SOT arises from the view that the cranium is "a collection of very upper cervical segments."[7] It would follow, according to SOT practitioners, that cranial dysfunction alters either dural function or the flow of cerebrospinal fluid, resulting in central nervous system dysfunction and body-wide disturbances.

HISTORY

Major Bertrand DeJarnette, DC and DO, although universally known as "The Major," bore no military commission. While working as an engineer, he sustained severe injuries in an explosion, which led to both a consultation with an osteopath and eventually osteopathic college.[8,9] There he met and became very friendly with Garner Sutherland, inventor (perhaps coinventor with Cottam) of cranial manipulation.[9] After receiving an osteopathic degree in 1922, DeJarnette obtained a chiropractic degree in 1924, motivated in part by a chance encounter with a senior chiropractic student. He was arrested for practicing medicine without a license in 1929.[9] Collaboration with

Randolf Stone (bloodless surgery) eventually led to the development of CMRT.[9] His 1983 claim that SOT was in its 58th year would assign its invention to the year 1925.[10]

Although DeJarnette was aware that osteopathic craniopathy developed beginning in 1929, by both Sutherland in osteopathy and Cottam in chiropractic, he did not introduce his own version of craniopathy until 1967. Apparently, "This flow from full body adjusting to specific cranial adjusting was developed over many years by Dr. DeJarnette."[11,12] Apart from the osteopathic input, it is very likely that DeJarnette was influenced by the work of John Hurley, Palmer Chiropractic graduate of around 1919, who developed a light-touch chiropractic technique that incorporated, among other things, acupuncture analysis. Hurley and Sanders published *The Aquarian Age of Healing* (see Further reading) in 1932, 2 years before DeJarnette's *Reflex Pain*.[2] The title of the book is most informative: this book is about reflex technique. The pelvic blocks were introduced in 1962.[9] In 1957, DeJarnette founded the Sacro Occipital Research Society International (SORSI),[13] which publishes *The Source*.[14] He passed away in 1992 at the age of 92, the author of some 140 books on SOT.[5,8] At the current time there are two primary SOT organizations: SOTO-USA and SOTO.

DEFINITION OF TECHNIQUE-SPECIFIC TERMS

SOT, not unlike other "reflex techniques" in chiropractic,[15] has evolved a large lexicon of jargon. A chiropractic reflex technique purports to examine or treat the patient by means of physiological pathways that tend to lie outside what has been established by normal science. Such techniques often claim undocumented connections between body parts and functions. Most of the definitions that follow make reference to other definitions, so that the list should be read in its entirety to make sense of the individual terms.

- Mind language: according to DeJarnette:[10] "We use the right arm as the testing mechanism and the left index finger as the finder, or pointer, finger ... We simply contact the point of pain or complaint and test the

- arm for strength or weakness. Weakness shows that area to be the problem area"
- Blocks: padded wedges used as fulcrums to correct intrapelvic torsion in either the prone or supine position
- Steffensmeier board: padded platform used to underlie the patient during blocking procedures
- Category I: "A disturbance in the cranial sacral system in its distribution of the cerebrospinal fluid, the tension of its dural membranes and the function of the cranial/sacral structures to promote these qualities"[12]
- Category II: "A complex of anatomical, physiological and symptomatic findings associated with ligament sprain and laxity, with resultant hypermobility of the Sacro-Iliac joint … [and] a loss of weight-bearing pelvic stability."[16] There is said to be an associated disturbance of the "cranial weight-bearing sutural systems"[12]
- Category III: "A lumbar joint failure resulting in discogenic involvement and nerve root compression or stretching … a failure of the pyriformis muscle."[12] "Category III relates to the cartilaginous system of man"[6]
- Arm fossa test: "A challenge of multiple stimuli calling on the upper motor neuron system to coordinate function with the lower motor neuron function."[12] The examiner exerts mild pressure at either the superior-lateral or inferior-medial aspects of the inguinal ligament, looking for a potential weakening of the shoulder girdle musculature. This weakening, when present, is thought to confirm the presence of a Category II presentation (post-traumatic sacroiliac dysfunction), and instability of the sacroiliac joint[17]
- UMS: Category II finding of Upper fossa active, Medial knee pain, and Short leg on the ipsilateral side to the weak fossa
- LLL: Category II finding of Lower fossa active, Lateral knee pain, and Long leg on the ipsilateral side to the weak fossa
- Soft-Tissue Regional Orthopedics (STO): developed by Mervyn Lloyd Rees, as described in Heese,[18] STO purports to diagnose musculoskeletal and organ dysfunction,[12] as a further development of

the temperosphenoidal reflex work discovered by DeJarnette[5]
- Cranial-sacral respiratory mechanism (CSRM): "A combination of integrated functions that support, nourish and enhance the performance of the nervous system as it controls bodily functions."[12] According to Getzoff, it involves each of the following entities: cranial motion, sacral weight-bearing motion, dural tension, cerebrospinal fluid pulsation and flow, ventricular respiration, and several other functions that relate to cranial development[12]
- Occipital fiber analysis: SOT practitioners believe that thoracolumbar subluxations are accompanied by both an organ reflex and occipital fiber involvement. Occipital nodules in precisely defined locations are thought to correspond to blockage in either pre- or postganglionic neurons. Occipital fibers are generally involved in Category I patterns and serve as CMRT indicators as well
- Trapezius fiber analysis: this involves the palpation of seven areas on the trapezius, between the acromioclavicular joint and the spinous process of C7. A palpable nodule is said to indicate a specific vertebral subluxation and point toward a particular CMRT technique that should be performed. Trapezius analysis addresses subluxations not resolved by other procedures, most often as a follow-up in stubborn Category II presentations
- Basic I and Basic II cranial adjusting: the cranial procedures that are associated with treating the Category I and Category II syndromes, respectively
- Heel tension: a Category I indicator, occurring on the short-leg side. It is detected as a unilateral "difference in relative resistance in one of the heels in response to being stretched," with some degree of dorsiflexion, or as tenderness of the Achilles tendon to pinch.[5] When present, it is thought to reflect atlas adaptation to tension in the dura[17]
- Crest sign: relative hypotonus of the erector spinae and quadratus lumborum muscles at the level of L4, that corrects during blocking. The normal contralateral side is called the "crest sign side." It is seen in Category I presentations. Balanced muscles are thought

to indicate reciprocal function of the temporal bone and the innominate[17]

- Dollar signs: relative hypotonus of the gluteal muscle (at junction of piriformis, gluteus medius, and gluteus maximus) in an area the size of a silver dollar, 3 in. (7.5 cm) inferior and 2 in. (5 cm) lateral to the posterior superior iliac spine, that corrects during blocking. The normal contralateral side is the "dollar sign side." It is seen in Category I presentations. The muscle's relative tone is thought to indicate reciprocal function of the sacrum and occiput[17]

- Posterior iliofemoral technique: restriction in medial rotation of the hip in the Category I or Category III patient, corrected by a double-thumb thrust on the posterior aspect of the greater trochanter

- Anterior iliofemoral technique: restriction in medial rotation of the hip in the Category II supine patient, corrected by a patient-resisted internal rotation and a lateral-to-medial thrust on the ligament

- Sacral base + and sacral base –: with the examiner's thumb placed lightly on the spinous process of L5, the patient gives a light cough. An upward bounce of the thumb indicates SB+, and a cephalad drag SB–. Each situation requires a specific blocking technique to reduce the sacral component of craniosacral subluxation. The findings are indicative of the extension or flexion fixation of the dural system[17]

- Vasomotor technique: following identification of the SB+ or SB– Category I patient, this breathing and traction procedure may evoke blanching over various spinous processes. In this case, the involved segments are adjusted using an inferosuperior line of drive

- Cervical stairstep and figure 8 adjusting: caudal pressure on the cranium of the supine patient should cause the skull to glide inferoanteriorly in four discrete steps. If this is not the case, the clinician moves the head and neck in a "figure 8" motion at the point of restriction in gliding

- SOTO (step out, turn out): a method of stretching the piriformis muscle, especially when sciatica is present,[5] by abducting and externally rotating the leg, part of the Category I procedure. Getzoff uses it to

monitor Category III pelvic distortions,[17] and describes how the SOTO procedure can be used to identify the category that is present, in addition to treating Category III[19]

- R + C factors: the letters stand for "resistance" and "contraction," and relate to the fact that DeJarnette felt that each member of a pair of vertebrae could affect each other, and that atlas related to L5, and axis to L4, and so on.[20] This is comparable to the Lovett brothers' relationships described by the Applied Kinesiologists[21]

- Pre- and postganglionic technique: preganglionic work is said to address cholinergic vagal function proximal to the ganglion, whereas postganglionic work would address adrenergic vagal functions distal to the ganglion. The preganglionic reflex involves a contact on the sternum, thought by virtue of its marrow functions to be especially important for nerve conduction. The postganglionic work involves a contact on the anterior aspect of the C5 transverse processes, the approximate site of the carotid reflexes

- Chiropractic Manipulative Reflex Technique (CMRT): SOT specialty that is said to normalize somatovisceral function and somatospinal reflexes.[22] It involves a series of procedures intended to "improve organ circulation and normal vagal impulse conduction"[3] through postganglionic technique, vertebral adjusting, and "manual stimulation of the organs."[12] CMRT supposedly enables identification of visceral problems and thereby enables the prescription of nutritional support for the compromised organs

- Cranial sutures: hard and soft tissues of adjoining cranial bones, comparable to other joints of the body.[17]

PHYSIOLOGICAL MECHANISMS AND RATIONALE

From the beginning, DeJarnette believed that if the innominate bones could be balanced, then the sacrum, lodged between where it forms an integral part of the pelvic kinematic chain, would also achieve a balanced position (see Box 25.1). Interestingly enough, this is the obverse of Logan's

Box 25.1   DeJarnette's view of subluxation

Subluxations, like any other abnormality, are corrected when the thing is corrected that is causing them. To empirically keep pounding on a vertebra just because it feels malpositioned is Correspondence School tactic and merits no praise whatsoever. Every subluxation has a cause, be that cause in its own segment or some outlying segment. If the sacrum is causing the atlas to be subluxated, adjust the sacrum. If the atlas is causing the sacrum to be subluxated, adjust the atlas. A subluxation is as much a diseased condition as is a boil. Subluxations, as we have tried to show you, may be the result of conditions, just as they are the cause of conditions that are abnormal.[2]

position, in that he believed the sacral subluxation primary, and that sacral subluxation would lead in turn to pelvic torsion (Ch. 21). Later on, DeJarnette evolved the analogous concept of head-on-spine balance.[18,22] The very term "Sacro-Occipital" confirms the kernel idea of SOT: if the sacrum and occiput are both balanced, then the spine in between can function normally, hopefully eliminating the perceived need for the doctor to "adjust the vertebrae of the spine traumatically."[23]

The pelvic complex is stated to accomplish three tasks: (1) the posterior ligamentous aspect of the sacroiliac joint is weight-bearing; (2) the anterior fibrous aspect of the sacroiliac joint functions in the craniosacral respiratory mechanism; and (3) the pelvic complex must allow normal lumbosacral function.[24] Pelvic torsional dysfunction is thought to interfere with these functions, predisposing to and aggravated by associated cranial dysfunction.

SOT practitioners ascribe much importance to the controversial view that the cranial sutures are mobile, and can attain dysfunctional states. According to Sarkin, "It has been demonstrated that the cranial bones possess flexibility, both within the individual bones themselves and within the sutures that join them. Misalignment of the cranial bones and distortion of the dura attached to them can adversely affect the cranial nerves and blood vessels, cerebrospinal fluid circulation, and temporomandibular joint (TMJ)."[25] He goes on to attribute cranial dysfunction to birth trauma, subsequent trauma (including whiplash, given the occipital attachments of the trapezius

and sternocleidomastoid muscles), malocclusion of the teeth, and spinal (especially upper cervical) misalignment.[25] More recently, Pick found that external cranial manipulation can produce measurable magnetic resonance imaging changes in brain dimensions.[26] Blum and Curl wrote a two-part article describing SOT cranial techniques and their rationale, the first covering the relationship between the category system and sphenobasilar symphysis positioning,[27] and the second covering how SOT procedures affect category distortions when the sphenobasilar symphysis is treated.[28]

SOT practitioners believe that cranial and sacral subluxations are intimately associated, so that a hypermobile anterior sacrum would be associated with an ipsilateral compensatory hypomobile and contralateral hypermobile occiput.[29] The indications for cranial adjusting are partly derived from the category being treated, and partly from other "cranial needs and disturbances."[12] Craniopathic procedures are thought to address the problems of "patients with seizures, dyslexia, memory loss, chronic migraine, hearing problems, emotional disorders and most important of all, cranial technique unleashes the greatest instrument innate used to heal, the human brain."[3]

The adjustment of thoracolumbar subluxations is necessary, but not sufficient. The vertebral adjustment may realign facets and improve motion, but "it does not remove the anterior ganglionic complex, which, as a result of pre- or post-ganglionic stasis, produces viscus fixation and disease."[30,31]

DIAGNOSTIC/ANALYTIC PROCEDURES

The core of the diagnostic process consists in assigning the patient to one of the three categories. The differential diagnostic criteria include, but are not necessarily limited to, the detection of antero-posterior (AP)/lateral sway through plumb-line analysis, patient symptoms, first rib head palpation, cervical indicators, and mind language.

- Category I findings: the plumb-line analysis indicates AP sway. There might also be bilateral rib head tenderness, spinal pain, a visceral syndrome, unilateral heel tension, and the involvement of occipital fibers. The arm fossa test is negative. The Category I patient is further examined for the presence of either SB+ or SB– sacral subluxation, which, when present, further funnels the patient into the vasomotor diagnostic regimen. In addition, the Category I patient is examined for heel tension, dollar or crest signs, and active occipital fibers.

- Category II major findings: the plumb-line analysis indicates lateral sway in excess of ¼ in. (60 mm), mostly toward the more hypomobile side, a tendency also seen during ambulation. Other findings would include leg-length inequality, sacroiliac or lumbosacral pain, TMJ dysfunction, unilateral tenderness of an upper rib head, tenderness and spasm at C4, tenderness of the left mastoid process, and involved occipital fibers. The arm fossa test, which defines the primary side of subluxation, would be positive. It further classifies the Category II patient into either the UMS (posterior-inferior ilium major) pattern or the LLL (anterior-superior ilium major) patterns. The examiner checks for active trapezius fibers as well. The characteristic radiological finding is "a widening of one SI [sacroiliac] joint line of the AP pelvic view."[16]

- Category III major findings: typical findings include sciatica, severe lumbosacral pain, a rigid posture lacking sway in the plumb-line analysis, fixation of the first rib heads, and negative findings in the arm fossa test and for heel tension.

The cervical stairstep procedure attempts to detect blockage of cervical gliding motions, indicating the figure 8 maneuver when present. The cervical compaction test investigates whether compression of the cervical spine in the supine patient interferes with elevation of the lower extremities. It is thought to distinguish between sacroiliac stability and instability. (One might suppose that when positive it might indicate a cervicogenic low-back problem, as described by Kabat.[32])

The CMRT procedures, drawing on information supplied by occipital fiber and trapezius fiber examination and other indicators, are said to identify organs that are in need of manual and reflex stimulation. These procedures are also said to identify subluxations and are mostly associated with Category I patient presentations.

Detailed description of the cranial mechanism and examination procedures is beyond our scope, but it might be mentioned that Basic I and Basic II cranial adjusting is organically wed to the respective Category I and II treatment regimens. There are entire volumes written on more complex cranial patterns and their detection, such as Miles' *A Study Guide to Cranial Procedures.*[33]

Cooperstein describes[34] how padded wedges may be used for diagnostic purposes, even though they are typically used for treatment purposes. His method involves provocation testing, and which blocking positions increase and which decrease tenderness at a lumbopelvic monitoring point. This method has been further explored, as described below in the Outcome assessment section. Klingensmith[35] found that pelvic block placement could in fact create or affect distortions of the pelvis, possibly rationalizing the procedure Cooperstein describes.

TREATMENT/ADJUSTIVE PROCEDURES

SOT practitioners strongly prefer a block-assisted shifting of the pelvis to manual high-velocity, low-amplitude thrusting on the sacroiliac joints, which they believe introduces more of the microtrauma that supposedly led to the problem in the first place. In their opinion, thrusting on the innominate "tries to move a bone without supporting its opposing side … . The blocks are so constructed that they correct by respiratory motion."[10] The mechanics appear straightforward. Supine blocking (Category II) would be expected to approximate the sacroiliac joints, given the posterior to anterior pressure of the blocks on the innominate bones, while gravity tugs on the sacrum from anterior to posterior. Categories I and III prone blocking procedures, on the other hand, would be expected to distract the sacroiliac joints, given the anterior-to-posterior pressure of the blocks on the innominate bones, while gravity tugs on the sacrum in a posterior-to-anterior direction.

The use of pelvic blocks (padded wedges) as fulcrums to reduce intrapelvic torsional stress is arguably the central mechanical innovation of SOT. The blocks are inserted under the prone or supine patient to reduce pelvic torsion (Categories I and II) and/or minimize symptomatology (Category III). Blocking is not only thought to effect a more relaxed and easy correction from the patient's point of view, but to constitute a tremendous ergonomic innovation for the doctor, whose "effort is primarily lifting 1½ lb [0.65 kg] wedges to position them."[10]

Category II supine blocking attempts to reapproximate distended sacroiliac joints,[17] whereas Category I blocking would mobilize a fixated sacroiliac joint. Category III prone blocking intends to affect primarily the lumbar facetal and interbody joints. Although block placement in Categories I and II is quite specific and invariant, in Category III the clinician is expected to vary the position and angle of the blocks until there is maximal amelioration of the patient's symptoms. Indeed, according to Unger, "Very often it is found that rotating a block as little as one-eighth of an inch [3 mm] will make all of the difference."[36] Although the SOT literature does not seem to make much of the possibility, one assumes that the blocking procedures would effect viscoelastic creep of the sacroiliac and other pelvic connective tissues.[1]

Despite the multiplicity of possible procedures, the essence of the SOT regimen involves Category I prone blocking along with Basic I craniopathy, and Category II supine blocking with Basic II craniopathy.[6] There is more variability in prone Category III blocking with Basic III craniopathy. Category I also includes crest and dollar sign adjusting, vasomotor technique, CMRT, cervical stairstep and figure 8 technique, and intraoral cranial technique. Category II treatment also includes psoas technique, anterior iliofemoral treatment, cervical stairstep and figure 8 technique, and sutural cranial work. Category III also includes posterior iliofemoral treatment, lumbar/sacral adjusting, supine psoas technique, SOTO technique, and the sagittal spread procedure. It has also been claimed to benefit cervical problems like torticollis.[36]

SOT practitioners believe that successful balancing of the pelvis is crucial for an easy and lasting correction of the cranium.[29] As a barometer of how important the blocks were to DeJarnette himself, he once stated: "80% of all correction is accomplished by use of the DeJarnette mechanical wedges."[37] The preferred protocol involves first ruling out the Category II entity, which must be completely resolved prior to undertaking treatment of any Category I complex. In the best of cases, the examination findings in Category II presentations, for both UMS and LLL presentations, are internally consistent. However, when the examination findings are not congruent,[6] the doctor is required to engage in one or more of the following treatment and/or diagnostic procedures, listed here roughly in order of importance: diaphragm release, psoas technique, iliofemoral technique, upper cervical correction, superior-inferior innominate correction, sacral segmental subluxation correction, trapezius fibers, organ dysfunction as given by occipital fiber analysis, and extremity correction.

After a thoracolumbar subluxation is adjusted, the doctor palpates to find whether the anterior trigger point of C5 or the sternum is more tender. The pre- or postganglionic work that follows, depending on which is more tender, involves a simultaneous sternum/viscus or C5 trigger point/viscus contact, until some type of anticipated organ reflex (e.g., a gurgling sound) is detected.

Ancillary procedures

Craniopathy, CMRT, spinal ("articulative") adjusting, extremity adjusting, nutritional support, and activities of daily living/ergonomic advice would all have to be considered to varying degrees as somewhat external to the SOT core substrate of cranial-sacral balancing. Saxon regards occipital and trapezius fiber work and cervical stairstepping technique to be "extra-categorical."[5] Getzoff provides instructions for doctors wanting to get started in cranial manipulation.[38]

Given the importance that SOT clinicians attach to cranial diagnosis and treatment, it may seem unjustified to regard craniopathy as "ancillary." Nevertheless, DeJarnette did remark that "Craniopathy is not a total system of healing but is used as an addition to SOT because we believe that any block within the brain substances prevents the recovery of the patient ... You have to learn SOT before you can understand the Cranial Technique."[10] Miles wrote an illustrated manual of cranial adjusting[35] which credits many of its points to DeJarnette's own 1979–1980 *Cranial Manual.*[39]

Getzoff considers "CMRT, a system of organ function analysis and treatment as it relates to the spine and the trapezius and occipital muscles"[12] to be an important addition to the core cranial sacral work. Spinal and extremity adjusting would also be considered ancillary procedures, performed when such procedures would be expected to improve the function of the craniosacral mechanism.

Nutritional support and counseling are well within the purview of the SOT practitioner, as is advice regarding exercise, recreation, ergonomics, and the activities of daily living.[16] Cryotherapy is recommended for acute and swollen sacroiliac joints, and moist heat and/or ultrasound for chronic Category II presentations.[5] The patient with a persistent Category II subluxation wears a trochanteric belt around the pelvis just inferior to the anterior superior iliac spine for 4–6 weeks. This is thought to augment the role of blocking in reducing sacroiliac instability.

OUTCOME ASSESSMENT

Not surprisingly, the amelioration of the diagnostic findings that indicate the need for particular treatment procedures also confirms treatment success: "By observing the indicators, you also will know when the adjustment has been successful."[12] The DeJarnette four-footplate distortion analyzer, which features two plumb-lines, is used to assess the patient's clinical course. Heese describes the mechanics and terminology for some of the more common patterns that are seen.[18] Perhaps the most unusual case he describes is that of the symptomatic patient who does not show distortion in the plumb-line analysis. In such a case, the patient's "defense mechanism is not adapting to the patient's problem ... Your main objective is to initiate the body into some type of defense by moving the spine toward some type of distortion ... The patient could feel worse after this adjustment," but this would be acceptable.[18]

SAFETY AND RISK FACTORS

There are few contraindications to SOT care that differ from those that contraindicate spinal manipulative therapy in general. On the contrary, the light forces applied in most of the procedures are believed to be safer than more aggressive manipulative procedures. "Often patients that have failed to respond to general low back manipulation, yet fall clearly out of the realm of the medical scope of practice, have responded very favorably to SOT Category II procedures."[16] Getzoff advises limiting cranial care in acute Category IIIs "due to the effects of over-stimulation of the cerebrospinal fluid."[4]

EVIDENCE OF EFFICACY
Reliability studies

Leboeuf et al, who have done a number of reliability and validity studies on typical SOT examination findings, found satisfactory intraexaminer reliability for a single examiner in a single-blind study.[40] In this study, 45 subjects found to exhibit fossa failure by examiner one were randomly assigned to one of three treatment modalities by examiner two: (1) "correct" Category II supine blocking, (2) "incorrect" Category I prone blocking, or (3) a control regimen of no treatment. In post-check arm fossa testing, 73% of "correctly" blocked subjects had converted to arm fossa-negative, whereas only 37.5% of "incorrectly" blocked subjects had made this conversion. Only 14% of untreated subjects converted to arm fossa-negativity, indicating good intraexaminer reliability.

Leboeuf et al[41] also investigated the relationship between the findings of one investigator, who had already demonstrated "satisfactory" intraexaminer reliability in arm fossa testing, and those of a second examiner, who (1) had patients identify the location of their own pelvic region pain; (2) identified fixation in the sacroiliac joints; and (3) elicited pain responses through digital palpation of the spinous process of L5, the tip of the S2 tubercle, the iliolumbar ligaments, the posterior sacroiliac ligaments, and the gluteal muscles. There were no statistically significant correlations except between right iliolumbar ligament tenderness and right-sided fossa failure. The investigators readily admit that this study was limited in the fact that, among the examination procedures tested, the only procedure of known reproducibility was the arm fossa test. Nevertheless, they felt that the study reproduced the clinical situation well enough to warrant calling the adequacy of certain SOT examination procedures into question.

A third study by Leboeuf[42] investigated whether the results of arm fossa testing would correlate with seven orthopedic tests, either singly or in combination, for the lumbosacral area. Although the arm fossa test did not correlate with any of the orthopedic tests, it was also the case that none of them, with the exception of the heel–buttock test (positive in 44% of symptomatic vs 17% in asymptomatic subjects), could significantly distinguish symptomatic from asymptomatic controls. The arm fossa test was also somewhat able to make this distinction (positive in 54% of symptomatic vs 31% in asymptomatic subjects).

Leboeuf also reports on the results of four multisection interexaminer reliability studies and one validity study, all in one somewhat confusing paper.[43] Across the four multisection reliability studies, the following examination procedures were tested, 10 of them more than once: mind language, AP/lateral sway, moving first rib, bilateral supine leg raise, bilateral supine leg raise with cervical compaction, arm fossa test, supine leg length, prone leg length, knee pain, Category I/II discrimination, heel tension, right thenar pad pain, arm length for contracted psoas, calf pain, diaphragm pain, hiatal hernia reflux, hamstring pain, and the final diagnosis as to category. As may be expected, there are many results to report. According to the investigator, "only one test (bilateral supine leg raise with cervical compaction) had at least fair reliability more than once ... whereas six tests obtained poor agreement in more than one study ... One examiner out of two had a number of excellent and fair intra-examiner values, whereas the other examiner generally had poor results ... It appears unlikely that SOT tests can be reproduced to a sufficiently high degree to constitute useful clinical procedures."[43]

Unger tested the before and after strength of eight muscles upon 16 patients who received pelvic blocking procedures, all of whom were blocked until their Category II indicators had been cleared. In all but one of the cases, the muscles improved in their strength, and the results were statistically significant.[44] The study was non-controlled.

Although it is not a reliability study, the study by Lisi et al[45] is relevant. The purpose of this project was to determine if lumbosacral tenderness measured by algometry would change in response to varying positions of pelvic wedges under a prone subject. It was found that low-back tenderness did change in response to various positions of pelvic wedges, and a preferred pattern could be determined. Blocking positions that increase or decrease tenderness tend to be diametrically opposed; that is, directional preference can be shown. The investigators concluded that pelvic wedges could be used for provocation testing of low-back tenderness and assessment of directional preference in asymptomatic or minimally symptomatic subjects. A follow-up study is in press.[46]

We are aware of two intriguing studies in press at the time of this publication,[47] but we are not able to report on any of the data:

Thompson et al[48] sought a possible correlation between lateral pelvic sway, as determined by a device called a postural analyzer, and the amount of pressure it took to elicit pain along the inguinal ligament, as measured by a pressure algometer. They reasoned that a positive arm fossa test for Category II, which involves touching the inguinal ligament, and lateral sway, believed to be a Category II indicator, would predict such a correlation. Statistical analysis failed to confirm the hypothesis.

Outcome studies

Cook and Rasmussen,[49] in a rather esoteric article, report on the treatment of uterine fibroids in two chronic cases using a manual method known as the "total mesenteric apron" in conjunction with SOT chiropractic adjustments. Although the authors acknowledge that it was difficult to determine which of the utilized procedures had the largest impact, they felt there was no doubt that visceral manipulation did in fact have a beneficial impact in this case.

Hospers[50] reports on a case study involving a chiropractic student suffering from chronic headaches, who was studied with computerized electroencephalography (CEEG) before and after treatment of a Category II subluxation. Colorized brain maps recorded 10 and 60 min after treatment showed normalization of preadjustment frequency spectra in the brain. In an apparently overstated summary remark concerning this $n = 1$, non-controlled study, the investigator concludes that "subluxation in a remote member of the craniosacral pump mechanism, specifically unilaterally in the sacroiliac joint, can induce abnormal frequency spectra in cerebral cortical activity, which can return to normative values when this subluxation is removed."[50]

Gregory presents an interesting case of a woman with temperomandibular disorder whose symptoms reduced with pelvic blocking (without treatment directly aimed at the jaw), and whose low-back complaints were made worse by the replacement of a crown.[51] He goes on to present a model for the biomechanical interdependence of the TMJ and sacroiliac sprain (dental malocclusion and Category II sacroiliac dysfunction.[51]

Chinappi (orthodontist) and Getzoff (chiropractor) present two case reports illustrating successful integration of dental–orthopedic and craniochiropractic care, one a case of a woman with temperomandibular and cervical problems,[52] and the other a case of a woman with temperomandibular and lumbosacral pain.[53]

Getzoff and Gregory report on the successful treatment of a case of arthrogryposis multiplex congenita, a disease in which there is congenital lack of muscular development that results in multiple joint contractures and deformities.[54] The treatment procedures used included SOTO, iliofemoral abduction and external rotation, goading the iliofemoral joint, occipital line interventions, the figure 8 maneuver in the cervical spine, cranial adjustments, and home exercises.[54]

Blum reported[55] on the case of a child with Down syndrome, who had been scheduled for heart surgery. In addition to nutritional and supplementation advice, the primary manipulated care rendered consisted of craniopathic procedures as commonly performed by SOT practitioners. The child markedly improved, and the surgery was cancelled. Blum also reported on the successful treatment of a case of tinnitus using SOT "chiropractic/cranial care," although he hardly discusses the specific treatment measures used.[20] Blum provides a rationale for the SOT treatment of asthma, but no data are presented.[56]

Connelly and Rasmussen provide a case series of 3 patients with hypertension who improved after receiving SOT-related cranial technique procedures, apparently focusing on spreading the occipitomastoid suture, to provide more space for the vagus nerve where it exits the cranial vault.[57] An earlier small randomized trial by Unger et al[58] ($n = 6$ experimental group, $n = 4$ control group) showed a statistically significant reduction in blood pressure, following a cranial manipulative procedure that seems similar to that described by Connelly and Rasmussen.[57]

Blum et al[59] presented a case series of 3 cases of lumbar herniated discs each treated by prone blocking with padded wedges. In each of the cases, pre and post magnetic resonance images (MRIs) were available, although the imaging protocols varied from case to case. The investigators concluded that there were both symptomatic and structural improvements, as determined by the advanced images, in each of the 3 patients.

CONCLUSIONS

- Many, if not most chiropractors, although aware that most of their clinical interventions directly address somatic structures, nevertheless intend to treat visceral conditions, meaning organ disease, through purported somatovisceral reflexes. Their idea is that removing subluxations allows the body to heal itself – not just the musculoskeletal system but the entire body. It is in that indirect sense that they claim chiropractic treats diseases; they help the nervous system heal the rest of the body. SOT practitioners go one step further, by claiming to treat diseases *directly*, even going so far as to treat viscera manually as part and parcel of the CMRTs. They call it visceral manipulation.

- The mind language test bears an obvious resemblance to therapy localization used by Applied Kinesiologists (Ch. 11), as described by Walther.[21]
- DeJarnette was distinctly unimpressed with the Palmers' simple "bone-out-of-place causing nerve pressure" model, and seemed to direct some pointed criticism at a related Pettibon model (Ch. 27) that was quite current at the time of a 1982 interview: "A theory that cannot be proven … is that if a vertebra is a given distance from alignment to misalignment and if the adjustment moves the vertebra a measurable distance, we can then by a process of mathematics predict how many adjustments will be required for perfect alignment."[23] DeJarnette did not support the primacy attached to atlas by upper cervical

practitioners (Chs 32 and 33), who he felt neglected the role of atlas as a compensatory segment that could easily balance the cranium without allowing cord pressure.[10] Adopting a position resembling that associated with Nimmo's Receptor-Tonus Technique (Ch. 24),[56] DeJarnette described the "vertebral subluxation as being the effects of muscular contractions as often as it is the cause of the stimulus producing the muscular contractions."[57]
- With the possible exception of Applied Kinesiology, none of the major techniques attaches as much significance nor devotes as much attention to the cranial bones as SOT. It should be stated that the view that the cranial sutures can permit movement is not as ostracizing today as it was in times past.

REFERENCES

1. Cooperstein R 1996 Technique system overview: Sacro Occipital Technique. Chiropractic Technique 8 (3): 125–131
2. DeJarnette M B 1934 Reflex pain, p. vi, 89. DeJarnette, Nebraska City, NE
3. Koffman D M 1984 Technical excellence: the next key to our survival. Digest of Chiropractic Economics (July/August): 53, 128
4. Getzoff H I 1993 Technique assessment outline: S.O.T. report to advisory council to ACA panel on technique (private report).
5. Saxon A 1985 Participant guide. SOT: a seminar for technical excellence (date approximate). SORSI
6. Unger J F 1991 Category II congruency concept. American Chiropractor (April): 10–17
7. Hochman J I 1992 Analysis of the cervical spine. Today's Chiropractic 21 (4): 15–19
8. Unger J F 1995 The legacy of a chiropractor, inventor and researcher: Dr. Bertrand DeJarnette. In: Cleveland III C, Gibbons R (eds) Conference proceedings of the Chiropractic Centennial Foundation, pp. 35–36. Chiropractic Centennial Foundation, Davenport, IA
9. Heese N 1991 Major Bertrand De Jarnette: six decades of Sacro Occipital Research, 1924–1984. Chiropractic History 11 (1): 12–15
10. DeJarnette M B 1983 Sacro occipital technic: 1983. Self-published, Nebraska City, NB
11. Kotheimer W J 1993 Applied chiropractic in reflex analysis of the cranium. Digest of Chiropractic Economics (November–December): 14–19
12. Getzoff H 1990 Sacro Occipital Technique (S.O.T.): a system of chiropractic. American Chiropractor (August): 9–10, 41
13. Kaye R J 1987 Bringing Sacro Occipital Technique to greater heights. American Chiropractor (August): 4–8

14. SORSI. The official publication of the Sacro Occipital Research Society International. SORSI International Headquarters, Sedan, KS
15. Cooperstein R 1999 Chiropractic Technique. In: Gardner S, Mosby J S (eds) Chiropractic secrets, p. 325. Hanley & Belfus, Philadelphia, PA.
16. Buddingh C, Galinis M R 1980 A brief overview of the stubborn low back and category II. Digest of Chiropractic Economics (July/August): 72–73
17. Getzoff H 1999 Sacro-Occipital Technique categories: a systems method of chiropractic. Chiropractic Technique 11 (2): 62–65
18. Heese N 1988 Distortion patterns involving plumb line analysis. American Chiropractor (April): 32–34
19. Getzoff H 1998 The step out-toe out procedure: a therapeutic and diagnostic procedure. Chiropractic Technique 10 (3): 118–120
20. Blum C 1999 Spinal/cranial manipulative therapy and tinnitus: a case history [sic]. Chiropractic Technique 10 (4): 163–168
21. Walther D S 1981 Applied Kinesiology, vol. I. Systems DC, Pueblo, CO
22. DeCamp N Jr 1994 The TMJ and dysfunction of the lumbo-pelvic complex. Today's Chiropractic (July/August): 20–25
23. DeJarnette M B 1982 Cornerstone: Interview with M B DeJarnette. American Chiropractor (July/August): 22–23, 28, 34
24. DeCamp O N 1992 Pelvic subluxation patterns in the Sacro-Occipital Technique. Today's Chiropractic 21 (4): 32–36
25. Sarkin J M 1989 SOT cranial technique: an introduction. Digest of Chiropractic Economics (January–February): 12
26. Pick M G 1994 A preliminary single case magnetic resonance imaging investigation into maxillary

frontal-parietal manipulation and its short-term effect upon the intracranial structures of an adult human brain. Journal of Manipulative and Physiological Therapeutics 17 (3): 168–173

27. Blum C, Curl D D 1998 The relationship between Sacro-Occipital Technique and sphenobasilar balance. Part one: the key continuities. Chiropractic Technique 10 (3): 95–100

28. Blum C, Curl D D 1998 The relationship between Sacro-Occipital Technique and sphenobasilar balance. Part two: sphenobasilar strain stacking. Chiropractic Technique 10 (3): 101–109

29. DeCamp N 1990 Cranial sacral dysfunction and sacral segmental subluxations. American Chiropractor (November): 13, 16–17

30. Heese N 1988 Viscerosomatic pre- and post-ganglionic technique. American Chiropractor (March): 16–22

31. Heese N 1989 Viscerosomatic pre- and post-ganglionic technique. Digest of Chiropractic Economics (July–August): 67–70

32. Kabat H 1980 Low back and leg pain from herniated cervical disc. Warren H Green, St Louis, MO

33. Miles B J 1985 A study guide to cranial procedures. Tri-State Cranial

34. Cooperstein R 2000 Padded wedges for lumbopelvic mechanical analysis. Journal of the American Chiropractic Association 37 (10): 24–26

35. Klingensmith R D 2002 The relationship between pelvic block placement and radiographic pelvic analysis. In: Owens E (ed.) 10th annual vertebral subluxation conference. Sherman College of Straight Chiropractic, Hayward, CA

36. Unger J F 1991 Precision block placement indicator. American Chiropractor (March): 8–11

37. DeJarnette B 1977 Sacro Occipital Technic. In: Kfoury P W (ed.) Catalog of chiropractic techniques, p. 39. Logan College of Chiropractic, Chesterfield, MO

38. Getzoff H 1996 Cranial mandibular motion technique. Chiropractic Technique 8 (4): 182–185

39. DeJarnette M B 1979–1980 Cranial manual. Self-published, Nebraska City, NE

40. Leboeuf C, Jenkins D J, Smyth R A 1988 Sacro-occipital technique: the so-called arm fossa test. Intraexaminer agreement and post-treatment changes. Journal of the Australian Chiropractors' Association 18 (2): 67–68

41. Leboeuf C, Jenkins D J, Smyth R A 1988 Sacro-occipital technique: an investigation into the relationship between the arm fossa test and certain examination findings. Journal of the Australian Chiropractors' Association 18 (3): 97–99

42. Leboeuf C 1990 The sensitivity and specificity of seven lumbo-pelvic orthopedic tests and the arm fossa test. Journal of Manipulative and Physiological Therapeutics 13 (3): 138–143

43. Leboeuf C 1991 The reliability of specific Sacro-occipital Technique diagnostic tests. Journal of Manipulative and Physiological Therapeutics 14 (9): 512–517

44. Unger J F 1998 The effects of a pelvic blocking procedure upon muscle strength: a pilot study. Chiropractic Technique 10 (4): 150–155

45. Lisi A J, Cooperstein R, Morschhauser E 2002 A pilot study of provocation testing with pelvic wedges: can prone blocking demonstrate a directional preference? Journal of Chiropractic Education 16 (1): 30–31

46. Lisi A, Cooperstein R, Morschhauser E 2003 An exploratory study of provocation testing with padded wedges: can prone blocking demonstrate a directional preference? [In press]

47. http://www.soto-usa.org/frames.html

48. Thompson D M, Vrugtman R P, Johnson K M et al 2003 Correlation of lateral pelvic sway to variances of pain along the inguinal ligaments. Journal of Chiropractic Education 17 (1): 76–77

49. Cook K, Rasmussen S A 1992 Visceral manipulation and the treatment of uterine fibroids: a case report. ACA Journal of Chiropractic (December): 39–41

50. Hospers L A 1992 Brain mapping (CEEG) before and after SOT category II blocking of the sacroiliac joint. Today's Chiropractic 21 (3): 47–52

51. Gregory T M 1993 Temporomandibular disorder associated with sacroiliac sprain. Journal of Manipulative and Physiological Therapeutics 16 (4): 256–265

52. Chinappi A S Jr, Getzoff H 1995 The dental-chiropractic cotreatment of structural disorders of the jaw and temporomandibular joint dysfunction. Journal of Manipulative and Physiological Therapeutics 18 (7): 476–481

53. Chinappi A S Jr, Getzoff H 1996 Chiropractic/dental cotreatment of lumbosacral pain with temporomandibular joint involvement. Journal of Manipulative and Physiological Therapeutics 19 (9): 607–612

54. Getzoff H, Gregory T 1996 Chiropractic Sacro-Occipital Technique treatment of arthrogryposis multiplex congenita. Chiropractic Technique 8 (2): 83–87

55. Blum C 1999 Cranial therapeutic treatment of Down's syndrome. Chiropractic Technique 11 (2): 66–76

56. Blum C 1999 Chiropractic and Sacro Occipital Technique in asthma treatment. Chiropractic Technique 11 (4): 174–179

57. Connelly D M, Rasmussen S A 1998 The effect of cranial adjusting on hypertension: a case report. Chiropractic Technique 10 (2): 75–78

58. Unger J F, Sweat S, Flanagan S, Chudkowski S 1993 An effect of Sacro-Occipital Technique on blood pressure. In: Seater S R (ed.) International Conference on Spinal Manipulation, p. 87. FCER, Montreal, Canada

59. Blum C S, Esposito V, Esposito C 2003 Orthopedic block placement and its effect on the lumbosacral spine and discs. Three case studies with pre and post MRIs. Journal of Chiropractic Education 17 (1): 48–49

60. Nimmo R L 1963 The Receptor-Tonus Method. Self-published, Granbury, TX

61. DeJarnette B 1986 Sacro-Occipital Technique. Today's Chiropractic (May–June): 97–98, 115

FURTHER READING

Hurley J, Sanders H 1932 The Aquarian age of healing for you, Vol I. Haynes, LosAngeles, CA

26

Soft-Tissue Techniques: the case of Active Release Technique (ART)

INTRODUCTION

The inclusion of soft-tissue techniques in this book is something of a, well, stretch. After all, these methods are not so much technique systems as adjunctive techniques, methods that exist to complement adjustive techniques rather than serve as standalone technique systems. On the other hand, we cannot dismiss the fact that many chiropractors and chiropractic students regard soft-tissue technique seminars as on an equal footing with technique system seminars, whatever distinction we may care to make. Moreover, were we to omit soft-tissue techniques, we would be hard-pressed to rationalize the inclusion of Nimmo's Receptor-Tonus Technique (Ch. 24). It is distinguished from medical trigger point work largely by virtue of being indigenous to chiropractic, and is thus born of a different philosophy but convergent in its methods.

Rather than review the wide assortment of generic soft-tissue methods that chiropractors use (Box 26.1), many of which are shared with allied health professionals, we elected to review ART

merely as a case in point, which happens to be particularly well-described and packaged on the seminar circuit.

OVERVIEW

ART's Soft-Tissue Management system is a hands-on soft-tissue manipulative technique aimed at identifying and removing fibrous adhesions that are thought to be interfering with the proper biomechanical function of other tissues. In the context of ART, soft tissues include muscles, tendons, ligaments, and peripheral nerves. Spinal subluxations or dysfunctions are not necessarily or primarily corrected by this technique per se; rather, ART can be used as a precursor or adjunctive therapy to many of the other technique systems described in this textbook.

HISTORY

ART developer Michael Leahy began his academic career by obtaining an engineering degree from the US Air Force in 1971. He graduated from the Los Angeles Chiropractic College in 1984, and entered private practice in Los Angeles, California. By his own account, he focused on managing patients with various athletic soft-tissue injuries.[1] He noticed that many of these athletes responded favorably to various types of myofascial techniques, and it seems he became more and more interested in this form of therapy.

In 1984, Leahy uprooted and moved to Colorado Springs, Colorado. As he tells it, he kept trying to apply the knowledge gained from

---

Box 26.1 Generic soft-tissue techniques commonly used in chiropractic

Transverse frictional massage
Proprioceptive neurofacilitation (up to eight components)
Origin-insertion work
Strain–counterstrain/positional release
Myofascial trigger point
Myofascial release technique

his courses in engineering to the human body, especially concepts such as friction, dampening fields, and single-loop negative-feedback control systems (see below for definitions). Leahy had codified his approach into what he termed "neuromuscular reeducation," although by 1985 he had revised the name of this therapy to "myofascial release." Leahy remained unsatisfied with this appellation, as he believed it did not convey important features of his technique. In particular, he felt the title "myofascial" unnecessarily locked him into the muscles and tendons, whereas he believed 50% of the benefits derived from his technique dealt with peripheral nerve entrapments. Secondly, the term had a somewhat nebulous and generic connotation to him.[1] Finally, a key protocol of the therapy involved active motions on the part of the patient. Upon further consideration, Leahy settled on the name Active Release Technique Soft-Tissue Management, although it is usually referred to simply as ART.

His time in Colorado was well spent. Leahy recounts that his success rate in managing patients with soft-tissue injuries jumped from 50% to 90%. According to Leahy, his reputation became such that several professional athletes sought out his clinic, and he became a consultant for several national teams, ranging from basketball to swimming to weight lifting to triathlon.[1] According to Leahy, many of these patients experienced tremendous improvements in their abilities after only a few treatments, even if they had had the problem for years.

The seminal event in the public recognition of ART took place in 1990. During a conference discussing carpal tunnel syndrome, Leahy suggested that the doctors in attendance send him their "five worst cases" of carpal tunnel. Leahy writes that the patients referred to him had been under medical care for at least 2 years. Three had already undergone surgery, and all of them were adversely affected by their ailment at work. According to Leahy, all five cases were resolved within three visits, and all five patients returned to full-time, pain-free duties at work.[1] ART proponents quickly developed a module for the treatment of conditions affecting the upper limb.

Over the past few years, modules for the lower limb and spine have been developed.

DEFINITION OF TECHNIQUE-SPECIFIC TERMS

- Cumulative injury cycle (CIC): a mechanism used to explain the effect on tissue and subsequent development of fibrous adhesions as the result of injury, repetitive use, or constant pressure
- Fibrous adhesions: a product of inflammation from overuse or trauma, these are noxious soft-tissue structures that are thought to cling to and diminish the proper function of other soft tissues. In essence, these entities predispose a patient to biomechanical impediments that ultimately lead to syndromes, notably of the peripheral nerve roots
- Law of repetitive motion: a mathematical formula developed to express the relationship between the characteristics of a repetitive force and injury or insult to tissue
- Single-loop feedback control mechanism: a concept borrowed from aeronautical engineering, the characteristic appearance of an object's position over time as a function of the various internal factors.

PHYSIOLOGICAL MECHANISMS AND RATIONALE

The rationale behind ART is quite simple. Based on anatomical proximity, fibrous adhesions formed by physical injury are thought to interfere with the proper function of affected structures, be they muscles, tendons, ligaments, or peripheral nerves. For example, a fibrous adhesion may prevent the normal, smooth movement of a large muscle by increasing the amount of friction between it and surrounding structures, such as fascial planes. Similarly, a nerve root may be irritated, compressed, or otherwise affected by the close proximity of an adhesion, particularly during movement. Leahy pays particular attention to the effect of fibrous adhesions on neurological structures, going into great detail of how a nerve may become entrapped anywhere along its course from origin to termination.[2]

Several simple mathematical equations are applied to the body in motion under ART. The single-loop feedback control mechanism can visually explain how a muscle under increased friction from adhesions cannot achieve the same degree of excursion as a muscle not so affected. For example, in the case of throwing a ball, the individual pushes outward in front of his or her body in order to propel the ball forward (a forcing function). This motion is normally limited by the damping coefficient of the combined effect of the resistance to the motion by inertia and the action of antagonistic muscles, thus keeping the action under control. However, as Leahy describes it, "a fibrous adhesion in a nerve will increase the damping coefficient and leave the negative feedback system unchanged."[2] (p. 142) In order to perform the same task (throwing a ball) at the same level of skill, the participant would have to increase the forcing function (the throw) in order to try and overcome the increased damping coefficient. This will result in a prolonged period of time required to perform the task[2] but the forcing function may exceed the anatomical integrity of the structures used, resulting in injury.

Similarly, the CIC is a simple and straightforward conceptual model.[1,2] An injury or repetitive sprain results in an inflammatory process or decreased circulation, either of which subsequently leads to the development of fibrous adhesions. These adhesions, in turn, can result in a muscle becoming weak and tense, resulting in friction and increased tension. This can itself result in further inflammation and edema. The cycle self-perpetuates, culminating in decreased function of the tissue affected by the adhesion. In chronic cases, fibrous adhesions may become fibrotic scars.[2] Depending on the tissue entrapped, the patient may experience radicular signs and symptoms (tingling, loss of grip strength, difficulties in performing coordinated activities) or decreased range of motion.

Lastly, Leahy has developed the law of repetitive motion, which he describes as:

$$I = \frac{NF}{AR}$$

where I is the insult to the tissue, N is the number of repetitions, F is the force of tension used in each repetition as a percentage of maximum muscle strength, A is the amplitude of each repetition, and R is the relaxation time between each repetition.

For example, vibration results in a high N value, a low A value, and a low R value. This creates an equation with a high numerator and low denominator, and thus a high I value, or greater injury to tissue.[1] Many different scenarios can be inserted in this equation in order to calculate a rough estimate of the degree of injury a tissue may sustain.

DIAGNOSTIC/ANALYTIC PROCEDURES

The appeal of the technique to the chiropractor rests on its exclusive reliance on palpatory skills for diagnosis. The reproduction of the patient's chief complaint (pain, neurological signs, limited motion, and so on) would be considered pathognomonic for the diagnosis. More sophisticated equipment could certainly be used in conjunction with this technique to identify involved soft tissues, but it is seldom warranted.

ART practitioners are instructed to identify three components of a soft-tissue injury: the nature of the lesion (tear, crush, adhesion), the exact tissue involved, and the causative syndrome (rotator cuff syndrome, tennis elbow, and so on). Furthermore, four features of an involved structure should be assessed. These are tissue texture (indicative of the stage of inflammation), tissue tension (basically the equivalent to motion palpation of spinal joints), tissue movement (the degree to which one structure slides in relation to surrounding structures), and function (essentially a standard orthopedic examination entailing sensory, motor, and reflex testing).[1]

TREATMENT/ADJUSTIVE PROCEDURES

Again, because of its exclusive hands-on and anatomic-based approach, the therapeutic interventions of ART are relatively simple to envision. Once identified, the offending structure is worked on by the clinician in such a way as to remove or "break up" the fibrous adhesions. Several straightforward rules have been developed for the therapy; for example, the examiner is to work longitudinally along muscle or fascial planes to break down fibrous adhesions more optimally. The examiner should move slowly and within patient pain tolerance, and the stretching action imparted should be in the direction of venous and lymphatic flow. At first glance ART may seem similar to other soft-tissue techniques, such as Nimmo Receptor-Tonus Technique or massage. However, ART differs in that there is active involvement of the patient during treatment.

There are four basic levels of ART treatment. The first three are similar to those used in other soft-tissue release techniques, in that the patient is passive and the clinician moves the affected tissue without tension, moves the affected tissue with tension, or lengthens the affected tissue.[2] It is the fourth level that distinguishes ART from some other soft-tissue techniques. In Level 4, the patient is required actively to perform various movements as instructed by the clinician, while the clinician applies either a constant pressure (letting the offending tissue slide under the contact), or a pressure along the tissue as it moves. The ART practitioner combines low-compression/high-tension muscle stripping with a variety of active patient motions, such as using antagonist muscles to the ones being treated, which causes the muscle being treated to move under the clinician's fingers. In general, the patient is instructed to uncoil the muscle from its shortest position to its longest length. Significant results should be obtained within three or four treatment visits, according to ART practitioners.

OUTCOMES ASSESSMENT

As with most technique systems, the absence of diagnostic findings indicates a successful clinical encounter. In the case of ART, the diminishment or abolition of pain or other patient symptoms, with a restoration of normal function and motion, is the primary outcome goal. Other goals include improved muscular strength, negative response to provocative orthopedic testing, normalization of neurological findings, and absence of adhesions or nodules upon palpation post treatment.

SAFETY AND RISK FACTORS

There are no significant contraindications to ART, beyond obvious signs of blunt trauma (bleeding injuries, fracture, and the like) and active inflammation. Patients may experience local pain at the point of contact, but ART practitioners write that this may be described by the patient as "good pain."[2] The treatment frequency should not exceed every other day.

EVIDENCE OF EFFICACY

There is considerable anecdotal evidence for successful outcomes using this approach. Endorsements from high-performance athletes and celebrities are often cited as proof of ART efficacy. However, apart from such anecdotal reports, there seems to have been little clinical research investigating the effectiveness of this technique per se. The ample literature on related soft-tissue methods, such as proprioceptive neurofacilitation (PNF) and various active stretching methods must be considered relevant and is quite supportive of the clinical effectiveness of such methods.

Most articles on ART follow the same basic structural design. The author chooses a particular clinical condition to discuss, provides a review of the relevant anatomy, describes typical entrapment points, explains the standard ART therapeutic approach, and presents a representative case study as an example.[2,16] A few studies compare the results of ART to surgery, but not to other noninvasive approaches. We are unaware of any studies measuring the interrater reliability of palpation by ART practitioners to identify the offending tissue, nor have any prospective population-controlled studies been conducted. However, in the year 2000 Leahy wrote that there was a clinical trial in progress with the University of California San Diego Medical School on cumulative trauma disorders.[3] To date, however, no data have been published, at least to our knowledge.

CONCLUSIONS

- ART is a straightforward approach to soft-tissue injuries, firmly based on anatomy and physiology. The reliance on palpation for both diagnostic and therapeutic applications is appealing to chiropractic practitioners in general. It can be used as a standalone technique, or as an adjunct to other chiropractic technique systems primarily concerned with the correction of spinal subluxation, however defined. In addition, ART may aid a practitioner wishing to use spinal manipulation in that this technique may loosen up the holding elements surrounding the joint prior to the manipulative application. The net result may be the need for less force to accomplish a successful adjustment than might otherwise be required.

- Beside local discomfort, there are no significant contraindications to ART. In particular, for patients suffering neck pain or headaches, this approach may quell the anxiety some patients have with respect to cervical manipulation, in particular. In addition, radiography is not required, nor are any of the other diagnostic methods used by chiropractors that are controversial (leg check, thermography, and so on).

- ART is primarily a pain-based approach to care, which is all the more relevant due to the fact that 80–90% of chiropractic patients present with spinal pain. Diagnosis is based on the reproduction of physical symptoms, and outcome measures focus on the diminishing of these symptoms. Since advocates of this technique insist that results should be obtained within a few treatment visits, in our view this intuitive pain-based approach, coupled with an expectation of quick results, might be looked on favorably by both condition-based chiropractors and managed care organizations.[3]

- Unlike with most other therapeutic approaches, chiropractic or otherwise, patients are required to become involved in their care, providing feedback on the reproduction of symptoms and actively performing different muscular movements. It is widely believed that the more a patient is an active participant in his or her own healthcare, the better the outcome.

- Since ART practitioners claim such a high rate of recovery, we would welcome substantive evidence, such as would place ART on a firmer evidentiary base. Despite the lack of clinical trials, Leahy contends that some insurance companies are specifically asking that ART be utilized as a component of a patient's therapeutic regimen.[3] A recent review of the relevant literature by a group of senior chiropractic students concluded that, using the Kaminsky model,[17,18] ART should be granted "provisional acceptance" status.[19] Apparently, some senior students are comfortable dispensing with a firm evidentiary base when presented with a technique that makes sense to them.

- Currently, ART is offered in seminars throughout Canada and the USA. The cost for a spine module and materials is US $1590 and an extremity module US $1990. A practitioner must attend a seminar yearly (US $595) in order to retain ART certification.

REFERENCES

1. Leahy M P 1996 Active Release Technique soft-tissue management for the upper extremity. Seminar manual. Self-published, Colorado Springs, CO
2. Leahy M P, Mock L E 1992 Myofascial release technique and mechanical compromise of peripheral nerves of the upper extremity. Chiropractic Sports Medicine 6 (4): 139–150
3. Leahy M P 2000 How to build a practice with fewer patient visits. Canadian Chiropractor 5 (2): 6–7
4. Agios P, Crawford J W 1999 Double crush syndrome of the upper extremity. Journal of Chiropractic and Sport Rehabilitation 13 (3): 111–113
5. Baer J 1999 Iliotibial band syndrome in cyclists: evaluation and treatment: a case report. Journal of Chiropractic and Sport Rehabilitation 13 (2): 66–67
6. Browne W, Goodman J E, Berkson M 1999 Chiropractic soft tissue management of bilateral failed surgical decompression of the carpal tunnel: a case presentation. Journal of the American Chiropractic Association (Feb) 36 (2): 18–23
7. Buchberger D 2000 Posterior-superior glenoid impingement of the throwing shoulder: evaluation and treatment. Journal of Chiropractic and Sport Rehabilitation 14 (2): 5–12

8. Buchberger D 2000 Shoulder impingement in the overhand athlete: a chiropractic approach. Journal of Sports Chiropractic and Rehabilitation 14 (2): 5–14

9. Buchberger D, Rizzoto H, McAdam B J 1996 Median nerve entrapment resulting in unilateral action tremor of the hand. Sport Chiropractic Rehabilitation 10 (4): 176–179

10. Buchberger D 1993 Scapular dysfunctional impingement syndrome as a cause of grade 2 rotator cuff tear: a case study. Chiropractic Sport Medicine 7 (2): 38–45

11. Ger E, Letz R, Landrigan P J 1991 Upper extremity musculoskeletal disorders of occupational origin. Annual Review of Public Health 543–566

12. Goss K 2000 How to bounce back from training injuries ... fast. Muscle Media 113–118

13. Leahy M P 1995 Improved treatments for carpal tunnel and related syndromes. Chiropractic Sport Medicine 9 (1): 6–9

14. Leahy M P 1992 Synoviochondrometaplasia of the shoulder: a case report. Chiropractic Sport Medicine 6 (1): 5–8

15. Leahy M P 1991 Altered biomechanics of the shoulder and the subscapularis. Chiropractic Sport Medicine 5 (3): 62–66

16. Schiottz-Christensen B, Mooney V, Azad S 1999 The role of active release manual therapy for upper extremity overuse syndromes – a preliminary report. Journal of Occupational Rehabilitation 9 (3): 201–211

17. Kaminsky M 1990 Evaluation of chiropractic methods. Chiropractic Techniques 2 (3): 107–112

18. Kaminsky M, Boal R, Gillette R G 1987 A model for the evaluation of chiropractic methods. Journal of Manipulative and Physiological Therapeutics 10 (2): 61–64

19. Adams S, Boudreau G, McDonald D, Posein P 2000–2001 Active Release Technique, literature review. Student Investigative Project. Canadian Memorial Chiropractic College

27

Spinal Biomechanics (Pettibon) Technique

INTRODUCTION

In 1941, JF Grostic walked into RR Gregory's office; at the time Gregory was going through Wernsing's *The Atlas Specific*,[1] seeking an effective upper cervical adjustment. In 1956, Burl Pettibon took the first seminar in Upper Cervical technique to be conducted by JF Grostic. Although Pettibon would later extend that exacting upper cervical analysis (Chs 32 and 33) to the entire spine, we think he still feels himself upper cervical at heart, although full-spine in fact. Pettibon was not the first chiropractor to see subluxation as a matter of full-body distortion, as a matter of postural dysfunction; the Carver brothers, Hurley, Logan, and others preceded him. Pettibon was not the first chiropractor to use exacting X-ray analysis to measure spinal distortion; BJ Palmer had already used such methods for the upper cervical spine, and Hugh Logan had used such methods for the pelvis. But Pettibon was the first chiropractor to apply such exacting methods to the entire spine.

Rosenthal[2] distinguished the structural from the segmentalist approach in chiropractic:

The structural approach to chiropractic analysis held that the human spinal column was a gravity-adapting, weight-supporting structure. Its potential areas of weakness and breakdown, when studied using mechanical engineering concepts, could be readily determined, its advocates claimed. In contrast, the segmental school espoused that vertebrae subluxate in an independent autonomous fashion. The curves of the spine and distortionary patterns were adaptive, natural and normal unless the result of a subluxation which disturbed body balance, its practitioners held.

Although Rosenthal felt in 1981 that chiropractic structuralism had just about disappeared with the death of Willard Carver in 1943, he did not seem aware of the efforts of Burl Pettibon, a very important neostructuralist. In 1972, Pettibon wrote: "We must now discuss the concept of the neck, functioning, not as seven individual bones, but together as a unit of the spine. These bones are intimately related, and thus anything that affects one, affects all."[3] Writing in 2001, Pettibon stated: "Relating the subluxated spine optimally to its environment has to affect the entire spine and not just a pair of displaced vertebrae."[4]

Structuralism entails this emphasis on *posture*; indeed, all of the Pettibon Chiropractic Biomechanics (PCB) procedures are directed at defining what constitutes a normal posture, and devising methods to attain and maintain that posture. Apart from the emphasis on posture, PCB marks perhaps the first serious and comprehensive effort to rationalize and enhance its adjustive methods based on biomechanical principles, not to mention rehabilitation methods based on the science of the inflammatory response and its application to wound healing.

OVERVIEW

PCB is a full-spine technique. From an analytic point of view, it studies "normal spinal joint position, function, and neurology, as well as neuropathies that result from their abnormal position and function."[5] Subluxation identification depends heavily on X-ray analysis, which also constitutes the primary outcome measure. The tissues adversely affected by vertebral subluxations, that will need to be rehabilitated, are said to be ligaments, muscles, vertebrae (which remodel in accordance with abnormal stress), and nerves. From an adjustive point of view, the PCB procedures include high-velocity, low-amplitude adjusting, therapeutic and vectored exercises, stretching, and ergonomic interventions. Some of the hand thrusting procedures are augmented by the use of drop tables and handheld or floor-mounted adjusting instruments, as well as blocks and wedges to improve mechanical advantage. The rehabilitative procedures include the use of novel traction devices, and weights that may be suspended from various parts of the body. Exercises are prescribed, usually unilateral and vectored so as to assist in attaining an improved posture.

HISTORY

Originator Burl Pettibon received his chiropractic degree from Cleveland Chiropractic College in 1955. By 1956 he had become immersed in the upper cervical milieu that was developing around Grostic and Gregory. He later used the methodology that upper cervical analysis had applied to the upper cervical spine to the more caudad parts of the spine. This included an exacting X-ray technique. Although the Pettibon methods became – and remain – full-spine, the imprint of the upper cervical origin remains clearly visible in the extra attention given to the atlanto-occipital configuration and treatment. In the late 1960s and early 1970s, Pettibon founded an organization named Burl R Pettibon, DC, and Associates Inc., which was later recast as the Pettibon Biomechanics Institute Inc., and granted 501(C)(3) status with the IRS.[6] A series of monographs emerged in 1981,[7,9] followed by a textbook in 1989.[10]

In the mid-1960s, Pettibon patented a mechanical adjusting instrument, which now has versions that are floor-mounted and handheld.[11] His first Ferguson projection lumbar view was taken in 1970. He has designed adjusting tables, in-line X-ray frames, head clamps for exacting cervical X-rays, and X-ray chairs. For a brief period of time, Pettibon and Vernon Pierce (of Pierce–Stillwagon Technique, Ch. 23) combined their systems,[11] until

the time of Pierce's unexpected death. Don Harrison associated himself with Pettibon in the late 1970s, providing a substantial mathematics and mechanics input. He then broke with Pettibon in the early 1980s to found his own similar technique, Chiropractic Biophysics Technique (Ch. 14), which remains structuralist in the same sense as PCB.

In 1984, the Leading Edge Research Symposium was convened in St Louis, a gathering of technique system experts that was to devise, once and for all, a common definition of subluxation.[12] The result was almost entirely inspired by Pettibon concepts: "A subluxation is any relative malposition of a joint that produces consistent misalignment of its articular surfaces. A subluxation's physical definition: The physical subluxation is the distance a vertebral unit or units are displaced from their zero or optimum position or origin, multiplied by the amount of resistance that holds it displaced, the formula being $D \times R = S$ (distance times resistance equals subluxation)." This consensus definition is more of historical interest than anything else, in that it has had no impact on subsequent development of consensus definitions of subluxation. What it does tell us is how influential Pettibon's ideas, or at least his biomechanical approach, were, one day in St Louis.

DEFINITION OF TECHNIQUE-SPECIFIC TERMS

There are several terms adapted from Upper Cervical technique X-ray line marking.

- Lower angle: the angle between a line representing the center of mass of the functional cervical spine (center of the neural canal) and a line transversely through the atlas in the frontal plane
- Upper angle: the angle between a line representing the head, which has been "divided" using a special mensuration tool, and a line transversely through the atlas in the frontal plane
- Into the angles, against the angles, head subluxation: terms adapted from Upper Cervical work (Gregory), referring to cervical distortion patterns

- Vertebral subluxations: individual vertebrae or groups of vertebrae that are a measurable distance from their normal position
- Compensated, uncompensated subluxations: compensated subluxations are pain-free at the lesion site, while *uncompensated* or *overcompensated* subluxations are usually pain-expressive
- Frontal/lateral headweighting: suspension of a weight from a harness worn around the skull, to sagittal and frontal plane cervical postural distortions.[13]

PHYSIOLOGICAL MECHANISMS AND RATIONALE

Optimal spinal position is required for normal spinal function and the prevention of pathology. All Pettibon adjustive, rehabilitative, exercise procedures are designed to move the spine toward that mathematically defined optimal structure. Normal sagittal curves are thought to represent arcs of circles in which the radius of the circle equals the chord length of the arc.[14,15] The resulting arcs then measure 60° for the cervical, thoracic, and lumbar spines. When these lordotic or kyphotic curve angles are not present, the result is thought to be suboptimally functioning, including energy waste and nerve interference as a result of distorted osseous position and attendant piezoelectric effects (electromagnetic nerve interference). Returning spinal structures and related tissues to normal positions is said to result in more normal physiological functioning of these tissues, especially the nervous system.[16]

Pettibon regards the head as a vertebra,[16] the only one that has neural tissue – the eyes – controlling its position and, via righting reflexes, the position of all the other vertebrae. When the body is injured, righting reflexes level the head, injuries notwithstanding, resulting in compensatory vertebral subluxation complexes in the neck and lower spine. These, therefore, should be understood in this context as necessary evils. In the Pettibon system, there is always a keen sense of subluxations and their compensations: "When any part of the spinal system is misplaced relative to its upright environment of gravity, a like amount of opposing compensating displacements must occur."[4]

The *initiating event* subluxation is said to be the loss of atlanto-occipital flexion movement,[17] which leads immediately to an asymmetric loss of atlanto-occipital lateral flexion movements. The next alteration would be subluxation of the head on the cervical spine. The righting reflex will keep the head level, but at the expense of spinal subluxations and biomechanical alterations that may extend as far caudad as the feet. Once the adaptations have set in, correcting the initiating subluxation may not adequately correct the caudad problems, which will require rehabilitation of the affected spinal structures and ligaments. There will be changes in the soft tissues, such as fibrosis, ligamentous shortening, and faulty neurological responses. According to Pettibon, "Strong, repetitive and sustained forces on injured spinal soft tissues are necessary for those tissues to heal and remodel properly so that they function optimally. Such tissues must heal in line with their functional stresses in order to be clinically stable."[17]

DIAGNOSTIC/ANALYTIC PROCEDURES

In the Pettibon system, diagnosis begins and ends with X-rays and X-ray line-marking procedures: "The only objective, accurate method for determining vertebral displacements, was and is X-ray, followed by scientific marking and measuring procedures."[4] The Pettibon full-spine X-ray series consists of five somewhat non-standard views: (1) lateral cervicothoracic; (2) anteroposterior (AP) cervicothoracic with central ray in the atlas plane line (nasium); (3) sitting AP lumbosacral-dorsal (Ferguson sacral base projection); (4) sitting lateral lumbosacral-dorsal; and (5) vertex cervical X-ray. If there has been trauma, then the Davis series and/or lumbar oblique and stress views would be added to the Pettibon five-view series. Post X-rays are fairly routine, taken at intervals of care.[16] PCB practitioners, in addition to these *static* (i.e., conventional) X-rays, also take *dynamic* X-rays, generally known as stress X-rays.[18] That is, the patient is forward or side-flexed, or extended, during the radiographic procedure. Excessive or diminished participation of one or more vertebrae can then be seen in these stress X-rays.

Showing his derivation from the Grostic Upper Cervical work, Pettibon developed fairly abstruse formulas for calculating the optimum line of drive in adjusting the upper cervical spine, based on X-ray line-marking procedures adapted from Grostic. The exact numbers that were calculated determined the stylus position on the cervical adjusting tool, which was far more easily achieved when the doctor used a floor-mounted adjusting instrument. Thus, these adjusting formulas were discarded when the handheld tool was used instead. Apparently, these mathematical formulas are not used at this time, at least not by Pettibon himself. A leg check may be performed to detect neurological imbalance; as is typical in a classic Upper Cervical setting, it is performed with the patient supine.

TREATMENT/ADJUSTIVE PROCEDURES

Although PCB is a Full-Spine technique, there is a pervasive Upper Cervical feeling about it, in the sense that the upper cervical unit (and we note that, for Pettibon, this includes not only atlas, but the skull and the temporomandibular joints) is considered of paramount importance. Thus we read: "The position of the head relative to gravity takes precedence over the position of the lower spine ... the lower spine cannot be corrected and/or remain corrected until the head's position is first stabilized front to back and side to side."[19] Restoration of a normal cervical lordotic angle, estimated to be 43–45°, is also considered very important, and, according to Pettibon, does not take as much time as one would think: he claims that Pettibon Cervical Lordosis Restoration Procedures produce correction within 1–6 weeks.

The patient is prestressed toward correction prior to the administration of the thrust.[20] The adjusting instrument is usually used in the upper cervical area, but can be used anywhere. The lower cervical, thoracic, lumbar, and pelvic adjustments are done using thrusting procedures. Long-lever contacts are taken on the innominate bones to alter the angle struck by the lumbar

spine with the sacrum in the frontal plane.[20] The preferred adjustment for the thoracic spine is the anterior thoracic maneuver. Diversified-like procedures are often used in the lower cervical spine.

When the spinal entity to be corrected is considered regional (not segmental), then the adjusting force is correspondingly multisegmental; thus, it is not specific in the usual sense of that word, although it is carefully *vectored*. For example, a patient with a right lateral curvature of the lumbar spine may be placed in side-posture with the convex side up, and an adjustive force applied to the apex of the curve, with an attempt to reduce (flatten) the lateral curvature. In the practice of structural chiropractic, the word "specificity" takes on a new meaning, wherein it refers not to the patient contact point or segmental level addressed, but the specific vectors that are chosen to reverse a multisegmental postural distortion.

Therapeutic exercises and stretching programs are mentioned below as ancillary procedures, but they are critical enough to the Pettibon program to be considered in this paragraph as well. PCB practitioners believe that exercises, when indicated, should be specific, unilateral and usually isotonic, designed to correct the posture (and not just to cause general muscle hypertrophy).[21]

Pettibon practitioners describe four stages of care: (1) acute care aimed at pain reduction; (2) subacute care aimed at restoration of duties; (3) corrective care for restoration of optimal spinal structure; and (4) maintenance care to keep the spine in its optimum condition.[16] PCB believes that, without rehabilitation, the benefits of adjusting, such as improved range of motion and pain relief, would be lost within a week.[19] Rehabilitative exercises would be doomed to failure minus the adjusting components of PCB, while the adjustments themselves would result in only short-term improvements in pain and range of motion minus the rehabilitative procedures.[22] "The building of muscle strength and the endurance necessary to maintain the correction often takes an additional 90 days of corrective-rehabilitation care."[19]

In recent years, PCB practitioners have been using weights, suspended from the patient's head, shoulder girdle, and pelvic girdle, to effect changes in the spine, mediated in their view by righting reflexes.[19] Lateral headweighting, with 2–10 lb (0.9–4.5 kg) suspended from the head on the side of tilt, is used to provoke the contralateral lateral flexors of the neck into compensatory hypertonus, to correct lateral frontal plane postural distortion.[23] Frontal headweighting is utilized to correct what appears to be occiput–C1 hyperextension, forward head, and cervical hypolordosis.[13]

Pettibon's idea is that the body's isometric effort to achieve balance, confronted with these loading stresses, can be used to strengthen and retrain muscles so as to normalize posture. Although it is beyond our scope to explore these protocols beyond what has already been stated, suffice it to say that the details on how this is done depend on whether "the spine is compensated, uncompensated, or spine is compensated,"[19] and whether there is an inference of ligamentous damage to some degree. X-rays with and without the weights in place are used to determine the appropriateness of the protocol and the prognosis for postural correction.

Ancillary procedures

- The patient does warm-up exercises prior to being adjusted.
- The patient may be placed on pelvic blocks prior to being adjusted.
- During the acute phase of care, the patient may receive deep massage.
- Cervical traction in extension is an important part of the treatment plan in many cases.[24]
- Cervical collars and lumbosacral supports may find a role in trauma cases.
- Cervical pillows and other orthopedic devices may be used, mostly in an attempt to introduce and/or maintain lordosis in the secondary curves.
- Asymmetric exercises are prescribed that reverse the patient's spinal distortions. Special fulcrums assist the patient to maintain lordosis during the performance of these exercises, for both the neck and the lumbar spine.
- Nutritional advice is given – nothing particularly esoteric, e.g., vitamin C for collagen repair, B vitamins for the nervous system, etc.

- Physical therapy modalities such as ultrasound are apparently not used.

OUTCOME ASSESSMENT

Post X-ray plays a critical role in assessing the outcome of care.[4] Symptom (pain) relief is not considered to be of major significance.

SAFETY AND RISK FACTORS

None is listed other than the usual contraindications to adjustive care. The use of extension traction is contraindicated when extension is contraindicated for a particular patient.

EVIDENCE OF EFFICACY

Jackson et al found very good reliability in Pettibon-like upper cervical X-ray marking procedures:[25] "The Pettibon technique appears to have both temporal stability for individual practitioners and equivalence across practitioners."[26] Harrison et al,[27] in their review article on the reliability of various chiropractic line-marking systems, came to the same conclusion.

Venditti et al[28] assessed five different home-use supine traction devices, looking at the amount of mechanical separation achieved and the degree to which surface electromyogram recordings from the posterior cervical and masseter muscles changed. The Pettibon device was clearly the least favored of the devices among the subjects tested.

West et al[29] performed a non-controlled study on 177 patients, the "worst of the worst" in that they had not responded well to other treatments for their spinal complaints. All of the patients received manipulation under anesthesia (MUA), followed by 4–6 weeks of spinal manipulation, physical therapy modalities (including traction[24]), and active resistance rehabilitation. The spinal manipulation is described as "osseous," in addition to which "some patients required the use of Pettibon's specialized spinal biomechanical technique."[29] This apparently included a prone drop move on the occiput and "percussive technique" on offending cervical vertebrae. On average, cervical range of motion improved by 47%, and pain levels as reported using the visual analog scale (VAS) reduced by over 60%.

CONCLUSIONS

- Even though Pettibon and his followers developed a full-spine system of care, in a larger sense it remains unquestionably an Upper Cervical technique. Any and all adjustments apart from the atlas adjustment seem to be considered, in a sense, spinal hygiene: preparation for the primary adjustment of atlas. Months of care may go by without atlas being adjusted even once, in order that all the other spinal problems be cleared out so that the atlas adjustment will "hold."
- Pettibon's most unique contribution may have been to extend the Grostic/National Upper Cervical Chiropractic Association chirometric analysis inferiorward, developing a series of lines akin to their upper and lower angles (referring to the orientation of both the head and the cervical spine to the atlas), all the way to the sacrum. These collectively constitute the Pettibon line-marking system.
- We read comments by Pettibon implying that extensive research has been done, for example:"Digital analysis was performed on more than 25 000 sets of pre- and post-care X-rays";[22] and "During our eight year research program, all existing chiropractic clinical procedures were tested."[22] We are unaware of any of this research having been published, at least not in a formal sense, and therefore from our point of view it cannot be presumed to exist. We also read sweeping statements with a research bent, such as: "97.3% of the patients analyzed had the following posture and/or posture-caused problems: Forward head posture (16 more structural pathologies, several listed as having sub-pathologies)."[22] Again, we are unable to interpret such remarks minus the supportive evidence.
- Although we, as chiropractic college teachers, do not share Pettibon's view, we note that he

paints a rather bleak situation in the chiropractic colleges today,[i] colored by his particular take on the importance and clinical utility of X-ray procedures:

> The examination, X-ray and clinical procedures taught in all chiropractic colleges do not detect and/or correct spinal displacements of any kind, in fact, they do not detect and/or correct anything. Therefore, by definition, chiropractic colleges are therapy and most chiropractors are practicing a therapy rather than a separate and distinct science.

- Although Pettibon invokes the West et al study[29] in support of the clinical utility of PCB procedures,[30] going so far as to state the investigators had "performed clinical trials on 200 patients using the Pettibon Adjusting and Spinal Rehabilitation methods,"[30] we must note that the authors themselves considered this a study of MUA. In the post-MUA phase of their care, the patients received fairly generic "osseous" spinal manipulation, consisting of side-posture manipulation of the low back and pelvis, the anterior thoracic maneuver, and supine (i.e., Diversified) cervical move. Some, but not apparently all, also received maneuvers specifically described as Pettibon procedures. In its entirety, it is difficult to interpret this study as having much to do with the clinical effectiveness of PCB.
- We confess to being intrigued by Pettibon's observation that "In order to keep the skull upright, innate intelligence often must subluxate the lower spine below the skull front to back and side to side."[22] Imagine that, *the spine must become subluxated, to correct subluxation.* Pettibon is, of course, not the only chiropractor to have observed that some subluxations are compensatory to others, but more than anyone else he discusses this process as an intelligent choice by the neuromusculoskeletal system, a component of normal function in an abnormal postural environment.
- The Pettibon work brings to the fore an issue which chiropractors will some day have to face definitively: is there really a "normal spine," that is, normal for everybody? Or, is my spine normal for me, given my history of accidents, my genes, my mode of using my body, my

handedness, my congenital musculoskeletal variants and developmental tendencies, my fetal birth presentation, my personality, my whatever?

- In the History section above, we comment that the Leading Edge Research Symposium of 1984 adopted a Pettibon-like consensus definition of subluxation. Following remarks by Drs Pettibon and Morter in apparent support of the definition, cancer researcher and chiropractic advocate Dr. Ronald Pero, sitting in the audience and possibly reflecting the sentiments of other non-chiropractic professionals, remarked "Yeah, well, uh, not really feeling this passion over the definition of 'subluxation,' maybe that gives me a little more freedom to just ask a simple question. Maybe some value would be taken in not only defining what a subluxation is but really defining what 'normal' is. I mean, when you say that it's a matter of when you don't have any misalignment, what is 'normal'? I mean, that's a very important philosophical point here. How do you do that?" Although the audience laughed, we still think that is an excellent question. Pettibon, and after him Harrison, have spent most of their careers attempting to answer that question, through the elaboration of spinal models.

REFERENCES

1. Wernsing A A 1941 The atlas specific. Oxford Press, Hollywood, CA
2. Rosenthal M J 1981 The structural approach to chiropractic: from Willard Carver to present practice. Chiropractic History 1 (1): 25–29
3. Pettibon B R 1972 The concept of cervical unit subluxations. Digest of Chiropractic Economics (March/April): 48–49
4. Pettibon B 2001 Posture correction and spinal rehabilitation. http://www.worldchiropracticalliance.org/tcj/2001/feb/feb2001pettibon.htm: WorldChiropracticAlliance.org
5. Pettibon B R 1995 Pettibon Chiropractic Bio-mechanics Procedures for detection and correction of the vertebral subluxation complex – Part I. Chiropractic Products (October): 120–122, 124–126, 128–130
6. Pettibon B 2001 The science of postural correction and spinal rehabilitation. http://www.worldchiropracticalliance.org/tcj/2001/jan/jan2001pettibon.htm: WorldChiropracticAlliance.org
7. Pettibon B, Harrison D 1981 Pettibon Spinal Bio-Mechanics: theory and implications. Pettibon Biomechanics Institute, Vancouver, WA
8. Pettibon B 1981 Bio-Mechanics and bio-engineering of the cervical spine with X-ray analysis and instrument adjusting, 6th edn. Pettibon Biomechanics Institute, Vancouver, WA
9. Pettibon B, Harrison D 1981 True plane spinography: an introduction to Pettibon X-ray procedures, 2nd edn. Pettibon Biomechanics Institute, Vancouver, WA
10. Pettibon B 1989 Introduction to Spinal Bio-Mechanics. Pettibon Spinal Biomechanics Institute, Tacoma, WA
11. Hochman J I 1991 Pierce and Pettibon combine their systems. Today's Chiropractic (July/August): 84–86
12. Cooperstein R 1996 Guidelines in chiropractic: our own private Bosnia? Dynamic Chiropractic (March 11): 16, 32–34
13. Pettibon B 2001 Neuro-physiology of spinal subluxation and correction. http://www.worldchiropracticalliance.org/tcj/2000/jan/jan2000pettibon.htm: WorldChiropracticAlliance.org
14. Pettibon B R, Loomis W P 1973 Biomechanical research by Pettibon & Associates #5. Today's Chiropractic (April–May): 12–15
15. Pettibon B R 1972 Biomechanical research by Pettibon & Associates #2 in a series. Today's Chiropractic (August–September): 12–13
16. Pettibon B 1991 Upper cervical care and functional leg length inequality. In: Hansen D (ed.) Sixth Annual Conference on Research and Education, pp. 114–116. Consortium for Chiropractic Research, Monterey, CA
17. Pettibon B 2001 Detection and correction of the spinal system's subluxation complexes. http://www.worldchiropracticalliance.org/tcj/1997/apr/apr1997pettibon.htm: WorldChiropracticAlliance.org
18. Pettibon B 2001 Detection and correction of the spinal system's subluxation complexes. Part 6 in a series. http://www.worldchiropracticalliance.org/tcj/1996/nov/nov1996pettibon.htm: WorldChiropracticAlliance.org
19. Pettibon B 2001 Neuro-physiology of spinal subluxation and correction. Part 4 in a series. http://www.worldchiropracticalliance.org/tcj/2000/mar/mar2000pettibon.htm: WorldChiropracticAlliance.org
20. Pettibon B 2001 Detection and correction of the spinal system's subluxation. http://www.worldchiropracticalliance.org/tcj/1997/mar/may1997pettibon.htm: WorldChiropracticAlliance.org
21. Pettibon B 2001 Delivering the promise by re-inventing chiropractic. Part 7 in a series. http://www.worldchiropracticalliance.org/tcj/2000/jun/jun2000pettibon.htm: WorldChiropracticAlliance.org
22. Pettibon B 2001 Posture correction and spinal rehabilitation (cont'd.). http://www.worldchiropracticalliance.org/tcj/2001/apr/apr2001pettibon.htm: WorldChiropracticAlliance.org
23. Pettibon B 2001 Delivering the promise by reinventing chiropractic. Part 11 in a series. http://www.worldchiropracticalliance.org/tcj/2000/oct/oct2000pettibon.htm: WorldChiropracticAlliance.org

24. Pettibon B 2001 Detection and correction of the spinal system's subluxation complexes (part 2). http://www.worldchiropracticalliance.org/tcj/1997/oct/oct1997pettibon.htm: WorldChiropracticAlliance.org

25. Jackson B L, Barker W, Bentz J, Gambale A 1987 Inter- and intra-examiner reliability of the upper cervical X-ray marking systems: a second look. Journal of Manipulative and Physiological Therapeutics 10 (4): 157–163

26. Jackson B 1988 Reliability of the upper cervical X-ray marking system: a replication study. Journal of Chiropractic Research 1: 10–13

27. Harrison D E, Harrison D D, Troyanovich S J 1998 Reliability of spinal displacement analysis of plain X-rays: a review of commonly accepted facts and fallacies with implications for chiropractic education and technique. Journal of Manipulative and Physiological Therapeutics 21 (4): 252–266

28. Venditti P, Rosner A, Lettmer N, Sanders G 1995 A basic evaluation of home-use supine cervical traction devices. Journal of the Neuromusculoskeletal System 3 (2): 89–92

29. West D T, Mathews R S, Miller M R, Kent G M 1999 Effective management of spinal pain in one hundred seventy-seven patients evaluated for manipulation under anesthesia. Journal of Manipulative and Physiological Therapeutics 22 (5): 299–308

30. Pettibon B 2001 Delivering the promise by reinventing chiropractic. Part 8 in a series. http://www.worldchiropracticalliance.org/tcj/2000/jul/jul2000pettibon.htm: WorldChiropracticAlliance.org

28

Stressology
Spinal Stressology

INTRODUCTION

Sometimes in poring over the writings germane to a particular chiropractic technique system, it seems that the concepts, terminology, and technique procedures are so out of the ordinary that we are dealing with something that feels *oddly unchiropractic*. Lowell Ward's Spinal Stressology (SS) gives us that feeling, but not for long. Compared with Applied Kinesiology and Network Spinal Analysis, some of whose practitioners seem rather indifferent to the chiropractic umbilical cord that gave them life, SS always remains at least *chiropractically odd*.

SS is a full-spine technique, in the tradition of chiropractic structuralism, making heavy use of pre and post X-rays, and applying a myriad of adjustive and adjunctive treatment methods. It features a heavy dose of mind–body emphasis – but not lay psychotherapy, at least according to Ward.[1,2] We are going to do our best to describe SS, but the reader is warned that the terminology, and what's more, the concepts behind the terminology, are so unusual that most of the time we thought it best to let the technique speak for itself, lest we sow confusion by interpreting it incorrectly. The reader is urged to seek out the original articles to clarify that which we cannot.

OVERVIEW

SS aims at identifying and reducing structural stress in the spinal-pelvic-meningeal system, in order to prevent breakdown and ensure health. Various critical points that are regarded to be key areas for spinal column-pelvic stability and function are located radiographically, and compared with measurements derived from a critical stress analysis of the patient. The result demonstrates the behavioral habits and holding patterns of the unit. The finding may be that there is abnormal axial hyperelongation of the unit (over-stretching), which puts tension on the meningeal system. Meningeal tension may adaptatively tighten up a destabilized spine, perhaps following trauma. Treatment involves normalizing spinal structure, which sometimes requires analyzing and working with personality disorders.

HISTORY

Ward[3] tells the story of his son Stephen, who was a premature baby and also severely affected by the Hong Kong flu at the age of 6. Ward noticed that when he flexed his son's heels to his buttocks, the right one was 1.5 in. (3.75 cm) shorter than the other. Fitting a 1.5-in. (3.75 cm) heel lift apparently resulted in a dramatic improvement. This turned out to be a breakthrough case for Ward, who continues to emphasize structural balance in his practice. As for Stephen Ward, he is now a chiropractor as well.

Ward was heavily influenced by the writings of Selye, and found his three-stage theory of stress response (alarm, resistance, and exhaustion) very applicable to chiropractic. Working with an engineer named Fulkerson, Ward developed the means to measure the existence and progression of spinal structural disorders, analogous to the progression of stress that Selye had described. Later, much impressed with the work of Breig[4,5] on mechanical tension in the central nervous system, Ward and other Spinal Stressologists came to regard the meninges as one of the most important physiological systems in the body, and worked out means to normalize tension in the meninges. Eventually, they noted that when patients failed to improve, there tended to be a personality disorder. This observation led to their work on relating personality types to types of spinal structure, so that eventually they were able to derive personality profiles from spinal column-pelvic-meningeal measurements.

DEFINITION OF TECHNIQUE-SPECIFIC TERMS

SS uses few traditional chiropractic terms, and even questions the value of the venerable term "subluxation."[6] Ward says that, although the term should be retained for some purposes, by and large it is not helpful.[1] He finds it hard to document, and proposes using the term "biomechanical dysfunction."[7]

There are so many terms that are either unique to or atypically used by SS that the following list should be considered just a *sampling*. Most of these terms do not occur among any of the other technique systems. In some of the other sections we provide direct quotations, to enable the reader better to decode these terms.

- Spinal column-pelvic-meningeal unit: the subluxation entity treated by SS
- Stress: the rate of wear and tear in a biological organism
- Syntropy: ideal process of reorganizing or putting back together
- Stress dominant side: side of body opposite that of brain dominance, thought more prone to breakdown
- Synchronicity: the interconnectedness of all the spinal-pelvic regions
- Retracing (both emotional and structural): temporary worsening on the way to recovery
- Breakdown factors: these cause systemic structural collapse, either by trauma or insidiously

- Defense factors: these result from overutilization of energy, and can be determined or measured as degenerative changes seen on X-ray
- Reactive spinal abnormalities: compensations
- Entrophic, syntrophic: bad, good, respectively
- Intermittent force correction (IFC): procedure in which the patient walks with the shoe on one foot, first on the defense side, then on the breakdown side
- Entropic chaos: temporary worsening of the patient after care begins[2]
- Compustress: computerized disk stress evaluation system that apparently can be installed in doctors' offices[8]

PHYSIOLOGICAL MECHANISMS AND RATIONALE

SS practitioners say that stress may be defined as "an adaptive response to one's environmental situation" from a medical point of view, and as "forces per unit area" in an engineering context.[9] The frontal plane spinal configuration has to do with stability, and the sagittal view configuration has to do with functional flexibility. They claim that stress breaks down the spinal-meningeal unit and may also cause an overreactive defense mechanism that increases the damage. Ward even suggests that meningeal tension can produce diseases like Alzheimer's.[2]

Emotional stresses are thought to have profound effects on the spinal-meningeal system.[2] Conscious emotional patterns are said to show in standing X-rays, and unconscious patterns in sitting (sedentary) X-rays.[2] The spinal-meningeal unit is though to assume a pathological holding pattern (i.e., posture) that resembles the body's position at the time of injury.[10]

The following quotation is a representative statement pertaining to the physiological rationale of Spinal Stressology.[11]

HYPOTHESIS
The structure of the cranium, spinal column, pelvis, meninges and related tissues constitutes an integral thermodynamic system that follows thermodynamic process as it changes in internal energy as a result of

the energy consuming process of striving for homeostasis through adapting to stressor exposures ...

THEORY

The adaptive mechanisms in the body follow a thermodynamic process. Each adaptive mechanism is internally synchronous (spatially and temporally compensatory). The adaptive mechanisms in the body are synchronously interrelated.

SOME RAMIFICATIONS OF THE THEORY

Stress and strain of biological systems can be modeled according to a thermodynamic process. Adaptation coefficients can be determined for biological systems. Biological systems strain predictably in response to stress. The pathophysiology of the adaptive process is sequential. The sequence of events in the pathophysiology of the adaptive process is predictable ...

DIAGNOSTIC/ANALYTIC PROCEDURES

A new patient receives each of the following:

- comprehensive case history
- physical examination (in addition to the usual orthopedic/neurological examination, the Spinal Stressologist performs an *intrarectal* spine-meningeal systems tension stress examination)
- X-ray (singular unit spinal column-pelvic-meningeal radiograph)
- documented systemic evaluations (apparently, lab analysis).

Stressologists believe they can identify various health conditions from mere spinal measurements.[9] Emotional stress influences would have an impact on the spine, creating meningeal stress. Stressologists claim that such emotions can be identified through inspection of the radiograph. Full-spine films are obligatory, to permit measurements of the length of the neural canal. Indeed, "radiographic examination is one of the most important aspects of the Stressology model,"[12] and pre and post films are taken after 12–15 visits or sooner.[13] Sitting films are also taken, because Ward believes a "sedentary X-ray" is more likely to show injuries that most likely occur while the patient is in a sitting or flexed position. Faulkner says the stress breakdown process shows best on sitting views, whereas the resisting or reactive defense process shows best in standing X-rays; hence the need for both of them.[12]

What follows is a representative statement on the rationale for the routine radiographic examination, by Van Koten and Ward:[11]

SINGULAR UNIT, FULL-SPINE X-RAYS AND THEIR RATIONALE

A solution oriented, problem-solving, structural healing approach for any complaint ... demands that the System be radiographically examined ... The primary purpose of making singular unit radiographs of the System is to provide various integral System stress measurements and assess their inherent stress force classifications and intensities. Specialized singular radiography of the System, such as lateral bending views or sedentary views, may provide important additional information relative to the patient's condition and treatment needs relative to that position. When used, the doctor in charge should record his/her rationale for ordering such procedures and the findings in the patient's records.

Spinal Stressologists feel it is possible to use radiology for early detection of systemic disorders such as cardiac problems, not by visualizing the heart or blood vessels, but by assessing the spinal structure.[6,14-16] Van Koten and Ward add: "The diagnostic focus of this methodology is evaluating gross, abnormally configured, holding patterns of the System and their dysfunctional component inter-relationships."[11] Furthermore, it works both ways: Ward believes it is possible to predict which X-rays are likely to show degenerative changes by the finding of "blood pressure problems."[15]

Although it is possible to find contrary statements in the voluminous SS literature, pain is by and large *not* regarded as an indicator of systemic crisis, and does not provide a rationale for care. Ward feels that, even when a patient has achieved pain relief, there may be injury to the spine-meningeal system that could be life-threatening,[7] and, further, that this situation is radiographically visible as biomechanical "exhaustion or degeneration."[1] He also believes that he can develop a psychological profile of the patient from viewing radiographs, and that "it is a scientific break through."[1]

A procedure called *digital (synchronous) testing* is explicitly distinguished from the Applied Kinesiology vertebral challenge as described by Walther.[17] Digital testing involves pressure on a vertebra, and an outcome involving an occipital response, whereby it either stays level at the external occipital protuberance (EOP) (indicating a no-adjust) or dips (adjustment indicated). Great importance is attributed to the finding of a functional short leg. It does not indicate a "misalignment" somewhere, but rather some sort of general spinal-meningeal tension.[18,19]

TREATMENT/ADJUSTIVE PROCEDURES

In an interview with Sehi, Ward says that patients generally get worse before they get better, proceeding from baseline to "entropic chaos" to recovery.[2] Part of the treatment plan involves addressing psychological issues, in that Ward believes that failure to do so impedes biomechanical improvement.

Amongst the plethora of SS writings, descriptions of actual adjusting and other concrete treatment methods are not common. None the less, the following list of procedures has been gleaned from the literature:

- High-velocity, low-amplitude procedures are used between C7 and L5, and the sacrum, using an anteroposterior line of drive ("anteriors").
- The femoral head, ilium and ischium fixations are treated using a "large 50 ounce [1.4 kg] toggle gauge."[20]
- A thrusting procedure is also used on the occiput. "All 'popping' is intra-cranial (none in Cervical area)," and the "Patient feels immediate 'Meningeal Tension Release.'" The "intracranial meningeal adjustment" supposedly "reduces or eliminates need for Cervical adjusting."[20]
- Some, perhaps most, of the adjustments are made using compression gauges with 21 and 51 oz [588 and 1428 g] settings.[21]
- Heel lifts are supported, and a case involving a 36 mm lift is described.[18]
- A procedure is described in which one doctor intrarectally holds the sacrococcygeal area of a side-lying patient, while an assistant moves the torso about in different positions. Ward says this can relieve back pain.[18]

Each of the following is described as "adjunctive care":[11] shoe alterations (heel lifts), other orthopedic supports (cervical collars, lumbosacral supports, counterstressing sedentary wedge), therapeutic exercises, IFC, physical therapy, nutritional intervention, and "mental-emotional-structural profiling." At the Ward Chiropractic website, we read: "Application of the cervical collar and seat wedge is appropriate with sitting exhaustion patterns that show an anterior forward displacement at C2 and an anterior forward displacement of the thoracic apex. To reduce abnormal forward spinal curvature, counterstressing devices such as shoe lifts, seat wedges, and cervical collars can be used."[22]

Mental-emtional structural profiling is at once a diagnostic and a treatment procedure, but for convenience it is presented in the treatment section of the review. It is best that Van Koten and Ward's description[11] of the procedure be cited in its entirety.

MENTAL-EMOTIONAL-STRUCTURAL PROFILING

Mental-emotional-structural connections are established through measured and documented structural Systemic stress patterns. The combined measurement complex reflects quantitatively the behavior of adaptation and holding patterns of the mental-emotional-structural System. Once the Systemic structural analysis, evaluation and diagnosis are completed a mental-emotional-structural (MES) profile consultation may be performed. The profile informatively acquaints patients with the interrelatedness of their MES problem. Such awareness is an extremely important tool in solution-oriented, problem-solving health care. When used successfully, it reduces the spine-meningeal stress impact and reduces prominent physical findings and pain syndromes ... The Systemic structural stress pattern locking mechanisms are released at a much greater rate when the mental-emotional aspects are included with the structural Systemic profile. Total structural care, which includes MES profiling, achieves a greater recovery and can usually be achieved with 30 to 70% less treatment.

According to Stauth,[21] Ward believes that "With our structural measurements we are able to obtain a cursory personality profile of the patient. We can use this to confront the patient with his or her psychological blocks."

OUTCOME ASSESSMENT

All of the procedures used for diagnosis are also used for outcome assessment, principally, the post X-ray. "An objectively documented evaluation and report of findings is primarily a comparative radiographic evaluation."[23] Ward says that pain reduction is one of the goals of care, and can be achieved with about 10% of biomechanical change, compared with restoration of function that requires 10–25% change.[24] Ward believes that patients only rarely recover completely.[1]

SAFETY AND RISK FACTORS

SS is strictly X-ray-dependent,[12] so the biohazard of ionizing radiation must be noted. When asked about radiation hazards, Ward remarked: "Patients having high risk biomechanical stress intensities become ill, diseased, and die at a far more frequent rate than could ever be heretofore appreciated. Comparatively speaking, the diagnostic radiation factor is a minimal risk."[13]

Several comments are made regarding various common adjustive procedures. Posteroanterior adjustments are discouraged, because they "stress-load the meningeal System axially and may result in a meningeal constriction or stenosis on the brain center, precipitating immediate or delayed cardio-respiratory or cerebro-vascular effects." A variety of conditions are listed that contraindicate manipulation of the cervical spine above C7, especially using rotary or highly leveraged procedures. Axial tensions of the System may have to be released prior to performing anteroposterior ("anteriors") adjustments on the supine patient.[11, 14]

A careful history of rectal diseases, conditions or surgeries should be made and consulted prior to any intra-rectal Systemic intervention. Recent hemorrhaging may not preclude the need for treatment if no medical causation was detected. Recent surgery for hemorrhoids, fissures, polyps, cancer, etc. will probably preclude recommendation for treatment.[11]

EVIDENCE OF EFFICACY

Bahan claimed in 1991[25] that there are "over 30 000 cases documented and proven on Spinal Stressology's data base." Unfortunately, we are unable to retrieve any through standard literature retrieval procedures. Anecdotal descriptions of SS miracles are presented by Stauth.[21]

Koren and Rosenwinkel[26] published a study in which SS radiographs successfully predicted findings of the Minnesota Multiphasic Personality Inventory (MMPI). Observing that it is not uncommon that people with emotional problems adopt characteristic postures, they go on to ask if certain postures can directly "have a feedback effect on emotional experience?"[26] Certain of the personality scales apparently correlated with certain of the X-ray findings, such as pelvic torsion and sacral angle. For example, the atlas angle strongly predicted hypochondriasis and paranoia.

A rather large collection of what are billed as *Documented Case Studies*[27] is almost completely non-interpretable, at least to us. No information whatsoever is provided to make any sense of the various tables, legends, graphs, and symbols. Most of Ward's writings include several anecdotal case descriptions, that cannot really be considered case reports; for example, five are presented in an article on risk factors for strokes.[14]

CONCLUSIONS

- SS is situated within what has been called the *structural approach* to chiropractic technique,[28] in which regional concerns are more important than segmental considerations. "Total spinal column stress seemed more logical to him than localized areas of nerve impingement. From then on, Dr. Ward saw the spinal column acting and reacting as a single unit rather than a column of segmented, unconnected parts."[22] Indeed, at the limit, Ward and Koren are capable of commenting: "We found the entire spine subluxated."[29] As another example, Bahan points out that a cervical lordosis may appear normal when considered alone, but could be found abnormally situated anterior to the rib cage, thus afflicted with meningeal tension.[28]

- SS practitioners seem to find themselves under pressure to defend their heavy reliance on X-rays. This would explain Ward's four-part interview on the matter,[1,12,13,24] in which he discusses measures taken to reduce patient exposure to radiation, while rationalizing the 14 × 36 in. (36 × 90 cm) view.

- In an article purporting to support the view that personality is to a large extent determined genetically, Ward describes the case of a girl referred to him for the treatment of migraine headaches. He writes: "The source of the child's migraines was traced back psychogenetically through her MES profile to a great, great grandfather who was a murderer."[30] He goes on to explain that the girl got better once she realized her hostility actually belonged to the murderer.
- Ward feels that inherited dysfunctional experience can be transmitted through as many as five generations, causing impenetrable subluxation patterns. This, of course, amounts to the inheritance of acquired characteristics. Ward explains that a child afflicted with Duchenne muscular dystrophy had "inherited the hostility of his mother's two prior abortions."[31]
- Ward's theory of what may be called the *psychogenetic inheritance* of personality traits, although he believes it is consistent with modern understanding of hardwired personality, is merely a revisitation of Lamarck's discredited theory of the inheritance of acquired characteristics. In confirmation, Ward writes: "We have discovered that inherited dysfunctional experience can be passed on to three, four, or five generations, causing an impenetrable subluxation pattern."[32] Obviously, there can't be *any generational limit* on true genetically inherited traits. In 1990, Ward boasted "Psychogenetic profiling will eventually play as major a role in legal processing as fingerprints. Count on it!"[30]
- Ward claims to be able to identify "various forms of murder experiences from documented structural patterns in patients."[31] These experiences may include having murdered someone, having planned to commit murder, having had a family member murdered, having had some type of abortion experience – but not apparently having actually been murdered. Ward writes: "You know, I just lost a son-in-law, 35 years old, whose X-rays showed, back in 1986, that he inherited death wishes."[33] Less dramatically, according to Stauth[21] Ward claims that right lateral curvatures are associated with hypersensitive, overemotional people, and left lateral curvatures with overly pragmatic,

excessively rational people. Ward suggests that spinal fixation and personality fixation go together.[30]
- The SS practice of developing psychological profiles from X-rays is controversial. Ward does not feel that this type of analysis intrudes into the practice of psychiatry.[2] Ward also suggests that not all practitioners of SS support or need support the practice of reading radiographs for psychological problems.[1] Stauth, on the other hand, says: "Another treatment adjunct used by Dr. Ward is psychological counseling" and further says that Ward routinely conducts group therapy sessions.[21]
- It would be easy to overinterpret and sensationalize Koren and Rosenwinkel's finding that personality traits and radiographic findings may correlate.[26] No causality is proven, and certainly not any directionality for any possible causality. Koren and Rosenwinkel's speculation that X-rays may provide objective evidence for changes brought about through psychiatric care is reasonable, and their comments do not approach Ward's extremism: "With our structural measurements we are able to obtain a cursory personality profile of the patient. We can use this to confront the patient with his or her psychological blocks."[21]
- For all the discussion about measurement and documentation,[7,23,34] Stressologists are surprisingly sparse in their descriptions of how they measure things. As a technique that heavily depends on X-ray findings, SS claims to have determined "a systematically related set of normal values."[23] However, we are aware of no discussion on how these normals were established.
- We are unable to determine how or if Spinal Stressologists have established the reliability or validity of their X-ray line-marking procedures. What, for example, does it mean to say that "pelvic torsion" is seen on a Stressology radiograph, when there is no definition of what that is, how it can be seen? Cooperstein has reviewed some of the problems involved in the radiographic identification of pelvic torsion.[35–37]
- Ward takes some amazing liberties with numbers. He describes, for example, how he had

measured a 50 mm functional short leg in a son who eventually developed cancer and passed away. In another passage, Ward and Koren explain that a basketball player's height could change by 3 in. (7.5 cm)[29]

- Since in SS patient changes ostensibly for the worse may actually be good, and for the better may actually be bad, it seems that a positive spin could be attached to virtually any clinical outcome. For example, Ward has come to believe that the patient *has to* get worse before getting better, and uses the well-known concept of "retracing" (somehow the patient re-experiences the sequence of prior traumas during recovery) as a prerequisite.[32] Ward found that "some spinal abnormalities were beneficial," to the point that attempted "correction" might expose the patient to serious iatrogenesis: stroke, heart attack, etc.[14]

- The spinal-meningeal unit is thought to assume a pathological holding pattern (i.e., posture) that resembles the body's position at the time of injury.[10] This reminds us of Walker's Neuro-Emotional Complex,[38,39] as described in Chapter 12.

- No proprietary chiropractic technique is entirely free from loose ends and unsupported assertions, but SS does seem to stand out – indeed, may set the standard. Ward often asks unanswered and probably unanswerable questions. For example, in an article that is ostensibly about how doctors might best engage in problem solving,[40] we are asked: "Would a doctor give the same treatment for a male left sciatica as for a right sciatica? Under what circumstance will a female react to a heel lift?"[40]

- The "thousands of well-documented case studies" Ward alleges to have at his disposal[34] are not as useful as one case report that conforms to the usual standards for scientific reporting. Although Ward and colleagues were for a time prolific in the trade journals and self-published texts, it is a matter of some concern that apparently they have only one peer-reviewed publication.[26] There are no barriers to SS practitioners publishing in research journals, except their reluctance truly to join the community of chiropractic scholars. In 1990, Ward wrote: "There is far more to our science than just the publishing in peer review journals. Such will come when the time is right and our people become open."[30] With the elapse of another decade without SS representation in the peer-reviewed literature, one supposes the time is still not right, for some reason.

- "Since an emotional induced spine-meningeal compression is seldom accompanied by gross pathological damage, solving the emotional problem involved can often produce 'miraculous' spine-meningeal recoveries."[16] One wonders how much of what goes on in an SS practice resembles lay psychological counseling, as implied by the quote?

REFERENCES

1. Faulkner T A 1986 Confronting Dr Ward's Stressology radiographic examination procedures – part IV. An exclusive interview with Dr Lowell E Ward. Digest of Chiropractic Economics (January/February): 40–41, 43

2. Sehi T, Proetz J F 1986 New answers for old stress problems – part 2. An exclusive interview with Dr Lowell Ward. Digest of Chiropractic Economics (March/April): 36, 38–39, 41

3. Ward L. Origin of Stressology. http://chiroman.com/ward02.htm

4. Breig A 1960 Biomechanics of the central nervous system. Almqvist & Wisekll, Stockholm, Sweden

5. Breig A 1960 Adverse mechanical tension on the nervous system. John Wiley, New York, NY

6. Ward L 1986 High risk heart attack and stroke, part III. Today's Chiropractic (Jan–Feb): 75–81

7. Ward L E 1986 Documentation for objective evaluation procedures: an exciting new era – parts I–IV. American Chiropractor (October): 14–32

8. Ward L 1990 A revolutionary new chiropractic development in stress management technology. American Chiropractor 12 (2): 29–34

9. Sehi T, Proetz J F 1986 New answers for old stress problems – part 1. An exclusive interview with Dr. Lowell Ward. Digest of Chiropractic Economics (January/February): 68, 70–71, 120

10. Ward L E 1981 Harmful sedentary stress effects cited. Digest of Chiropractic Economics (November/December): 136–137

11. Van Koten R J, Ward L E 1990 Manual of practice standards for intact spinal column-pelvic-meningeal unit integral system disorders. 3rd edn. SSS Press, Long Beach, CA

12. Faulkner T A 1986 Confronting Dr. Ward's stressology radiographic examination procedures, part I. An exclusive interview with Dr. Lowell E. Ward. Digest of Chiropractic Economics (July/August): 76, 78–79, 81

13. Faulkner T A 1986 Confronting Dr. Ward's stressology radiographic examination procedures, part II. An exclusive interview with Dr. Lowell E. Ward. Digest of Chiropractic Economics (September/October): 60, 62, 64–65

14. Ward L 1985 High risk heart attack and stroke profiles, part I. Today's Chiropractic (July–August): 35–38, 58, 62, 79–80

15. Ward L 1985 High risk heart attack and stroke profiles, part II. Today's Chiropractic (September–October): 17–20, 39, 101

16. Ward L 1986 High risk cardio-respiratory and cerebro-vascular cases, part IV. Today's Chiropractic (March–April): 87–88, 103

17. Walther D S 1981 Applied Kinesiology, vol. I. Systems DC, Pueblo, CO

18. Ward L E 1993 Solving the mystery of the short leg syndrome, part I. Digest of Chiropractic Economics (March/April): 18, 20–21

19. Ward L E 1993 Solving the mystery of the short leg syndrome, part II. Digest of Chiropractic Economics (May/June): 25–27

20. Ward L E 1995 Systemic chiropractic. 37th edn. Spinal Stress Seminars, Long Beach, CA

21. Stauth C 1984 Spinal stress. The startling new concept in structural therapy. Journal of the Nutritional Academy 2 (1): 16–23

22. Ward L The beginning. http://chiroman.com/stress03.htm

23. Ward L 1986 Stressology's documented classification of biomechanical stress forces: a synchronous biomechanical stress model – parts V–VII. American Chiropractor (November): 12–26

24. Faulkner T A 1986 Confronting Dr. Ward's stressology radiographic examination procedures. Part III. An exclusive interview with Dr. Lowell E. Ward. Digest of Chiropractic Economics (November/December): 78, 81, 115–116

25. Bahan J R 1991 Spinal column stressology: a concept pioneering its way into the structural health care profession. Digest of Chiropractic Economics (November/December): 46, 98

26. Koren T, Rosenwinkel B A 1992 Spinal patterns as predictors of personality profiles: a pilot study. International Journal of Psychosomatics 39 (1–4): 10–17

27. Ward L E 1990 Documented case studies, p. 67. CSE, Long Beach, CA

28. Rosenthal M J 1981 The structural approach to chiropractic: from Willard Carver to present practice. Chiropractic History 1 (1): 25–29

29. Ward L E, Koren T 1987 Spinal column stressology. American Chiropractor (July): 16–21

30. Ward L 1990 Chiropractic's major scientific breakthroughs – (MES) mental–emotional–structural stress pattern profiling. American Chiropractor 12 (9): 4–13

31. Ward L E 1992 Important psychosomatic connections – diagnosing hostile processes and murder from their associated x-ray findings. American Chiropractor (June): 22–30

32. Ward L E 1993 Chiropractic stressology: exploring new frontiers. Today's Chiropractic (September/October): 74–78

33. Lowell D C, Ward D C Stressology pioneer (interview) http://www.chiroweb.com/archives/11/10/09.html

34. Ward L E 1991 Personal injuries most doctors and lawyers miss. American Chiropractor (September): 15–19

35. Cooperstein R 1990 Innominate vertical length differentials as a function of pelvic torsion and pelvic carrying angle. In: Jansen R D (ed.) Proceedings of the 5th Annual Conference on Research and Education, pp. 1–14. Consortium for Chiropractic Research, Sacramento, CA

36. Cooperstein R 1992 Roentgenometric assessment of innominate vertical length differentials. In: Hansen D (ed.) 7th Annual Conference on Research and Education, pp. 273–277. Consortium for Chiropractic Research, Palm Springs, CA

37. Cooperstein R, List A 2000 Pelvic torsion: anatomical considerations, construct validity, and chiropractic examination procedures. Topics in Clinical Chiropractic 7(3): 38–49

38. Walker S 1996 Disobedient vertebrae: are they (neuro)emotionally disturbed? Chiropractic Products (October): 22–26

39. Walker S 1992 Ivan Pavlov, his dog and chiropractic. Digest of Chiropractic Economics (March/April): 36–46

40. Ward L E 1994 Does your technique provide solution-oriented, problem-solving chiropractic care capabilities? Digest of Chiropractic Economics (July/August): 33–34, 89

29

Thompson Technique
Thompson Terminal Point Technique

This chapter is partially based on previously published material, and is printed with the permission of the National University of Health Sciences

INTRODUCTION

It would be hard to exaggerate the pioneering nature of J Clay Thompson, beginning with the invention of the drop table and the high-velocity, low-amplitude adjusting style now known as drop-assisted. In addition, he had a lot to do with the reintroduction of full-spine adjusting at the Palmer College where he taught; there is an old home movie that shows BJ Palmer adjusting on a drop table near the end of his life. Although Thompson did not invent the Derifield leg check (Ch. 4), so integral to so many practitioners across multiple technique systems, he did assemble the contributions of several individuals into a leg-checking system. Thompson also emphasized the importance of trigger points before they had become in vogue, outside the practice of Nimmo (Ch. 24). Besides having inspired other drop-table technique systems, such as Pierce–Stillwagon (Ch. 23), his technique manuals[1,2] led to the development of at least two other drop-table manuals[3,4] that closely follow his own.

There is a sense in which the Thompson Technique is the prototype of today's technique systems, in that it features particularly well-developed algorithms connecting specific examination findings to specific adjustive procedures: if the short leg stays short, do this, but if the short leg becomes long, do that. Rules like that may seem simplistic, worthy of castigation as "cookbook chiropractic," or they may seem to be invaluable clinical gems that guide the path from examination findings to clinical interventions, a form of systematized knowledge. Although it is impossible not to associate J Clay Thompson first and

foremost with the drop table he invented, we believe he should also be credited for pioneering the use of protocols in chiropractic. We may approve or disapprove of his particular implementation, but there can be no doubt that protocols of care are at the center of modern chiropractic technique development.

OVERVIEW

The Thompson Technique is a full-spine adjusting technique that emphasizes high-velocity, low amplitude, and some low-force procedures, using a drop table as an indispensable adjunct.[5] At the heart of the analytic component of the Thompson Technique is the Derifield leg check, adapted from the original work of Dr. Romer Derifield.[3,6,7] The Derifield–Thompson leg-check analysis enables the differential diagnostic distinction between primarily cervical and pelvic involvement, as well as distinguishing among the various subentities within these primary diagnostic categories. The procedure in all its parts allows the doctor to know "where to begin and what specific areas to adjust."[6] The leg-check procedure purports to detect neurophysiological imbalance, resulting from subluxations, as manifested by a "contractured leg." Thompson's "terminal points" amount to trigger points, a term he himself uses in his seminar workbook.[1]

The Thompson Terminal Point® drop table aims not only to protect the patient from being overadjusted, but to promote the clinical longevity of the doctor.[8] The adjustments themselves are considered by Thompson practitioners to be "low force, high velocity,"[8] in that a light thrust triggers the drop section release mechanism. Lumbodorsal and extremity problems are afforded less attention, but also need to be addressed after the primary cervical and lumbar areas have been addressed.

HISTORY

Like several other technique innovators, Thompson's passion for chiropractic stemmed from a dramatic experience in his youth.[9] As the story goes, young Clay developed diabetes mellitus after a severe blow to the back of his head while unloading lumber from a truck in the 1920s. The company physician gave Clay less than 2 weeks to live after he failed to respond to the traditional medical treatment available at that time. On the suggestion of his father, Clay sought out the services of a chiropractor, Dr. James Dick, who had helped the senior Thompson years earlier. Dick adjusted Clay for 16 consecutive days, after which time he demonstrated no signs or symptoms of the disease. This episode in Clay's life prompted him to enroll at the Palmer College at the age of 37.

At the current time, drop tables are so taken for granted that it is difficult to realize how central the invention of the Terminal Point table was to the development of the Thompson Technique, and hard to imagine a time when there were no such things. According to Moulton,[8] J Clay Thompson headed research and development at the Palmer College for over 10 years, working closely with BJ Palmer in the development of the first drop headpiece in 1952. Dr. Quigley brought the headpiece to his Clearview Sanatorium, where he used it with great results on his mental patients. Thompson obtained a patent on the drop table in 1956,[10] and constructed the first table incorporating cervical, dorsolumbar, and pelvic drop pieces in 1957.

If the drop table is central to Thompson's technological innovations, then the leg-check procedure is analogously central to his analytic contributions. He adapted it from the work of Dr. Romer Derifield, who first worked out the case of the positive Derifield result. Later, Derifield discovered quite fortuitously that prone

leg lengths occasionally changed when the patient rotated the head, and so developed the concept of cervical syndrome. As Thompson recounts the story,[7] Derifield, who was working for a railroad in Detroit at the time, was having trouble treating a difficult case. One day the phone rang for the patient while his legs were being checked. As he turned his head to speak, the legs suddenly and unexpectedly evened. Further investigation by Derifield into this case and others revealed that thrusting into tender nodules in the (mostly upper) cervical spine would not only reduce the patients' symptomatology but ameliorate prone leg-length inequality. Thompson credits a Dr. Alvin Niblo with the discovery of the negative Derifield.[7] By the early 1960s, Pierce and Stillwagon had developed their own version of Thompson Technique (Ch. 23), and, indeed, dedicated their seminar manual to J Clay Thompson.[11]

DEFINITION OF TECHNIQUE-SPECIFIC TERMS

- Terminal Point: refers to the table's drop piece, which is thought to correct vertebral subluxation at the "terminal point" – the endpoint – of its travel distance once having been set into motion
- Spastic muscular contraction: also known as contractured muscle, the process by which neurophysiological imbalance results in leg-length inequality. The short leg is said to be *contracted*
- Involved side: the side of the patient ipsilateral to the side of the short leg
- Derifield leg check: the Thompson leg check is patterned after the work of Romer Derifield and others, and is described in Chapter 4. The behavior of the prone subject's legs, with the knees either extended or flexed, as various test conditions are altered, gives rise to Thompson Technique listings
- Negative Derifield: the posterior superior iliac spine (PSIS) of the ipsilateral innominate subluxates posterior-inferior, the innominate rotating about an axis through the *sacroiliac* joint. The prone short leg with the knees

extended remains short when the knees are flexed

- Positive Derifield: the PSIS of the ipsilateral innominate subluxates posterior-inferior, the innominate rotating about an axis through the *hip*. The prone short leg with the knees extended crosses over to become the long leg when the knees are flexed
- X-Derifield: with knees flexed to approximately 90°, the patient's head is rotated to one side. If one of the legs shortens, or a previously short leg remains short, the X-Derifield syndrome is present. Turning in the opposite direction may even the legs, in which case the direction of rotation that evens the legs identifies the side of the syndrome, e.g., a "left X-Derifield"
- Posterior ischium: the ischium of the ipsilateral innominate subluxates posteriorly, as seen on an X-ray. The innominate rotates about an axis through the *sacroiliac joint*
- Unilateral cervical syndrome: with knees *extended*, the patient's head is rotated to a given side. If a leg shortens or a previously short leg remains short, the unilateral cervical syndrome is present. Turning in the opposite direction may even the legs, in which case the direction of rotation that evens the legs identifies the side of the syndrome, e.g., "left unilateral cervical syndrome"
- Overcompensated cervical syndrome: this is a condition of spinous process laterality, diminishing from C2 through C7, as seen on X-ray
- Bilateral cervical syndrome: refers to a bilateral occiput fixation. With the patient's knees extended, the head is turned from side to side. In *each* direction, the leg ipsilateral to the side of head rotation shortens
- Reversal syndrome: following correction of either a positive or negative Derifield syndrome, the post-check indicates that the patient has reversed to the other syndrome, presumably as a result of a shift in the interinnominate axis of rotation between the hip and the sacroiliac joint
- Sacral leg check: the prone patient is asked to extend one leg, then the other, off the table. The side of greater limitation (slower ascent,

less elevation, painful or jerky movement) is thought to indicate an anterior-inferior subluxation of the sacral base, with accompanying contralateral deviation of the sacral apex.

PHYSIOLOGICAL MECHANISMS AND RATIONALE

The emphasis is on disturbed proprioceptive input to the cerebellar and cortical areas, which would somehow *inhibit the inhibition* of facilitation influences on the spastic musculature. Neurological imbalance, the result of subluxation, is said to cause overstimulation of the spinal extensor muscles, resulting in a "contracted" leg. The neurology is not spelled out in great detail, but there is a suggestion that subluxation causes nerve impingement, which is manifested by muscle imbalance and finally leg-length inequality. Likewise, reduction of said subluxation would cause neurological balance and symmetry of leg lengths under all conditions.

A rather cursory invocation of "Newton's laws" purports to explains the manner in which the drop table facilitates the following result: "The free drop-through space and sudden concussion at the bottom of the stroke [allows] an element of correction not found in any other table."[7]

Apart from the interpretation of the leg-check results, and invocation of whatever mechanical consequences arise from the use of drop-table technology, the Thompson Technique does not really distinguish itself from other adjustive techniques that seek to identify and correct subluxations and related nerve interference.

DIAGNOSTIC/ANALYTIC PROCEDURES

The Derifield–Thompson leg check is a multistep procedure, that begins with a prone examination for leg-length inequality. In the next step, the doctor flexes the patient's knees to 90° or slightly more, again ascertaining the presence or absence of leg-length inequality in this flexed position. In the third and final step, the doctor returns the legs to the knees-extended position, and then has the patient rotate the head to the left and to the right, while looking for changes in the leg positions. There is another leg-check procedure that would be performed only if legs that were even in the knees-extended position became uneven in the knees-flexed position: the doctor has the patient turn the head left and right in the knees-flexed position, looking for leg-length responsiveness. Although the interpretation of most of these phenomena appears in the terminology section above, the reader should refer to one of the three Thompson technique manuals that we have seen.[1,3,4]

Although the leg check is central, there are several junctures at which the doctor assesses soft-tissue properties. These include the detection of hard and tender nodules, tenderness at specific body locations, and hypertonic musculature. In addition, the doctor assesses bony asymmetry, such as spinous process deviation, lateral curvatures of the spine, and abnormal sagittal curves (especially, thoracic "saucering," or hypokyphosis).

At different points, in various of the writings pertinent to the Thompson technique milieu, there are references to the value of X-ray and thermography, but the Thompson manuals we have seen[1,2] contain no relevant analysis of these diagnostic procedures. Thompson, in a 1992 article (said to be reprinted from his 1983 manual), affirms the importance of thermography in the chiropractic setting.[12] X-rays are "recommended ... are a great help" but do not appear absolutely mandatory.[1] Indeed, he stresses that X-ray cannot distinguish between positive and negative Derifield listings, which remain mechanically distinct and require different types of adjustive strategies.

Zemelka[3] indicates that X-ray is part of a routine examination, but his perfunctory mention makes it appear almost as an afterthought. Like Thompson, he finds that analytic pelvic radiography, unlike the leg-check procedure, cannot distinguish between negative and positive Derifield presentations. Hyman[4] opines that the "most effective chiropractor will employ radiographic studies in the management of the patient," but again, X-ray remains rather peripheral to the Thompson leg-check analysis. Indeed, the listed indications for analytic radiography all

involve situations (some rather extreme) where the leg-check analysis is difficult or impossible: amputation of one or both lower extremities, knee conditions that prevent flexion, cervical conditions that prevent rotation, and an anatomic short leg. The radiographic analysis itself is distinctly Gonstead-like in its character.[4] Hyman reiterates the traditional maxim that "instrumentation" (more precisely, thermography) identifies *nerve interference*, indicating not so much where as *when* to adjust.[4]

TREATMENT/ADJUSTIVE PROCEDURES

This is a drop-table technique, emphasizing high-velocity, low-amplitude adjusting, or thrusting procedures. The drop table serves three primary functions: (1) it reduces wear and tear on the doctor; (2) it enables relatively low-force adjustments to be delivered safely and effectively; and (3) it permits fine-tuning of the forces applied by means of adjusting the tension on the drop pieces. There are specific adjustments for each of the listings listed above. All are performed on a drop table, with both supine and prone versions for the pelvic listings. The cervical moves essentially amount to the Diversified "cervical break," performed prone. There are also moves for occipital subluxation, rotated ribs, the anterior thoracic subluxation,[13,14] and an elevated rib cage. Zemelka's manual[3] describes some "advanced" adjustments that lie outside the Thompsonian core repertoire, for the rotator cuff, the knee, the temporomandibular joint, and more.

OUTCOME ASSESSMENT

Thompson states: "By eliminating spinal subluxations in an organized, orderly fashion, from "top down and inside out," the Thompson practitioner will begin to verify the corrections he is making on the patient's spine."[1] The Thompson Technique assesses its outcomes in the same way that it derives its listings: through the use of the Derifield–Thompson leg check. A normal patient, whether at the intake examination, following a chiropractic treatment, or during an ongoing period of chiropractic care, is found to be subluxation-free when the legs are even in both the knees-flexed and knees-extended positions, and there are no changes when the head is rotated. Although symptom reduction is desired, the criteria for the presence and absence of subluxation take precedence, and are essentially orthopedic in nature; that is, they are based on the leg check.

CONTRAINDICATIONS TO CARE

Zemelka lists some contraindications to using the Derifield–Thompson leg analysis system.[3] These include: aneurysm, osteoporosis, congenital short leg, history of a serious broken leg, prosthesis in the hip or knee, and acetabular degenerative joint disease. Hyman[4] is more specific about which moves are contraindicated in given conditions, e.g., the internal (IN) ilium and anterior thoracic adjustments in severe osteoporosis, the spondylolisthesis move in Grade 3–5 spondylolistheses and aortic aneurysm, and the positive Derifield correction in cases of a lumbar herniated disk. Apart from these and a very few other considerations, there appear to be no published contraindications to drop-table maneuvers that are different from the generally established contraindications to spinal manipulative therapy.

EVIDENCE OF EFFICACY

Many studies on the diagnostic reliability of Thompson-like leg-check procedures have failed to show much interexaminer reliability, especially in the knees-flexed position.[15-22] The study by Rhudy and Burk[22] is especially notable, for the simple reason that Thompson himself and two "experts" (so designated by Thompson) were used as examiners in this reliability study, the results of which were poor. Cooperstein[23] provides a kinesiological interpretation of the Derifield pelvic leg check, but this otherwise interesting work is data-free.[24]

The forces involved in applying a specifically Thompson-like drop-table thrust were measured by Adams and Wood,[25] who found the following: (1) men applied stronger thrusts then women; (2) the doctors could not estimate very well how much force they were generating; and (3) handedness did not seem to be a factor in determining the forces generated. We are aware of no studies of clinical effectiveness, although there are some studies supporting the value of the closely related Pierce–Stillwagon technique (Ch. 23).[26,27] Comprehensive studies by Cooperstein et al and Gatterman et al found virtually no clinical trials using drop-table methods.[28, 29] This did not prevent the expert panel in that study, convened to rate chiropractic treatment procedures for low-back conditions, from giving drop-table procedures a high rating.[30]

In 1990, Hessell et al[31] measured the forces produced by two chiropractors on each of six patients lying prone on a drop-table, intending to thrust upon the PSIS using an adjustive procedure attributed to the Thompson Technique. Each subject received three thrusts from both chiropractors (a total of six), with 2 min between thrusts and 20 min between chiropractors. The investigators measured five parameters: (1) preloading force; (2) peak force; (3) duration of manipulation; (4) impulse of manipulation; and (5) point of application of the peak force. Although all the data were interesting and mostly consistent with the results of previous studies, we would like to draw attention to just one of the experimental findings: "The location of the point of application of the peak force relative to a low back reference system appeared to be very consistent. However, it was not on the posterior superior iliac spines (PSIS) as expected, but always slightly medial to this point."[31] Cooperstein draws out the implications for chiropractic theories pertaining to the notion of specificity in analyzing the patient and in applying adjustive forces.[32]

CONCLUSIONS

- Chiropractors and other allied healthcare professionals who employ leg-checking procedures well understand that the leg that appears to be short is not necessarily short in a structural sense, but may just be "functionally" shortened by postural imbalance. For that reason, the use of the term "contracted leg" is misleading.
- Thompson Technique theorists freely indulge in neurological explanations of the functional short leg, but generally present no data, nor do they cite relevant authorities beyond textbooks.

The neurology is not spelled out in enough detail to criticize, and therefore cannot really be made to explain adequately the rationale for the Thompson analysis.

- The Hessell study,[31] showed that neither of the two chiropractors could successfully land even one of their 12 thrusts on the PSIS of the research subjects, winding up on the sacral base instead. This may turn out to be reflective of a generic problem in adjustive specificity, common to many, if not most, technique procedures. Therefore, we should draw no conclusions from this study that pertain any more to the Thompson Technique than to any other thrusting technique. If these findings are relevant to technique procedures in general, there being little evidence that patients are routinely made worse by such procedures, then further discussion on the importance of segmental specificity is warranted.

- Very little is known on the biomechanics of drop-table adjusting, despite occasional vague references to Newton's laws[33] in some of the writings of Thompson authorities. We really don't know how it affects patients differently compared with non-drop-table methods of intervention. The relatively small distance through which the table drops when actuated, as compared with how far the patient's low back may be moved through space while lying in side-posture, may suggest that drop-table low-back interventions may be relatively safer than side-posture manipulations. However, even if this were true, it would certainly not mean that side-posture manipulations or other adjustive procedures have ever been shown to be unsafe for the great majority of patients.

- Apart from the impact on patients, it seems reasonable to suggest that methods such as these may be kinder and gentler for the doctor's own spine, especially if there has already been an injury, compared with side-posture manipulation techniques.

REFERENCES

1. Thompson C 1984 Thompson technique reference manual. Thompson Educational Workshops, Williams Manufacturing, Elgin, IL
2. Thompson C 1974 Thompson technique reference manual, 1st edn. Thompson Educational Workshops, Williams Manufacturing, Elgin, IL
3. Zemelka W H 1992 The Thompson Technique. Victoria Press, Bettendorf, IA
4. Hyman R C 1991 The Thompson Chiropractic Technique. Publisher unknown
5. Cooperstein R 1995 Technique system overview: Thompson Technique. Chiropractic Technique 7 (2): 60–63
6. Jackson D R 1987 Thompson terminal point technique. Today's Chiropractic 16 (3): 73–75
7. Thompson J C 1977 Thompson Terminal Point Technique. In: Kfoury PW (ed.) Catalog of chiropractic techniques, pp. 89–92. Logan College of Chiropractic, Chesterfield, MO
8. Moulton J P 1985 The terminal point drop principle. American Chiropractor (April): 28–29
9. Noyman B 1996 The Thompson technique: a low-force, high velocity approach. Today's Chiropractic 25 (2): 68–73
10. Wells D 1987 From workbench to high tech: the evolution of the adjustment table. Chiropractic History 7 (2): 35–39
11. Pierce W V, Stillwagon G 1976 Pierce–Stillwagon seminar manual. Self-published, Monongahela, PA

12. Thompson C 1992 Paraspinal thermography. American Chiropractor (July/August): 32
13. Fligg D B 1986 The anterior thoracic adjustment. Journal of the Canadian Chiropractic Association (4): 211–213
14. Zachman Z J, Bolles S, Bergmann T F, Traina A D 1989 Understanding the anterior thoracic adjustment (a concept of a sectional subluxation). Chiropractic Technique 1 (1): 30–33
15. Fuhr A E, Osterbauer P J 1989 Interexaminer reliability of relative leg-length evaluations in the prone, extended position. Chiropractic Technique 1 (1): 13–18
16. Shambaugh P, Scoltani L, Fanselow D 1988 Reliability of the Derifield–Thompson test for leg-length inequality, and use of the test to determine cervical adjusting efficacy. Journal of Manipulative and Physiological Therapeutics 11 (5): 396–399
17. Danelius B D 1987 Letter to the editor: inter- and intra-examiner reliability of leg-length measurement: a preliminary study. Journal of Manipulative and Physiological Therapeutics 10 (3): 132
18. Haas M, Peterson D 1989 Interexaminer reliability of relative leg-length evaluations in the prone, extended position [letter, comment]. Chiropractic Technique 1 (4): 150–151
19. DeBoer K F, Harmon R O, Savoie S, Tuttle C D 1983 Inter- and intra-examiner reliability of the leg-length differential measurement: a preliminary study. Journal of Manipulative and Physiological Therapeutics 10 (3): 61–66

20. DeBoer F F 1987 In reply: inter- and intra-examiner reliability of leg-length measurement: a preliminary study. Journal of Manipulative and Physiological Therapeutics 10 (3): 133

21. Falltrick D R, Pierson D S 1989 Precise measurement of functional leg length inequality and changes due to cervical spine rotation in pain-free subjects. Journal of Manipulative and Physiological Therapeutics 12 (5): 369–373

22. Rhudy T R, Burk J M 1990 Inter-examiner reliability of functional leg-length assessment. American Journal of Chiropractic Medicine 3 (2): 63–66

23. Cooperstein R 1990 Innominate vertical length differentials as a function of pelvic torsion and pelvic carrying angle. In: Proceedings of the 5th Annual Conference on Research and Education, pp. 1–14. Consortium for Chiropractic Research, Sacramento, CA

24. Hestbaek L, Leboeuf-Yde C 2000 Are chiropractic tests for the lumbo-pelvic spine reliable and valid? A systematic critical literature review. Journal of Manipulative and Physiological Therapeutics 23 (4): 258–275

25. Adams A A, Wood J 1984 Forces used in selected chiropractic adjustments of the low back: a preliminary study. Research Forum 1 (1): 5–9

26. Stump J L 1979 Efficacy of the Pierce-Stillwagon chiropractic technique in clinical application of the sacroiliac syndrome. ICA International Review of Chiropractic 33: 42–44

27. Kesten B S 1991 Multiple case study of five patients with pelvic unleveling. Chiropractic Research Journal 2 (1): 51–56

28. Cooperstein R, Perle S M, Gatterman M I et al 2001 Chiropractic technique procedures for specific low back conditions: characterizing the literature. Journal of Manipulative and Physiological Therapeutics 24 (6): 407–424

29. Gatterman M I, Cooperstein R, Lantz C et al 2001 Rating specific chiropractic technique procedures for common low back conditions. Journal of Manipulative and Physiological Therapeutics 24 (7): 449–456

30. Gatterman M I 2002 Rating specific chiropractic technique procedures for common low back conditions [reply]. Journal of Manipulative and Physiological Therapeutics 25 (3): 198

31. Hessell B W, Herzog W, Conway P J, McEwen M C 1990 Experimental measurement of the force exerted during spinal manipulation using the Thompson technique. Journal of Manipulative and Physiological Therapeutics 13 (8): 448–453

32. Cooperstein R 1999 Specificity failure and petrified thought. Dynamic Chiropractic 17 (13): 20–21, 50–51

33. Kontz H 1991 Thompson Technique (manual long and short lever mechanically assisted procedure). In: Hansen D (ed.) 6th Annual Conference on Research and Education: emphasis on consensus, pp. 65–69. CCR, Monterey, CA

30

Toftness Technique

INTRODUCTION

Given the widely perceived importance of identifying the chiropractic subluxation, and the unsatisfactory nature of purely subjective examination methods that purport to do so, it is not surprising that in different times and places chiropractors designed and implemented technologies intended to identify vertebral subluxations. X-ray worked well enough for many chiropractors, but IN Toftness, who saw subluxation more as spinal stress than mere misalignment, went on to develop a particularly unique *subluxometer*: the Toftness Radiation Detector (TRD) (Box 30.1). It is this device that specifically lends Toftness Technique its unique character, rather than anything having to do with its treatment procedures.

The innards of the TRD do not concern us much, since that is less important than the use to which Toftness put the instrument. We have no problem seeing it as a mysterious black box,

---

Box 30.1 Abstract of patent for the Toftness Radiation Detector

A housing embodying a lens system, the lenses of said system being comprised of components providing a clear window for a radiation on the order of 69.5 gHz, the lower of said lenses having a greater lens area and a greater focal length than the upper of said lenses to collect a wide spherical angle of said radiation to focus the same upon a detection plate carried by said housing for sensory detection of said radiation, and means carried by said housing for adjustably positioning said detection plate to focus said radiation thereon. (From original patent application #3626930, published 12/14/71)

---

the clinical utility of which is unknown, but not different in that regard from subluxation detectors that are better understood and widely accepted. The TRD uses a unique tube-shaped instrument with a series of lenses that help detect the area of subluxation and neurological disturbances. This instrument is said to detect minute radiation and electromagnetic disturbances that exist with spinal subluxations. The technique uses a light non-force adjustment, similar to that used in Logan Basic Technique (Ch. 21), in conjunction with this instrument to make all corrections.

OVERVIEW

The Toftness Technique system aims to correct spinal subluxations, as identified by a device that putatively detects a certain electromagnetic radiation frequency said to be characteristic of subluxated spines. Toftness credits himself with the discovery that "abnormal" radiation is created by stress in the spine, and that it can be detected by mechanical/electronic means.[1] He further discovered that low-force adjustments can correct subluxations. The unique aspects of Toftness Technique center on the invention and marketing of the aforementioned radiation detection device, which is used to detect subluxations and indicate the outcome of spinal adjustments.

HISTORY

After a successful chiropractic treatment for a "lazy eye" at the age of 12, IN Toftness, 1909–1990, entered the Palmer College in 1928, where he studied under BJ Palmer. He entered into practice in

Cumberland, Wisconsin, in 1932, where he was arrested in 1935 for practicing chiropractic without a license (it was difficult to become licensed in that state at that time). The jury found him not guilty. Although at first Toftness was a Hole-In-One (HIO) Upper Cervical technique practitioner (Ch. 32), by the late 1930s he had become heavily influenced by Hugh Logan's emphasis on the sacrum, and the technique that devolved from that (Ch. 21). He changed his whole practice to Logan Basic at that time.[1]

Noting that some patients responded better to the HIO of Palmer, whereas others responded better to the sacral technique of Logan, Toftness eventually came to the conclusion that more information was required to predict what would result in the best outcome. That insight led to his own Toftness system of chiropractic.[1] He claimed: "a resistance was encountered whenever my hands passed over areas of the spinal column that were problem areas."[2] Reasoning that a detection instrument could improve upon his bare hands in palpating for this phenomenon, Toftness invented what came to be called the Toftness Radiation Detector (TRD), and patented it in 1971. However, in 1984, after winning a lengthy court battle initiated by the Food and Drug Administration (FDA), the Justice Department ordered chiropractors who still possessed a Toftness device to return it. IN Toftness' son, David Toftness, following graduation from the Logan College, joined up with his father in developing the Toftness system, and took over the Foundation for the Advancement of Chiropractic Research (the Toftness Technique research arm) upon the death of IN Toftness in 1990.

DEFINITION OF TECHNIQUE-SPECIFIC TERMS

- Toftness Radiation Detector (TRD, Sensometer,[3] or Toftness Electromagnetic Radiation Receiver): a tube containing a series of lenses that serve to focus the radiation emitted by the body on a diaphragm that distorts in the presence of said radiation[4]
- Aberrant nerve impulses: also known as nerve stress, meaning essentially nerve interference.[4]

PHYSIOLOGICAL MECHANISMS AND RATIONALE

Toftness believed that the ends of the spine – the upper four cervical vertebrae and the sacral area – were of primary significance, leaning on the work of Palmer and Logan,[2] respectively.

Jenness and Toftness originally theorized that microwave radiation is abnormally emitted from the body due to sensory overload of the brain.[4] They further speculated that emission of radiation from the body is the result of aberrant nerve impulses called "nerve stress".[4] Other authors working with the Toftness system have suggested that segmental spinal joint dysfunction, rather than brain overload, causes the putative microwave emission.[5,6]

Any form of stress on the body – physical trauma, emotional trauma, sudden temperature changes – causes an "uncontrolled" volley of nerve impulses to be transmitted to the brain. This results in a sensory overload shock to the brain, which is theorized to be the primary causal factor in many disease processes.[4,7] The Toftness adjustment is able to "clear" this sensory overload by sending a "controlled" volley of nerve impulses to the brain, thereby enabling the brain to restore health to the body.[4]

Gemmell has suggested that the mechanism of action of the Toftness adjustment is related to a stimulation of muscle spindle receptors, which affects gamma and alpha motor neurons, ultimately leading to relaxation of hypertonic muscles and improved joint function.[8,9] It is also stated that the adjustment may relax ligaments (such as the sacrotuberous) directly.[10]

There have been basic science discoveries put forth in the biomedical literature regarding the presence of electromagnetic fields in the human body. Some authors point to such discoveries as evidence supporting the Toftness theory.[11]

DIAGNOSTIC/ANALYTIC PROCEDURES

The TRD is the primary diagnostic tool. Although a patent was originally obtained in 1971, the device was once banned from healthcare use by the FDA (Box 30.2).[12] The device is essentially a tube containing a series of lenses that serve to focus the radiation emitted by the body on a diaphragm that distorts in the presence of said radiation.[4] As the examiner moves the device over the exposed spine of a prone patient, the distortion of the diaphragm may be palpated by the examiner's fingers, indicating that the corresponding level is subluxated. A confirmatory measure for the examiner is to challenge the vertebra in question with digital pressure on the spinous process. When such a challenge decreases the perceived distortion, it is thought to be reducing the subluxation, and thus indicates the level and direction for adjustment.[5, 13]

A further description of the device is provided by Schimp and Schimp,[14] who describe the Toftness Sensometer as "a cone shaped instrument with a thin diaphragm," that can be distorted by microwave radiation to the point that a clinician can feel this distortion by drawing his or her fingers across the diaphragm.[6] The instrument supposedly provides information on the "specific line of drive, depth, and duration of treatment as assessed by decreasing levels of diaphragm distortion."[14]

Toftness practitioners also take X-rays, and believe the lateral view is the most important view to obtain, since there are supposedly five times as many subluxations identified on lateral as compared with anterior-posterior views.[2]

A caliper is used to measure the length of the spine on X-rays.[2]

TREATMENT/ADJUSTIVE PROCEDURES

Treatment consists of adjustments using light force (2–32 oz: 56–896 g), delivered by a spring-loaded stylus instrument. The pressure is sustained for a specific period of time, ranging from 10 s to 10 min.[5, 15] Toftness believed that a light force held for a long time achieved an outcome similar to a larger force applied for a smaller amount of time.[2]

OUTCOME ASSESSMENT

As with many other chiropractic techniques, Toftness practitioners expect there to be a reduction in patient symptoms. Beyond that, they expect reduction in subluxation, as evidenced by elimination of radiation findings via the TRD. Toftness practitioners also claim that their methods bring about before-and-after X-ray changes,[2] and several are published on the worldwide web.[1] The claim is made that many such X-rays are published in a book[16] that we have not seen.

SAFETY AND RISK FACTORS

The TRD is essentially an inert device,[4] and as such poses no known risk to patients. Toftness adjustments, due to their low-force nature, could be considered safer than thrusting adjustments,[9] although the latter are not shown to be unsafe.

EVIDENCE OF EFFICACY

There are several studies on the reliability and validity of the Toftness instrument, and also on the clinical value of the care itself. One study found 43% interexaminer agreement in detecting regions (cervical, thoracic, or lumbar) of highest spinal stress using the TRD.[10] Other studies have been somewhat less satisfactory. Two examiners seeking an upper cervical subluxation with the TRD yielded a kappa of 0.30 (fair) for interexaminer reliability,[17] insufficient for confidence in using it for clinical practice. Poor to fair inter- and intraexaminer reliability was found for the TRD in detecting spinal joint dysfunction in subjects with low-back pain.[18] The authors suggested that determining joint dysfunction in low-back pain patients by chance may be more reliable than by using the TRD.

Gemmell found moderate interexaminer reliability (kappa = 0.52) for determining the presence of a sacral reading, but poor reliability (kappa = 0.06) for determining side of lesion.[19] He stated that the lack of reliability shown in this and other studies suggests that the TRD instrument lacks validity. More recently, Gemmell and Jacobson found no significant difference between palpation for tenderness and TRD in determining subluxation level.[6] They also found no significant correlation between acute spinal pain intensity and amount of sustained pressure needed to perform a Toftness adjustment,[5] although Gemmell also found that sacroiliac hypomobility as measured by joint palpation was decreased after Toftness adjustments.[10]

Among the other treatment studies, Jenness and Toftness[4] reported a decrease in frontalis muscle activity greater in treated patients than sham-treated controls. Although the patients were blinded, the outcome assessment was not. A non-blinded, non-randomized subgroup of patients demonstrated decreases in the frequency and intensity of headache, neck pain/stiffness, shoulder pain, mid dorsal pain, and low-back pain.

Gemmell,[20] using a time-series design, described three patients with low-back pain who improved with Toftness care. Hawkinson et al[13] randomized 14 subjects with acute musculoskeletal pain into Toftness and sham-treated groups. After 12 days or 10 adjustments, there was a statistically significant positive change with the Toftness group, and a non-significant change in the sham group, as measured by the visual analog scale. Both the patients and the outcome assessors were blinded, although the doctors delivering the treatment were not blinded.

Gemmell et al[21] tested the effect of a Toftness sacral adjustment on palpatory fixation findings. Twenty patients with sacroiliac joint fixations were randomized to a Toftness or a sham group. Patients and outcome assessments were blinded as to group assignment. There was no difference between the treatments upon post-treatment assessment of sacroiliac joint fixation. The author mentioned the possibility of a type II (false-negative) statistical error. It should be noted that Hawkinson and Snyder expressed concerns about this study, as to (1) whether a true Toftness adjustment was used as compared with a version of a Logan Basic adjustment; (2) whether a reasonable protocol had been used; and (3) whether the outcome measure had been appropriate.[22] Gemmell's response indicated that he stood by his work as published.[8]

Gemmell described a case report of a migraine patient who failed to improve with prior trials of Activator and Diversified adjustments, but improved with Toftness adjustments.[9] Studying three different groups, Snyder and Sanders found improvement in chronic back pain subjects and in chronic tension headache subjects, but not in primary dysmenorrhea subjects.[23] Snyder et al enrolled 14 subjects into a study on the effectiveness of the Toftness system for the treatment of mechanical low-back pain.[24] The mean pain scores and the Oswestry scores for 9 experimental subjects were significantly improved compared with the scores of 5 subjects who received sham adjustments.

Schimp and Schimp successfully treated a 7-year-old boy suffering from post-traumatic hemiparesis, who did not have any pathology seen on computed tomography scan, with low-force (Toftness-style) adjustments to the atlanto-occipital joint.[14] They diagnosed the problem and monitored the outcome of care using a TRD. There is a testimonial from a satisfied Toftness patient who had been under care for some 50 years.[25]

Snyder[3] divided 20 subjects with low-back pain into two groups. All the subjects received a real Toftness adjustment, but 10 were adjusted at locations identified as appropriate by the Sensometer, whereas the other 10 were adjusted in different places. Thermographic instrumentation showed that 80% of the "correctly" adjusted subjects had a significant before-and-after difference in their thermographic findings, whereas none of the 10 "incorrectly" adjusted subjects experienced such a change. Zhang and Snyder[26] were able to demonstrate that Toftness adjustments produced a measurable reduction in the electromagnetic radiation from the bodies of an adjusted group but not in a control group. Troyanovich[27] thought there should have been a clinical side to the study, but the investigators did not accept his criticism.

CONCLUSIONS

- Hugh A Gemmell, the Toftness Technique's most prolific researcher, states that "[the] studies suggest that the instrument lacks adequate reliability as a clinical tool for the determination of putative subluxations."[19] On the other hand, although the device and its use are, to say the least, unusual, there are at least some studies showing some possible degree of reliability, if not concordance with other examination findings.
- A further point of contention is the validity of the TRD. There is little evidence that the device can detect microwave radiation of any source, let alone that purports to be emitted from a region of joint dysfunction. It seems that one of the most basic requirements for Toftness practitioners is to demonstrate that the device measures up against a gold standard for microwave detection. On the other hand, it is interesting to note that thermographic findings changed in a group receiving the "right" adjustment compared with the "wrong" one,[3] in an interesting study design in which the examination procedure was in effect the target of inquiry. Nevertheless, we must be cautious about overinterpreting this study, since the thermographic findings were of unknown accuracy or clinical relevance.
- Gemmell states that the Toftness system should be considered investigational rather than a valid chiropractic technique.[9] However, when stripped of the TRD, Toftness is essentially a system of low-force, sustained-pressure treatments, not entirely unlike Logan Basic Technique.[28] Minus the part about the alleged radiation emissions, these treatments may be compared to acupressure, ischemic compression, or other low-force chiropractic techniques.

ACKNOWLEDGMENT

Dr. Anthony Lisi coauthored an early version of this chapter.

REFERENCES

1. Toftness D I N Toftness. http://www.airstreamcomm.net/~toftness/page3.html
2. Toftness I N 1977 The Toftness system of chiropractic. In: Kfoury P W (ed.) Catalog of chiropractic techniques, pp. 93–97. Logan College of Chiropractic, Chesterfield, MI
3. Snyder B J 1999 Thermographic evaluation for the role of the Sensometer: evidence in the Toftness System of chiropractic adjusting. Chiropractic Technique 11 (2): 57–61
4. Jenness M E, Toftness I 1981 Validation of the Toftness/Jenness system of chiropractic. Digest of Chiropractic Economics (Sept/Oct): 22–26, 126–129
5. Gemmell H A, Jacobson B H 1993 Association between level of acute spine pain and level of sustained pressure used in the Toftness adjustment. Chiropractic Technique 5 (4): 150–151
6. Gemmell H, Jacobson B 1998 Comparison of two adjustive indicators in patients with acute low back pain. Chiropractic Technique 10 (1): 8–10
7. Toftness I N 1977 A look at chiropractic spinal correction. I N Toftness, Cumberland, WI
8. Gemmell H 1990 Effectiveness of Toftness sacral apex technic (letter). American Journal of Chiropractic Medicine 3 (3): 133–134
9. Gemmell H, Jacobson B, Sutton L 1994 Toftness spinal correction in the treatment of migraine: a case study. Chiropractic Technique 6 (2): 57–60
10. Gemmell H, Heng B 1987 Correction of sacroiliac fixation by a low force sustained pressure method. American Chiropractor (Nov): 28–32
11. Bell F B, Foster M D 1988 The energy within. American Chiropractor (March): 58, 64–66
12. Oregon Board of Chiropractic Examiners (OBCE) OBCE's guide to policy and practice questions. http://www.obce.state.or.us/pdfs/pp-section1.pdf
13. Hawkinson E J, Snyder B J, Sanders G E 1992 Evaluation of the Toftness system of chiropractic adjusting for the relief of acute pain of musculoskeletal origin. Chiropractic Technique 4 (2): 57–60
14. Schimp J A, Schimp D J 1992 The neuropathophysiology of traumatic hemiparesis and its association with dysfunctional upper cervical motion units: a case report. Chiropractic Technique 4 (3): 104–107

15. Toftness I N 1987 The phenomenon of neurological analysis. Today's Chiropractic (Nov/Dec): 77–78
16. Toftness I N 1977 A look at chiropractic spinal correction. Self-published, Cumberland, WI
17. Gemmell H A, Heng B J, Jacobson B H 1990 Interexaminer reliability of the Toftness Radiation Detector for determining the presence of upper cervical subluxation. Chiropractic Technique 2 (1): 10–12
18. Gemmell H, Jacobson B, Edwards S, Heng B 1990 Interexaminer reliability of the electromagnetic radiation receiver for determining lumbar spinal joint dysfunction in subjects with low back pain. Journal of Manipulative and Physiological Therapeutics 13 (3): 134–137
19. Gemmell H A 1994 Interexaminer reliability of the Toftness instrument for determining need and side of sacral adjustment. Chiropractic Technique 6 (1): 16–18
20. Gemmell H A 1992 Treatment of chronic low-back pain with low force manipulation. Chiropractic Journal of Australia 22 (2): 54–59
21. Gemmell H A, Jacobson B H, Heng B J 1990 Effectiveness of Toftness sacral apex adjustment in correcting fixation of the sacroiliac joint: preliminary report. American Journal of Chiropractic Medicine 3 (1): 5–8
22. Hawkinson E, Snyder B 1990 Effectiveness of Toftness sacral apex technic [letter]. American Journal of Chiropractic Medicine 3 (3): 133–134
23. Snyder B, Sanders G 1996 Evaluation of the Toftness system of chiropractic adjusting for subjects with chronic back pain, chronic tension headaches, or primary dysmenorrhea. Chiropractic Technique 8 (1): 3–9
24. Snyder B, Hawkinson E, Sanders G 1993 Effectiveness of the Toftness system of chiropractic adjusting for the treatment of subjects with chronic pain of musculoskeletal origin. In: Seater S R (ed.) Proceedings of the International Conference on Spinal Manipulation, p. 88. FCER, Arlington, VA
25. DeLane M H L 1989 A patient speaks out: in praise of Dr. Toftness. Today's Chiropractic 18 (5): 32
26. Zhang J, Snyder B 2001 The effect of chiropractic adjustment on body surface electromagnetic field. Journal of Chiropractic Education 15 (1): 42–43
27. Troyanovich S J 1999 Thermographic evaluation for the role of the Sensometer: evidence in the Toftness system of chiropractic adjusting [comment]. Chiropractic Technique 11 (4): 186
28. Logan H B 1950 Textbook of Logan Basic Methods. Logan Chiropractic College, Chesterfield, MI

31

Torque Release Technique (TRT™)

INTRODUCTION

Christopher Kent wrote[1] that Cooperstein had "described two broad approaches to chiropractic technique, the segmental approach and the postural approach", citing Cooperstein.[2] Then, citing D Murphy, he adds a third, the tonal approach:

In 1910, DD Palmer wrote, "Life is an expression of tone. Tone is the normal degree of nerve tension. Tone is expressed in function by normal elasticity, strength, and excitability ... the cause of disease is any variation in tone." Tonal approaches tend to view the spine and nervous system as a functional unit. Tonal approaches emphasize the importance of functional outcomes, and acknowledge that clinical objectives may be achieved using a variety of adjusting methods. Examples of tonal approaches include Network Spinal Analysis and Torque-release Technique.

TRT™ claims direct lineage from DD Palmer, whose 1910 work[3] contains the quotation above, providing animus to Kent's classification of TRT™ as a tonal approach to chiropractic. As we see it, this concept is captured in the term "Cranial-Spinal Meningeal Unit (C-SMFU)," a form of which also occurs in Network Spinal Analysis as the SMFU (spinal meningeal functional unit) (Ch. 22).

OVERVIEW

TRT™ was first presented by Holder at Life College's 20th anniversary homecoming in 1994. It is described by the developers Jay Holder and Marvin A Talsky as a vitalistic, tonal-based, non-linear and non-mechanistic approach to health care.[4-6] They state that both TRT™ and the Integrator™ adjusting device were born out of a research study ("the largest in the history of chiropractic") monitoring the effects of this technique on patients with drug addictions.[4] TRT™ incorporates elements from several other technique systems, all the subject of other chapters in this book, including Hole-In-One (HIO) Upper Cervical, Directional Non-Force Technique, Sacro-Occipital Technique, Toftness, Thompson, Gonstead, Logan, Pierce–Stillwagon, and Network.[4-6]

HISTORY

According to a brochure published by the Holder Research Institute,[7] "At the age of 14 Dr. Holder began his experience in research in neurotoxins at the University of Miami School of Medicine." He obtained his degree in chiropractic from National College, and at some point began his work with Marvin A Talsky, a 1963 Palmer College graduate[5] and cofounder of TRT™.[8]

According to Holder, during his presentation at Life College, faculty member Lasca Hospers questioned the concepts of TRT™ and thought that the brain reward cycle model would not hold up under intense scrutiny.[4] She challenged Holder to allow her to perform an electroencephalogram (EEG) reading of a person in attendance who suffered from attention-deficit hyperactivity disorder (ADHD).[4] According to the anecdote, the patient's abnormal "prefrontal EEG spiking" was gone after he was adjusted with the Integrator™,[4] apparently normalizing the EEG readings and demonstrating the clinical efficacy of the technique.

DEFINITIONS OF TECHNIQUE-SPECIFIC TERMS

- Abductor technology/adductor resistance: an examination procedure that determines the tendency of one or both legs of a prone patient to remain in abduction, and resist being adducted when moved into that direction by the examiner. Thought to be indicative of a C2 subluxation, usually on the side of greater resistance[6]
- Brain reward cascade: mechanism by which the TRT[TM] is thought to operate. A 1997 advertising brochure[7] describes the cascade as: "a scientific model that provides an understanding of the neurophysiological mechanisms of how the meso-limbic system expresses a state of well-being. The vertebral motor unit and the dorsal horn are the common denominators." The absence of a properly maintained brain reward cascade cycle is said to result in a deficiency in the state of well-being[6]
- Cranial-Spinal Meningeal Functional Unit (C-SMFU): the composite of the brain, spinal cord, meningeal layers, bones of the cranium, vertebral column, and pelvis, thought to function as an integral unit[5]
- Foot flare: foot inversion/eversion [sic], thought to be indicative of torsion of the spinal cord and meninges.[6] [We note that, although foot flare herein seems synonymous with internal/external foot rotation, that is not what is usually meant by the terms inversion/eversion]
- Integrator[TM]: a handheld device that can be used to perform adjustments. It is self-releasing (producing a recoiling effect) and can produce clockwise or counterclockwise torque and recoil[5,9]
- Non-linear: a principle of TRT[TM] that informs practitioners that they should not adjust the same vertebral segments in or with the same vector, in the same order, in any three visits in a row[9]
- Non-mechanistic: proponents of TRT[TM] state that their technique operates in the realm of quantum mechanics, non-mechanistically, unlike other chiropractic techniques such as Diversified, Gonstead, or Thompson that utilize the principles of Newtonian mechanics of force, momentum, acceleration, and mass

- Reward deficiency syndrome: a lack of state of well-being, resulting from disruption in the brain reward cascade cycle
- Subluxation: considered in TRT[TM] to be "separation from wholeness," but also (more conventionally) "a condition of one or more spinal segments that have lost their ability to move freely or completely throughout their range of motion that physically interfere with the spinal cord and/or spinal nerves and their function"[6] (p. 13)
- Torque: distortion of the neuraxis, as well as the torque component of the adjustment used to correct spinal subluxation.[5,6]

PHYSIOLOGICAL MECHANISMS AND RATIONALE

"Chiropractic being a deductive philosophy," says Holder, "[it] has a fundamental premise called 'the major premise' which states: 'there is a universal intelligence which is constantly giving matter it's [sic] qualities and characteristics, thus maintaining all matter in existence.'"[9] He continues: "[the] basis of chiropractic and it's [sic] practice are not primarily Newtonian physics and mechanics, nor energy work, it is the communication of intelligence through touch. Intelligence gives direction to energy and organization to matter."[9]

The brain reward cascade cycle is said to explain the neurophysiological difference between a state of subluxation and a state of well-being that may be achieved with TRT[TM].[4–6] According to Holder, this model stemmed from early research conducted at the Holder Research Institute in 1994 that found that only vertebrates have an opiate receptor site brain reward system.[4] According to TRT[TM] practitioners, an interruption of the precise sequence of chemical changes, resulting in what is termed a "reward deficiency syndrome," will prompt an individual to seek mood-altering substances or activities.[9] According to this line of thought, neurotransmitters must be released in the proper sequence in order for a person to "feel good." The neurochemical dopamine is accorded particular importance in this model. The subluxation, or misalignment of the back, impacts on this process because "emotions and feelings are felt not just in your head, but in your spine as well,"[9] presumably via the nervous system. The mechanism at work here, according to this line of thought, is that spinal misalignments can interfere with the proper operation of the limbic system and the flow of reward chemicals in the brain. The chiropractic adjustment "gets the dopamine flowing again, balancing the brain reward cycle."[9]

In addition to the involvement of neurochemicals, the adjustment is thought to remove nerve interference, allowing innate intelligence to adjust the body by "giving it permission and time to process."[6] There is also reference to the importance of touch between the practitioner's intelligence and the patient's innate intelligence, using the nervous system as a transmission medium.[6]

ANALYTIC PROCEDURES

Several examination procedure tests are used, most finding their roots within the parent tonal-based techniques that led to TRT™. Holder states that TRT™ is not simply another leg-check system, but rather a method to determine which specific vertebral segment is subluxated. There are 14 examination procedures that can be used to detect spinal subluxation, or disease.[6] Examination procedures include: palpation, functional leg-length assessment (a modified Derifield check), the determination of abductor tendency/adductor resistance, foot flare, heel tension, abnormal breathing patterns, "congestive tissue tone," postural analysis, cervical syndrome (Derifield cervical check), bilateral cervical syndrome, Derifield leg checking, and using various devices to detect abnormal head and energy radiations from the body (including thermography, the neurocalometer, and the Insight 7000 Subluxation Station). Despite the claimed link to HIO Upper Cervical technique, an X-ray-intensive system, we are aware of no discussion of the clinical utility of X-ray in TRT™.

ADJUSTIVE PROCEDURES

TRT™ practitioners have developed several rules that they believe should be applied during a clinical intervention. As an example, since TRT™ is said to be non-linear, a practitioner should "never adjust the same segment in or with the same vector in the same order, any three visits in a row."[6] Likewise, non-linear timing implies that, at any moment, there is only one most appropriate subluxation to adjust. The doctor's task is to find the appropriate "window," which seems to refer to the practitioner's ability to determine which segment should be adjusted in order to gain optimal access to the patient's nervous system at that particular time.

TRT™ practitioners state that only one, two, or three – but never more than three – segments be adjusted each visit, and never more than three contacts per segment.[6] (p. 1) The concept of "nonlinear testing priorities" is the practice of checking segments in a specified sequence. This starts with the lateral sacrum-coccyx or a cranial segment, especially the occiput or sphenoid. In fact, the TRT™ system considers the sphenoid as a "very upper" cervical segment. Following this pairing, the clinician would then adjust atlas or C5, then the anterior sacral base or pelvis, including the pubes. The next level to adjust would be axis or C3, then C7, L3 spinous, L5 spinous, double upper and lower contacts, and lastly any other segment requiring correction.[5,6]

Preferring to avoid high-velocity, low-amplitude thrusting procedures, especially those with a rotary character, such as master cervicals or lumbar rolls, TRT™ practitioners advocate low- or minimal-force techniques.[5,6] The preferred method of intervention is through the use of the Integrator adjusting instrument. According to its proponents, years of development, testing, and design resulted in the production of the Integrator™ (also referred to as the Torque Adjustor™), a device said to be capable of producing an adjustment in as little as 1/10 000th of a second.[6,9] In the literature, it is stated that the Integrator™ is trademarked, and Food and Drug Administration (FDA) approved. (See remarks in Ch. 38 on the significance of the term "FDA approval".)

Holder suggests that one need not use an Integrator™ for adjustive corrections, although it is placed at the top of the preferred adjustive method hierarchy. Nadler et al[5] suggest that a practitioner is free to integrate any adjustive technique he or she may want to use into the TRT™ protocol of care. In descending order after the Integrator™, a practitioner can use sustained contacts with "positional ease," padded wedges, a toggle-recoil manual thrust, a drop-table adjustment, another adjusting instrument, and, lastly, non-rotary cervical breaks or thumb moves.[5,6]

At some point the use of auriculotherapy (the use of acupuncture on ear meridians) was incorporated into TRT™ protocols. This form of therapy now appears to be at the forefront of TRT™, and seminars are offered throughout Canada and the USA on the use of TRT for treating addiction.

OUTCOME ASSESSMENTS

The lack of specific findings on examination following treatment with TRT™ appears to indicate that the patient is not subluxated and is therefore in a state of "ease" and well-being. With the exception of addiction, symptom resolution is not mentioned as an important outcome measure, although it is suggested that subluxation of the coccyx may be related to a long list of clinical conditions, including migraine headaches, dysmenorrhea, compulsive disorder, Tourette's syndrome, impotence, infertility, dyslexia, vertigo, epilepsy and ADHD.[6]

CONTRAINDICATIONS TO CARE

Since it appears to be a relatively low-force technique, TRT™, like other low-force techniques, might be considered a relatively safe technique. We have not noted any listed contraindications to TRT™ in the articles we consulted.

EVIDENCE OF EFFICACY

According to Holder, the original randomized, placebo-controlled, and blinded study using TRT™ on patients with drug addictions was supported in part by a grant from the Florida Chiropractic Society. He states it was designed by the University of Miami School of Medicine and the Holder Research Institute.[4-6,9] Patients receiving chiropractic care purportedly experienced a 100% retention rate within the 30-day residential model, as well as statistically significant improvements in anxiety, depression, and need for nursing station visits.[6,10]

A similar study reported on the retention rates among chemically dependent individuals in a residential setting using auriculotherapy and the TRT™ system.[11] The study had two arms: (1) it monitored the progress of a group of patients receiving either auriculotherapy or a capsule placebo; and (2) it monitored the progress of a group of patients receiving TRT™ using an Integrator™ ($n = 35$), placebo TRT™ using an Integrator™ set to zero force ($n = 32$), or usual care (no Integrator™). The researchers reported that upon completion of a 10-day trial period, all patients receiving auriculotherapy without concurrent medications were more likely to complete the 30-day residential program than were the patients in the placebo group. Similarly, Holder et al reported that all patients in the Integrator™ group (active treatment) completed the 28-day program, compared to only 75% of the placebo group and 56% in the usual care group. It was also reported that patients in the active treatment group scored better on anxiety scales than did patients in the placebo groups, and active treatment patients tended to visit the nurse less often than either the placebo group or usual care group.[11] The inference drawn was that the completion of the 28-day program would be associated with better rates of addiction recovery.

CONCLUSIONS

- TRT™ is said to be a tonal-based chiropractic technique system, developed out of research on patients with addictions. TRT™ combines traditional theories that date back to the Palmers with modernist concepts such as quantum mechanics: "Utilizing The Integrator™, a torque and recoil release adjusting instrument combines the best of existing chiropractic techniques and principles, quantum physics and the body/mind connection."[4] Reference is often made to the field of quantum mechanics, but the exact manner in which it is applied to this technique is not clear. We have also seen quantum mechanics invoked by Network (Ch. 22).

- The TRT™ system can be easily integrated into many current private practices in that it strives to use as many examination procedures as possible, while avoiding the dogmatic insistence that a practitioner should use its preferred method of adjustive correction, the Integrator™ adjusting instrument. Instead, TRT™ emphasizes the importance of its model rather than its adjustive methods.

- TRT™ developers seem to go to great lengths in order to appeal to as wide an audience as possible, particularly among very traditional chiropractors.
- While the results gathered from the study on patients with addictions are interesting and encouraging, in the authors' view it is regrettable that these studies were not published in the much more widely disseminated peer-reviewed chiropractic or medical literature. We have not seen enough evidence to conclude that TRT™ does or does not occupy a unique position, among chiropractic adjustive techniques, in the treatment of addiction.

REFERENCES

1. Kent C 1996 Vertebral subluxation: a review. Journal of Vertebral Subluxation Research 1 (1) (no page numbers available, online pdf file reprint)
2. Cooperstein R 1995 Contemporary approach to understanding chiropractic technique. In: Lawrence D (ed.) Advances in chiropractic, vol. 2, pp. 437–459, Mosby Year Book, Chicago, IL
3. Palmer D D 1910 The chiropractor's adjuster, the science, art and philosophy of chiropractic, p. 7. Portland Printing House, Portland, Oregon
4. Holder J M 1995 Torque Release Technique™: a subluxation-based system for a new scientific model. Today's Chiropractic (Mar/Apr) 62–66
5. Nadler A, Holder J M, Talsky M A 1998 Torque Release Technique™ (TRT): a technique model for chiropractic's second century. Canadian Chiropractor: Focus on Technique 3 (1): 30–37
6. The Holder Research Institute 1998 The Torque Release Technique™: special illustrated review section. Holder Research Institute, Miami, FL
7. The Torque Release Technique™ 1997 Advertising brochure. Self-published
8. Holder J M 1966 New technique introduced ... EEG confirms results. International Chiropractors Association of California Journal (May): 10
9. www.TorqueReleaseTechnique™.com (accessed 8 July 2003)
10. Blum K, Braverman E R, Holder J M et al 2000 Reward deficiency syndrome (RDS): a biogenic model for the diagnosis and treatment of impulsive, addictive, and compulsive behaviors. Journal of Psychoactive Drugs 32 (suppl)
11. Holder J M, Duncan R C, Gissen M et al 2001 Increasing retention rates among the chemically dependent in residential treatment: auriculotherapy and subluxation-based chiropractic care. Molecular Psychiatry 6 (suppl. 1): 88

32

Upper Cervical Technique (UCT)

INTRODUCTION

The American Chiropractic Association Council on Technique conducted several multitechnique symposia in the mid-1990s. Well-known figures representing several of the technique systems were asked to describe how each in turn would address various patient presentations, while the moderators and observers tried to incite the technique spokespeople to butt heads over adjustive strategies. Cooperstein recalls being present at one of these in which the late John D Grostic, Upper Cervical practitioner and educator, described the UCT approach to a low-back case being presented. He said he would provide upper cervical care. This was not shocking. Someone then asked him what he would do if the case failed to resolve with UCT care alone, whereupon he responded: "Then I would refer the patient to a full-spine chiropractor who would specifically address the low back."

Although in retrospect that seems to have been an obvious response, one to be expected of a conscientious chiropractor, this was before the idea of "patient-centered care" had taken hold in the chiropractic profession. It was at a time when Cooperstein would have expected a dyed-in-the-wool UCT advocate to have answered: "Although I am always pleased when the patient's symptoms resolve, my job is to correct the atlas subluxation, so the body can heal itself. If I am unable to do so, I might best refer the patient to yet another UCT practitioner who can. If symptoms persist, despite the atlas subluxation having been corrected, I must explain to the patient that if one must have low-back pain, it is better not to have atlas subluxation as well!"

We think this recollection says a lot about the inappropriateness of the derision, the typecasting, that is sometimes leveled at the UCT practitioner. Like the surgeon who comments that "the surgery was a success, but the patient died," the stereotypical UCT practitioner says: "We successfully corrected the atlas subluxation, so the persistent low-back pain is not our concern." That was not Grostic's position, that's for sure.

It is hard to believe, given that for over two decades the Palmer College was exclusively upper cervical in its program, that at this time only 1.7% of modern practitioners, according to a survey conducted by the National Board of Chiropractic Examiners, claim to be upper cervical.[1] On the other hand, we have reasons to believe that this select population of chiropractors is far more likely not to respond to a survey mailed them by the National Board, so that the survey result may understate their numbers, perhaps dramatically. Sherman College and Life University (although the latter is imperiled at the time of this writing) continue to emphasize the UCT concept in their chiropractic programs, and several other colleges continue to offer UCT courses in their core curricula. Whatever the number of UCT practitioners, they make up in zeal whatever they may lack in numbers, and thus continue to exert a big impact on this profession.

There are and have been historically many UCTs. Despite notable differences in their adjustive methods and equipment, they tend to be similar in their analytic methods and, of course, in their fervent loyalty to UCT (in its most extreme form, "atlas only") concept. Therefore, we have elected to combine – not without some degree of unease – the primary UCTs, Hole-In-One (HIO) and Grostic/National Upper Cervical Chiropractic Association (NUCCA), in one chapter. We draw out their primary differences, particularly in the adjustive procedures and equipment, in the section below on Treatment/adjustive procedures.

OVERVIEW

UCT intends to correct the atlas subluxation in one adjustment, so as to eliminate nerve interference at the only location BJ Palmer thought it could really arise, as the result of cord pressure, a point Kale echoed.[2] Innate intelligence, so it is said, is thus freed to be in complete control of the nervous system, which heals the entire body in all of its functions. The original HIO UCT is a carefully conceived and highly coordinated "concussion of forces," applied by the hands, which attempts to reduce or correct multiplanar structural disrelationships of the atlas and axis vertebrae. From a philosophical point of view, the thought is that only in the upper cervical spine could nerve interference block the communication of mind and body.[3] Apart from its use among a general population of chiropractic patients, there are also claims for the special value of UCT in a select population, such as pediatric cases[4] and geriatric cases.[5]

The Grostic/NUCCA wing of the upper cervical chiropractic community uses a lighter, more measured force than that used in the HIO method of BJ Palmer and his descendants. On the other hand, from an analytic point of view, the Grostic/NUCCA community agrees with the HIO adherents that the specific adjustment of atlas profoundly affects the central nervous system, and through it, the mechanical and visceral functioning of the entire body. They add that the atlas subluxation affects the reticular formation in the brainstem, so that a disinhibition of caudal structures is brought about. The resulting spasticity can only be corrected by reducing the atlas subluxation, as confirmed by the post X-ray, monitored from visit to visit using the anatometer.

HISTORY

According to Dye,[6] the upper cervical concept was in the air at the Palmer College in the late 1920s, something of a *Weltanschauung*. BJ Palmer introduced the concept of the primacy of the upper cervical subluxation, apparently emphasizing axis at first, to his contemporaries in the early spring of 1930.[6] He felt by this time that it was only here that there could be interference with the neurological connection between the brain and rest of the body. Not all of the chiropractors who had previously followed BJ Palmer every step of the way were equally enthused to learn that "Every case you and I ever got well through adjustment was an accident." HIO in BJ Palmer's hands required four items for an analysis: the neurocalometer, the spinograph X-ray, the toggle-recoil-innate adjustment to put the vertebra in motion, and the knee–chest table.[7] The toggle-recoil adjustive approach, although originally used in full-spine adjusting,[8] was adapted for atlas adjusting by BJ Palmer himself.[9]

Around 1932 AA Wernsing, in connection with some personal health problems, began developing his own UCT concepts in conjunction with GP Loomis. In 1934, Wernsing, having become convinced that it was atlas and not axis that should be emphasized, and that atlas side-slips were more likely than atlanto-occipital rotational misalignments, took his work to the Palmer College.[10-12] This included his revolutionary UCT radiographic series,[13] the forerunner to the atlas orthogonal X-ray techniques of today. Wernsing also invented the light-force technique that led directly to the Grostic/NUCCA practitioners:

In making correction in any case, I do not advise a heavy thrust. The heavy thrust many times will accomplish less than a light force given with greater speed. Having available an accurate analysis, and proper placement of the patient being made according to the analysis in degrees, with proper care having been taken in palpation of the transverse process of the atlas, and correct contact being made on the transverse process of the atlas, a greater degree of correction can be accomplished with a light, speedy thrust.[13] (p. 59)

Modern practitioners who practiced in the tradition of BJ Palmer have included Kale[2,14-18] and

Mears, as well as their adherents. Dr. Donald Mears, who passed away in 1991, developed his Mears Technique,[19,20] starting from the proposition that others of the HIO practitioners had inadequately identified primary occiput problems, that is, X-ray methods and adjustive approaches for thrusting upon the occiput as compared with the atlas. Mears' contemporary William Blair also sought to correct what he believed to be an inadequacy in the HIO analysis, having to do with congenital asymmetry in the upper cervical spine.[21] According to modern-day Blair practitioner Addington, "Despite the proliferation of orthogonally-based upper cervical techniques deriving from the work of John F. Grostic and ultimately from BJ Palmer, the Blair Technique remains the only non-orthogonal precision spinographic and adjustive technique for the cervical spine in the chiropractic profession."[22] Blair altered the thrust, eliminating the recoil, and also performed his adjustments in side-posture using a cervical drop piece, rather than on a knee–chest table with the head turned, as in BJ's style. JC Thompson also used a side-posture, drop-assisted atlas adjustment starting around 1952.[23]

Apart from HIO, a whole other style of upper cervical care developed out of Wernsing's original contribution, using a lighter contact. In 1941, JF Grostic walked into RR Gregory's office; at the time Gregory was going through Wernsing's *The Atlas Specific*,[13] seeking an effective upper cervical adjustment. That date marked the beginning of a collaboration that lasted until Grostic's death in 1964.[24] JD Grostic wrote that his father's analytic innovations, mostly having to do with the radiography and its interpretation, were first presented in 1946.[25] The original HIO high-velocity, low-amplitude toggle-recoil thrust of BJ Palmer was replaced by a "closed stance, lighter contact, and a shallower thrust" around 1952. Gregory was present at Grostic's first upper cervical teaching seminar, and so were several other chiropractic pioneers at various times: Cecil Laney attended his first Grostic seminar in 1951, Roy Sweat in 1952, and Burl Pettibon in 1956.

Low-force upper cervical practitioners like JF Grostic, his son JD Grostic, and Gregory accepted the upper cervical thesis on the primacy of atlas subluxation, but developed a gentler and more measured adjustive approach.[25,26] Harrison comments that JF Grostic leaned heavily on the original atlas-specific technique of Wernsing, appropriating from him much of the X-ray series, the use of the Vernier side-posture table, his cervical measuring instruments, the triceps pull atlas adjustment, and his post X-ray procedures.[27] Although, according to Sweat, Grostic introduced the post X-ray into chiropractic in 1946,[28] we find that Wernsing had advocated taking such radiographs in his 1941 text.[13]

Following Grostic's death, there was a schism in this low-force, highly measured upper cervical milieu,[24] which led Gregory to found NUCCA, a fraternal organization, on 16 April 1966. The National Upper Cervical Chiropractic Research Association (NUCCRA) was incorporated for research purposes only on 6 October 1971. It received tax-exempt status from the federal government, and Daniel C Seemann of the University of Toledo was appointed research advisor in 1971.

The earliest atlas adjusting instruments (Ch. 33) were developed by Arden Zimmerman[29] in the 1930s with the goal of duplicating the manual toggle-recoil adjustment.[9] Several types of adjusting instruments have been devised. Some of the cervical adjusting instruments are hand-held, others are mounted on devices that sit on the floor, and still others are mounted on adjusting tables.

Summing up the diversity that developed from BJ Palmer's original upper cervical concept, we count as HIO descendants the NUCCA adherents (Gregory, etc.), the milieu that developed around Life Chiropractic College (JD Grostic, Roy Sweat, Cecil Laney, etc.), DB Mears, William Blair, and HIO practitioners Kale (recently deceased) and Kessinger. Grostic wrote that the orthospinology taught at Life Chiropractic College was a variant of the Grostic methods.[25] We must also classify Pettibon and Harrison as HIO descendants, given that their full-spine techniques retain a distinctly upper cervical cast. According to Tiscareño,[30] although this does not seem entirely accurate, the practice of upper cervical chiropractic remained essentially unchanged after the closing of the BJ Palmer Research Clinic in 1951. More recently, he goes on to say, there have been advances in spinography, thermography, fiberoptics, and neurophysiological research which promise a "new paradigm" for upper cervical specific chiropractic.[30]

According to Dr. Ed Owens[31] (Table 32.1), research director at Sherman College of Straight Chiropractic, which retains a strong emphasis on UCT, the offshoots of Grostic work (NUCCA and Atlas Orthogonal) are having more success building numbers than the followers of the original HIO work of BJ Palmer. He also comments that Advanced Upper Cervical Biomechanics (AUCB) is taught by the International Upper Cervical Chiropractic Association, a group doing and teaching a form of HIO in California. Finally, according to Dr. Owens: "There are two types of HIO … The older HIO is done on a knee chest table with a posterior arch contact. Kale and AUCB both derive from that kind of HIO. In 1954, BJ added the drop head piece and went to a side-lying posture with a Transverse Process contact. Grostic and Blair derive more from that kind of HIO. Life College only taught the side posture version of HIO, but Sherman teaches both".[31]

Table 32.1 Upper Cervical Technique today (from information gathered by Owens[31])

Upper cervical technique	Current practitioners	Source of estimate
Atlas Orthogonal	350	Roy Sweat
NUCCA	800	Monograph mailing list
Orthospinology/Grostic	120	Kirk Eriksen
Kale Upper Cervical	100	Owens
Advanced Upper Cervical Biomechanics	500 practitioners worldwide, 200 in USA	International Upper Cervical Chiropractic Association
HIO/toggle recoil	Many (taught in chiropractic college curricula)	

NUCCA, National Upper Cervical Chiropractic Association; HIO, Hole-In-One.

DEFINITION OF TECHNIQUE-SPECIFIC TERMS
Primarily related to HIO, toggle recoil

- Subluxation and misalignment: in Palmer Upper Cervical Specific technique, subluxation refers only to atlas and axis, whereas misalignment is used to refer to the caudad segments
- Specific chiropractic: confines all adjustments to C1 and C2[16]
- HIO: acronym for Hole-In-One, a synonym for Palmer Upper Cervical Specific technique. It refers to the idea that a perfect listing, given a perfect thrust, using perfect technique, will clear the atlas subluxation in one stroke (thrust)
- HIO listings: a typical four-letter listing would be ASRA. The first A stands for atlas, the S refers to an excessively steep atlas plane line in the sagittal plane, the R refers to atlas laterality to the right, and the second A refers to an anterior rotation of the atlas transverse process (relative to the occipital condyles) on the right, the side of atlas laterality
- Toggle recoil: the HIO adjustive style, using a reinforced pisiform applied to either atlas or axis, delivered in a rapidly accelerated thrust, with torque, followed by a so-called recoil. It is believed that the atlas is thus moved with respect to both the segment above and below,[32] provided enough speed is generated[2]
- Blair Toggle-Torque adjustive thrust: the Blair adjustment[22] is essentially a toggle-recoil adjustment, minus the recoil.

Primarily related to Grostic/NUCCA

- Central skull line, atlas plane line: representative terms drawn from the UCT X-ray line-marking system, referring to a vertical line representing head tilt and a horizontal line representing atlas inclination
- NUCCA: an acronym for National Upper Cervical Chiropractic Association; the technique system associated with founder Gregory and that organization
- Atlas subluxation complex (ASC): denotes in NUCCA the "extensive and detrimental effects

of a C1 subluxation on the CNS [central nervous system] and the spinal column"[33]

- Head subluxation, into the kinks subluxation, and against the kinks subluxations: typical NUCCA X-ray listings. In the head subluxation, the head is tilted by more than the cervical spine has lost vertical alignment. In the into and against configurations, the head and neck are oblique to the gravity line, on the same side as the gravity line (the into configuration) or the opposite side from the gravity line (the against configuration).[34] The against configuration is said to be the most common of the three[34,35]
- Relatoscope, cephalometer: these tools and their descendants are transparent plates with various slots and line markings, used in NUCCA and other UCT-inspired techniques (e.g., Pettibon's Spinal Biomechanics, Harrison's Chiropractic Biophysics) to perform line marking on the C1 and skull areas, respectively
- Anatometer: a device used primarily by NUCCA practitioners to measure postural deviations and leg-length inequalities said to result from C1 subluxations
- Approach, settle-back, turn-in, arch, roll-in, conversion, triceps pull: terms referring to the sequence of events or phases in the NUCCA adjustment
- Triceps pull: the actual NUCCA adjustment, described below in the paragraphs under Treatment/adjustive procedures.

PHYSIOLOGICAL MECHANISMS AND RATIONALE

According to JD Grostic,[26] there are four ways in which atlas subluxation can result in nerve interference:

1. Trauma to the upper cervical area may result in splinting of cervical muscles, which produces direct mechanical irritation to the nerves passing through these muscles.
2. Tissue edema surrounding the vertebrae can produce direct mechanical irritation of the nerves, arteries, and veins passing through the intervertebral foramen and the superior cervical ganglia.

3. Upper cervical extreme rotatory subluxations may reduce or occlude the vertebral arteries, reducing blood flow to the brain and upper cervical cord. They may also cause the cervical cord and medulla to be displaced laterally away from the direction of rotation, allowing the tip of the dens to compress the medulla.

4. The denticulate ligaments may directly exert traction on the spinal cord, interfering with the long nerve tracts by (1) direct mechanical irritation and by (2) closing the small veins of the spinal cord, producing a blood flow stasis and a resultant loss of nutrients necessary for normal nerve conduction.

This last mechanism is JD Grostic's dentate ligament, cord distortion hypothesis. He felt that, given the attachment of the dentate ligaments to the osseous structures of the upper cervical spine, upper cervical misalignment would distort and irritate the spinal cord.[36,37] Moreover, the hypothesis also states that venous occlusion and resulting anoxia may compound the cord distortion.[38]

NUCCA practitioners believe that the atlas subluxation produces neurological imbalance of the central nervous system, resulting in spastic contracture of the skeletal muscles,[39] because the atlas subluxation would affect the reticular formation in the brainstem. This would in turn bring about a disinhibition of caudal structures, resulting in postural distortion and displacement of the body's center of gravity, one outcome of which could be pelvic distortion and "leg disparity."[40] Likewise, the atlas subluxation would interfere with the normal function of the central reticular formation of the brainstem, resulting in decreased inhibition of caudal muscles, and thus spastic contracture. Neural imbalance in the extrapyramidal connections is thought to be the primary pathology.

Turning now to the upper cervical correction, adjustments in the areas of local spasticity will not be effective unless the subluxation of C1 is addressed. The adjustment, once made, is thought to reduce cord pressure in the upper cervical spine, allowing the brain to control the function and structure of the body more effectively. Why use a light force, as in the NUCCA and Grostic systems? "The contact must be light enough to be non-threatening to the patient."[11]

There is a rather metaphysical twist in the way HIO explains how the technique results in atlas realignment. The doctor doesn't apply a force that repositions the vertebra. Rather, the adjustment happens only after the doctor's hand is withdrawn from the patient: the thrust reduces nerve interference, which allows innate intelligence to make the adjustment. Let's let Kale make the point in his own words:[4]

To us, adjusting a vertebra, the adjustment with that extra something is what happens after the hand has left the back. It is the reaction that occurs after the adjustment when the INNATE responds in the body of the patient now that the vertebra, in the natural position, has assisted Innate to keep the nerves at work as they were intended. The body, with its Innate knowledge, is the hero.

DIAGNOSTIC/ANALYTIC PROCEDURES

Given the diversity of UCTs, we cannot describe the examination and analytic systems in a way that would apply similarly to all UCT advocates, but we may list several procedures that tend to be used. Indeed, the differences among UCTs tend to show up in the adjusting area, not the subluxation theory, analysis, X-ray protocols, or other examination procedures. The principal analytic (i.e., examination) procedures include thermography (generally using a dual-probe instrument resembling the original neurocalometer of BJ Palmer's time), a supine leg check, palpation of the upper cervical area, and an upper cervical specific X-ray series.

The patient's work-up also includes standard orthopedic/neurological testing, but not much, if any, motion palpation, even though Sweat does recommend palpating the cervical spine for soft-tissue changes and the like.[42] Some UCT practitioners, not unlike Logan technique advocates, assess the standing patient's bilateral weight distribution,[43] and some would also analyze the full-body posture using any of a number of devices, such as the Gravity Stress Analyzer[41,43] or the anatometer.[44,45] Kale did not believe it would be necessary even to talk to the patient, in that purely

chiropractic "analytical procedures" would allow just that adjustment that would cure him or her of any problem, whether identified or not.

Killinger[46] succinctly described the means by which typical patients at the BJ Palmer Chiropractic Clinic were examined and their progress monitored:

A daily spinal examination also was administered to each subject. This examination included spinal palpation and a repeat graph of spinal skin temperature using the neurocalometer. Each subject recorded notes on their perceived daily progress in a patient diary. Weekly physical examinations, blood, urine, vision and audiometric tests were administered to monitor the presence of any confounding conditions. Follow-up X-rays were taken on each subject.

In NUCCA, after a case history is taken, a supine leg check is performed to determine if the patient is a candidate for chiropractic care. A short leg is thought to indicate atlas subluxation. The anatometer, a multiplanar device that measures postural distortion using plumb-lines and adjustable horizontal cables, is used to detect "leg disparity" and pelvic distortion in the standing patient. Following this, the doctor performs a standard orthopedic/neurological examination. Only then would an X-ray be taken. That stated, it must be said that NUCCA is a very X-ray-intensive technique, in that the primary diagnostic method is the determination of atlas misalignment through the use of upper cervical X-rays, as pioneered by Wernsing.[13,27]

The upper cervical X-ray series includes at least three views that are mutually perpendicular (Box 32.1). A neutral lateral film establishes the sagittal atlas plane line. Then, the nasium view is taken from anterior to posterior, with the tube tilted so as to be parallel to the atlas plane line established by the neutral lateral film. Either a base posterior or vertex view is obtained, perpendicular

---

Box 32.1 Typical upper cervical X-ray series

- Lateral cervical
- Nasium
- Base posterior or vertex
- Anteroposterior (AP) open-mouth (usually)

to the nasium, depending on whether a superior to inferior or vice versa tube tilt is preferred.[43] An anteroposterior open-mouth view may also be obtained. Grostic assessed the atlanto-occipital joint by comparing the horizontal atlas plane line to an upright line representing the inclination of the skull, unlike the HIO practitioners who represent the skull as a horizontal line like that of atlas.[25] In Grostic's method, careful measurement of the upper cervical area enables the distinction of four basic subluxation types: the first basic type involves C1 laterality on the side opposite angular rotation; the second basic type has the head turning inward on the side of atlas laterality; the third basic type has the head moving in the frontal plane and causing a subluxation in relation to a horizontal C1; and the fourth basic type is a combination of types 1 and 2.[47]

TREATMENT/ADJUSTIVE PROCEDURES

There are significant differences among UCT practitioners when it comes to how the adjustment is applied, despite their striking similarity in subluxation theories and analytic procedures. Here are the primary distinctions to be drawn among the various UCTs (Fig. 32.1):

- Atlas only and "mostly atlas" techniques: some UCT practitioners are strict and adhere strictly to adjusting atlas, whereas others may identify and correct axis subluxations, or apply adjustive forces to the cranium.

- High-velocity and low-velocity hand techniques: although UCT was originally developed as an HVLA procedure, it did not take long for light-force varieties, as exemplified by Grostic and NUCCA practitioners, to come into existence.

- Instrumented and hand adjusting: some UCTs use adjusting instruments to apply the force, whereas others use manual forces only (see Ch. 33, on instrumented UCTs).

- Table-mounted, floor-mounted, and hand-held instrumented techniques: there are both table-mounted adjusting devices, featuring a stylus whose line of drive is adjustable and measurable in three planes, and handheld devices. These latter may be as simple as the Activator Adjusting Instrument (AAI), or more complicated and bulky, to the point of resembling an electric drill and allowing non-linear stylus travel or a rotating stylus. There are also floor-mounted adjusting instruments, although these are generally used for full-spine-adjusting applications.

In HIO, the archetype manual, high-velocity UCT, the primary, and even exclusive, treatment is the toggle-recoil adjustment with body drop (Fig. 32.2). Patients are positioned on a table on

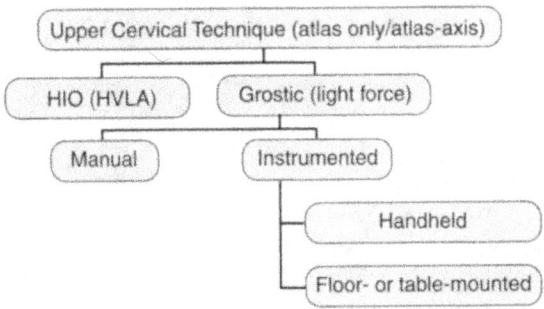

Figure 32.1 Family tree of Upper Cervical technique. HIO, Hole-In-One; HVLA, high-velocity, low-amplitude.

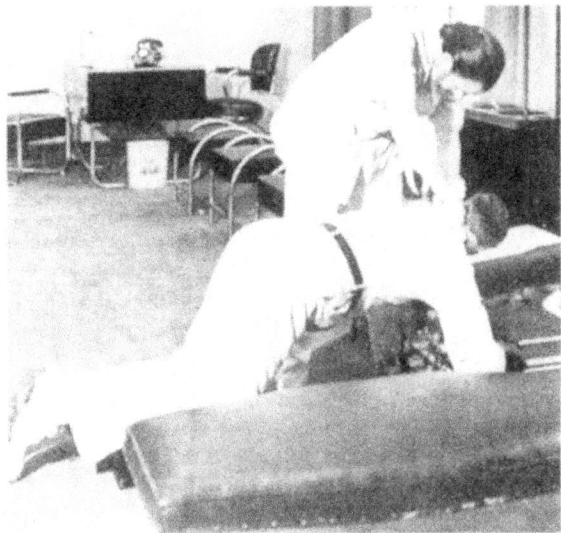

Figure 32.2 BJ Palmer performing a toggle-recoil atlas adjustment on a knee-chest table, although modern togglers are more likely to use a side-posture setup.

their side, with the side of atlas laterality facing upward. The head is placed on a drop piece that has a travel distance of about 1/2 in. (1.25 cm). Kale used a knee–chest table with a solid head piece.[15] Tiscareño said, citing BJ Palmer himself, that this was the preferred method for achieving patient relaxation.[30] Some doctors use side-posture patient position and a cervical drop piece. The customary segmental contact points are the transverse process of the atlas and the lamina of the axis. Kale prefers the lateral posterior portion of the posterior arch of atlas for the segmental contact. The thrust itself is applied by an extremely rapid contraction of the doctor's pectoralis and triceps muscles, which brings the pisiform of the contact hand into abrupt contact with the segmental contact point. The hands and the arm effect a quick "recoil" away from the patient, minimizing patient discomfort. (Blair omits the recoil.) Nelson and De Visscher-Nelson describe the triceps pull as "traction impulse type thrust" and found that it generates 4–6 lb (1.8–2.7 kg) of pressure over 0.5 s.[43]

Killinger,[46] in presenting a case series of 7 chronic headache patients successfully treated at the BJ Palmer Chiropractic Clinic from 1949 to 1951, provides a particularly concise but thorough description of the toggle-recoil adjustive procedure:

All chiropractic adjustments were administered using the Palmer Upper Cervical Specific (Toggle-Recoil) technique. These adjustments were performed with the subject lying, with the involved side up, on a Toggle-Recoil table. This type of table, designed specifically for the technique, allowed the headpiece to be positioned to eliminate rotation, flexion, extension, or lateral flexion of the subject's neck. The doctor's stance was always in front of and facing the subject, with shoulders centered over the subject's involved spinal segment. The thrust was delivered through the pisiform of the doctor's left hand on all left side adjustments (right pisiform for right side adjustments). The doctor's other hand grasped the adjusting arm's wrist for stabilization of the thrust. The doctor delivered a quick shallow thrust in the direction appropriate for the correction of the subluxation. Contact points were the subject's transverse process of the involved side of C-1 for atlas subluxations. For axis subluxations, the contact point was just lateral to the spinous process on the involved side of C-2.

In Grostic/NUCCA, the archetypal manual low-velocity UCTs, the atlas is restored to its normal position through the application of a specific force vector, calculated from a detailed analysis of the upper cervical X-rays. The NUCCA atlas adjustment is called the triceps pull. The doctor assumes a procedure like that assumed in the toggle-recoil adjustment, in a position over the atlas transverse to be contacted, arranging his or her hands and body in a manner consistent with the X-ray line-marking information. The patient is prepositioned carefully on the table in a side-posture position. The triceps muscles are then "pulled" from a point about 1/4 in. (0.6 cm) below the center of the glenoid cavity, resulting in a slight extension of the arms that delivers a very light but carefully focused thrust. At some point, some of the doctors who developed within this milieu became interested in developing instrumented equivalents of their light-force manual adjustments; some of their work is reviewed in Chapter 33.

Ancillary procedures are sparse among most UCT practitioners. In HIO, patients are advised to rest following a typical adjustive procedure. A common-sense regimen of exercise and a balanced diet are suggested as part of the treatment plan. According to Kale, "there will be no room for modalities."[17] In NUCCA, "As a general rule no supplementary measures, adjuncts, or appliances are used."[35]

OUTCOME ASSESSMENT

In HIO, the postchecks following an upper cervical adjustment center on thermographic analysis and a supine leg check, with a post X-ray from time to time. Reduction of symptomatology is not an important component of outcome evaluation. In Grostic/NUCCA UCT, X-ray, anatometer, and thermographic postchecks are used to assess the outcome of care. Although a leg check is done following an adjustment, the anatometer is preferred, because leg checks are considered too subjective to be useful for this purpose. The post X-ray series consists of the nasium and vertex views. On the following visit, if the anatometer and other instruments show no body distortion, no adjustment is given. Symptom assessment is not considered to be reliable.[48]

SAFETY AND RISK FACTORS

HIO practitioners generally believe that seeing the patient too frequently is the primary cause of a patient not progressing or even worsening. Their thought is not so much that subluxations would be overadjusted, but that subluxations would be *created* by overaggressive care.[14] Given the propensity most HIO practitioners have for taking post X-rays, it is good that NUCCA authors describe methods to ensure that the patient-absorbed X-ray dosage is minimal. They advocate using state-of-the-art X-ray equipment, filtration, and films to minimize patient exposure to ionizing radiation.[25,49]

EVIDENCE OF EFFICACY

Analytic efficacy

Seemann has presented data supporting the reliability of NUCCA X-ray marking, anatometer measurements, atlas laterality, and postadjustment reduction in atlas laterality.[45] Most of these data are from case reports or retrospective chart reviews and were self-published in the NUCCA *Upper Cervical Monograph*. Seemann also found decreased bilateral weight differential and decreased leg-length inequality, as measured by anatometer, following NUCCA atlas adjustments.[50] However, Addington found low coefficients of reliability for certain anatometer measurements.[51]

Harrison et al,[52] in their review article, discussed substantial evidence that upper cervical X-ray line-marking methods, like other line-marking methods, are quite reliable. We are aware of few, if any, data, however, on the *validity* of NUCCA X-ray marking or anatometer measurements. Hart[53] looked at the interexaminer reliability of upper cervical X-ray line marking, and of upper cervical palpation, and the correlation of the two. There was some reliability (reproducibility) in the line marking, but not the palpatory procedures. There was no agreement between the X-ray and palpatory methods.

Adjustive efficacy

Case reports

Without question, the most abundant evidence on efficacy of HIO would be found in the records of the BJ Palmer Research Clinic, which operated from 1935 to 1951. Killinger,[46] in what amounts to a chiropractic research archeological dig, presents a case series of 7 chronic headache patients who were successfully treated at the BJ Palmer Chiropractic Clinic from 1949 to 1951. She also assembled a report on a case of infantile colic,[54] another case of asthma,[55] and four cases of multiple sclerosis.[56]

Pistolese[57] identified no less than 17 case reports of patients with epilepsy who received chiropractic adjustive care, upper cervical in 15 cases, and all improved (he does not describe what style of UCT was administered in each case). One of the reports did describe how a light-force, manual upper cervical adjustment relieved symptoms in the case of a patient with a seizure disorder.[58] Similarly, in a review of the literature on the chiropractic care of children with autism, one of us (Gleberzon) found several case studies[59] and one clinical trial[60] that reported favorable clinical outcomes principally using upper cervical adjustments.

Thomas reports on a case where a mentally handicapped 14-year-old girl had improved mental and motor function following NUCCA adjustments.[61] A patient with a herniated cervical disk showed both subjective and objective improvements following the administration of Grostic manual procedures.[62] There is a case series of 3 patients with cervical torticollis who improved after receiving upper cervical care, in the toggle-recoil tradition.[63]

There is a case report describing improvement in Parkinson's disease, subjectively and objectively measured, following intervention with a Kale adjustment – a toggle-recoil-type upper cervical adjustment, on a knee–chest table.[64] The same investigator also provides a case series of 10 Parkinson's disease patients,[65] and another of five multiple sclerosis patients.[65] There is a report of the successful treatment of two cases of Bell's palsy using knee–chest HIO technique.[66]

Grostic (light-force) procedures were used in a case where a patient suffering from widespread complaints – fatigue, dizziness, facial numbness, ataxia, headaches, difficulty speaking, and diffuse arthralgias – and thought to have an unrelated Arnold–Chiari type I malformation, achieved resolution of her symptoms.[67] Likewise, Grostic procedures were accompanied by improvement in a case of constipation.[68] There is also a case report showing postural improvements.[69] Knutson[70] provides a case series of three patients who showed reduced low-back pain with low-force upper cervical care.

Kessinger and Boneva[5] provide an interesting case report of a 75-year-old female whose vertigo, tinnitus, and hearing loss were presumed to be caused by Ménière's disease. After the patient was analyzed with both upper cervical thermographic and X-ray procedures (including atypical flexion–extension views), she received a series of three HIO adjustments on a knee–chest table. Not only were there radiographic improvements, but there was also an improvement in hearing function. The same investigators[71] used the same analytic and adjustive methods in a case of a motor vehicle accident victim who developed cervical kyphosis and instability, associated with complaints of pain, vertigo, tinnitus, and confusion. There were both objective and subjective indicators of improvement during 10 weeks of care and 22 office visits, featuring seven HIO-style knee–chest atlas adjustments.

Larger studies

A multiple baseline study demonstrated a decrease in blood pressure among six of eight hypertensive subjects after NUCCA treatment.[58] Using Kale-style HIO (toggle-recoil) adjusting, another non-controlled study involving 67 patients showed pre–post improvement in visual acuity – not only in people with visual acuity below the norm prior to upper cervical care, but also in those with normal and above-normal vision as measured on Snellen charts.[72] Still another showed both objective and subjective improvements in pulmonary function among 55 patients, also using a simple non-controlled pre–post study design.[73] A non-controlled headache study showed significant improvement in 26 patients receiving toggle-recoil upper cervical adjustments.[74]

A practice-based research project was conducted on 311 patients who received upper cervical care, mostly for pain complaints. After 4 weeks of care, there was significant improvement, as measured using both the Rand SF-36 Health Survey and a global well-being score (GWBS) as primary outcome measures.[75] A report too brief to interpret looked at the effect of NUCCA-type low-force adjustments on diabetes.[76]

There is a non-controlled, retrospective study showing improvement in low-back pain in patients receiving Grostic, low-force care.[77] There are also case studies supporting the hypothesis that upper cervical adjustments can improve low-back pain, such as a case series of three presented by Knutson.[70] However, there appear to be no blinded, controlled, or randomized studies testing the clinical value of upper cervical care for low-back pain.[36] There is a brief report that upper cervical care, presumably HIO-style, improved lumbar range of motion in an experimental group, compared with a non-adjusted control group.[78] In addition, there is a study in which 26 patients were divided into three groups, one of which received upper cervical care, another of which received full-spine care, and a third a combination of the two. This last group, receiving the combination of methods, showed the most improvement in their pain scores[79] and SF-36 scores, but not in their low-back flexibility.

A double-blind, randomized clinical trial was conducted to determine whether a single toggle-recoil (HIO-type) adjustment would affect the subject's reaction time to images appearing on a computer monitor, as a surrogate measure for cortical processing time.[80] There were 18 treated subjects and 18 controls, all selected for the study based on static and motion palpation findings. Although both groups showed improvement in their processing times, the larger improvement occurred in the experimental group (15% compared to 9%). In a study aimed at determining if upper cervical care (not otherwise defined in the study) would influence athletic performance in baseball players,[81] it was found that the group receiving upper cervical care, but not the control group, showed a trend toward decreased resting blood pressure and pulse rate. By comparison, trends in these same measures showed increases within the control group. The group receiving upper cervical care also showed a relative increase in their capillary count.

Knutson[82] investigated the effect of a single, manual upper cervical adjustment (probably low-force, although this is not stated) on pulse rate and blood pressure in both hypertensive and normotensive groups. There were two components to the study, one in which the results of 40 treated patients were compared to those of a non-treated control group, and another in which each of 30 similar patients was used as his or her own control. About the same result occurred in each of the study components: although pulse rate and diastolic pressures did not change, the systolic pressure of the treated patients dropped by about 10 mmHg (test 1) and 7.5 mmHg (test 2). The results were statistically significant.

Changes in objective measurements

Grostic and DeBoer[83] published retrospective data showing that patients found to be misaligned using the Grostic X-ray system of measurement tended to be more neutrally aligned following a single upper cervical adjustment. The study is marred by the fact that the person or persons who did the line marking were not masked; that is to say, blinded. In some cases, UCT advocates have correlated the degree of patient improvement with reduction in the amount of atlas subluxation, as radiographically measured.[84] Pre–post changes have been reported in thermographic findings as well, which are too numerous to cite.

CONCLUSIONS

- Considering that the focus of UCT intervention exclusively concerns occiput, C1, and C2, it is surprising how many permutations of upper cervical misalignment are said to exist – 274 in all.[2]
- UCT practitioners almost always use supine leg checks, whereas full-spine doctors tend to use prone leg checks. We are not aware of any definitive justification or rationalization for these practices.

- Although at this time the toggle-recoil method of adjusting is almost synonymous with HIO-inspired methods of atlas adjusting, it is interesting to note that this thrusting technique was also deployed by Carl Cleveland to be used in full-spine adjusting. It is still taught as such in the Cleveland Chiropractic Colleges, as part of the Meric Technique (Ch. 19).
- Since correcting the upper cervical subluxation is said to restore balance and normal function to the entire body, some UCT practitioners consider their practice to be "full-spine." This usage of the term, however, is not what full-spine generally conveys: the application of forces to multiple spinal regions, anywhere from the occiput to the pelvic girdle. Although UCT practitioners typically eschew adjusting other spinal levels, at least one of them recommends that full-spine adjusters take up careful atlas adjusting, using typical UCT analytic methods.[85]
- Since UCT doctors, through atlas adjusting, profess to treat ("correct") somatic and systemic (visceral) conditions, it must be a matter of some concern that patients suffering from such complaints might be found to be suffering from atlas subluxation as something of a default option, and might receive inappropriate care.
- Grostic/NUCCA adherents, more than even HIO practitioners, consider their thrust to be a *precise* vectored adjustment. Such an adjustment requires a combination of two components: exact patient positioning and delivery of a precise rectilinear force by the doctor.[86,87] The clinical feasibility of achieving this type of specificity in either patient positioning or force delivery has been questioned,[88,89] with a rejoinder as well.[90] An error of 1/16 in. (0.15 cm) in placement of the head on the adjusting table can result in a 1° change in the position of the atlas. This could drastically change the purported direction of some NUCCA adjustments, resulting in some adjustments that are delivered in exactly the opposite direction from what was intended. Additionally, it has been suggested that the human body is virtually unable to deliver the required rectilinear force, much in the same way that it is virtually impossible to hit a pool ball successfully with one's pisiform rather

than a cue stick.[89] There is no evidence that the NUCCA precise, linear, vectored adjustment – the primary rationale for the NUCCA X-ray series – is physically possible to perform.

- UCT practitioners' propensity for X-ray evaluation cannot be ignored, relative to the biohazards of ionizing radiation. (Unfortunately, we have known doctors who take upper cervical X-rays without protecting the patients' eyes, for fear that shielding would interfere with performing their line-marking analysis.) It may be inappropriate to expose patients to excessive ionizing radiation unless the information derived from that radiation provides a clear clinical benefit.

- In writing about UCT, sometimes we forget that upper cervical-*only* advocates do not own the cervical spine. In gathering literature for our review, we came across an article called "Upper cervical technique" by D Bruce Fligg,[91] which is mostly about motion palpating the upper cervical spine. We were in the process of tempering our comment that UCT does not employ much motion palpation, when we realized that Fligg was a full-spine guy who happened to write about the upper cervical spine. As another example, Dr. George W Such wrote a detailed paper on examining and treating the

occipitoatlantal joint.[92] His approach is entirely integrative, combining both high-force and low-force methods of several professions that employ manual procedures for somatic complaints, and not upper cervical at all, in our sense of the term. Finally, Pollard and Ward showed that a high-velocity, low-amplitude upper cervical thrust (not using the toggle-recoil method) improved hip flexion more than a sacroiliac adjustment did, in a clinical cohort study involving 52 subjects,[93] providing rare evidence of an upper cervical impact on extremity function.

- Depending on how one feels about the concept of the primacy of upper cervical subluxation, the practitioners of UCT may be seen as either a bizarre cult to be avoided, or a sage group of visionaries who are tuned in to the essence of chiropractic. We would recommend that anyone attempting to formulate a seasoned evaluation of what UCT has to offer should ignore these twin stereotypes, which are opposite sides of the same coin, and pay more attention to the relative abundance of clinical research on the effect of upper cervical care. In writing this chapter we were astounded by how much we came across. Hey, one of us may even toggle the next patient that walks in!

REFERENCES

1. Christensen M G 2000 Job analysis of chiropractic. A project report, survey analysis and summary of the practice of chiropractic within the United States. National Board of Chiropractic Examiners, Greeley, CO
2. Kale M 1989 How the toggle is used in adjusting. Today's Chiropractic (July/August): 54–58
3. Vear H J 1981 Introduction to chiropractic science. Western States Chiropractic College, Portland, OR
4. Prax J C 1999 Upper cervical chiropractic care of the pediatric patient: a review of the literature. Journal of Clinical Chiropractic Pediatrics 1(4): 257–263
5. Kessinger R C, Boneva D V 2000 Vertigo, tinnitus, and hearing loss in the geriatric patient. Journal of Manipulative and Physiological Therapeutics 23(5): 352–362
6. Dye A A 1969 The evolution of chiropractic – its discovery and development. Photo reprint of 1939 edition, published by the author. Richmond Hill, NY
7. Montgomery P D, Nelson M J 1985 Evolution of chiropractic theories of practice and spinal adjustment, 1900–1950. Chiropractic History 5: 71–77

8. Cleveland C S I 1992 The high-velocity thrust adjustment. In: Haldeman S (ed.) Principles and practice of chiropractic, 1st edn, pp. 459–482. Appleton & Lange, Norwalk, CT
9. Grostic J D 1988 The adjusting instrument as a research tool. Chiropractic Research Journal 1 (2): 47–55
10. Wernsing A A 1959 Origin of the atlas specific (part I). American Chiropractic Association Journal 1 (4): 2–3
11. Wernsing A A 1959 Origin of the atlas specific (part II). American Chiropractic Association Journal 1 (5): 5–12
12. Wernsing A A 1960 Origin of the atlas specific (part III). American Chiropractic Association Journal 1 (6): 6–10
13. Wernsing A A 1941 The atlas specific. Oxford Press, Hollywood, CA
14. Kale M 1984 The upper cervical specific. Today's Chiropractic (July/August): 28–29
15. Kale M 1984 The upper cervical specific. Part two of two. Today's Chiropractic (September/October): 27–30
16. Kale M 1995 Dr. B J Palmer's upper cervical specific: the final test of greatness. Today's Chiropractic (January/February): 28–31

17. Kale M 1987 Reviewing the HIO technique. Today's Chiropractic (July/August): 53, 55, 95

18. Kale M 1986 The HIO technique. Today's Chiropractic (May/June): 69

19. Mears D B 1977 The Mears Technique. In: Kfoury P W (ed.) Catalog of chiropractic techniques, p. 27. Logan College of Chiropractic, Chesterfield, MO

20. Mears D B J 1999 The Mears Technique. Journal of Vertebral Subluxation Research 3 (3): 130–131

21. Addington E 1991 Blair cervical spinographic analysis. In: Hansen D (ed.) Proceedings of the Sixth Annual Conference on Research and Education, pp. 117–120. Consortium for Chiropractic Research, Monterey, CA

22. Addington E A 1995 Overview of Blair Cervical Technique. http://www.chiro.org/LINKS/blair.html

23. Grostic J 1991 Upper cervical adjusting and short lever specific contact procedures. In: Hansen D (ed.) Sixth Annual Conference on Research and Education, pp. 258–260. Consortium for Chiropractic Research, Monterey, CA

24. NUCCA/NUCCRA 2002 NUCCA-NUCCRA historical highlights. National Upper Cervical Chiropractic Association. http://www.nucca.org/histhigh.html

25. Grostic J D 1991 The Grostic procedure. Today's Chiropractic (July/August): 51–52

26. Grostic J D 1998 The origins of the Grostic procedure. International Review of Chiropractic (March): 33–35

27. Harrison D D 1985 History of scientific chiropractic and spinal correction. Digest of Chiropractic Economics (January/February): 20–22

28. Sweat R, Sweat M Guidelines for pre- and post-radiographs for care documentation. http://www.atlasorthogonality.com/papers/guidlines.htm

29. Green B N 1998 Improving historical research reports: a case report format and example in Arden Zimmerman, D C. Journal of Chiropractic Humanities 8 (1): 43–54

30. Tiscareño L H 1993 HIO: a new paradigm? Today's Chiropractic (September/October): 70–72

31. Owens E F Jr 2002 Re. modern upper cervical technique practitioners. Personal communication

32. Kale M 1988 Upper cervical chiropractic: who's responsible? Part II. Dynamic Chiropractic (January 1): 20–21

33. Gregory R R 1977 The atlas subluxation complex and its correction technique. In: Kfoury P W (ed.) Catalog of chiropractic techniques, pp. 73–77. Logan College of Chiropractic, Chesterfield, MO

34. Nelson C R, De Visscher-Nelson I 1982 Pilot study part 2. Deviations in bodily posture and center of gravity as possible indicators of certain upper cervical subluxation complexes. Digest of Chiropractic Economics (July/August): 88–89, 92, 134–135

35. McAlpine J E 1986 Nasium and vertex X-ray survey. Today's Chiropractic (March/April): 37–39

36. Olivero A 1993 A review of the literature: adjusting only the cervical spine and its effect on low back pain. Chiropractic Research Journal 3 (1): 3–6

37. Grostic J D 1988 Dentate ligament – cord distortion hypothesis. Chiropractic Research Journal 1 (1): 47–55

38. Vaillancourt P J, Collins K F 1993 Case report: management of post-surgical low back syndrome with upper cervical adjustment. Chiropractic Research Journal 2 (3): 1–15

39. Gregory R 1983 Biomechanics of the upper cervical spine. Digest of Chiropractic Economics (September/October): 14–18

40. Seemann D C 1982 The biomechanics and neurological aspects of the atlas subluxation complex. Digest of Chiropractic Economics (November/December): 20–23

41. Grostic J D 1987 Reflections on the past, present, and future of research. Today's Chiropractic (May/June): 87–90

42. Sweat R 1985 Scanning palpation. Today's Chiropractic (January/February): 23–24

43. Nelson C R, De Visscher-Nelson I 1982 Pilot study part I. Deviations in bodily posture and center of gravity as possible indicators of certain upper cervical subluxation complexes. Digest of Chiropractic Economics (May/June): 20–21, 24–25, 121

44. Hoiriis K T, Hinson R H, Elsangek O et al 2000 Baseline characteristics of chiropractic patients: correlation of anatometer readings with supine leg length inequality. Journal of Vertebral Subluxation Research 3 (3): 2–3

45. Seemann D C 1990 Exploring the relationship between anatometer measurements and X-ray listings. Upper Cervical Monograph 4 (9): 1–2

46. Killinger L Z 1995 A chiropractic case series of seven chronic headache patients. Palmer Journal of Research 2 (2): 48–53

47. Gregory R R 1987 Updating the four basic types. Digest of Chiropractic Economics (January/February): 68–71, 116–117

48. Gregory R R 1982 Some comments regarding the concept of normal. Digest of Chiropractic Economics (September/October): 14–15, 17, 139–140

49. Dickholtz M 1989 Comments and concerns re X-ray radiation (a guide for upper cervical X-ray). Upper Cervical Monograph 4 (8): 7–9

50. Seemann D 1993 Bilateral weight differential and functional short leg: an analysis of pre and post data after reduction of an atlas subluxation. Chiropractic Research Journal 2 (3): 33–38, 65

51. Addington E A 1982 Reliability and objectivity of anatometer, supine leg length test, ThermoScribe II, and Derma-Therm-o-Graph measurements. Upper Cervical Monograph 3 (6): 8–12

52. Harrison D E, Harrison D D, Troyanovich S J 1998 Reliability of spinal displacement analysis of plain X-rays: a review of commonly accepted facts and fallacies with implications for chiropractic education and technique. Journal of Manipulative and Physiological Therapeutics 21 (4): 252–266

53. Hart J 2000 Comparison of X-ray listings and palpation listings of the upper cervical spine. Journal of Vertebral Subluxation Research 4 (1): 30

54. Killinger L Z, Azad A 1998 Chiropractic care of infantile colic: a case study. Palmer Journal of Research 3 (1): 203–206

55. Killinger L Z 1995 Chiropractic care in the treatment of asthma. Palmer Journal of Research 2 (3): 43–47

56. Killinger L Z, Azad A 1997 Multiple sclerosis patients under chiropractic care: a retrospective study. Palmer Journal of Research 2 (4): 96–100

57. Pistolese R A 2001 Epilepsy and seizure disorders: a review of literature relative to chiropractic care of children. Journal of Manipulative and Physiological Therapeutics 24 (3): 199–205

58. Goodman R 1992 Hypertension and the atlas subluxation complex. Chiropractic: The Journal of Chiropractic Research and Clinical Investigation 8 (2): 30–32

59. Gleberzon B J, Rosenberg-Gleberzon A R 2001 On autism: its prevalence, diagnosis, causes and treatment. Topics in Clinical Chiropractic 8 (4): 42–57

60. Aguilar A L, Grostic J D, Pfleger B 2000 Chiropractic care and the behavior of autistic children. Journal of Clinical Chiropractic Pediatrics 5 (1): 293–304

61. Thomas M, Wood J 1992 Upper cervical adjustments may improve mental function. Manual Medicine 6 (6): 215–216

62. Eriksen K 1998 Management of cervical disc herniation with upper cervical chiropractic care. Journal of Manipulative and Physiological Therapeutics 21 (1): 51–56

63. Bolton S P, Bolton P S 1996 Acute cervical torticollis and Palmer upper cervical specific technique: a report of three cases. Chiropractic Journal of Australia 26 (3): 89–93

64. Elster E L 2000 Upper cervical chiropractic management of a patient with Parkinson's disease: a case report. Journal of Manipulative and Physiological Therapeutics 23 (8): 573–577

65. Elster E L 2000 Upper cervical protocol for five multiple sclerosis patients. Today's Chiropractic 29 (6): 76–92

66. Kessinger R, Boneva D 1999 Bell's palsy and the upper cervical spine. Chiropractic Research Journal 6 (2): 47–56

67. Smith J L 1997 Effects of upper cervical subluxation concomitant with a mild Arnold–Chiari malformation: a case study. Chiropractic Research Journal 4 (2): 77–81

68. Eriksen K 1994 Effects of upper cervical correction on chronic constipation. Chiropractic Research Journal 3 (1): 19–22

69. Reynolds C 1998 Reduction of hypolordosis of the cervical spine and forward head posture by specific upper cervical adjustment and use of a home therapy cushion. Chiropractic Research Journal 1 (5): 23–27

70. Knutson G A 1999 Rapid elimination of chronic back pain and suspected long-term postural distortion with upper cervical vectored manipulation: a novel hypothesis for chronic subluxation/joint dysfunction. Chiropractic Research Journal 2 (6): 57–64

71. Kessinger R C, Boneva D V 2000 Case study: acceleration/deceleration injury with angular kyphosis. Journal of Manipulative Physiological Therapeutics 23 (4): 279–287

72. Kessinger R, Boneva D 1998 Changes in visual acuity in patients receiving upper cervical specific chiropractic care. Journal of Vertebral Subluxation Research 2 (1): 43–49

73. Kessinger R 1998 Changes in pulmonary function associated with upper cervical specific chiropractic care. Journal of Vertebral Subluxation Research 1 (3): 43–49

74. Whittingham W, Ellis W B, Molyneux T P 1994 The effect of manipulation (toggle recoil technique) for headaches with upper cervical joint dysfunction: a pilot study. Journal of Manipulative and Physiological Therapeutics 17 (6): 369–375

75. Hoiriis K T, Owens E F O Jr 1999 Changes in general health status during upper cervical chiropractic care: a practice-based research project update. Chiropractic Research Journal 2 (6): 65–70

76. Webster S K, Dickholtz M, Woodfield C, Bakris G L 1999 Acute effect of Nucca Upper Cervical adjustment on patients with diabetes type II. Chiropractic Research Journal 7 (2): 81

77. Robinson S S, Grostic J D, Collins K F 2003 A retrospective study: patients with chronic low back pain managed with specific upper cervical adjustments. Chiropractic Research Journal 2 (4): 10–16

78. Kessinger R 2000 The influence of upper cervical specific chiropractic care on lumbar range of motion. Chiropractic Research Journal 7 (2): 80

79. Hoiriis K, Pfleger B, Elsangak O et al 1999 Clinical trial comparing upper cervical and full spine chiropractic care for low back pain. Journal of Chiropractic Education 13 (1): 67–68

80. Kelly D D, Murphy B A, Backhouse D P 2000 Use of a mental rotation reaction–time paradigm to measure the effects of upper cervical adjustments on cortical processing: a pilot study. Journal of Manipulative and Physiological Therapeutics 23 (4): 246–251

81. Schwartzbauer J, Kolber J, Schwartzbauer M et al 1997 Athletic performance and physiological measures in baseball players following upper cervical chiropractic care: a pilot study. Journal of Vertebral Subluxation Research 1 (4): 1–7

82. Knutson G A 2001 Significant changes in systolic blood pressure post vectored upper cervical adjustment vs resting control groups: a possible effect of the cervicosympathetic and/or pressor reflex. Journal of Manipulative and Physiological Therapeutics 24 (2): 101–109

83. Grostic J D, DeBoer K F 1982 Roentgenographic measurement of atlas laterality and rotation: a retrospective pre- and post-manipulation study. Journal of Manipulative and Physiological Therapeutics 5 (2): 63–71

84. Eriksen K, Owens E F Jr 1997 Upper cervical post X-ray reduction and its relationship to symptomatic improvement and spinal stability. Chiropractic Research Journal 4 (2): 10–17

85. Forest T J 1980 Upper cervical chiropractic in a full spine practice. Digest of Chiropractic Economics (January/February): 89, 111

86. Gregory R R 1983 A kinesiological basis for the C-1 adjustment – part 1. Digest of Chiropractic Economics (January/February): 23–27, 122

87. Gregory R 1983 A kinesiological basis for the C-1 adjustment – part 2. Digest of Chiropractic Economics (March/April): 41–44

88. Molthen D A 1980 Vectored adjusting: a critique. Digest of Chiropractic Economics (November/December): 73

89. Molthen D A 1981 Vectored adjusting: further comments. Digest of Chiropractic Economics (November/December): 58–61

90. Gregory R R, Seemann D C 1981 A critique of a critique of vectored adjusting. Digest of Chiropractic Economics (July/August): 14–18

91. Fligg D B 1985 Upper cervical technique. Journal of the Canadian Chiropractic Association 29 (2): 92–95

92. Such G W 1999 Upper cervical synthesis: integrative manual care of the occipitoatlantal joint. Chiropractic Technique 3 (11): 116–124

93. Pollard H, Ward G 1998 The effect of upper cervical or sacroiliac manipulation on hip flexion range of motion. Journal of Manipulative and Physiological Therapeutics 21 (9): 611–616

33

Upper Cervical Instrumented techniques

INTRODUCTION

One surreal evening, about 1995, Cooperstein met with a table manufacturer in Woodside, Georgia, visiting the factory and place of business that fabricated a table patterned after his own design. The so-called "friction-reduced table"[1-3] was a smart table optimized for the detection and measurement of leg-length inequality. Purely by chance, another chiropractor walked in, to discuss a table based on his own design, which mounted at the head of the table a cervical adjusting device called the Torque Cervical Instrument. That other chiropractor was Dr. Cecil Laney, famed Upper Cervical doctor and pioneer in instrument adjusting. Anyway, he and Cooperstein started talking, and agreed that Cooperstein's table could be just the right thing to investigate his concept of how upper cervical subluxations might relate to leg-length inequality. So they laid the table-maker down on the table, whereupon Dr. Laney administered a series of upper cervical adjustments with a hand-held adjusting instrument, while Cooperstein carefully scrutinized the position sensor mounted between the table-man's legs. What happened? Well, Cooperstein will never tell … except to mention the pleasure of having met Dr. Laney, who presented him with a down-home measuring device for estimating upper cervical subluxation that he treasures to this day.

HISTORY

The earliest atlas adjusting instruments were developed by Arden Zimmerman[4] in the 1930s with the goal of duplicating the manual toggle-recoil adjustment.[5] In essence, according to McAlpine,[6] the original goal of instrument adjusting was to duplicate the hand adjusting of John D Grostic. Williams et al, in rationalizing its use, stated: "the use of adjusting instruments allows precise and repeatable thrusts to be delivered with little physical effort and shifts the emphasis of training to analysis for the determination of adjusting direction factors."[7] Several types of adjusting instruments have been devised, beginning with the earliest flywheel/crankshaft 1930s devices, followed by solenoids like those devised by Laney around 1956, to dental hammer derivatives like that used by JK Humber in 1967 and Activator doctors today, and cam-stylus devices like the Pettibon device.[5] Some of the cervical adjusting instruments are handheld, others are mounted on devices that sit on the floor, and still others are mounted on adjusting tables.

THE CASE OF ARDEN ZIMMERMAN[4]

The whole idea of making machine adjustments on the human neck by mechanical means is completely revolutionary. It is not to be considered lightly, and only after proper preparation and care can this work be done with the miraculous results described in this article. The machine is not a toy and any person who wishes to investigate its possibilities must bear this in mind for it really moves a vertebra. In proper hands, it opens up a field for practice with absolutely no competition."[8]

Dr. Arden Zimmerman graduated from the Engineering School of Stanford University in 1931. Always of poor health, he was carried in to the BJ Palmer Clinic in Davenport, Iowa, on a stretcher in 1937. After some partial improvement at the hands of BJ Palmer's atlas adjustments, he entered the Palmer Chiropractic College and graduated in 1939. He eventually came to believe that side-slips of atlas under the occipital condyles and rotational misalignment of atlas on axis were the only subluxations capable of producing nerve pressure, and that the intervertebral joints of the rest of the vertebrae are too tightly juxtaposed to allow such pressure, barring fracture-dislocations. Careful measurement of the speed, thrust, depth, and force of Zimmerman's hand adjusting led to the design and construction of a machine – the first adjusting machine ever – that could emulate hand thrusting, but in a more controlled and adjustable manner. Although Zimmerman took no post X-rays, he did use a thermographic device with a graphic output to confirm subluxation and monitor its resolution following adjustive care.[9] Zimmerman claimed, following statistical analysis of the charts of 48 000 of his own patients, that a properly performed atlas adjustment would hold on average for *19 months* (!).

LIFE UPPER CERVICAL: ROY SWEAT AND CECIL LANEY

JD Grostic wrote that the orthospinology taught at Life Chiropractic College, and associated with the name Roy Sweat (faculty), was a variant of the Grostic methods.[10] Cecil Laney has also been a prominent fellow-traveler, if you will, in the Life Upper Cervical milieu. Owens in 1987 provided a thorough description of Life Upper Cervical Technique (UCT),[11] emphasizing its research efforts. He described a novel cervical adjusting instrument with built-in force and position sensors.[11] Steinle wrote[12] that the purpose of Life UCT was threefold: to determine the patient's subluxation pattern, to deliver a precise adjustment through the use of the floor-mounted adjusting instrument, and to render that adjustment reproducible through the use of the instrument. In addition to the instrument itself, the way the table was used was also characteristic.[13]

Roy Sweat

R Sweat, having studied UCT under both BJ Palmer and JF Grostic, built his first adjusting instruments in the 1970s after 20 years of hand adjusting.[14] He describes having devised adjusting instruments with continuously decreasing depth settings, starting with a tool that could be set between 1/2 in. (1.25 cm) and 1/16 in. (0.15 cm), a tool that could be set between 1/8 in. (0.15 cm) and 1 mm, and finally "a percussion instrument with no forward excursion," driven by a 1.8 lb (0.8 kg) solenoid.[15] As an example of his intended precision, R Sweat explains that, since there is a 3/4 distance between the skin and the atlas transverse process, the segmental contact point, whether the thrust is delivered by a manual pisiform contact or through instrument adjusting, must be 1/2 in. (1.25 cm) superior to the palpated transverse process (assuming there is a superior-to-inferior line of drive).[16]

Sweat believes that the atlanto-occipital subluxation, usually described as atlas laterality, is better understood as a rotational subluxation, around the z-axis.[17] In a routine case, Sweat takes the standard three-view upper cervical X-ray series, and follows the adjustment with two more postadjustment views.[18] Frequency-of-visit guidelines are published, ranging from daily visits for 2 weeks for acute injuries to three to six visits per year for supportive care.[19] Pediatric care is supported,[20] as is geriatric care.[21]

Cecil Laney

To Cecil Laney are ascribed the terms "high and low adjusting factors," referring to how factors including the head piece of the table and the line of drive bear on how the adjustment is executed and the result obtained.[6] McAlpine wrote that Laney was "one of the earliest pioneers in instrument adjusting."[6] He has been developing various hand-held and table-mounted adjusting instruments since 1956 using solenoids, unlike the earlier punch-press devices that employed a flywheel coupled to a crankshaft.[5]

EVIDENCE OF EFFICACY

Although some publications simply state that instrumented Life UCT was used, others stipulate that the methods of Sweat, Laney, or someone else practicing orthospinology were used. There are case reports involving Life UCT showing remission of cervicobrachialgia,[22] of Tourette's syndrome,[23] knee pain,[24] and postsurgical low-back pain.[25] There are also cases of reduced post-surgical low-back pain[26] A case series, $n = 45$, showed reduction in low-back pain associated with instrumented (either Life UCT or Laney instruments used) with atlas adjusting. The most dramatic improvements occurred in cases where there was lumbar neurologic involvement.[27] Hospers et al provide case reports of the successful treatment of an epileptic female during a 6-week period,[28] a hyperactive teenager,[29] and of drowsiness and fatigue.[30] Sweat describes the successful treatment of a case of multiple herniated lumbar disks,[31] and there is another case report of C5 disk herniation being successfully treated using Sweat's Atlas Orthogonal Technique.[32]

A randomized clinical trial was conducted, in which 5 human immunodeficiency virus (HIV) positive patients received Laney-instrumented upper cervical care, while 5 controls received a sham "thrust" on the mastoid process with an inactive instrument. The treated group showed a 48% increase in their CD4 cell levels, while the controls showed an 8% decrease in their levels. Extreme caution must be exercised in interpreting this study, for a number of reasons: half of the initial recruits dropped out, no baseline showing possible stochastic fluctuations in CD4 cells was obtained, the absolute changes in CD4 levels were far less dramatic than the percentage changes, only one of the experimental group improvers showed both a relatively large absolute and percentage change in CD4 levels, no follow-up data were provided, and the study had very few subjects enrolled.

CONCLUSIONS

- Although instrumented cervical adjusting initially attempted to emulate hand adjusting in a more controlled, measured, and reproducible manner, at some point device designers realized that machine adjusting allowed forces with physical properties very different from hand adjusting to be generated and used in patient care. Adjusting instruments, such as the Activator Adjusting Instrument (AAI; Ch. 10) are used in full-spine chiropractic techniques as well.

- Instrumented adjusting has research implications. Randomized clinical trials generally require masking (blinding) the participants in various ways. This might include, for example, a doctor not knowing whether he or she is delivering the treatment under investigation or a sham/placebo treatment. For obvious reasons, this is difficult in manipulation studies. Williams et al[7] point out that instrument adjusting, because it so carefully separates out the analysis that determines the appropriate adjusting vectors from the actual thrust, allows these phases of an adjustive session to be entirely in the hands of different people, thus allowing for blinded studies to be conducted in a manner which is usually difficult or impossible in this profession. Williams et al write: "The doctor doing the adjusting can be different from the doctor who sets the actual adjusting parameters on the instrument. In this manner, the adjusting doctor is 'blinded' from knowing whether a real or a 'sham' adjusting vector or thrust is being used, and his bias is taken out of the experiment."[7]

- Although there are a number of publications concerning the design and use of various cervical adjusting instruments, there is not enough information available to conclude that any particular device design or clinical protocol is superior to any other.

REFERENCES

1. Cooperstein R, Jansen P 1996 Technology description: the friction-reduced segmented table. Chiropractic Technique 8 (3): 107–111
2. Cooperstein R 2001 What's going on with "the table"? Dynamic Chiropractic 19 (24): 16–19, 20, 41
3. Cooperstein R 1997 The reverse double whammy leg check. Dynamic Chiropractic 15 (16): 35–38
4. Green B N 1998 Improving historical research reports: a case report format and example in Arden Zimmerman, D C. Journal of Chiropractic Humanities 8 (1): 43–54
5. Grostic J D 1988 The adjusting instrument as a research tool. Chiropractic Research Journal 1 (2): 47–55
6. McAlpine J E 1987 Considerations in instrument adjusting. Today's Chiropractic (May/June): 91–93

7. Williams S E, Owens E F Jr, Hosek R S 1988 Will this new adjusting instrument change upper cervical adjustment techniques? Today's Chiropractic 17 (2): 83–84

8. Zimmerman A D 1986 An adjusting machine to correct subluxation. San Jose, CA

9. Harrison D D 1985 History of scientific chiropractic and spinal correction. Digest of Chiropractic Economics (January/February): 20–22

10. Grostic J D 1991 The Grostic procedure. Today's Chiropractic (July/August): 51–52

11. Owens E F Jr 1987 Life cervical technique. Today's Chiropractic 16 (3): 45–47

12. Steinle L 1986 Life cervical technique. Today's Chiropractic (May/June): 67, 41

13. Sweat R 1987 Atlas orthogonal table placement. Today's Chiropractic (March/April): 83

14. Rainville G 1999 Atlas orthogonal technique. Canadian Chiropractor (February/March): 12–13

15. Sweat R W 1988 Minimum force vs. moderate force in the occipital-atlanto-axial subluxation complex (OCP-C1-C2). The American Chiropractor (February): 22–24

16. Sweat R 1985 Atlas transverse contact. Today's Chiropractic (March/April): 45–46

17. Sweat R, Sweat M, Johnston W, Douglass I 1991 Atlas laterality: a rotational movement. Today's Chiropractic 20 (1): 42–43

18. Sweat R, Sweat M 2002 Guidelines for pre- and post-radiographs for care documentation. http://www.atlasorthogonality.com/papers/guidlines.htm

19. Sweat R, Sweat M Practice guidelines for the Atlas Orthogonal Doctor. http://www.atlasorthogonality.com/papers/practice_guide.htm

20. Sweat R, Sweat M Atlas Orthogonal details. http://www.atlasorthogonality.com/papers/details.htm

21. Sweat R 1998 Chiropractic Atlas Orthogonal technique for the care of the senior citizen. Today's Chiropractic (May/June): 86–91

22. Glick D M 1989 Conservative chiropractic care of cervicobrachialgia. Chiropractic Research Journal 1 (3): 49–52

23. Trotta N 1989 The response of an adult Tourette patient to Life Upper Cervical adjustments. Chiropractic Research Journal 1 (3): 43–48

24. Brown M, Vaillancourt P J 1993 Case report: upper cervical adjusting for knee pain. Chiropractic Research Journal 2 (3): 6–9

25. Vaillancourt P J, Collins K F 1993 Case report: management of post-surgical low back syndrome with upper cervical adjustment. Chiropractic Research Journal 2 (3): 1–15

26. Hoiriis K T 1992 Case report: management of post-surgical chronic low back pain with upper cervical adjustment. Chiropractic Research Journal 1 (3): 37–42

27. Robinson S, Collins K F, Grostic J D 1993 A retrospective study: patients with chronic low back pain managed with specific upper cervical adjustments. Chiropractic Research Journal 2 (4): 10–16

28. Hospers L A, Sweat R W 1987 Response of a three-year-old epileptic child to upper cervical adjustments. Today's Chiropractic (December/January): 69–70

29. Hospers L A, Zezula L, Sweat M 1987 Response of a three-year-old epileptic child to upper cervical adjustments. Today's Chiropractic (December/January): 73–75

30. Hospers L A, Sweat R W 1987 EEG and EMG studies before and after Life Upper Cervical adjustment of a patient complaining of excessive drowsiness and fatigue while writing. Today's Chiropractic (March/April): 79–82

31. Sweat R 1993 Correction of multiple herniated lumbar disc by chiropractic intervention. Journal of Chiropractic Case Reports 1 (1): 14–23

32. Licata F, Miller M A 1995 The treatment of herniated nucleus pulposus in the cervical spine using atlas orthogonal technique. In: Cleveland III C, Gibbons R W (eds) Conference proceedings of the Chiropractic Centennial Foundation, p. 365. Chiropractic Centennial Foundation, Washington, DC

Issues in chiropractic technique

Section 4 discusses selected collateral issues germane to many of the topics surrounding the world of chiropractic technique. There can be little doubt that the determination of the chiropractic profession's past and present identity, and its role in the healthcare delivery system, impact upon the future role of technique systems, and much of Section 4 focuses on such and related matters. Chapter 34 explores some historical matters pertaining to chiropractic technique, focusing on the forces that have fragmented the profession and led to the development of so many different and often mutually exclusive technique systems. Chapter 35 provides utilization rates for the individual technique systems, and for chiropractic care in general. Chapter 36 addresses the fascinating allure of technique systems to both chiropractic practitioners and patients, and Chapter 37 the legal climate in which chiropractic care is administered. Section 4 concludes with chapter 38, a chapter that discusses matters pertaining to chiropractic research as well as CAM (Complementary and Alternative Medicine) providers in a more general sense.

34

Genesis of technique systems in chiropractic

TECHNIQUE SPAWNING

There is a vast number of technique systems currently in existence, and the process of gratuitous technique spawning shows no signs of diminishing. There is nothing new about this splintering of the chiropractic profession. In order to grasp the multitude of complex factors that led to the fragmentation of the profession, it is necessary to understand the historical and ideological background of the chiropractic profession.

Ironically, much of the impetus that led to this fragmentation can be directly attributed to the profession's staunchest supporters and earliest developers: DD Palmer and his son, BJ Palmer. Many of the Palmers' contemporaries became disgruntled with their attitude, behavior, and proprietary theories of chiropractic and branched out on their own, ultimately developing their own technique systems and, in some cases, even establishing their own competing chiropractic colleges. Some chiropractors have resisted attempts to modify or alter the founders' techniques, or make them contemporary in any way, remaining unwaveringly loyal to the tenets held by the Palmers and their interpretation of how the body works. On the other hand, other techniques have been developed showing little relation to the Palmers at all.

In essence, there is a common process that eventually leads to a chiropractic technique system, often beginning with some kind of creation event, a serendipitous clinical observation or outcome that led to an established technique. The classic example is the story told of Romer Derifield, developer of the leg-check method used in Thompson Terminal Point Technique.[1] According to the story, Derifield was in her office treating a patient, who was prone. The phone rang, and as Derifield went to answer it, the patient lifted her head to look at the ringing telephone. Apparently, as the patient turned her head, Derifield noticed that the patient's leg length appeared to change. Over time, that observation led to the development of the Derifield leg-checking procedure (Ch. 4), integral to many technique systems (including Activator Methods, Thompson, and Pierce–Stillwagon; Chs 10, 20, and 14, respectively).

Nelson satirized the process of technique system creation in an article entitled "Five steps to your own technique: the Nelson method".[2] In that article, Nelson suggested that any practitioner can develop his or her own technique by: (1) choosing a name that has "neuro" or other impressive-sounding words in it (energy, physio, quantum); (2) relying on science if it is nonsensical and understood by few, if any, people; (3) requiring practitioners to purchase expensive equipment; (4) invoking the names of DD and BJ Palmer; and (5) above all, not attempting to test the reliability or effectiveness of the technique procedures. Nelson implies, quite correctly in our opinion, that sometimes technique systems are developed by individuals with questionable scruples, motivated only by the prospect of monetary gain.

On the other hand, there is nothing wrong with attempting to systematize clinical observations. Empirical observations appropriately become the cornerstone of new explanations in matters of health and disease. In conjunction with peers who may have made clinical observations, a technique developer codifies these observations into a set of rules and procedural guidelines to account for these observations, and may look to the basic sciences for support. That's where the trouble often begins. Oftentimes, no rational explanations can be found within the realm of normal science, so proprietary and even bizarre theories are developed to fill the void. Sadly, much of this is entirely unnecessary, since explanations as to how treatments work are not as important as clinically confirming that treatments do in fact work. Research today is primarily outcomes-driven, as well it should be.

THE BONESETTERS AND MAGNETIC HEALERS

Spinal manipulation is one of the oldest and most widely practiced healing methods.[3] Manual and manipulative procedures have been depicted in the art and writing of most ancient cultures. References to spinal manipulation can be traced as far back as Hippocrates and Galen.[3] Although manipulation has been a part of orthopedic medical practice for centuries, the largest group of non-medical practitioners of spinal manipulation in the 19th century was known as the "bonesetters."[3,4] The bonesetters, who learned their skills primarily by apprenticeship and observation, rose to prominence during the mid 19th century in the USA by virtue of their willingness to fill a void in healthcare vacated by medical practitioners of the day.

At the end of the American Civil War, medicine was in a state of turmoil.[4] New scientific discoveries, coupled with the general ineffectiveness of allopathic treatment (which often included the use of toxic substances such as mercury or lead, and used other "heroic" methods such as bloodletting and purges), undermined the confidence of the public in medicine. More and more people were consulting "irregular" doctors. (In the 19th century, it was customary to describe medical physicians as "regular" and non-medical doctors as "irregulars"[4].) It should be noted that the popularity of these irregular doctors rivaled that of regular doctors, and the former group enjoyed a larger following and income level. At the same time, physicians started to place greater and greater importance on the nervous system, and

both osteopathy and chiropractic saw this organ system as the focal point of human disease.

In the mid 19th century, bonesetters, along with midwives, tooth-pullers and barber-surgeons, were often consulted by clients with healthcare problems that academically trained physicians of the time considered inconsequential or beneath their dignity to address.[4] For example, an article in the *British Medical Journal* in 1867 by Paget indicates that bonesetters often treated painful conditions caused by subluxation, which referred to "joint 'put out'; and the one method to cure [is] the wrench aid, the rough movement by which it is said that the joint is 'put in' again."[5]

Although bonesetting gave chiropractic its method, it was magnetic healing that provided the theory. Anton Mesmer was a pioneer in this area, and his research examined the (supposed) curative properties of magnetism in the late 1780s.[4,6] He believed that there was a fluid or force that filled the universe but was concentrated in an animal's nervous system and in magnets. Furthermore, he surmised that planets and stars exerted a magnetic influence on the cosmic fluids within each and every person. Aberrations of these forces would then result in disease. However, healers could be trained to use their hands or a magnet to correct these wayward forces, and thus the field of magnetic healing was born. Some time later in his career, Mesmer would place his patients in a state of trance or "somnambulic" state. Persons in this semi-conscious state were exceptionally responsive to instructions. These "mesmerized" patients could, they claimed, perceive light coming out of magnets, crystals, and the human body. Mesmer also began using the *baquet*, a large covered tub filled with water, from which iron rods projected. Patients would be tied together in a circle, and would have these iron rods applied to afflicted areas of the body, whereupon they might start to convulse, vomit, or cry, and were eventually declared to be cured.[6]

Magnetic healers posited that the unimpeded flow of energy accorded health, whereas obstructed flow resulted in disease. DD Palmer, who was predominantly a magnetic healer, directed these theories to the nervous system in his development of what would become chiropractic. In his words, "chiropractic was not evolved from medicine or any other method, except that of magnetic."[6]

The field of radionics also played a role in the development of early chiropractic theories.[6] Advocates of this approach theorized that all matter "radiated" at certain wavelengths. In particular, it was thought that living tissue emitted energy that was a reflection of its vitality and state of health. Thus, practitioners who were able to measure this radiation could arrive at a diagnosis and a treatment plan. Radiesthesia practitioners, such as Albert Abrams MD, claimed to be able to detect electromagnetic waves being emitted by patients.[6] According to Morgan,[6] Abrams enhanced this process by attaching a wire from a patient's spinal lesion to a healthy person's cervical vertebrae. Abrams went still further, claiming that by percussing the spine while facing the patient in an east or west direction, he could detect the presence of organic disease. Abrams believed that each disease had its own characteristic wavelength and devised a rheostat to measure patient emissions. Eventually, Abrams developed the Oscilloclast, better known as the "Black Box," a device with which Abrams believed he could diagnose a patient's disease and treat it by means of measured vibration. The Black Box was eventually prohibited under the 1976 US Pure Food, Drug and Cosmetic Act. We are unable to escape the temptation to compare all this to the supposed mechanism and fate of the Toftness Radiation Detector (Ch. 30).

Some researchers and historians suggest that advances in the field of electricity may have also influenced the chiropractic "nerve flow" theory.

DD PALMER: THE FIRST CHIROPRACTOR

There is evidence to suggest that DD Palmer had some training as a bonesetter, and his work as a magnetic healer is well established. Palmer revised the theory of traditional magnetism to "innate intelligence" (Ch. 2), which focused on the concept that the body possessed inherent healing abilities.[4] Palmer claimed that it was the nervous system, with particular emphasis on the spinal cord and nerve roots, that served as the pathway through which innate intelligence functioned. Palmer adopted the theory of magnetism and combined it with the bonesetter's definition of subluxation; the net effect was a model of health that theorized that misaligned spinal vertebrae impinged the flow of innate intelligence to cause illness. In addition, DD Palmer eschewed the use of drugs or surgery as an unnatural invasion into the body, instead focusing on the normalization of nervous function as the key to optimal health.[4] Some time later, DD's son, BJ Palmer, would develop this model further and suggested that specifically adjusting a patient's atlas would "emancipate the imprisoned rivulets of life force."

DD Palmer opined that disease had three general causes: mechanical, chemical, and psychic irritation (autosuggestion) of the nervous system.[7] Thus, the groundwork for the four components of a vertebral subluxation within Palmer's tonal-based model was laid. These were: (1) a vertebra is out of normal alignment in relationship with the segments above or below, resulting in (2) occlusion of the foramen (spinal or intervertebral) which (3) applies pressure on corresponding nerves, thereby (4) interfering with and interrupting the normal quality of mental impulses.[8] Given the advances in 19th-century science demonstrating the importance of the nervous system in human physiology, it is not surprising that Palmer would deduce that this cascade of events could detrimentally affect health.

In addition to merging the traditions of bonesetters and magnetic healing, Palmer also synthesized what was at the time orthodox science and popular health reform.[4] As early as the 1820s, medical physicians often cited "spinal irritation" as a cause of disease (although it is possible they were referring to what would be called "depression" today), and Palmer's adaptation of this theory to what would evolve into chiropractic gave the profession a firm scientific basis upon which to build. At the same time there was a blossoming of non-medical or irregular healers in the USA, including homeopaths, providers of herbal medicines and Christian Scientists. As is the case today, these early complementary and alternative medicine providers pointed toward the limitations of conventional medicine while simultaneously claiming that miraculous cures were, in fact, obtainable while under their care. Thus, chiropractic offered a unique blending of alternative, complementary

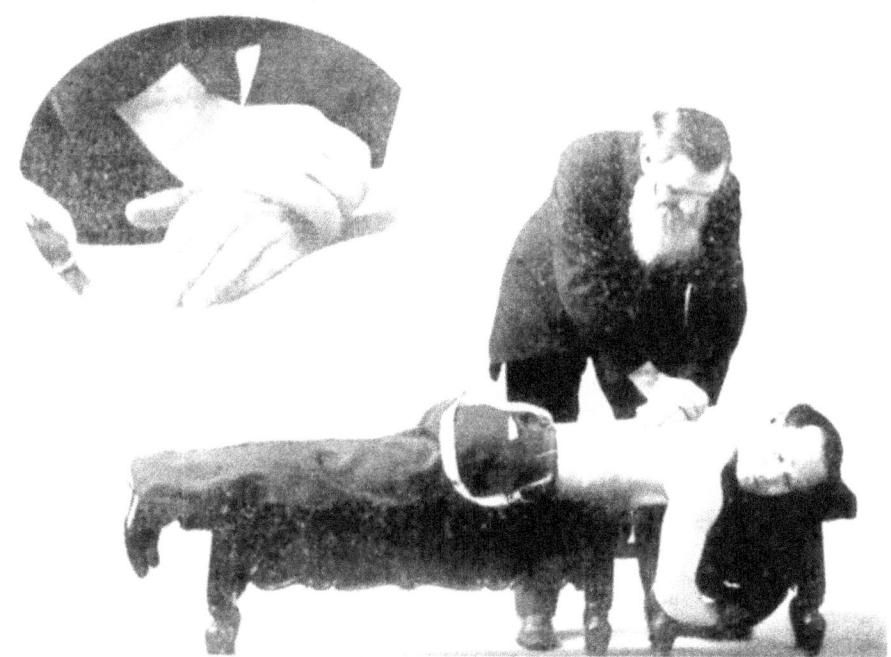

Figure 34.1 One of the few photographs of DD Palmer giving an adjustment. Reproduced from Palmer DD, Palmer BJ with permission.

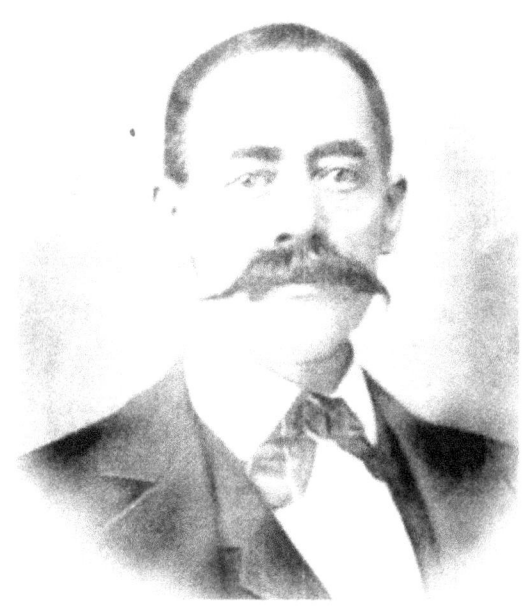

Figure 34.2 Harvey Lillard, an African-American who operated a janitorial service in the Ryan building, was DD's first chiropractic patient. Ironically, it would be over 50 years before the Palmer School would admit African-Americans. Courtesy of the Palmer College of Chiropractic Archives. Davenport, IA.

and contemporary approaches to health and healing, a formula still apparent in modern times.[4]

DD Palmer went still further in his thinking on the nervous system (Fig. 34.1). He theorized that the nervous system should have a normal or optimal tone, and that, by extension, any alteration in this tone was the cause of disease. As he stated in his book *The Chiropractor's Adjustor*:

Life is the expression of tone. In that sentence is the basic principle of chiropractic. Tone is the normal degree of nerve tension. Tone is expressed in functions by normal elasticity, activity, strength and excitability of the various organs, as observed in a state of health. Consequently, the cause of disease is any variation of tone – nerves too tense or too slack.[9]

DD Palmer's first patient was a deaf janitor named Harvey Lillard (Fig. 34.2). On 18 September 1895, so the story goes, Lillard related the story of his hearing loss to DD while cleaning his office. Lillard had lost his hearing 17 years earlier, as he stooped over in a cramped position trying to move an object. He felt something give way in his mid-back and immediately became deaf. Palmer examined Lillard's spine and found vertebral segments "racked" from their normal position. Theorizing that this was interfering with Lillard's nerve function, Palmer convinced Lillard to allow him to "rack" the vertebra back to its proper position. The adjustment was delivered, and Lillard's hearing was restored.[4,7]

Some of the facts of this event are often misinterpreted. For example, in an otherwise accurate and articulate article in the *Archives of Internal Medicine* discussing chiropractic's origins and controversies, Kaptchuk and Eisenberg[4] erroneously report that DD adjusted Lillard's atlas vertebra, whereas the historical truth is that DD probably adjusted Lillard's mid-back. The reason for this misunderstanding, and why the distinction between the two versions is important, will become apparent in the discussion below.

It is an important historical footnote that Palmer is credited as the founder of chiropractic not because he was the first to adjust the spine (he clearly was not, as bonesetters predated him by centuries), nor because he was the first to consider the nervous system as fundamental to human health (again, this was an adaptation from traditional magnetic healing). Instead, Palmer was the first healer to state that he was adjusting a vertebral segment by the method of using vertebrae as levers for the sole purpose of restoring nervous tone. In addition, Palmer is the father of the "bone-out-of-place" theory, or the later-renamed "segmental approach theory" that enjoys a measure of popularity even today.[7]

Despite these results, Palmer's transition from magnetic healer to chiropractor was slow. His new chiropractic practice became quite successful, and DD earned over $9200 in 1898, this at a time when the average medical doctor was earning between $1000 and $1500[10] (as referenced by Perle[11]). According to Wardwell,[12] DD was rather secretive about his discovery. Based on this success, DD founded the Chiropractic School of Cure in 1897 in Davenport, Iowa, although he initially did not accept any students into the program.[11] However, after a nearly fatal accident, Palmer was concerned that his discovery of chiropractic might die with him. Thus, he accepted the first five students into this school in 1898.[12] The 6-month $500 program taught students how

to adjust all the articulations in the body, with a particular emphasis on the spine.[12] Perle notes that it is an interesting historical footnote that the first 12 graduates from Palmer's school were either medical doctors or osteopaths.[11] In addition to learning how to correct anatomical misalignment, students were taught how to correct chemical imbalances and adverse mental thoughts (autosuggestion).[7]

BJ PALMER: CHIROPRACTIC'S DEVELOPER

An equally central figure in chiropractic history, BJ Palmer was trained by his father to be a chiropractor (Fig. 34.3). In 1906, partly because DD was charged with practicing medicine without a license and was jailed for a time, and partly because of ongoing financial difficulties with his school, a court agreement transferred directorship and ownership to BJ for $2196.79, a few dozen books, and some osteological specimens (Fig. 34.4).[11] BJ assumed the mantle of power, and renamed the college the Palmer School of

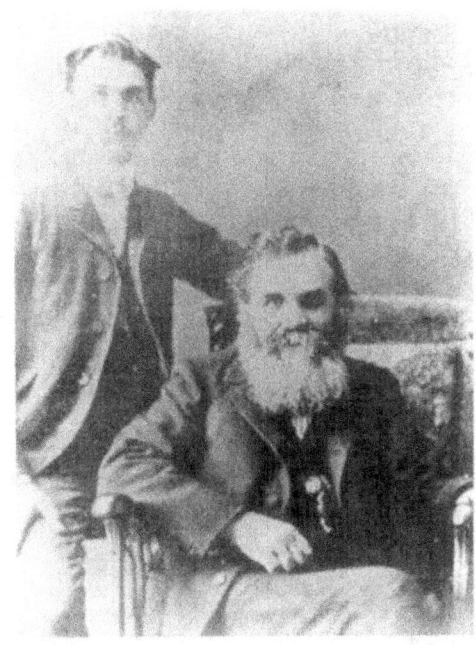

Figure 34.3 DD Palmer with his son, BJ, about the time BJ earned his degree in chiropractic. Courtesy of the Palmer College of Chiropractic Archives, Davenport, IA.

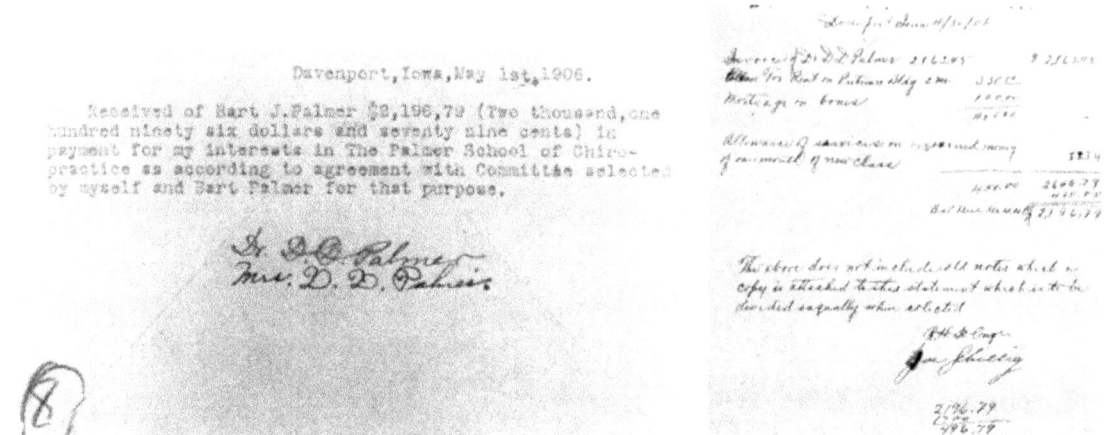

Figure 34.4 The purchase agreement whereby BJ Palmer purchased DD's half of the school for $2196.79. Courtesy of the Palmer College of Chiropractic Archives, Davenport, IA.

Chiropractic (PSC).[7] According to Gibbons,[13] (as cited by Perle[11]) such was the hegemony exerted by BJ at the PSC that any correspondence to the college could only be addressed to himself or to the college, not to any other individual.[13]

DD Palmer left Iowa somewhat broken-hearted, and continued until his death to denigrate his son.[11] DD eventually traveled to Oklahoma (where he established two chiropractic schools), Portland, California, and Oregon. In a recent article, Keating[14] describes DD's role in the complex evolution of the chiropractic colleges in the western continental USA, that would eventually become Western States Chiropractic College. During his sojourn, DD continued to develop the science of the profession, eventually moving away from the "foot on the garden hose" theory of nerve compression by misaligned vertebrae. While in Portland, DD wrote: "I doubt very much that nerves are pinched, squeezed or compressed anywhere. Nerves cannot be impinged between two bones, vertebrae or other joints."[14] (p. 46) Perhaps as a stab at his son, DD now rejected the bone-pinching-nerve concept and claimed that altered biomechanics (subluxations) changed the tension in nerves (making it too much or too little), thereby altering the neural messages reaching end-organs.[14] In essence, DD came to compare the functions of nerves to the vibrations of strings on musical instruments, asserting that: "The cause of

nearly all diseases is an over-supply of nerve force; therefore, we have fever."[9] (p. 60)

At least initially, BJ advocated the same philosophical model of chiropractic as his father. In his book *The Science of Chiropractic* (c. 1906), he stated that chiropractic was: "The science of cause of disease and art of adjusting by hand all sub-luxations of the three hundred articulations of the human skeletal frame, more especially the 52 articulations of the spinal column, for the purpose of freeing impinged nerves, as they emanate thro [sic] the intervertebral foramina, causing abnormal functions, in excess or not enough, named disease."[15] (p. xii) It is noteworthy that BJ felt that chiropractic was founded on mechanical adjusting and that the "pathology of therapeutics is not that of Chiropractors." Lastly, it was around this time that BJ's belief emerged that chiropractors do not treat the diseases of patients at all, but only their subluxations.[7]

In the later part of the 1910s, BJ instructed his students that they should restrict their adjustments to five or six of the "main" vertebrae, that adjusting any more might interfere with the innate ability to correct abnormal function.[7] He also believed that chiropractors should consider the possible effect of subluxation on the autonomic nervous system. This would eventually lead to the Meric system,[16] described in Chapter 19.

DISSENSION WITHIN THE RANKS: THE PROFESSION FRAGMENTS

Much of the fragmentation seen in the chiropractic profession in the early years can be traced to internecine fights, on the one hand between DD and BJ Palmer and, on the other hand, between the Palmers and their students, graduates, and faculty members. Many in the chiropractic profession were incensed with the dogmatic fundamentalism that emanated from the PSC, the "Fountainhead," and many founded chiropractic colleges in direct competition with it.

Even from the start, many of DD Palmer's first graduates saw flaws in his educational curriculum, especially in the area of his scientific theories. Three of these graduates, Oakley Smith, Solon Langworthy, and Minora Paxson, were so unhappy with DD's views that they founded the American School of Chiropractic and Nature Cure in 1903.[7] Interestingly enough, it was Langworthy who first used the term "subluxation" in chiropractic, and it was he who first emphasized the importance of the intervertebral foramen (IVF). According to Montgomery and Nelson,[7] it was Langworthy who theorized that subluxations at the IVF interfered with the "supremacy of the nerves." In addition, Smith, Langworthy, and Paxson, were the first chiropractors to publish a textbook of chiropractic theory, *Modernized Chiropractic* (1906),[17] which predated BJ Palmer's text by several weeks.

What is significant about *Modernized Chiropractic* is that the authors included elements of gait analysis, motion inspection, nerve traction, static and motion palpation, extremity adjusting, and postural analysis. Without doubt, their approach was inherently more dynamic and eclectic than DD's or BJ's model of chiropractic. However, because *Modernized Chiropractic* did not promote the same world-view held by BJ Palmer, he did not recognize their book as a chiropractic text and instead insisted that his own book, *The Science of Chiropractic*, had been the first published chiropractic text.[7]

Another early dissenter from the sway of the Palmers was Willard Carver (Fig. 34.5). A friend, patient, and lawyer to DD, Carver, upon graduation as a chiropractor, developed the *structural approach* to chiropractic technique, in which the

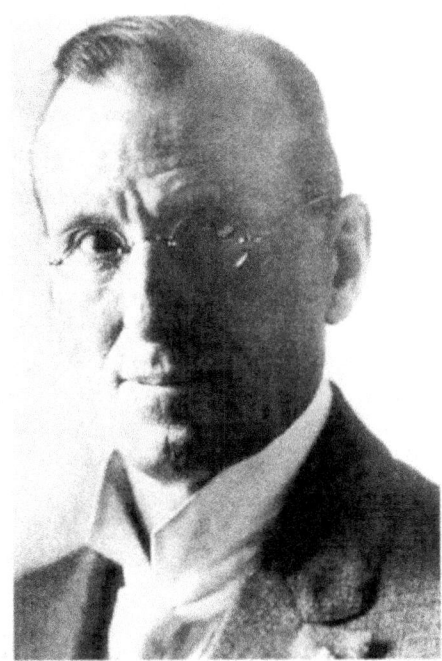

Figure 34.5 Willard Carver, a lawyer and close family friend of "Old Dad Chiro," was an important figure who influenced a number of early chiropractic leaders. Dr. Carver's lectures and books added a scientific dimension to the profession. A prolific writer, "The Constructor" established four separate schools of chiropractic in Oklahoma, Colorado, New York, and Washington DC. Courtesy of the Palmer College of Chiropractic Archives, Davenport, IA.

spinal column is a weight-bearing, gravity-resisting structure that adapts to different stressors on it, based on the laws of mechanical engineering. It was the breakdown of these adaptive strategies, Carver theorized, that led to subluxations, and ultimately disease. This structuralist (i.e., postural, or regional) approach to chiropractic technique greatly expanded upon the strictly segmental views of BJ Palmer.[16] It seems that Carver was given the derogatory epithet "mixer" from BJ,[16] largely because he displayed an open distaste for proprietary technique systems, for which reason he established the Carver Chiropractic College. This college extended the length of the curriculum from 9 months to 3 years, and promoted a greater grounding in the scientific basis of the health arts.[7] According to many historians, Carver referred to himself as the "Science Head" and "Constructor of Chiropractic", in contrast to BJ's titles of the

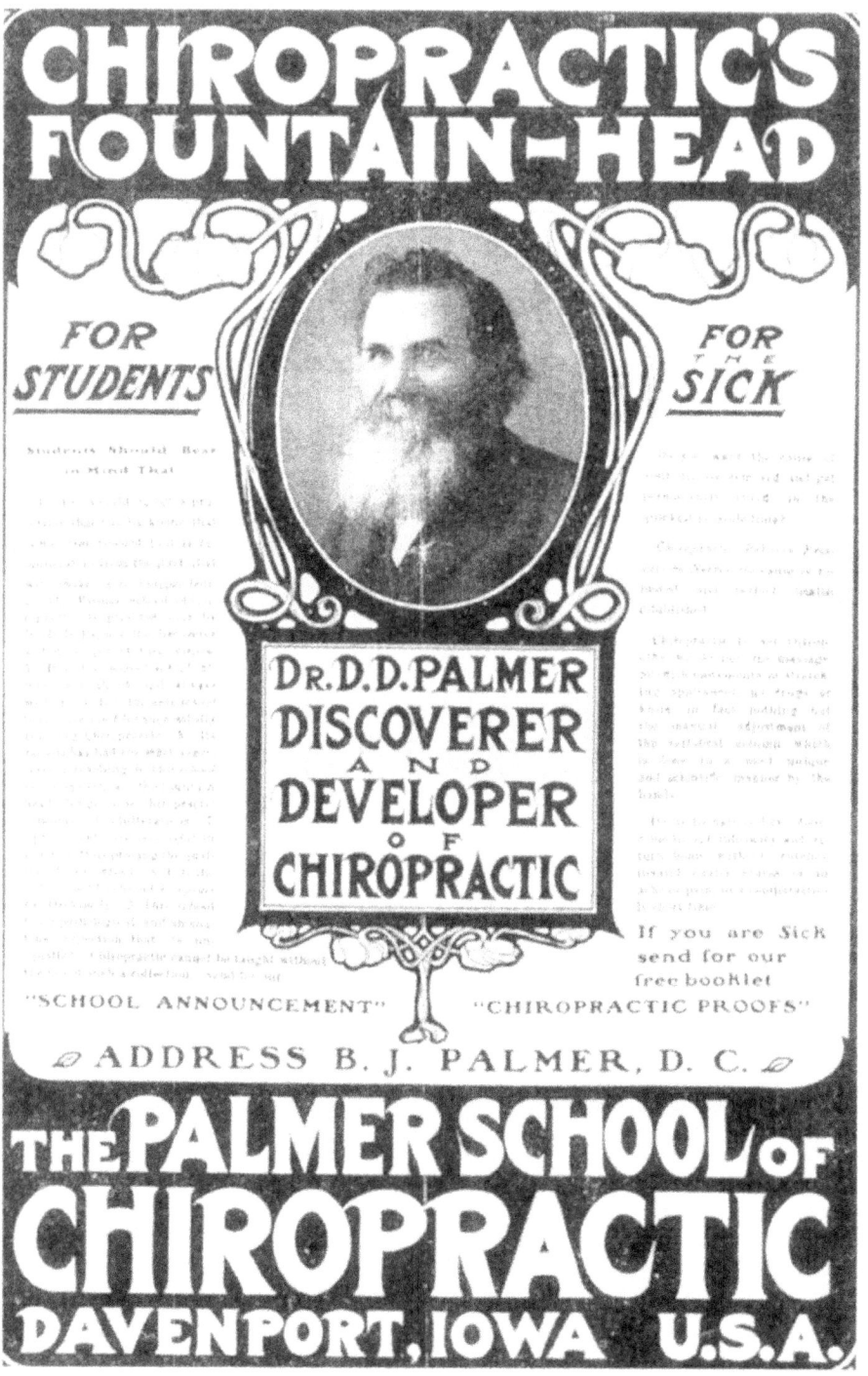

Figure 34.6   This example of DD Palmer's advertising of his Chiropractic Fountain-head was targeted at prospective students and patients. Courtesy of the Palmer College of Chiropractic Archives, Davenport, IA.

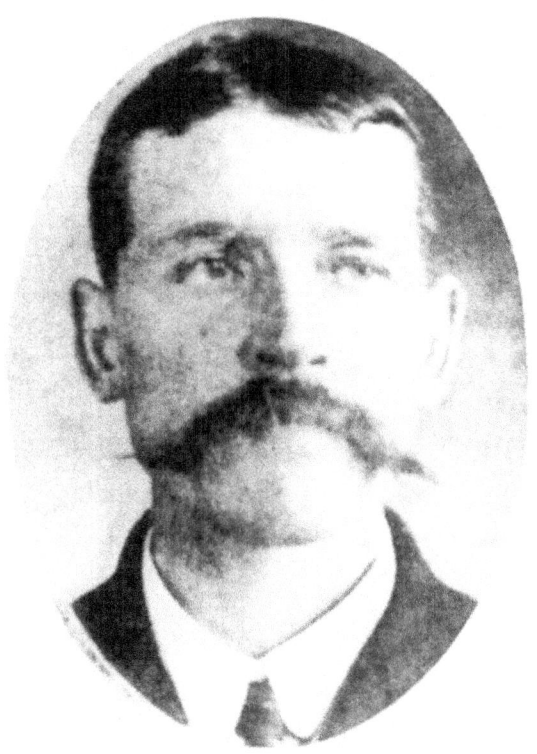

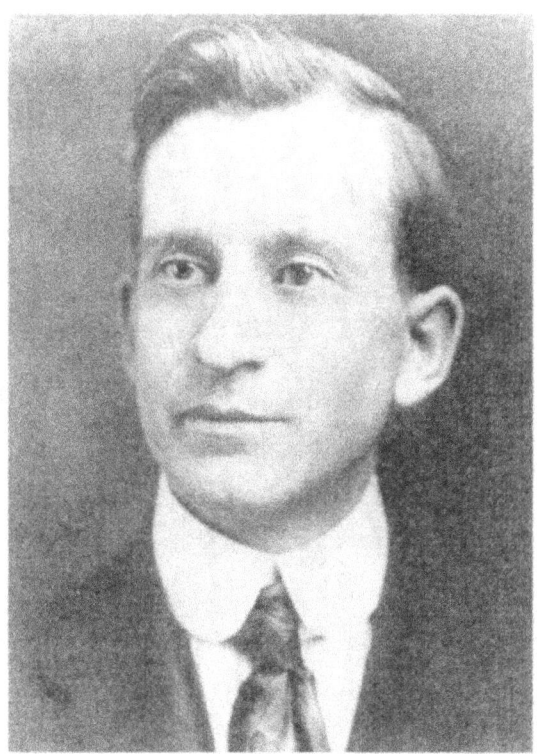

Figure 34.7 John FA Howard, DC (1876–1954), founder of the National School of Chiropractic, 1906. Reproduced from Palmer DD, Palmer BJ with permission.

Figure 34.8 Joy M Loban, a protégé of BJ Palmer's, was to leave the Palmer School of Chiropractic in 1910 and establish Universal Chiropractor College in Davenport, which moved to Pittsburgh, PA, in 1918. He was also the author of several textbooks, including *Textbook of Neurology*. Courtesy of the Palmer College of Chiropractic Archives, Davenport, IA.

"Fountainhead" and "Developer of Chiropractic (Fig. 34.6)."[18]

In 1906, John Howard (Fig. 34.7), a new graduate, disturbed by Palmer's reluctance to furnish cadavers for anatomy classes, suggested that BJ increase the amount and quality of human dissection in the curriculum. He also objected to BJ Palmer's blend of "Specific, Pure and Unadulterated" chiropractic.[16] "He became overzealous," said Howard. "He claimed that all disease is due to subluxations of the vertebrae and that all diseases could be eradicated by adjustment of the vertebrae. He derided all other forms of therapy, and persisted in his original views to the end."[19]

Unable to abide the behavior and actions of BJ, Howard started his own school, the National College of Chiropractic, and made what we see as important pedagogical improvements in chiropractic education.[7] The college eventually became more medically oriented when Howard formed

a partnership with a medical doctor, William Schulze, in 1910.[16] In addition to a greater emphasis on dissection, National College introduced training in physiotherapy and other ancillary techniques, including hydrotherapy, muscle techniques, massage, and remedies both internally and externally applied.[16] It was this use of "physiological therapeutics" that was at the core of the never-ending and bitter mixer-straight debate between Howard and BJ Palmer,[13, 16] and Howard was the particular target of much of BJ's vitriol.[11]

There were other challenges to BJ's reign at the Palmer College. Joy Loban (Fig. 34.8), chair of philosophy, objected to the introduction of X-rays to chiropractic by BJ in the early 1910s (Fig. 34.9); by then, BJ had established the first and finest X-ray laboratory of any healing institution.[7,13,16] Loban

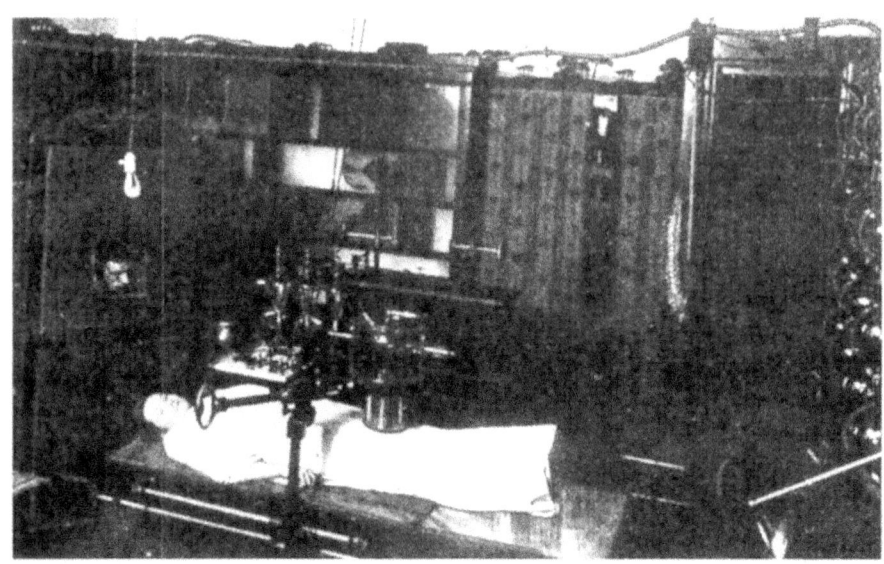

Figure 34.9   An early X-ray unit being used at the Palmer School of Chiropractic, 1911. Reproduced from Annual Announcement, Davenport, IA, 1911, Palmer School of Chiropractic.

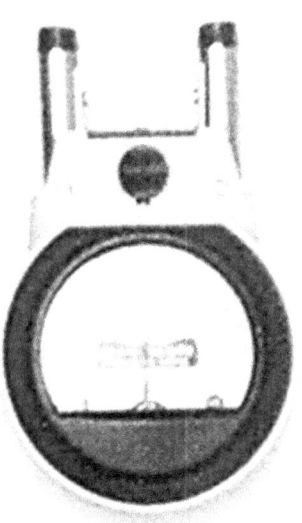

Figure 34.10   An early neurocalometer, which BJ Palmer introduced to the profession at the Palmer School of Chiropractic's August 1924 Lyceum. From Logan College of Chiropractic Archives, Chesterfield, MO.

felt that the use of X-ray was against the very principles of the profession, which he felt should be "hands only." Loban and BJ being unable to reconcile their differences, Loban gave a passionate and stirring oration before his philosophy class, after which he, along with 50 of his students, picked themselves up and left the Palmer campus. They established the Universal College of Chiropractic, and also located it in Davenport, Iowa.[7]

Although DD Palmer himself believed that nerve pressure would create "an increased amount of heat," the first measuring device was not built until 1924 by Dossa Evins (Ch. 8). Evins took his thermographic device, the neurocalometer (NCM: Fig. 34.10), to the Palmer College where it was used before and after adjustments to show that nerve pressure had been present and eliminated. BJ Palmer was so enamored with the device that he came to the conclusion that it was not possible to practice as a true chiropractic without using the device. For the 1924 Lyceum (essentially a homecoming for the PSC), BJ let it be known that his speech would have tremendous repercussions throughout the profession.[11] In his "The hour has struck" address, Palmer announced that chiropractors must start to use the NCM to determine the location of nerve interference, even though up to this very moment he had warned against using instrumentation of any kind. In BJ's words: "no chiropractor can practice chiropractic without a NCM ... no chiropractor can render an efficient competent or honest service without the NCM"[14] (referenced in Perle[11]).

BJ, ever the entrepreneur, insisted that chiropractors should henceforth use the NCM or essentially be excommunicated from chiropractic. This was distasteful for many in the field, since BJ owned the patent to the neurocalometer, and thus obtained tremendous financial gain by its lease.[16] The débâcle was so extreme that BJ Palmer lost much of his influence over the profession for decades, even though thermography continued to interest many practitioners. The NCM could not be purchased outright, and the $3500 NCM was leased to practitioners at a cost of $5 a month.[11] Many of PSC's leading faculty members were unimpressed by his coupling of narrow dogmatism and commercial motivation, and, according to Gibbons,[14] were also kept in the dark on the NCM research (although Keating sees this as hardly possible[20]). Many resigned, and four of them, notably James N Firth, Harry E Vedder, Stephen J Burich, and Arthur C Hendricks (the Big Four) founded the Lincoln Chiropractic College.[18] The new college was based on a diversity of adjustive techniques, and promoted a philosophy more in keeping with the traditions of DD Palmer. In this philosophy, nerve interference and interference with innate intelligence could occur anywhere a subluxation could be found in the body. The Big Four, in an effort to elude Palmer's autocratic position in the profession, developed what could be called a "proto-diversified" technique.[16]

Another major shift in BJ's thinking occurred when he evolved the Upper Cervical concept, which was in the air at the Palmer College in the late 1920s (Ch. 32). He left the realm of segmentalism and turned his attention exclusively to focus on the upper cervical region, now believing that the subluxations of the atlas were the cause of all disease.[7] BJ introduced the concept of the primacy of the upper cervical subluxation, apparently emphasizing axis at first, to his contemporaries in the early spring of 1930. He felt by this time that it was only here that there could be interference with

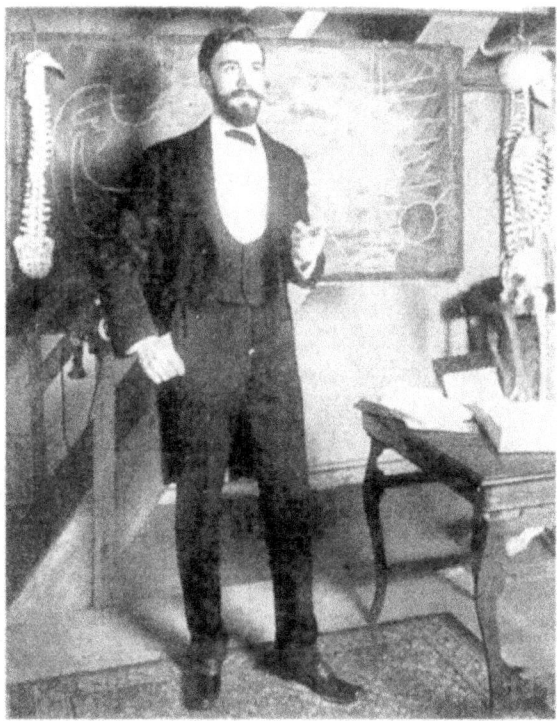

Figure 34.11   BJ Palmer (1882–1961) delivering lectures in the lecture hall of the Palmer School of Chiropractic. Courtesy of the Palmer College of Chiropractic Archives, Davenport, IA.

the neurological connection between the brain and the rest of the body. In his words:

no chiropractor has or ever will adjust a vertebral segment below the axis ... no person has ever gotten well because of any chiropractor ever having adjusted a subluxation below the atlas ... and it is impossible to have any misalignment with occlusion, with pressure, with interference at any intervertebral foramen anywhere else along the spinal column in lower cervical, thoracic or lumbar vertebrae.[15] (p. 67)

It was from this model that BJ pronounced "that everything within the chiropractic philosophy, science and art works from above-down, inside-out. Anything and everything outside that scope is medicine, whether you like it or not" (referenced in Wardwell[12]). BJ theorized that subluxation of the atlas or the axis led to disease, resulting from superior brain congestion, inferior body starvation, or a combination of the two (Fig. 34.11).[13] In his words: "The brain would become energy-clogged and the body energy-empty."[21] (p. 96)

Not all of the chiropractors who had previously followed BJ every step of the way were equally enthused to learn that "Every case you and I ever got well through adjustment was an accident." The toggle-recoil adjustive approach, although originally used in full-spine adjusting, was adapted for atlas adjusting by BJ himself. The practitioner applies a quick thrust and then quickly releases the contact, in theory creating a recoiling effect.[16] Palmer believed that this maneuver removed any nerve interference and allowed the body's innate intelligence to restore the vertebral segment to its proper anatomic position (Ch. 23). (This may explain why several articles on chiropractic, such as the one by Kaptchuk and Eisenberg[4] erroneously reported that DD adjusted Lillard's atlas, and not his mid thoracic spine.[7])

Some historians believe that BJ Palmer's sudden focus on upper cervical adjustments and the importance of the atlas to a person's health may have come from a conversation he had with AA Wernsing, a Palmer College faculty member.[7] Some historians go still further and suggest the entire Upper Cervical theory was Wernsing's concept, and not BJ's.[16]

In adopting Upper Cervical theory and practice, BJ wound up leaving himself without an explanation for the seminal case in the creation of chiropractic origin, the restoration of Lillard's hearing 40 years earlier when DD had adjusted the fourth thoracic segment, and not atlas. BJ simply suggested that it was Lillard's atlas that had been adjusted, and not the thoracic spine after all. According to Stowell, BJ's dogmatic adherence to the theory that all disease results from atlas subluxation prompted him to remove from the PSC curriculum "all learning and knowledge, all inquiry and scientific research which did not fit with this premise."[18] (pp. 75–76)

CONCLUSIONS

We have described how chiropractic technique fragmented during its first decade, a process that continues to the present. The model for technique bifurcations, often associated with considerable acrimony, accrues to the Palmers themselves, who by their example set the stage for all that was to follow. Despite the negative implications of these remarks, the news is not all bad. Out of the technique wars that were to come, the very competitiveness of chiropractic technique systems led to true innovations, of the type that rarely emerge from a complacent harmony. We describe this phenomenon in Chapter 36.

Ironically, as the years went by, Diversified Technique, the body of chiropractic methodology that had originated as a liberating, eclecticizing response to the myriad of narrowly defined and often cultistic technique systems of the day, found itself more than occasionally arranged alongside, rather than alternative to them – as yet another technique system.[22] However paradoxically, it appears that modern Diversified Technique is chiefly distinguished from all of the others by its poor distinction from any one of them.

REFERENCES

1. Zemelka W H 1992 The Thompson Technique. Victoria Press, Bettendorf, IO
2. Nelson C 1993 Five steps to your own technique: the Nelson method. Journal of Manipulative and Physiological Therapeutics 16 (2): 115–117
3. Meeker W C, Haldeman S 2002 Chiropractic: a profession at the crossroads of mainstream and alternative medicine. Annals of Internal Medicine 136: 216–227
4. Kaptchuk T J, Eisenberg D M 1998 Chiropractic. Origins, controversies and contributions. Archives of Internal Medicine 158: 2215–2224

5. Paget J 1867 Cases that bonesetters cure. British Medical Journal 1: 1–4, 15
6. Morgan L 1998 Innate intelligence: its origins and problems. Journal of the Canadian Chiropractic Association 42 (1): 35–41
7. Montgomery D P, Nelson J M 1985 Evolution of chiropractic theory of practice and spinal adjustment, 1900–1950. Chiropractic History 5: 71–76
8. Boone W R, Dobson G J 1996 A proposed vertebral subluxation model reflecting traditional concepts and recent advances in health and science. Journal of Vertebral Subluxation Research 1 (1): 19–30

9. Palmer D D 1910 The chiropractor's adjustor', p. 60. Portland Printing House, Portland, OR

10. Keating J C 1997 BJ of Davenport: the early years of Chiropractic. Association for the History of Chiropractic, Davenport, IA

11. Perle S M 2000 Concept paper on chiropractic. Unpublished manuscript

12. Wardwell W I 1992 Chiropractic: history and evolution of a new profession. Mosby-Year Book, St Louis, MO

13. Gibbons R W 1992 Medical and social protest as part of hidden American history. In: Haldeman S (ed.) Principles and practice of chiropractic, 2nd edn, p. 15–28. Appleton & Lange, East Norwalk, CT

14. Keating J C 2002 Early chiropractic education in Oregon. Journal of the Canadian Chiropractic Association 46 (1): 39–60

15. Palmer B J 1906 The science of chiropractic. Palmer School of Chiropractic, Davenport, IA

16. Cooperstein R 1995 On Diversified Chiropractic Technique. Journal of Chiropractic Humanities 5 (1): 50–55

17. Smith O G, Langworthy S M, Paxson M C 1906 Modernized chiropractic. Lawrence Press, Cedar Rapids, MO

18. Stowell C C 1983 Lincoln College and the "Big Four": a chiropractic protest, 1926–1962. Chiropractic History 3 (1): 75–78

19. Forster A I. 1915 Principles and practice of spinal adjustment. National School of Chiropractic, Chicago, IL.

20. Keating J C 1991 Introducing the Neurocalometer: a view from the fountainhead. Journal of the Canadian Chiropractic Association 35 (3): 165

21. Palmer B J 1934 Subluxation specific – adjustment specific. Palmer School of Chiropractic, Davenport, IO

22. Cooperstein R 1995 Diversified technique. Core of chiropractic or "just another technique system"? Journal of Chiropractic Humanities 5 (1): 50–55

35

Current and future utilization rates and trends

According to many authorities who specialize in the field, demographics can explain two-thirds of everything.[1] Demographics can trace past trends and patterns of behaviors, it can access the current state of affairs, and it can often accurately predict events yet to come. For example, a review of the demographic profile of American and Canadian populations reveals the rectangularization (the increased probability of survival to older ages) of the population pyramid with the aging of the Baby Boomers, those individuals born between 1946 and 1963.[2] Government officials, administrators, and other social planners must be cognizant of this information to make long-term plans in the areas of healthcare, housing, transportation, and recreation. In much the same way, educators at chiropractic colleges, as well as both regulatory bodies and third-party payers, must know which techniques are being utilized more frequently by practitioners in the field in order to make more rational decisions in the areas of curricula content, reimbursement schedules, and professional practice guidelines (Ch. 37).

GENERAL UTILIZATION RATES OF CHIROPRACTIC SERVICES IN THE USA

Chiropractic is the third largest healthcare discipline in North America, following medicine and dentistry. It is the largest, most regulated and best recognized of the complementary and alternative medicine (CAM) providers, and the only system of healing indigenous to the USA.[3] Among CAM providers, chiropractors are consulted more often than any other group.[3] One need look no further than the media and popular culture to see that chiropractic is now firmly entrenched in mainstream USA. Television shows such as *Seinfeld*, *The Simpsons*, and *Sex and the City* have all aired episodes that revolved around the lead character's experience with chiropractors. Howard Stern, a popular icon of morning radio, described his experience with a chiropractor in his first best-selling book, *Private Parts* (see Further reading). If what chiropractors do were relatively unknown, the humor would be lost on audiences. In contrast, these satires did not describe the practice or existence of, for example, naturopaths or homeopaths, given their current relative obscurity in North American culture.

Utilization rates for chiropractic care have tripled in the past two decades from about 3.6% to approximately 11%.[3] Two studies by Eisenberg et al[4,5] are the most-cited references documenting the changes in utilization rates of chiropractic and other CAM providers during the 1990s. The second study by Eisenberg et al, from the year 1998,[5] reported that 50% of respondents had been to a CAM practitioner, an almost 50% increase from their original study published in the early 1990s.[4] The researchers calculated that this represented an increase from 427 million total visits in 1990 to 629 million visits (by 22 million people) in 1997, a number that exceeded the total visits to all US primary-care physicians.[5] The total cost for seeing CAM providers was conservatively estimated to exceed $21.2 billion in 1997, with over $12 billion paid for by patients out-of-pocket. Many third-party payers, such as Workers' Compensation, Medicare,

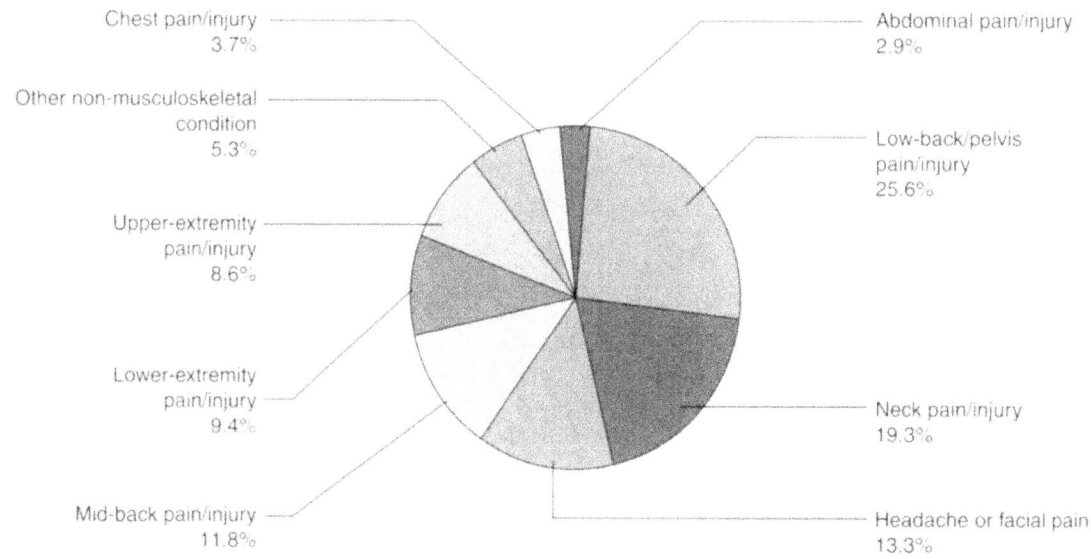

Figure 35.1 Chief complaints of chiropractic patients. Reproduced from *Job Analysis of Chiropractic 2000*,[8] with permission.

and all forms of managed care (including health maintenance organizations) pay for the services rendered by CAM providers.[3] In particular, 50% of health maintenance organizations and more than 75% of private health insurance plans now offer chiropractic services; and, under order of the US Congress, the military healthcare system has initiated a series of demonstration projects to investigate the feasibility of providing chiropractic services to military personnel.[3]

According to Eisenberg et al, the average demographic profile of a CAM user was that of a Caucasian, age 25–49 years, and of higher education and higher income than non-users of CAM services.[5] Women were more likely to consult with a CAM provider; African-Americans were the least likely. Usage of CAM therapies was more common than usage of conventional providers for 5 of the 10 most frequently cited medical conditions. The most common chief complaints that prompted patients to consult with a CAM provider were, in descending order: chronic low-back and neck pain, anxiety, depression, headache, fatigue, insomnia, arthritis, and sprains and strains, with one-third of patients presenting with more than one of these problems.[5] Patients with back problems, neck problems, headaches, and strains and sprains were more likely to seek out chiropractic care than other

CAM therapies. Not surprisingly, most clinical investigations into the effectiveness of chiropractic care have focused on these conditions, particularly spinal manipulation and low-back pain.[3,6] That said, there have been some studies that report that patients with more severe medical conditions, such as prostatic cancer, also consult a CAM provider in addition to their medical physician.[7] Lastly, visits to chiropractors and massage therapists accounted for nearly half of all visits to CAM practitioners in 1997.[5]

The *Job Analysis of Chiropractic 2000*, produced by the National Board of Chiropractic Examiners, (NBCE) reports that almost one-quarter of patients seeking chiropractic care present with low-back or pelvic pain or injury (Fig. 35.1).[8] In addition, approximately 20% of chiropractic patients present with neck pain or injury, and an additional 13% present with headache or facial pain.[8] The remaining chief complaints of patients to chiropractors are evenly distributed between mid-back pain (11%), lower-extremity pain or injury (9.4%), and upper-extremity pain or injury (8.6%); 11.9% of patients present with "other conditions" (such as non-neuromusculoskeletal conditions, chest pain, and abdominal pain).[8] The *Job Analysis of Chiropractic* also reports that the most common reasons for which individuals sought care were

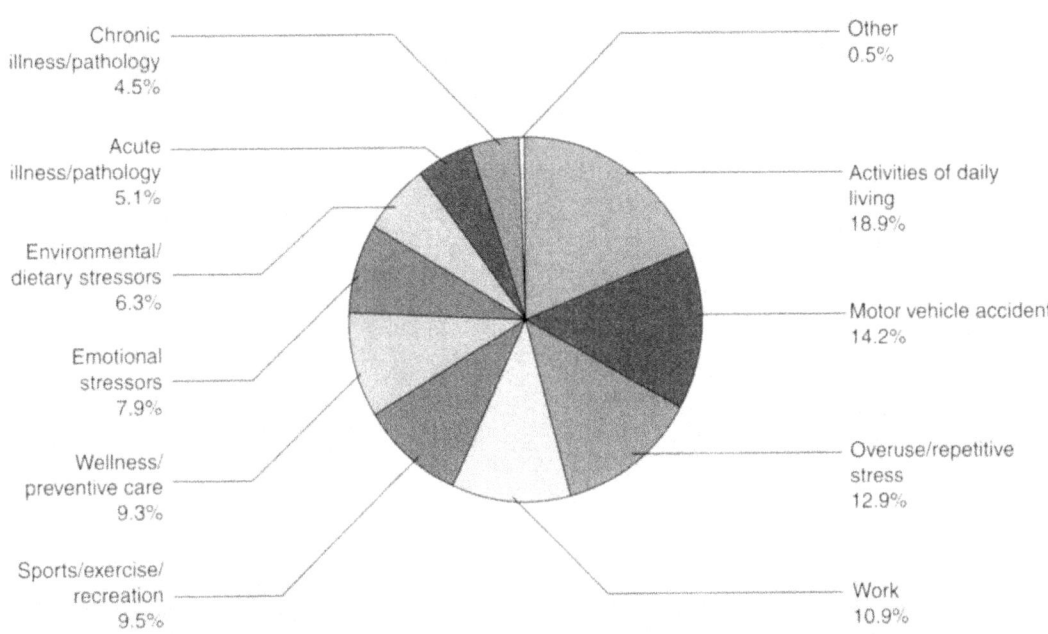

Figure 35.2 Primary etiology of patient conditions. Reproduced from *Job Analysis of Chiropractic 2000*,[8] with permission.

related to the activities of daily living (18.9%), motor vehicle accidents (14.2%), overuse and repetitive stress (12.9%), work (10.9%), sport/exercise/recreation (9.5%), wellness/prevention (9.3%), and emotional stress (7.9%; Fig. 35.2). Lastly, the *Job Analysis of Chiropractic* confirms the finding of Eisenberg et al,[5] in that the single largest group of persons seeking out chiropractic care (almost 32%) are Baby Boomers, those individuals between the ages of 31 and 50 years of age.[8]

National surveys conducted outside the USA suggest that CAM therapies are popular throughout the industrialized world. Studies have estimated that utilization rates of CAM providers are 10% in Denmark, 33% in Finland, and 49% in Australia.[5] Public opinion polls and consumers' associations suggest high utilization rates throughout the rest of Europe and the UK.[5] Other studies have estimated that 27 million Americans sought out chiropractic care in 1999.[9]

MEDICAL ATTITUDES ABOUT CAM

Another indicator of the increasing importance of chiropractic in the healthcare system is the apparent increase in interest in and acceptance of CAM

within the medical community. For example, of the 117 (of 125) medical schools in the USA that responded to a survey documenting information about CAM education within their curricula, 64% offered some type of CAM instruction.[10] Most classes offered were electives, although some institutions provided information within required courses. Common topics included chiropractic, acupuncture, homeopathy, herbal therapies, and mind–body techniques. In another study, when asked, 39% of medical physicians described chiropractic as a "legitimate medical practice"[10] – whether chiropractors appreciate that appellation or not.

Similar findings were recently reported with respect to Canadian physicians and their interest in CAM providers. In one study, 98 Canadian physiatrists were surveyed.[11] Seventy-two percent reported referring to a CAM therapist (12.5% referred often), 20% had training in, and 20% practiced some form of alternative medicine. According to the physicians in that study, the therapies most highly rated in terms of usefulness were acupuncture (85%), biofeedback (81%), and chiropractic (80%). Sixty-three percent of respondents thought alternative medicines had ideas and

Table 35.1 National Board of Chiropractic Examiners job analysis 1993

Adjustive technique	Percentage of American DCs using technique in past 2 years	Percentage of Canadian DCs using technique in past 2 years
Diversified	91.1	87.3
Gonstead	54.8	35.0
Cox Flexion–Distraction	52.7	22.3
Activator	51.2	43.6
Thompson Terminal Point	43.0	30.0
Sacro-Occipital Technique	41.3	44.2
Nimmo Technique	40.3	32.4
Applied Kinesiology	37.2	31.0
Logan Basic	30.6	25.9
Cranial	27.2	22.2
Palmer Hole-In-One	26.0	22.3
Meric	23.4	
Pierce–Stillwagon	19.7	
Pettibon	6.3	
Barge	4.1	
Grostic	3.4	
Toftness	3.3	
Life Upper Cervical	2.0	
Other	15.0	15.5

DC, doctor of chiropractic.
Adapted from Christensen et al.[8,14]

methods that would be beneficial to physiatrists. Less than 38.8% of respondents believed CAM worked via the placebo effect, and only 9% of this group thought CAM therapies were a threat to public health. This contrasts with an earlier 1990 study of Canadian family physicians that found that 21% felt CAM was a threat.[11] Of further interest, CAM referrals and utilization appeared to be higher in younger, more recently graduated physiatrists.[11]

NAME TECHNIQUE UTILIZATION IN THE USA

An unwaveringly simple historical pattern of utilization rates of chiropractic system techniques emerges within the USA, which can be captured by one word: fragmentation. As the previous chapter discussed, "chiropractors have been at war against themselves for 90 odd years,"[12] and "chiropractic techniques go on, with 'new' technics coming and going as frequently as women's fashions."[13] (p. 167)

The *Job Analysis of Chiropractic* of the NBCE[8] is the best source of data from which to draw information characterizing usage and practice patterns in the area of chiropractic technique systems. The

NBCE gathered data on what percentage of chiropractors use the primary technique systems, and in addition, what percentage of their patients actually receive each of these various techniques. On average, individual practitioners in the USA use seven different technique systems in their practices. The most commonly practiced technique was Diversified, practiced by 95.9% of respondents, who used it on 73.5% of their patients. Some 50–60% of respondents said they used Activator, Gonstead, Flexion–Distraction, Thompson, or Sacro-Occipital Technique (SOT); and about 40% used Applied Kinesiology or Nimmo Receptor-Tonus (Table 35.1). The percentage of patients receiving these last seven techniques ranged from 28.9% (Gonstead) to 14.5% (Applied Kinesiology).

A comparison of the results reported by the NBCE between 1993[14] and 2000[8] demonstrated an increased usage of the nine most commonly used techniques. For example, in 1993 (based on data collected in 1991), 51.2% of chiropractors used Activator Methods; in 1998, this number rose to 62.8% (Table 35.2). Similar trends of increased utilization rates are seen for Gonstead, Flexion–Distraction, Thompson, SOT, Applied Kinesiology, Nimmo/Receptor-Tonus, Cranial, and Palmer

Table 35.2   Percent and percent change of chiropractors using named techniques in 1991 and 1998

Adjustive procedure	Percentage of chiropractors using technique in 1991	Percentage of chiropractors using technique in 1998	Change in percentage (+ increase; − decrease)
Diversified	91.1	95.9	+4.8
Activator Methods	51.2	62.8	+11.6
Gonstead	54.8	58.5	+3.7
Cox Flexion–Distraction	52.7	58	+5.3
Thompson	43.0	55.9	+12.9
Sacro-Occipital Technique	41.3	49.0	+7.7
Applied Kinesiology	37.2	43.2	+6.0
Nimmo/Receptor-Tonus	40.3	40.0	−0.3
Palmer Hole-In-One	26.0	28.8	+2.8
Logan Basic	30.6	28.7	−1.9
Meric	23.4	19.9	−3.5
Pierce–Stillwagon	19.7	17.1	−2.6

Adapted from Christensen et al.[8]

Upper Cervical/Hole-In-One (HIO). There were slight decreases, probably insignificant, of 2% or less in the utilization rates of Logan Basic and Pierce–Stillwagon techniques.[8,14]

The popularity of technique systems is also apparent based on the current number of chiropractic colleges offering instruction in these techniques in either the core curriculum or as an elective program. In general, the chiropractic colleges in North America are about equally split between those colleges that emphasize generic technique, and those colleges that emphasize technique systems (Boxes 35.1 and 35.2). Chiropractic colleges that do not emphasize instruction in different technique systems in their core curricula often offer them as electives or as continuing education programs. Since prospective students often ask the admissions offices of chiropractic colleges "which techniques" are taught at the college, there is pressure on colleges that prefer teaching generic technique to find a way to teach technique systems in some way.

An example of the difficulty in determining which chiropractic technique is taught at which chiropractic college became apparent from a survey published in *Dynamic Chiropractic*.[15] Although much of the reported information was likely accurate, there were inaccuracies as well. For example, the survey inaccurately reported that Canadian Memorial Chiropractic College (CMCC) offers Activator and Gonstead in the postgraduate department. The article listed several techniques

Box 35.1   Chiropractic colleges emphasizing generic techniques

- Bridgeport Chiropractic College
- Canadian Memorial Chiropractic College
- Los Angeles Chiropractic College
- National Chiropractic College
- New York Chiropractic College
- Northwestern Chiropractic College
- Palmer College of Chiropractic
- Palmer College of Chiropractic-West
- Texas Chiropractic College
- Western States Chiropractic College

Box 35.2   Chiropractic colleges emphasizing technique systems in the core curriculum

- Cleveland (KC) Chiropractic College
- Cleveland (LA) Chiropractic College
- Life University
- Life West Chiropractic College
- Logan College of Chiropractic
- Parker College of Chiropractic
- Sherman College of Straight Chiropractic

that are "taught" at some colleges, whereas in fact they cannot be used in that college's outpatient clinic. This suggests that sometimes colleges briefly make students aware of particular technique systems, without really instructing in how to use them. We understand how a busy department chair may not make that distinction in responding to a survey, and also appreciate the pressures to exaggerate the extent to which specific technique systems are taught at some of the colleges.

NAME TECHNIQUE UTILIZATION IN CANADA

For those who study demographic trends, Canada offers a unique opportunity to observe how powerful demographic influences can be. This is because the pattern of technique system usage by Canadian chiropractors has followed a much different path from that of their American counterparts. Before World War II, chiropractors in Canada were trained in the USA, and returned to practice the various technique systems they were taught. However, in 1945, the CMCC was established, the only chiropractic college in Canada until Université du Québec à Trois-Rivières (UQTR) opened its doors to students in Quebec in the mid-1990s.

It is important to note that, for the first 30 years or so, CMCC taught a variety of techniques in the core curriculum, including Gonstead, SOT, Applied Kinesiology, and Logan Basic, in addition to Diversified Technique.[16] However, by the mid-1970s, the college faculty had shifted to a motion-based functional model, and decided to make Diversified Technique the sole technique taught at CMCC. Since through the mid-1990s most of Canada's chiropractors were educated at CMCC, it is not surprising that Diversified Technique remained the most commonly used technique system. However, several factors have changed this pattern, and while Diversified Technique is still the most widely and commonly used technique in Canada (as in the USA), other technique systems are experiencing a rise in popularity in Canada hitherto not observed. This can be attributed to the confluence of two epidemiological causes: (1) an increase in the interest and use of technique systems by Canadian field practitioners; and (2) the large influx of American-trained Canadians back to Canada, who bring with them the technique systems they were taught abroad.[16]

It has been predicted that the number of Canadian chiropractors will have doubled in the decade following 1995, from 5000 to 10 000.[17] CMCC consistently graduates 150 students every year. Thus, in a 10-year span, 1500 new practitioners in Canada will have been CMCC graduates. The balance of 3500 will therefore graduate from primarily American chiropractic colleges. This assumption is supported by information from the Canadian Chiropractic Examining Board (CCEB).[18] The CCEB reports that 608 candidates sat for the Canadian Board Examinations (CBE) in 1999, compared to only 186 in 1992. In total, 1812 candidates sat for the CBE between 1995 and 1999. Of these candidates, only 730 were CMCC graduates (40%). The other candidates were graduates of Western States ($n = 194$), National College ($n = 155$), Palmer College West ($n = 150$), Northwestern College ($n = 102$), Palmer College ($n = 100$), and other chiropractic colleges ($n = 381$).[18]

TECHNIQUE SYSTEMS USED IN CANADA BY FIELD PRACTITIONERS

In 1993, the NBCE released its findings of a job analysis of chiropractors in Canada[14] reporting that 87.3% of Canadian chiropractors use Diversified Technique. In addition, 44.2% used SOT, 43.6% Activator, 37.7% Meric, 35.0% Gonstead, 32.4% Nimmo/Receptor-Tonus, 31% Applied Kinesiology, 30% Thompson, 25.9% Logan Basic, 22.4% Cox Flexion–Distraction, 22.3% Palmer HIO, 22.2% "cranial" techniques and 15.5% were listed as "other" techniques[14] (Table 35.1).

These numbers differed substantially from those collected for the Canadian Chiropractic Resource Databank (CCRD) by Kopansky-Giles and Papadopoulos in 1997.[17] The authors of that study conducted a practice pattern survey of Canadian chiropractors in 1995 ($n = 2587$). Seventy-two percent of respondents reported using Diversified on 76–100% of their patients, indicating up to one-quarter of Canadian chiropractors use other techniques as well. In addition, respondents reported using Activator (31.4%), SOT (18.8%), Thompson (14.3%), Gonstead (10.9%), Craniosacral (8.3%), and Palmer HIO (6.9%).[17]

It is not known why the utilization rates of technique systems by Canadian chiropractors reported by Kopansky-Giles and Papadopoulos are lower than those reported in the NBCE 1993 *Job Analysis of Chiropractic*. A more recent study indicated that utilization rates of system techniques by CMCC graduates tended be somewhat higher than those reported for the CCRD. Watkins and Saranchuk[19] conducted a survey of CMCC interns and recent graduates that sought to compare professional practice activities with the educational programming at CMCC. Their study sought to gather information pertaining to the techniques *primarily* and *regularly* utilized by CMCC graduates ($n = 325$) between 1993/4 and 1997/8 as well as techniques that fourth-year students ($n = 95$) thought they might primarily or regularly use after graduation. The survey revealed that 84.5% of students thought they would use Diversified Technique upon graduation. However, the same group of students also reported that they thought they would regularly use Activator (21.6%), Applied Kinesiology (15.5%), Craniosacral Therapy (14.4%), Thompson Terminal Point (12.4%), Motion Palpation Institute (MPI) (11.3%), Gonstead (11.3%), and other techniques (13.6%).[19]

The second part of this survey reported that utilization rates of technique systems among CMCC alumni were higher than those predicted by fourth-year student surveys. While 86.7% of CMCC graduates reported that they primarily used Diversified Technique in their clinical practices, 33.3% reported regularly using Activator Technique, 22% MPI, 20.7% Thompson Terminal Point, 11.3% Gonstead, 9.7% Craniosacral Therapy, 9.1% Palmer HIO, and 13.6% other technique systems[19] (Table 35.3).

INTEREST IN TECHNIQUE SYSTEMS AMONG CMCC STUDENTS

An examination of the interest in technique systems specifically among students at CMCC serves as a microcosm for demographic trends in this area, and may help to illustrate how the fluidity of the interest in technique system use impacts the profession as a whole.

Between 1996 and 2001, one of us (Gleberzon) has collated the data from an ongoing project that asks students to list and defend which, if any, of the different system techniques they would like to receive greater instruction in while at CMCC.[20] Over this 6-year period, 1250 students have submitted 595 reports. In general, students express the most interest in learning those techniques that would best integrate with the Diversified Technique currently taught at CMCC. In particular, almost 94% of student reports expressed interest in learning Thompson Terminal Point, 93% Activator Methods, 90% Gonstead, and 89% Active Release Therapy in the core curriculum, as an elective program, or in the continuing education program.[20]

HEEDING LESSONS LEARNED FROM DEMOGRAPHICS

This ongoing increase in utilization rates of chiropractic services, coupled with increased acceptance of chiropractic both within and without the

Table 35.3 Survey by Watkins and Saranchuk,[19] on the utilization rates of chiropractic techniques primarily and regularly utilized by Canadian Memorial Chiropractic College (CMCC) alumni (graduates from 1993/4 to 1997/8) ($n = 325$)

Adjustive technique	Technique primarily utilized by CMCC graduates (%)	Technique regularly utilized by CMCC graduates (%)
Diversified	86.7	11.1
Activator	17.8	33.3
Thompson Terminal Point	14.9	20.7
Motion Palpation Institute	10.7	22
Gonstead	6.1	11.3
Applied Kinesiology	4.2	6.5
Craniosacral	1.9	9.7
Palmer Hole-In-One	1.0	9.1
Other	9.7	13.6

medical community, underscores the importance of characterizing chiropractic treatment methods clearly. In the recent editorial previously mentioned, Philips implored the profession to, in his words, "bring order to our techniques."[15] The concern from Philips is that, since chiropractic is arguably the least standardized of all the health-care systems, a patient or referring doctor does not know what techniques a practitioner may use in his or her practice. Philips quite poignantly articulates that one problem of this non-standardization within the profession is that a patient may consult with a chiropractor who fails to meet his or her expectations based on previous care, and become disillusioned with the chiropractic profession as a whole. He also quite accurately argues that all accredited chiropractic programs do not teach the same adjustive techniques, nor do they necessarily teach the same ones equally well. The fault, he contends, is with the Council on Chiropractic Education (CCE), which neither sets appropriate guidelines for what technique courses are to be taught in the colleges, nor stipulates a minimum number of hours of training that should be given in any particular technique, so as to ensure competency. We are not entirely sure that the CCE should be getting down to that level of detail in defining standards for teaching chiropractic technique.

WHAT IS THE DIFFERENCE BETWEEN MAINSTREAM AND FRINGE CHIROPRACTIC TECHNIQUES?

This is a question that many individuals and organizations would like answered, and answered now. We have attended meetings of chiropractic technique groupings that are routinely approached by the various states and provinces, seeking an opinion on what defines a legitimate chiropractic technique, what is mainstream compared with fringe. Patients, managed care organizations, attorneys, state licensing boards, and governmental bodies all have a stake and an avid interest in this. No doubt most chiropractors have a sense of what is mainstream and what is fringe, and many recognize that techniques most would consider fringe

continue to attract glaring negative attention and do the profession harm. However, few individuals and organizations are willing to take public positions on what is mainstream and what is fringe. Everyone wants someone else to do it, and for good reason.

Since there is very little evidence that "mainstream" diagnostic and treatment procedures are safer or more effective than "fringe" procedures, there can be legal repercussions from commenting publicly and negatively on a technique in a manner that could cause material harm to its practitioners. What's more, potential critics probably do not relish the thought that their own non-validated mainstream methods could become subjected to the same critical standards they might set for the fringe procedures. The same logic that drives a particular state or province to reject some techniques will one day point the finger at its own favored techniques. It is not clear whether regulators should be defending practice rights for all but the most obviously eccentric "doctors," or enjoining the nascent profession-wide attack on quackery.

There can be no doubt that techniques taught in the majority of the chiropractic colleges, especially within their core curricula (as opposed to the elective and continuing education programs), must be considered mainstream. This comment refers to both generic technique procedures like motion palpation and spinal manipulation, and some system techniques, like Gonstead and SOT, since about half of the American chiropractic colleges feature technique systems in their core curricula. All we can say for sure about the other techniques is that they are more likely than the college core techniques to be considered fringe – by somebody, somewhere.

IS CAM STATUS DESIRABLE FOR CHIROPRACTIC?

The widely-based acceptance of chiropractic by the public and the medical establishment, along with the impressive accrual of evidence of its clinical effectiveness, presents an unusual problem for the chiropractic profession: can chiropractic still be considered a CAM therapy? That is, have the lobbying efforts of chiropractors been so successful that their profession is now seen as mainstream, perhaps a subspecialty of medicine, not unlike dentistry? On the one hand, chiropractic could realize tremendous political and economic gains by being embraced by conventional medicine. No longer barred from hospitals or long-term facilities, chiropractors could become more firmly entrenched in the healthcare delivery system in general, and could develop a stronger rapport with individual medical practitioners in particular. Moreover, the elusive goal of university affiliation could be more easily obtained by those colleges that seek it. On the other hand, there is an alluring mystique to being labeled an alternative to medicine. Many patients are looking for a distinctly non-medical solution to their healthcare problems and management. Further-more, many funding agencies, such as the National Institute of Health, are awarding large research grants into projects examining CAM approaches. Ironically, if chiropractic is eventually thought of as "mainstream," this source of funds could become unavailable to them and, after championing so many battles for acceptance, chiropractors could find themselves outside the CAM movement, enviously looking in.

REFERENCES

1. Foote D 1998 Boom, bust and echo. Profiting from the demographic shift in the new millennium. MacFarlane, Walter & Ross, Toronto
2. Gleberzon B J 2001 Geriatric demographics. In: Gleberzon B J (ed.) Chiropractic care of the older patient, pp. 13–21. Butterworth-Heinemann, Oxford, UK
3. Meeker W C, Haldeman S 2002 Chiropractic: a profession at the crossroads of mainstream and alternative medicine. Annals of Internal Medicine 136: 216–227
4. Eisenberg D, Kessler R, Foster C et al 1993 Unconventional medicine use in the United States. New England Journal of Medicine 328: 246–252
5. Eisenberg D, Davis R, Ettner S et al 1998 Trends in alternative medicine use in the United States, 1990–1997. Journal of the American Medical Association 280: 1569–1575
6. Cooperstein R, Perle S M, Gatterman M I et al 2001 Chiropractic technique procedures for specific low back conditions: characterizing the literature. Journal of Manipulative and Physiological Therapeutics 24 (6): 407–424
7. Ko G D, Devine P 2000 Use of complementary health practices by prostate carcinoma patients undergoing radiation therapy. Cancer 88: 615–619
8. Christensen M, Kerkhoff D, Kollasch M W et al 2000 National Board of Chiropractic Examiners. Job analysis of chiropractic. A project report, survey analysis and summary of the practice of chiropractic within the United States, p. 129. National Board of Chiropractic Examiners, Greeley, CO
9. Presented at the Association of Chiropractic Colleges, San Antonio, Texas, Mar 16–19, 2000 (unpublished)
10. Meeker W C 2000 Public demand and the integration of complementary and alternative medicine in the US health care system. Journal of Manipulative and Physiological Therapeutics 23: 123–126
11. Ko G D, Berbrayer D 2000 Complementary and alternative medicine: Canadian physician's attitudes and behavior. Archives of Physical Medicine and Rehabilitation 81: 662–667
12. Diggett D M 1987 Commentary: the chiropractic wars. Journal of Manipulative and Physiological Therapeutics 10 (2): 71–77
13. Homola S 1963 Bonesetting, chiropractic and cultism. Critique Book, Panama City, FL
14. Christensen M, Kerkhoff D, Kollasch M W et al 1993 National Board of Chiropractic Examiners. Job analysis of chiropractic. A project report, survey analysis and summary of practice of chiropractic within the United States, p. 84. National Board of Chiropractic Examiners, Greeley, CO
15. Philips R 2002 We need to bring order to our techniques. Dynamic Chiropractic 20 (1): 1,28–31
16. Gleberzon B J 2001 Name techniques in Canada: current trends in utilization rates and recommendations for their inclusion at the Canadian Memorial Chiropractic College. Journal of the Canadian Chiropractic Association 44 (3): 157–168
17. Kopansky-Giles D, Papadopoulos C 1997 Canadian Chiropractic Resource Databank (CCRD). A profile of Canadian chiropractors. Journal of the Canadian Chiropractic Association 41 (3): 155–191
18. www.CCEB.ca
19. Watkins T, Saranchuk R 1999 Analysis of the relationship between educational programming at the Canadian Memorial Chiropractic College and the professional practices of its graduates. Journal of the Canadian Chiropractic Association 44 (4): 230–244
20. Gleberzon B J 2002 Chiropractic name techniques in Canada: a continued look at demographic trends and their impact on issues of jurisprudence. Journal of the Canadian Chiropractic Association. 46 (4): 241–256

FURTHER READING

Stern H 1993 Private parts. Simon & Schuster, New York, NY

36

The allure of technique systems

TECHNIQUE SYSTEMS ARE SUPPOSED TO LIMIT THOUGHT

The result, if not the purpose, of a technique system is to limit thought, and this is not always a bad thing. Clinical reasoning that is too expansive does not result in effective care, because the clinician becomes overburdened with knowledge that has not been properly refined, and distilled down to manageable proportions. In order to render care, it may be necessary to avoid being blinded by details that obfuscate, rather than illuminate, the way. If we were to take into account all the diagnostic possibilities that are consistent with a given patient's presentation and consider all conceivable treatments, we might never know where to begin. A technique system culls selected items from the plethora of detail which is presented when a patient walks in the room, settles upon a treatment plan specific to its desired outcome, and defines the outcome assessment parameters accordingly.

Therefore, a technique system is a set of rules that limits the diagnostic inputs and range of therapeutic options open to the doctor. It is a series of on/off switches and if/then decisions, admittedly often unsubstantiated, that guide the doctor virtually automatically (and even thoughtlessly) to the therapeutic intervention. The naked truth is that we chiropractors eventually get used to the fact that we operate on a very uncertain terrain. Although it would be foolish to commit immediately to a narrow diagnosis and treatment plan, based on technique system rules that are too limiting, it is equally important not to become paralyzed by an overabundance of diagnostic findings

and treatment options; hence the allure of technique systems.

Although reliance on a technique system may result in missing important clinical information from the history and/or the examination procedures, the saving grace is that treatment is not an act but a process, a dialogue between the doctor, the patient, and the patient's unconscious neuromusculoskeletal system. By means of interacting with the patient over time, the doctor transforms the clinical impression into a diagnosis, gradually honing in on a commensurate treatment plan. Chiropractic care is an iterative process, a process in which the repetition of a sequence of operations produces results which become increasingly accurate. Clinical chiropractic procedures do not so much discover the truth of a patient's condition as converge upon its essence in a trial-and-error, empirical fashion. The technique system, if its initial findings do not result in a good therapeutic outcome, must be wise enough to get out of the way and allow clinical iteration to take over the course of care, which may involve altering the technique substantially, "breaking the rules."

Chiropractic students are possessed with an understandable anxiety, and even terror, when they look ahead to the time when they will enter into clinical practice. They wonder how they will know what to do, and sometimes make the rash decision to "learn one technique" before they enter clinic. Students in this frame of mind are susceptible to overly emphasizing the chosen technique system, thus depriving themselves of the opportunity to learn others, including how to pick, choose, and combine their elements (i.e., practice a diversified technique). Those interns who enter the chiropractic college clinic with a technique already "up their sleeves," as it were, often remain totally preoccupied with closed systems of thought and action. They deprive themselves of the great wealth and diversity of what chiropractic has to offer its patients, preferring to hang on to what they already know, as an infant does its security blanket. Conversely, less experienced entry-level interns tend to be the ones who complete the clinic experience bigger than when they arrived.

WHY THERE ARE SO MANY TECHNIQUE SYSTEMS

The bewildering array of mutually exclusive chiropractic technique systems, many claiming to be the legitimate pretender to the medical throne, requires some explanation. Although much of this competition is of little redeeming value, it remains entirely possible that where back care languishes for lack of imagination, even chaos has its advantages. It is easy to point an accusatory finger at the custodians of technique systems – yes, they confuse the public, make insupportable claims, and may ignore standard scientific methods – but these same technique mavens, past and present, are the ones who have reduced to practice much of what is evolving into the more responsible generic technique just on the horizon. The world of technique systems, past and present, deserves no less than a healthy admixture of constructive and destructive criticism.

Development at the margin

Chiropractic today displays just the sort of methodological diversity that one would expect of a discipline that developed on the fringes of the organized healthcare profession. It is always at the margins of society that freedom of experimentation commingles with reckless adventurism, that lack of regulation breeds simultaneously bold innovation and abject quackery. The phenomenon is not unlike the explosion of new life forms that is seen when existing species rush in to exploit a new biological niche that suddenly opens up following

a geological catastrophe or other rapid and major environmental change.

Hopefully, human society can exercise more restraint than natural selection, which, while ensuring survival of the fittest, undoubtedly discards many promising biological innovations that are unfortunately coupled to environmentally unsuccessful strategies, what amount to failed genetic experiments. It would be unfortunate if, under the guise of bringing order to the house of technique, the chiropractic profession were to throw out the kernels of analytic truth and clinical utility that surely reside in some of its dirtiest bath water. This fear is acknowledged, in both the chiropractic and medical settings, when every measure to standardize the delivery of healthcare evokes the same refrain: cookbook healthcare will stifle research and innovation.[1] Of course, it is equally true that continued technique chaos will risk excluding chiropractic from national healthcare and worsen its position in a managed-care environment.

Lack of market penetration

Revolutionaries without a revolution always do the same thing. When their messianic zeal to transform society stumbles in the face of the predictable establishment backlash, their movement fragments into an assortment of political sects that have no option left except to transform each other (e.g., the American "New Left" c. 1975). Rage against the status quo transmutes into multilateral civil war, which flares up from time to time in direct proportion to the magnitude of the lost opportunities. Chiropractic, which has always behaved like and regarded itself as something of a movement, cannot escape the internal consequences of long-term marginalization.

Although chiropractic is the nation's third largest primary healthcare profession, with more than 50 000 practitioners in North America alone, only one in 20 Americans obtains chiropractic treatment in any one year.[2] Given that the point prevalence of low-back pain alone is 5–30%, and that 80% of all people suffer from low-back pain at some time in their lives,[3–5] it does not appear that chiropractors have been able to take their case effectively to the public. No doubt medical and media chiro-bashing have compounded the problem. For an entire century chiropractic has struggled to become a mass movement, but has been unable to attract suitable numbers of adherents (patients). Although failed movements go away, and victorious movements immediately close ranks, the frustrations of partial success sow disunity and foster internecine struggle. Such is the situation of chiropractic today, as it always has been.

The economic advantage of retaining several techniques

Consumers are presented with a bewildering array of choices in the healthcare market: medicine, chiropractic, acupuncture, nutritional supplements, biofeedback, etc.[6] Healthcare providers, just like the vendors of other sorts of goods and services, are subject to market forces that drive them to strive for product diversification and the establishment of brand names.

To some extent consumer choice is governed by pure geography, the amount of space occupied on the shelf by given brands, say, of healthcare professions. Assume the simplest competitive case imaginable: that consumers are constrained to choose between medical and chiropractic care. Let us suppose that the choice is purely dichotomous, that the public is indifferent between the two, and that both chiropractic and medicine end up with half of the market. Now, have some chiropractors segment themselves into a number of well-defined, mutually exclusive techniques – technique 1, technique 2, and technique 3. Classic microeconomic theory predicts that the market share for chiropractic as a whole will probably increase relative to medicine, because the consumers' choice is no longer purely dichotomous, medicine vs chiropractic, but multilateral: medicine vs chiro-technique 1 vs chiro-technique 2 vs chiro-technique 3.

Although chiropractic technique systems are not literally brands on the shelf, consumer choice is still partially governed by such psychogeographic considerations. The chiropractic alternative to medicine occupies a larger psychic space in the consumer's mind to the extent that it is divided into several technique systems. Of course, there is no net benefit to any existing individual chiropractic producer when a new brand of technique is invented, since his or her market share may decline even if chiropractic as a whole were to increase its share relative to medicine. As for the newcomer, he or she is bound to observe Boulding's principle of minimum differentiation: "Make your product as like the existing products as you can without destroying the differences."[7]

Technique proliferation may reach a point where the variety of techniques itself becomes confusing, especially if some of the brands are of questionable quality. In such a case, each new product introduction risks engendering what economists call a "negative externality," a kind of backlash effect. The public may eventually develop a preference for healthcare services sold in a more stable and coherent market. We all know how hard medicine has worked to be that preferred market, but not without some deep misgivings about sacrificing market share to a suite of more exciting "unconventional" therapies.[6]

The chiropractor as generalist

The chiropractor who wishes to distinguish him- or herself from another – and there are always purely commercial reasons to do so – usually does so on the basis of the particular type of technique used, rather than conditions or types of patients treated. This accrues to the simple fact that most chiropractors claim to be generalists treating a great variety of diseases, even though most patients present with musculoskeletal complaints.[2] By comparison, the vast majority of medical doctors are specialists, distinguishing themselves from one another by the organ systems addressed, and the range of patients and diseases treated.

On the other hand, there does seem to be increasing interest in the advent of chiropractic specialists: chiropractic neurologists, orthopedists, radiologists, nutritionists, and so on. A technique system that purports to have particularly good outcomes treating diseases and conditions where medicine (or other technique systems) commonly fails (e.g., fibromyalgia, gastroesophageal reflux disease, autism, and so on), may increase its slice of the healthcare pie.

Mercantile bent of the founders

There is no need to harp on the fact that both of the Palmers, especially the son, were susceptible to purely commercial considerations, and were not averse to lurid, sensationalist advertising claims for the advantages of chiropractic care.[8] Chiropractors certainly have no monopoly on the possession of a certain human frailty by which entrepreneurial interests occasionally displace scientific and clinical concerns. The question isn't so much why overtly philistine technique vendors have been so numerous, but why they have gone so unchecked and even unopposed, until fairly recently.

Lack of knowledge

Given the contemporary importance of evidence-based care and best-practice development in healthcare (Ch. 38), one would assume that the actual data and substantive research would constitute the best potential check on chiropractic technique hyperbole. However, as with all healthcare disciplines, there is much that remains unknown within the chiropractic profession, and many phenomena germane to chiropractic techniques have so far defied explanation and resisted investigation. Throughout most of its history, chiropractic, not unlike other "soft sciences," has endured wild speculation concerning its basic phenomena. It has witnessed a plethora of hypotheses governing the nature of the chiropractic subluxation and the mechanism of the chiropractic adjustment. Such speculation is not only necessary but desirable, in so far as future knowledge takes root in the theoretical constructs of the present.

Although it is never true that "one opinion is as good as another," until the mid-1980s the research community was simply not up to the task of counteracting the endless unfolding of technique systems. In a word, the technique innovators, and purveyors of even exceedingly strange techniques, flourished *because they could*. Competition has been fierce. Although the fairly recent explosion of data

has narrowed down the field of legitimate conjecture considerably, not everyone has noticed. As teachers in chiropractic colleges, we have observed a significant minority of students, confronted with a research study that invalidates some cherished chiropractic procedure, respond: "Oh, those crazy researchers, there they go again." Such remarks are also common in the letters sections of our journals and other trade publications. A recent study at the University of Bridgeport College of Chiropractic showed that those students most uncomfortable with clinical uncertainty were the most likely to be attracted to the most dogmatic of the chiropractic technique systems, systems that claimed to treat the widest range of human ailments. On the other hand, Robert Jansen's large-scale survey on chiropractors' attitudes toward practice standards and the organizations developing them showed surprising support for research; for example, only 8% agreed with the statement that "chiropractic methods do not need to be validated."[9]

The quest for nerve interference

Since chiropractors have always emphasized the concept of "nerve interference" or equivalent, it should be noted that the consequences of a hypothetical subclinical neuropathy, occurring at the histological level, have been extraordinarily difficult to detect.[10] No one has any problem in diagnosing severe nerve damage, since there are obvious neurological deficits: anesthesia, muscle weakness, altered deep tendon reflexes. In the absence of so-called hard neurologicals, chiropractors have claimed to detect neuropathy by the presence of pain, tenderness, altered galvanic skin response, surface skin temperature asymmetry, peculiar electromagnetic radiations, and so-called "reflexes" of different kinds.

Since few of these have been particularly convincing, a perennial market has been created for the proclamation of new and increasingly outlandish indicators, which has greatly enriched the world of technique systems. If anything over the years has represented something of a chiropractic golden fleece, it would be the sustained effort to demonstrate "nerve interference" – that is, mild or even subclinical neuropathy – that would supposedly accompany minor articular misalign-ment and/or altered motion characteristics.

The allure of brand-name techniques[11]

Chiropractic science has developed to the point that, like other maturing sciences, it has been able to cast off the tiresome arrogance of the neophyte, having assumed instead a firm grasp on its limi-tations. Although this exercise in humility has been necessary and desirable, it has inadver-tently rendered chiropractors and chiropractic students increasingly vulnerable to the exploita-tion of technique charlatans. They offer us what a disabused appraisal of the state of the arts can-not: absolute conviction in the value of the tech-nique for sale, including the smoke and mirrors of its ideological accouterment. In the hands of an expert, mastery of a particular technique sys-tem and its particular psychomotor tools can be linked with a whole set of purely extraneous, unre-lated values: loyalty to chiropractic, staunch oppo-sition to medical expropriation, quality service to patients, and above all, the daily accomplishment of miracles.

The chiropractic colleges' pre-eminence in research and commitment to normal science has wound up undermining some of the confidence their students would have in their technique pro-grams. Some instructors unfortunately make a daily practice of mocking historically entrenched chiropractic ideas, only to conclude that at the current time we really have no better ideas to replace them. How much of the edifice of tradi-tional chiropractic thought and practice can be ripped down without being replaced, before the students become disenchanted with their future profession? Why would they be expected to sup-port a college which accepts their tuition but does not seem proud of the essence of what it offers?

This state of affairs mandates to the colleges the task of teaching their students how to function comfortably within a realm of clinical uncertainty, how to do without the outmoded pseudo-confidence and pseudo-science of technique char-latans. They must proudly tell the students that we now know enough about our craft to cast off

safely some of the tethers of technique systems, that their rules and methodologies are too narrow and constraining. This does not mean rejecting technique systems, but more carefully nurturing the concept of systematic thinking, without which efficient patient care cannot begin. Students and field doctors alike deserve the freedom to practice chiropractic technique in a more creative, eclectic way, always consistent with the dictates of nor-mal science. Hopefully, they will experience the thrill of participating in the most liberal period of chiropractic technique practice since its very inception, one in which the leanings of system techniques can be organized and enriched by the success of chiropractic research.

The glasshouse effect

There is no hard and fast line that separates what is known from what is not known, nor even sci-ence from myth. Rather, there is a continuum that defines the fabric of reality, stretching from abject nonsense to proven fact. Where an individual practitioner situates him- or herself on this very elastic fabric is to some degree a question of taste. In a science where so much remains "investiga-tional," traditionalist chiropractors seek comfort in the science of myth, whereas more contempo-rary practitioners seem more at home in the myth of science.[12]

Ideally, the chiropractic profession would weed from its garden those methods that stretch credibility to the point of incredulity, but there is a fundamental problem in doing so: only the thinnest of margins separates officially endorsed "mainstream" chiropractic methods from the others. These latter earn a variety of epithets, anything from "unorthodox" to "experimental" to "quackery," depending on the nay-sayer's degree of charity and sometimes professional rivalry. Admittedly, it may seem odd that Doctor X gets his listings from aura analysis, and adjusts the spine with forces not in excess of 25 g, but where is the evidence that Doctor Y, a motion pal-pator, possesses superior diagnostic acumen or gets better clinical outcomes? To apply an old adage, those who live in glasshouses shouldn't throw stones.

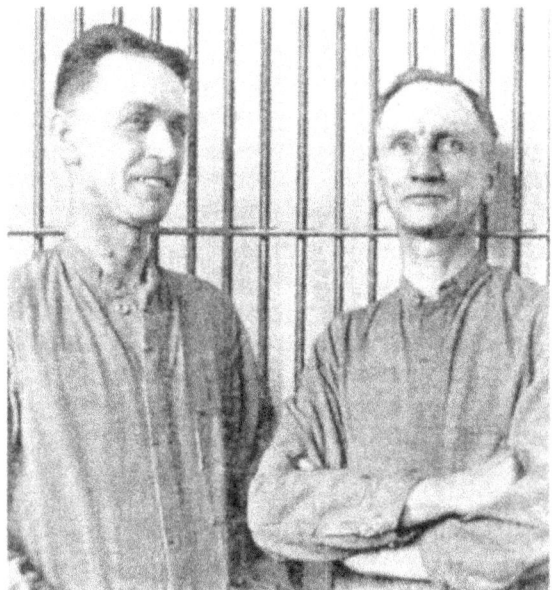

Figure 36.1   Chiropractors used their incarceration to gain the public's support against medical monopoly. Courtesy of the Palmer College of Chiropractic Archives, Davenport, IA.

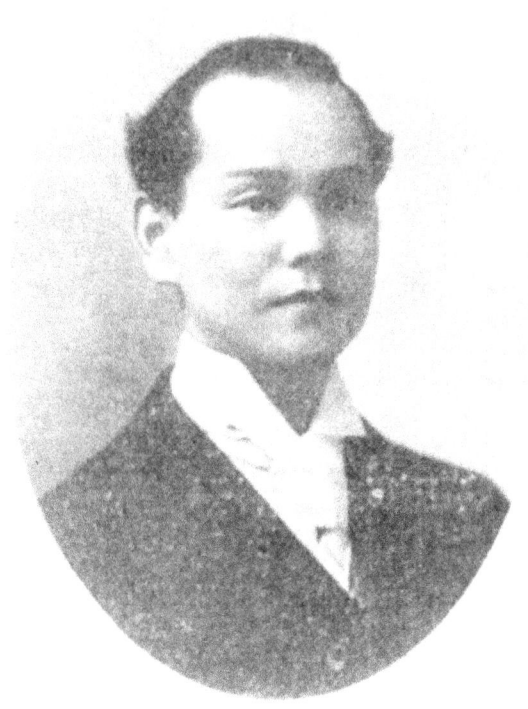

Figure 36.2   Shegataro Morikubo, DC, a 1903 graduate of DD Palmer's. This Japanese chiropractor was successfully defended against the charge of practicing osteopathy without a license in LaCrosse, WI. Courtesy of the Palmer College of Chiropractic Archives, Davenport, IA.

NOTE: MEDICINE VS CHIROPRACTIC

When we discussed the allure of brand-name techniques, we agreed that one of the historical impetuses has been the marginalization of the chiropractic profession to the fringes of healthcare. Clearly, some of the blame for being so positioned can be laid at the feet of chiropractic itself. However, many of the forces trying to drive chiropractic out of the healthcare delivery system have come from the orchestrated discriminatory behavior of medical doctors and their organizations.

THE FIGHT FOR SURVIVAL

Medicine throws down the gauntlet

Starting in the early 1900s, organized medicine had attempted to contain and prohibit the development of chiropractic, primarily by either blocking licensure of its earliest practitioners, or by charging them with practicing medicine without a license (Fig. 36.1). D D Palmer was jailed for a time in 1906 under this allegation. The next year, chiropractor Shegataro Morikubo (Fig. 36.2) was arrested in Wisconsin for practicing medicine, surgery, and osteopathy without a license, a case instigated by the chairmen of the State Medical Board as part of a concerted effort to eliminate chiropractic from the state.[1]

One of the earliest, and perhaps most vicious, of the profession's adversaries was Morris Fishbein, Secretary of the American Medical Association (AMA) and editor of the Journal of the American Medical Association (JAMA) from 1924 to 1949. He began a relentless campaign against the chiropractic profession, writing in one editorial that chiropractors were "rabid dogs, playful and cute but they're killers".[13] Elsewhere, Fishbein wrote that chiropractic arrived on the healthcare scene 'through the cellar ... besmirched with dust and grime"[14] (p. 98), quoted in Kapchuk and Eisenberg.[15]

The principal medical shot against the chiropractic bow was fired in 1963 when the AMA Board of Trustees established the Committee on Chiropractic, renamed the Committee on Quackery. In a 1971 report to the AMA Board of Trustees, H Doyl Taylor, Director of the AMA Department of Investigation and Secretary of its Committee on Quackery wrote: "… your Committee [on Quackery] has considered its prime mission to be, first, the containment of chiropractic and ultimately, the elimination of chiropractic".[13,15]

However, the primary weapon the AMA used to ensure the medical boycott of chiropractic was its Code of Ethics. From its inception in 1847, the AMA had a clause prohibiting its members from consulting with practitioners whose practice is based on an exclusive dogma.[16] In 1957, in reaction to the political and economic gains made by chiropractors, the AMA explicitly interpreted this clause to apply to the Palmers' theories of Innate Intelligence and forbad medical doctors from consulting or otherwise engaging in any interprofessional relationships with chiropractors[15]. To ensure compliance with this code, the Joint Commission of Accreditation of Hospitals' *Hospital Accrediting Manual* stated that the failure of medical staff or administrators "to take all reasonable steps to ensure adherence to [the AMA Principle of Medical Ethics] shall constitute grounds for non-accreditation".[13] In essence, any medical doctor who worked in any way with a chiropractor could have his or her hospital privileges revoked, and the hospital in which he or she worked could lose its accreditation standing.[13]

Chiropractic fights back

In 1976, chiropractor Chester A Wilk, along with four of his colleagues, filed a massive antitrust law suit under the Sherman Anti-Trust laws of the 1920s, alleging that the AMA and 11 other medical associations had illegally colluded to boycott the chiropractic profession. Much of the evidence for this suit was provided to the plaintiffs by a disgruntled AMA staff member, a doctor who called himself "Sore Throat", after the "Deep Throat" informant of Watergate fame[17] (referenced by Perle[18]).

The Wilk case came to trial in December 1980, and lasted for 2 months. At the end of January, the jury found for the defendants. The strategy employed by the AMA legal team was to describe some of the excesses and eccentricities of some chiropractors in the field.[13,16] However, the Seventh Circuit Court of Appeal remanded the case for a new trial in 1983, with a ruling that would disallow that legal stratagem from being used again. A few of the defendant associations settled out of court. After hearing all the evidence (including an allegation from the AMA that the only motivation behind the Wilk case was for monetary gain), Judge Susan Getzendanner found the AMA, the American College of Radiology, the American College of Surgeons, and the American Academy of Orthopedic Surgeons guilty of illegal boycott and conspiracy. Judge Getzendanner's Permanent Injunction Order against the AMA was published in the Jan 1, 1988 issue of the JAMA, and the Supreme Court Injunction Order was mailed to all members of the AMA. In her ruling, Judge Getzendanner noted that the need for injunctive relief was necessitated by the fact that, although the boycott of chiropractic ended in 1980 with an amendment to the AMA Code of Ethics, the AMA "never affirmatively acknowledged that there are and should be no collective impediments to the professional association and cooperation between chiropractic and medical physicians, except as provided by law".[19] In summary, Judge Getzendanner wrote that:

Most importantly, the court believes that it is important that the AMA members be made aware of the present AMA position that it is ethical for a medical physician to professionally associate with a chiropractor if the physician believes it is in the best interests of his patient, so that the lingering effects of the illegal group boycott against chiropractors finally can be dissipated.[19]

In 1990, the US Supreme Court let this decision stand without comment.[3]

REFERENCES

1. Chassen M R 1988 Standards of care in medicine. Inquiry 25 (winter): 437–453
2. Christensen M G 1993 Job analysis of chiropractic. National Board of Chiropractic Examiners, Greeley, CO
3. Manga P 1993 The effectiveness and cost-effectiveness of chiropractic management of low-back pain. Kenilworth Publishing, Richmond Hill, Ontario, Canada
4. Frymoyer J W, Pope M H 1980 Epidemiologic studies of low back pain. Spine 5: 419–423
5. Liebenson C S 1992 Pathogenesis of chronic back pain. Journal of Manipulative and Physiological Therapeutics 15 (5): 299–308
6. Eisenberg D M, Kessler R C, Foster C et al 1983 "Unconventional" medicine in the United States. New England Journal of Medicine 328 (4): 246
7. Boulding K 1966 Economic analysis. Harper & Row, New York, NY
8. Gibbons R W 1992 Medical and social protest as part of hidden American history. In: Haldeman S (ed.) Principles and practice of chiropractic, 2nd edn, pp. 15–28. Appleton & Lange, East Norwalk, CT
9. Jansen R D 1991 A survey of American chiropractors' attitudes toward practice standards and the organizations developing them. Palmer College of Chiropractic-West, San Jose, CA
10. Stonebrink R D 1990 Evaluation and manipulative management of common musculoskeletal disorders. Western States Chiropractic College, Portland, OR
11. Cooperstein R 1990 Brand name techniques and the confidence gap. Journal of Chiropractic Education 4(3): 89–93
12. Quine W V O 1964 Two dogmas of empiricism, 2nd edn. Harvard University Press, Cambridge, MA
13. Wardwell W I 1992 Chiropractic: history and evolution of a new profession. Mosby-Year Book, St Louis, MO
14. Fishbein M 1925 The medical follies. Boni & Liveright, New York, NY
15. Kapchuk T J, Eisenberg D M 1998 contributions. Archives of Internal Medicine Chiropractic: origins, controversies and 158: 2215–2224
16. Wilk C A 1996 Medicine, monopolies, and malice. Avery Publishing Group, Garden City Park, NY
17. Rothstein W G 1985 American physicians in the 19th century: from sects to science. Johns Hopkins University Press, Baltimore, MD
18. Perle S M 2000 Concept paper of chiropractic. Unpublished
19. Getzendanner S 1988 Permanent injunction order against AMA. Journal of the American Medical Association 250: 81–82

37

Name techniques and chiropractic jurisprudence

I will sell Chiropractic, serve Chiropractic and save Chiropractic if it takes me twenty life times to do it. I will promote it within the law, without the law, in keeping with the law or against the law in order to get sick people well and keep the well from getting sick (anecdotally attributed to BJ Palmer c. 1940).

It is impossible to separate any discussion of chiropractic in general, or technique systems in particular, from the overarching domain of the law. In addition to the usual and customary legal obligations required of a chiropractor (or any healthcare provider, for that matter) providing reasonable professional care, such as record keeping and ensuring patient confidentiality, there are unique concerns specifically related to the practice of technique systems. This chapter will describe some of these areas of jurisprudence that, at times, defy a simple solution, requiring instead a Solomonesque judgment, weighing the rights of the practitioner against the rights of the public to be protected from substandard practice.

STANDARDS OF CARE AND GUIDELINES

As a self-regulating profession, it is incumbent on chiropractic to develop standards of care and professional guidelines to which a practitioner must adhere. *Guidelines* are statements that seek to assist a practitioner with respect to patient care planning (often developed through consensus opinion), whereas *standards* are authoritative statements that set minimal levels or ranges of acceptable performance or results[2] (referenced in Gatterman et al).[3] The differences between guidelines and standards are, at times, obscured in the minds of practitioners; because of this, they may at times be ignored. As an example, consider the subtle differences between chiropractic adjustments and generic manipulations, especially in terms of outcomes. Understanding the different therapeutic goals of chiropractic care requires an appreciation of cultural or contextual differences among chiropractic practitioners. If standards and guidelines are developed without consideration of the different world-views within the chiropractic profession, some field practitioners may feel that these guidelines do not apply to them and may reject them out of hand, or may simply develop their own.

An example of this is the recent development of several sets of guidelines: Mercy, International Chiropractic Association (ICA), Glenerin, Wyndham, and Council on Chiropractic Examination (CCE) (Table 37.1).

The Wyndham and Mercy Guidelines were developed in the same year, 1993, representing essentially traditional (straight) and more moderate (less straight?) chiropractic constituencies, respectively. Individuals involved with chiropractic education were primarily responsible for the development of the Mercy Guidelines in the USA and the Glenerin Guidelines, their Canadian counterpart. However, some members of the chiropractic profession objected to the Mercy and Glenerin guidelines, criticizing not only the guidelines themselves, which they tended to find "too medical," but both the process that had led to them and the lack of follow-up. In response to these perceived shortcomings, the Council on Chiropractic

Table 37.1 Clinical guidelines in chiropractic

Title of guidelines	Year	Organization	Comments
Recommended Clinical Protocols and Guidelines for the Practice of Chiropractic	2000	International Chiropractic Association	
Guidelines for Chiropractic Quality Assurance and Practice Parameters (Mercy Guidelines)	1993	Congress of Chiropractic State Associations (COCA)	A commission of 35 chiropractors established by COCA
Guidelines for Straight Chiropractic (Wyndham Guidelines)	1993	World Chiropractic Alliance (WCA)	International Straight Chiropractic Consensus Conference in May 1992
Clinical Guidelines for Chiropractic Practice in Canada (Canadian Guidelines)	1993	Canadian Chiropractic Association	35 Canadian chiropractors, assisted by three facilitators and four staff members
Vertebral Subluxation in Chiropractic Practice	1998	Council of Chiropractic Practice (CCP)	CCP is registered as a non-profit organization, independent in its activities

Practice (CCP), which includes many of the same individuals who had been involved in the Wyndham Guidelines, was convened to develop a set of professional practice guidelines it thought more in keeping with traditional tenets of straight chiropractors. This included strong emphasis on vertebral subluxation. Membership of this Council was primarily derived from individuals who developed or championed many of the different technique systems. Among the CCP's principal recommendations was:

Adjusting procedures should be selected which are determined by the practitioner to be safe and effective for the individual patient. No mode of care should be used which has been demonstrated by critical scientific study and field experience to be unsafe or ineffective in the correction of vertebral subluxations.[4] (p. 147)

In this statement not only is there is an emphasis on combining scientific evidence with the experience and judgment of the practitioner, there is the overriding focus on choosing therapeutic procedures that would specifically correct *vertebral subluxations*, a therapeutic outcome not mentioned in either the Mercy or Glenerin Guidelines. However, it is noteworthy that the Council did indicate that many of the studies that have been conducted purporting to demonstrate the clinical efficacy of various technique systems have not passed the scrutiny of peer and editorial review.[4]

A recent review of the literature published on chiropractic name techniques by Gleberzon[5] reported that, of the 111 articles found, only 17 were clinical trials. The other 94 articles were discussions of the different techniques, case studies, case series, or investigations of a particular diagnostic procedure used by some technique systems (i.e., muscle testing or leg-length check). As mentioned in several letters to the editor, this article underscored the paucity of clinically based research in the area of chiropractic technique systems.

A recent article addressed this issue, opining that the poor differentiation of guidelines from standards of care contributes to mistrust of the guideline development process.[3] In essence, guidelines must allow for flexibility for individual differences, in terms of ideological principles, diagnostic and therapeutic preferences, and individual patient preferences, whereas standards of care are authoritative statements that establish minimum levels of acceptable performance. Thus, rather than being seen as a cookbook from which policy is built, legal restrictions imposed, or cost containment derived, guidelines must reflect the ideological differences that exist throughout the profession. As one group concluded: "to reduce barriers of acceptance and implementation, guidelines should be inclusive, patient-centered, and based on a variety of evidence and clinical experience."[3] (p. 14) This would allow guidelines to be used subsequently as an educational tool better to inform practitioners to make more rational decisions with respect to patient care.

SELF-REGULATION

Ironically, but similarly, legal strategies, once used to attack the chiropractic profession, are now being used to protect it. Whereas the medical community sought to use its legal influence and political clout to exclude chiropractors from healthcare, chiropractors now seek legal remedies to ensure no one intrudes upon their domain. By using clear definitions of what is and what is not a chiropractic technique, chiropractors are able to safeguard the public from would-be unlicensed practitioners; that is, individuals attempting to practice chiropractic without a license.

Just such a case was recently heard before the Supreme Court of Nova Scotia in Canada in 2001.[6] In that case, the Board of the Nova Scotia College of Chiropractors (NSCC) sought an interlocutory injunction against an individual (and his spouse) accused of practicing chiropractic without a license. Although the defendant did not have a license to practice chiropractic in Nova Scotia, he held himself to be a "spinologist," using the Blair Technique Correction on his patients. (The Blair Technique is a tonal-based technique comprised of a hybrid of Torque Release Technique (Ch. 31) and Upper Cervical Techniques (Ch. 32).) On the one hand, if a chiropractic technique procedure were regarded to comprise by definition a high-velocity, low-amplitude (HVLA) thrust into the paraphysiological space, then: (1) the Blair Technique, or at least its thrust, would not qualify as a chiropractic technique; (2) the defendant would not be found to be practicing chiropractic without a license; and (3) the injunction would probably be denied. On the other hand, if it could be shown that the Blair Technique was in fact a chiropractic technique, the injunction sought by the NSCS would be granted.

One of the authors (Gleberzon) was asked to offer an opinion in this case, and was sent the file for review. Several telling facts immediately became apparent. The Blair Technique purports to be based on the tenets of DD Palmer, following his tonal-based approach. The defendant referred to his therapeutic interventions as "adjustments," the people who presented to his office for care were referred to as "patients," and his primary outcome goal was "wellness." All these terms were in keeping with a tonal-based chiropractic technique approach. Succinctly put, it was Gleberzon's opinion that the Blair Technique met the equivalent of the duck test: if an animal looks like a duck, waddles like a duck, and quacks like a duck, it is reasonable to assume it is a duck. Similarly, since the Blair Technique was developed by chiropractors, uses chiropractic assessment procedures, uses chiropractic therapies and outcomes, and uses the same unique language, the Blair Technique could reasonably be classified as a chiropractic technique.

Based on the evidence submitted during the trial, the presiding judge of the Supreme Court of Nova Scotia decided that the Blair Technique was a chiropractic technique, and granted the injunction. This is an important landmark in Canadian chiropractic law because it demonstrated the importance, ability, and willingness of a chiropractic regulatory body to regulate and protect itself.[6] Incidentally, spinology experienced a similar demise, and for similar legal reasons, in the state of California during the mid-1980s.

INFORMED CONSENT

Any chiropractor, practicing a technique system or otherwise, must obtain informed consent from a patient prior to performing any assessment or therapeutic interventions. That stated, the practice of a technique system does raise some special issues and areas of concern. Some technique systems, such as Diversified Technique, are taught in some form at all accredited chiropractic colleges, while other technique systems, such as Gonstead, Thompson, Activator Methods and Palmer Hole-In-One, are taught at a number of accredited chiropractic colleges (Ch. 35). In addition to these techniques that are well-represented at the chiropractic colleges, a number of technique systems used by field practitioners are only taught at extracollegiate technique seminars. Thus, jurisdictions are confronted with the problem of techniques that are utilized according to practitioner (and patient) preferences, in which there has been potentially little or improper instruction, and often questionable quality assurance or guarantees of at least minimal practitioner competence.

After all, it is the chiropractic college community that is most familiar with designing evaluation instruments, with the administration of competency-based examinations and the collation of performance-based outcomes. The accredited colleges serve as the repository of much of the profession's knowledge, by employing skilled researchers, by funding or developing external funding for research projects, executing and publishing research, and by networking with other scholars and research organizations. By contrast, these pedagogical and operational skills are only rarely typical of those who conduct weekend technique seminars.[7]

In addition to issues related to minimal-competency performance, there are also concerns by third-party payers as to the appropriateness of many of these technique systems for patient care, in light of the fact that little, if any, evidence has been published on their clinical effectiveness in peer-reviewed journals. Third-party payers are understandably reluctant to pay for unproven therapies, especially if there exists evidence to support the clinical efficacy of other, alternative therapies (Ch. 38). Some regulatory boards, such as the College of Chiropractors of Ontario (CCO), are attempting to develop standards of practice to address these concerns.

Initially, the CCO proposed that a practitioner who plans on using a "technique, technology, device or procedure" that is not accepted by a "responsible and substantial segment of the chiropractic community" obtain written consent from the patient explicitly describing the intervention to be performed.[8] However, after consultation with several members of the profession (including Gleberzon), the CCO decided to tackle this issue from a different perspective. One proposal was to separate those therapies that, although used by some chiropractors in the field, are generally thought to fall outside of the realm of "normal" chiropractic care (for example, acupuncture, iridology, ear candling, and the use of botanical medicines). Another proposal was to leave the decision of what is an "acceptable"

chiropractic technique, device, or procedure to the chiropractic college community. In essence, the CCO is considering following, rather than leading, the chiropractic colleges, deferring to the judgment of chiropractor educators as to which techniques are reasonable for patient care, and which are not. The CCO is now proposing that any device or procedure considered for clinical use must "be taught in the core curriculum, postgraduate curriculum or continuing education division of one or more colleges accredited by the Council on Chiropractic Education (i.e., in a manner intended to achieve clinical proficiency) or approved by the CCO."[9] If a technique, device, or procedure does not meet these criteria, it would not be permitted for use in a clinical setting within Ontario.[9]

The practice of technique systems that are not well-represented at chiropractic colleges also raises concerns for malpractice carriers. Consider, for example, the case of a patient claiming to have been injured by a practitioner using a technique system that falls outside the core procedures taught and evaluated at a chiropractic college. The patient might reasonably state that he or she would not have consented to the procedure, knowing in advance that the technique had been learned at a weekend seminar. Conversely, if the patient had provided express written consent indicating that he or she had, in fact, been aware that the technique the chiropractor was going to use had not been taught within the college environment, the patient could not later claim ignorance in this regard. Lastly, there is also the issue of the technique falling within or outside the scope of practice in the jurisdiction where the doctor practices. If this determination is not made before the procedure is delivered, there could be issues of coverage eligibility should a civil suit be launched.[10]

Part of the issue of standards of practice and guidelines involves the determination of what constitutes "reasonableness" or, even more difficult to define, what professional practice activities are considered "professional." Many chiropractors are concerned that they will be judged by the odd behaviors, and even odder ideologies, of their peers. In general, reasonableness is rather an arbitrary concept: it is usually defined as those actions or activities that seven out of 10 chiropractors would consider acceptable. Professionalism is much more difficult to define. Perhaps we can borrow from the definition used by Supreme Court Judge Scalia when asked to define pornography. Paraphrasing, "We may not be able to define what professionalism is, but we know it when we see it … ."

GUIDING PROFESSIONAL PRACTICE STANDARDS OF CARE

It is self-evident that considerable divisiveness can result from standards of care produced by a regulatory body that are not congruent with the professional practice activities of its members or that are at odds with patient interests. A better understanding of the clinical effectiveness of the various technique systems, as well as their familiarity among both practitioners and patients, may help guide regulators to modernize their standards of care and guidelines. An example of this approach may be applied to a standard of care that we find particularly puzzling, having to do with the use of adjusting instruments. We explore the circumstances surrounding this case in some detail, not because instrument adjusting is more significant than any type of adjustive approach, but because the issues raised in this case are applicable to many others.

Currently, the use of an Activator Adjusting Instrument or any other mechanical device is prohibited in Saskatchewan. Specifically, the most recent professional standard states that:

No member shall use a machine or mechanical device as a substitute method of adjustment by hand of any one or more of the several articulations of the human body.[11]

Hypothetically, there may be justifiable reasons to prohibit the use of a mechanical device by a field practitioner. These may include: lack of evidence of clinical effectiveness, patient safety concerns, quality control concerns, and the lack of customary physical contact with the patients. However, in the case at hand, we find that there is good evidence suggesting that patients experience favorable and safe therapeutic outcomes while under the care of a chiropractor using an Activator Adjusting Instrument.[5]

Although a recently published article described three cases of adverse reactions experienced by patients treated with a mechanical assisted device (MAD),[12] there were issues in each case which were not unique to the use of non-manual procedures. One of these cases involved the eventual discovery of a rare tumor of the scapula which failed to respond to two different surgeries; another case involved a chiropractor who did not refer a patient for further investigations even after a lengthy period of non-responsiveness to care; and the third case involved a practitioner who did not obtain proper consent and had only minimal training in the proper use of the MAD.[12]

Defining what constitutes a quality therapeutic encounter seems to continue to challenge regulators. Many practice management coaches strive to teach chiropractors how to develop a high-volume practice, in which they see many patients per hour. However, how many patients can be seen in a finite amount of time before quality care can no longer be rendered? In general, if a practitioner is capable of gathering sufficient information to address the questions of SOAP (subjective, objective, action, and plan) record keeping, then the encounter is thought to meet minimal standards of care.[13] Thus, if practitioners are able to obtain this information, even if they have a high patient-volume practice, they have met minimum standards of care, regardless of the therapeutic method used.

Lastly, while one of the strengths of the chiropractic encounter rests on it being low-tech and high-touch,[14] there may be instances where the use of a mechanical device may be advantageous. These include adjusting an osteopenic patient or infant (one study reported that the activator generated a force of less than 50 N, compared to 120 N during spinal manipulative therapy of the neck);[15] circumstances of a large patient and a diminutive doctor; and cases involving patients who have been physically or sexually abused and may resist personal contact.

REFERENCES

1. Meeker W C, Haldeman S 2002 Chiropractic: a profession at the crossroads of mainstream and alternative medicine. Annals of Internal Medicine 136: 216–227
2. IOM Committee on Clinical Practice Guidelines provisional assessment instrument
3. Gatterman M I, Dobson T P, Lefevbre R 2001 Chiropractic quality assurance: standards and guidelines. Journal of the Canadian Chiropractic Association 45 (1): 11–17
4. Council of Chiropractic Practice clinical practice guidelines (number 1) 1998 Vertebral subluxation in chiropractic practice. Abbreviated version. Journal of Vertebral Subluxation Research 2 (3): 141–157
5. Gleberzon B J 2001 Chiropractic "name techniques": a review of the literature. Journal of the Canadian Chiropractic Association 45 (2): 86–99
6. The Board of the Nova Scotia College of Chiropractors v. Timothy Kohoot and Laura Kohoot no. 172528. Nov 2/2001
7. Gleberzon B J 2002 Chiropractic name technique in Canada: a continued look. Journal of the Canadian Chiropractic Association 46 (4): 241–256
8. CCO 2001 Experimental techniques, technologies, devices and procedures (draft). Standard of practice S-010 November. Chiropractic College of Ontario, Toronto, Ontario
9. CCO 2002 Experimental techniques, technologies, devices and procedures (draft). Standard of practice S-010 June. Chiropractic College of Ontario, Toronto, Ontario
10. Dunn G 2002 Oral presentation before the College of Chiropractors of Ontario's "Consultative day". Toronto, Ontario (unpublished)
11. Chiropractic Association of Saskatchewan 2001 Professional standards 19 (De amended October
12. Nykoliation J, Mierau D 1999 Adverse effects potentially associated with the use of mechanical adjusting device: a report of three cases. Journal of the Canadian Chiropractic Association 43 (3): 161–167
13. CCO 1999 Definition of a chiropractic visit. Guideline G-004 10 April. College of Chiropractors of Ontario, Toronto, Ontario
14. Coulter I D 2001 A philosophy for alternative health care. Butterworth-Heinemann, Oxford, UK
15. Kawchuk G N, Herzog W 1993 Biomechanical characterization (fingerprinting) of five novel methods of cervical spine manipulation. Journal of Manipulative and Physiological Therapeutics 16 (9): 573–577

38

Evidence-based practice

I believe, in fact know ... that our individualized, segmented spiritual entities carry with them into the future spiritual state that which has been mentally accumulated during our physical existence; that spiritual existence, like the physical, is progressive; that a correct understanding of these principles and the practice of them constitute a religion of chiropractic; that the existence and personal identity of individualized intelligences continue after the change known as death; that life in this world and the next is continuous – one of eternal progression (DD Palmer[1]).

Perhaps, in the early days of the chiropractic profession, authoritative statements such as the one above were all that was needed to reassure the chiropractic rank and file that "chiropractic works," as the phrase goes. However, in today's outcomes-driven market for healthcare services, neither unimpeachable testimony nor authoritative opinions convincingly demonstrate clinical and cost-effectiveness, or safety. This is true of all the healthcare professions, not just chiropractic, but special issues are raised for the technique systems in chiropractic. This chapter addresses some of these issues. We use the term "evidence-based care" (EBC) to convey the industry-wide move towards increased provider accountability and responsibility for practicing in accordance with *best-practice* procedures.

WHAT IS EVIDENCE?[2]

It has been traditional to depict levels of evidence in a hierarchical way, with those types that are considered lowly, such as anecdotal evidence and case reports, at the base of a pyramid whose apex is represented by randomized clinical trials (RCTs).

In recent years, it has become apparent that there are problems with representing types of evidence in this way, largely because it does not acknowledge the issue of *clinical relevance*. Practice-based research may not be very fancy, but its results are immediately applicable to typical clinical situations that arise in the day-to-day practice of the doctor. An RTC may be sophisticated and cost a lot of money, but it may have constructed a set of circumstances unlikely to occur in most cases. Given the limitations of RCTs (see below), we understand why many field practitioners (including ourselves) fear being tyrannized by research, in effect urged or even forced to use only those procedures that have withstood the artificial rigors of RCTs. This would be an overkill response to the obvious problem that some of the most popular technique procedures (both diagnostic and therapeutic) are largely unstudied outside case reports and clinicians' practice-based research.

The epidemiological profession has evolved its views in recent years, showing more sympathy for practice experience and less blind faith in the RCT. Sackett, a well-known proponent of EBC, defined evidence-based medicine as: "the conscientious, explicit and judicious use of the current best evidence in making decisions about the care of individual patients ... integrating clinical expertise with the best available external clinical evidence from systematic research."[3] After emphasizing that "Good doctors use both individual clinical expertise and the best available external evidence, and neither alone is enough," Sackett draws the conclusion that "without clinical expertise, practice risks become tyrannized by evidence, because even excellent external evidence may be inapplicable to or inappropriate for an individual patient."[3]

THE LIMITATIONS OF RCTS (Box 38.1)

The randomized, blinded, controlled clinical trial is generally regarded to be the gold standard for determining which treatments are best. Patients are randomly assigned to one or more treatment methods, to an untreated group, to a group that receives a sham treatment, or to a group that receives an alternative treatment that has been previously studied. Random assignation is actually more difficult than it sounds, and many otherwise well-executed studies are often discounted for having failed to describe or utilize defensible randomization procedures. Every effort is made to blind all the individuals involved, in various ways depending on the experimental design: the patient doesn't know whether he or she received the real or placebo adjustment; the person who assesses the result is not the same person who administers care; nor does this person know whether the patient received the real or placebo treatment, and so on.

Since there are several limitations to RCTs, no healthcare profession can exclusively rely on them to aid in the final determination of which diagnostic or therapeutic procedure to use[4-7] (see Box 38.1). Researching adjustive methods like manipulation presents a unique challenge in that it is exceedingly difficult to carry out a mock or sham manipulation. This is primarily because the presumed "placebo" hands-on treatment may have a substantial impact (compare with a patient in the medical research setting receiving a sugar pill as a placebo drug). Furthermore, in a real chiropractic clinic, the doctor often uses a mixture of treatments and only rarely one procedure, as is usually required in one of these RCTs. A specific treatment procedure, such as lumbar spine side-posture manipulation, may be of little value unless it is combined with ancillary procedures such as stretching, or manipulative procedures in other parts of the body, such as the feet or sacroiliac joints. The flip-side of the advantage in an RCT, of knowing exactly what treatment procedure is tested, is the disadvantage of not being able to generalize the outcome to a real clinical setting, where that treatment method is never used in isolation.

Along with the general challenges of conducting RCTs previously described, there are several obstacles to investigating the effects of chiropractic care on patients with spinal pain. These include: the generators of spinal pain remain poorly understood; the physiological and psychological mechanisms of pain are elusive in nature; there is heterogeneity of patients and ambiguity in diagnoses; there are indications that some subgroups seem to respond better to spinal manipulative therapy (SMT) than others; and there is difficulty in identifying or isolating the clinical target in need of therapeutic intervention.

Because RCTs are by design controlled, they do not necessarily represent clinical practice (which is fraught with confounding factors). Some types of patients, usually those at higher risk, are excluded from RCTs by design. For example, very few RCTs have been conducted in any area of geriatric healthcare, including chiropractic.[5] Rosner recently offered an example of the limitations of evidence-based medicine in the care of the older person when he opined:

Evidence-based medicine is not kind to the elderly. This movement trusts only the product of randomized, controlled trials or, preferably, meta-analyses of those trials. But subjects over the age of 75 years are rarely found in such trials thus

---

Box 38.1 The seven deadly sins: design flaws of randomized controlled trials (RCTs)

- Outcome of meta-analyses depends largely on input scales
- Corrupted comparison of two pharmaceutical agents (often one drug compared to another drug, which is administered in a knowingly less effective manner for a condition which is known not to respond well to that drug)
- Duplicate ("sausage") publication
- Fastidious interventions masquerading as clinical practice RCTs
- Inappropriate sham procedures
- Methodological scores overemphasize sham procedures and patient blinding
- Inappropriate generalization of RCTs

rendering this population invisible to scientific medicine. If we teach only what we know, and if we know only what we can measure in clinical trial, then we can say little of important resources required in caring for the very old – sufficient time and empathy – are not included in the critical pathways of managed care.[7]

More importantly, RCTs focus primarily on an a priori endpoint, often not monitoring other potentially important outcomes such as the prevention of the disease's progression, reduced impact on comorbid conditions, subjective improvements, and improvement in quality of life.[2-4] Vernon recently described some of the typical methodological deficiencies in RCTs.[5] These are: lack of full observer blinding; unacceptable dropout rates; failure to compare those patients who drop out of the study to those that complied with it; failure to reduce cointerventions; and inappropriate statistical testing.[5]

As Bolton recently wrote, because they have tried to take on the ability to determine cause and effect and to reduce potential sources of bias in the data, RCTs have become more and more divorced from the real world.[2] In other words, while RCTs may have *internal* validity, they do not necessarily have *external* validity. RCTs have been most successful in those cases in which both external and internal validity are high, in situations where the treatment under review is homogeneous and does not vary with either the patient or doctor, such as the administration of a drug by mouth.[2] These trials allow for sham treatment (use of sugar pill), variability of dosage, frequency of use; moreover, their outcome measures are most commonly objective. Ironically, the most invasive of therapeutic interventions, surgery, has the fewest number of RCTs, due to the difficulty of devising placebo surgeries, and gaining permission to perform placebo surgery from the institutional review board that oversees research.

We have already mentioned the difficulty in designing RCTs involving hands-on treatment methods, largely owing to the problem of devising sham treatments. That is not the only problem; chiropractic clinical practice is inherently complex and multifactorial, and that itself has implications. The clinical encounter is affected not only by the presenting chief complaint of the patient and the patient's response to it, but also by the interactions and rapport built between the patient and doctor. As mentioned, blinding is often difficult or impossible, the patient is often given multiple suggestions to augment the efficacy of the therapeutic intervention (instructions to apply ice or heat at home, stretches to perform, and so on), and the patient's cultural background and ethnicity also impact upon recovery. Given these issues, it is easy to see why many field practitioners choose not to rely exclusively on the results gleaned from RCTs for the purposes of patient care planning.

CHIROPRACTIC TECHNIQUE RESEARCH

Legitimate, sustained, scientific research in chiropractic is rather a recent phenomenon. However, throughout chiropractic's 100-year history, the terms "research" and "science" have been among the most popular in the literature of chiropractic and have often been used in ways that are unfamiliar to most scientists[8] (cited in Meeker et al[9]).

During the first half of the 20th century, research into chiropractic methods amounted to model building for claimed therapeutic successes,[9] bolstered by careful clinical observation in some cases. Prospective studies and randomized trials were as rare in chiropractic as they were in medicine. Whatever else may be said about BJ Palmer, the fact that he was a meticulous researcher cannot be denied. In 1935, Palmer created the BJ Palmer Chiropractic Clinic (sometimes simply referred to as the Research Clinic), in order to collect the data on the effects of chiropractic care. The Research Clinic had both medical and chiropractic facilities, and housed some of the most advanced diagnostic equipment of the time, representing an investment of hundreds of thousands of dollars.[10] The overall purpose of the Research Clinic was to document medically patient cases treated by chiropractors. Unfortunately, partly due to lack of formal training in research methods, the vast quantity of data collected was ultimately unusable.[10] As an exception to the rule, Killinger has been able to bring to life some of the upper cervical case reports.[11-15]

The clinical trials that have been conducted using different technique systems and procedures in chiropractic have usually been practice-based. For example, Hoiriis, Owens, and their colleagues have published the results of their ongoing study monitoring the response of patients under upper cervical care with the Rand SF-36 and Global Well-Being Scales.[16–18] The SF-36 measures changes in several different health domains, such as social well-being, physical well-being, pain, and mental well-being. These authors observe that measuring wellness as an outcome measure in healthcare is emphasized as important not only among complementary and alternative medicine providers, but also within the domain of conventional medicine. Further examples include studies on Bioenergetic Synchronization Technique[19] (Ch. 13) and Network Technique[20] (Ch. 22).

The Medical Outcomes Study Short Form-36 Health Survey, Rand modification 1.0 (Rand SF-36) is the most commonly used and most extensively tested instrument to measure changes in quality of life.[21] The SF-36 is self-administered and generic (meaning the measures are relevant to individuals generally and not to specific conditions). The SF-36 has been used in over 400 clinical trials in the USA, and its use in various projects, surveys, and organizations exceeds 4500.[22] According to Ware,[22] the SF-36 can be administered in 5–10 min with a high degree of acceptability and data quality to the general population, and normative values exist for the general population.

One of the first attempts to develop a chiropractic technique research agenda consisted of an intercollegiate association of the 18 accredited chiropractic colleges in North America at the time. In the late 1970s, Drs Herb Magee and Ted Shrader were instrumental in creating the Panel of Advisors to the American Chiropractic Association (ACA) Council on Technique.[23] Shortly thereafter, Dr. JR Campbell, then President of the ACA Council on Technique, suggested that the divisiveness within the chiropractic profession could be overcome by a detailed study of the "subluxation."[24] In response, the ACA Council on Technique conducted its first "Conference on Technique Fundamentals" in the fall of 1983 at

Cleveland College (Los Angeles). The Panel assembled many experts from chiropractic colleges to tackle this issue. From that time until the Panel conducted its last meeting in 1997, biannual meetings were conducted, hosted on a rotating basis at the different colleges.[23] By the spring of 1998, the Panel had given birth to the Technique Consortium, discussed below.

The first few meetings witnessed the International Chiropractic Association (ICA) and ACA people splitting into private camps[24] and poor representation from some member colleges.[23] Originally, working committees were developed to accomplish various tasks between meetings. Unfortunately, time constraints, academic obligations, and the distance between Council members prevented much committee work from getting done. Nevertheless, one of the important precedents the Council set was quite simply to meet on a regular schedule. This was not a trivial accomplishment, as it fostered strong personal and working relationships between Panel members, and it did much to demystify the culture of one college in the eyes of the others.

These meetings went well beyond simply gathering chiropractic educators from ideologically diverse institutions in a demilitarized technique zone. Agenda items from early meetings included: (1) identifying the most commonly used chiropractic techniques and indications of their use (biomechanical, radiographic, neurological, etc.); (2) improving terminology and listing methods; (3) developing a database of technique-related textbooks and articles; (4) changing postgraduate programs; and (5) changing requirements for technique instructors and examiners.[24] Minutes from the early meetings[25,26] indicate that discussions addressed the importance of research in chiropractic, perhaps foreshadowing the evidence-based practice movement currently in vogue throughout the profession. There was often a sharing of curricula and course outlines, including a list of expected competencies, evaluation methods, and resource materials. Several meetings tackled the "subluxation-question,"[27] and it appears there were early attempts to develop common definitions. These pioneering collaborative efforts anticipated that same perceived need for professional consensus that would eventually evolve into the 1996 Association of Chiropractic Colleges (ACC) paradigm statement.[28]

As is the case today in the Technique Consortium, the Panel purposely avoided any position statements that would contradict the philosophy or mission statement of any of the member chiropractic colleges, assuming instead consultative and advisory roles, attempting to reach consensus whenever possible. The Panel constantly reminded itself that, although the ACA, the parent organization, was indeed a political body, the Panel was not. There were times when one of the college presidents would decline to send a representative, not fully appreciating this subtle distinction.[24]

The Panel stressed that research should attempt to improve, not simply prove the value of, chiropractic technique procedures.[24,26] It noted that technique instructors are primarily clinically based and untrained in research methods, whereas researchers may be quite distant from chiropractic principles and practice. The Panel also pointed out that lack of research on the effectiveness of a technique should not result in the elimination of the technique from a college curriculum,[25] since lack of evidence is not evidence of lack. It also bemoaned the lack of funding to conduct clinical trials, and the lack of released time from their administrative responsibilities for faculty members to pursue research projects.[25] Algorithms to promote technique evaluation were published,[25] as well as minimal performance competency lists for student evaluation.[26] The Bartol classification system[29,30] (itself developed with the input of the Council) was used to characterize several of the chiropractic adjustive procedures. Upon compilation of this information, a number of review articles on techniques were published.[23]

Between 1993 and 1995, the Panel cosponsored three national multitechnique symposia to compare chiropractic technique system approaches to treating and managing cases presented by a moderator.[23] Invited guests, representing a cross-section of many of the more commonly used named technique systems, were asked to discuss their respective clinical diagnostic and therapeutic methods and outcomes. Not all of the Panelists

were equally enthusiastic about these multitechnique symposia; some felt they simply advertised technique systems in a non-critical way, even though the purported goal was to subject these techniques to constructive criticism. The last outstanding project of the Panel, the convening of an expert panel to rank the indications for specific adjustive methods for specific lowback conditions, has now been completed and published.[31,32]

In the fall of 1996, the Panel began intense deliberations on its organizational future, ultimately deciding to strengthen its ties with the ACC.[33] Despite the continuity, there would be important differences in focus between the Panel and the Consortium. The former was more concerned with field doctor issues, whereas the latter body has from its inception been more concerned with matters pertaining to the teaching of chiropractic technique. Developers of new technological innovations often use the Consortium as a preliminary stop prior to addressing chiropractic colleges, seeking the opinion of its members. The Consortium has devoted considerable time to discussing issues related to technique evaluation and instruction, as well as networking with other chiropractic organizations, including the National Board of Chiropractic Examiners and the Federation of Chiropractic Licensing Boards.[24]

Compared with the predecessor Panel on Technique, the Technique Consortium is somewhat more research-oriented. It has hosted several discussions on the friction that develops at the research/technique interface, including between the technique and research departments at the chiropractic colleges. Since many members of the Consortium work in both departments, and in some cases wear both of these administrative hats, they are able to discuss this interface first-hand. Another consequence of this convergence is that in some colleges current research has become more technique-related. The Consortium has recently developed recommendations for chiropractic technique in general, as follows:[34]

- Colleges, in deciding which techniques should be taught, should devise and adhere closely to process, involving as many faculty members as possible, and should not introduce arbitrary changes after the fact.

- As much as possible, decisions regarding the teaching of chiropractic technique should be evidence-based.
- As new information becomes available, and more studies are conducted, technique instruction should change in a commensurate fashion.
- At the same time, there must be respect for traditional chiropractic methods. Indeed, the highest measure of respect that can be shown lies in making them more contemporary by reflecting current scientific evidence.
- Discussion on chiropractic techniques should be method-driven, not name-driven. Therefore, the core procedures from the various technique systems should be identified and investigated as such.
- Specific technique procedures drawn from different technique systems may be used, but need not be used, in combination, depending on the needs and preferences of the individual patients and doctors.
- The Technique Consortium acknowledges that one can no longer simply say "it works" and expect to get away with it.
- Colleges, in determining which chiropractic techniques should be taught, should rely on evidence as much as possible, and less on tradition and convention. According to Cooperstein and Schneider, "Colleges today are confronting the challenges of charting a path between the Scylla of an initially disappointing run at technology assessment and the Charybdis of an anachronistic faith in chiropractic procedures."[23] (p. 47)

TECHNOLOGY ASSESSMENT

While some in the profession might superficially acknowledge the wisdom of accepting an evidence-based practice doctrine, they often fail to apply it for its intended purpose. While a noble goal, the concept of EBC remains just that: a concept, unless it is used to strengthen clinical decisions.

But how? The means by which healthcare providers such as chiropractors can best utilize the doctrines of EBC is technology assessment (TA). TA is a form of policy research that evaluates procedures, devices, and protocols for providing decision-makers with information on different policy options.[23] As Cooperstein and Schneider suggested, technology not only consists of the assessment tools and office procedures, but also includes the analytic engine that doctors use to formulate a diagnosis, design a treatment plan, select appropriate outcome measures, and choose reasonable therapeutic interventions to manage a patient's case in the best way.[23] A useful methodological tool for TA of chiropractic technique systems is the Kaminsky model.[35] This algorithm can systematically and objectively evaluate therapeutic and diagnostic procedures. In addition, the Kaminsky model can be used to determine whether a technique or procedure is unsubstantiated, provisionally acceptable, or fully acceptable.[35]

In medicine, newly developed procedures or approaches (particularly pharmacological agents) are usually subjected to intense research scrutiny prior to approval for use on the public (although we have seen how this system can be perverted). However, as described in Chapter 34, new chiropractic procedures and techniques typically arise from field doctors and technique entrepreneurs who seldom subject these new approaches to systematic scientific investigations prior to using them in private practice. The only evidence-based filter that typically exists is the chiropractic colleges, who do what they can to prevent the more outlandish procedures from taking hold of students through exploitation of their inexperience.[36] Technique system advocates have always had an unfair advantage over chiropractic colleges because the former are able to make virtually any unsubstantiated claim without fear of professional censure; technique promoters need only avoid being seen as so fringe, so out of line, that practitioners are barred from using their particular procedure.[23] In contrast, chiropractic colleges are accountable to public health agencies, the scientific community, student loan-granting agencies, alumni, students, faculty members, and accreditation boards.[23]

As long as the doctor remained the sole arbiter of what was and what was not acceptable for patient care, it did not matter that the technology used was unstudied and the science behind it was largely theoretical.[23] According to Cooperstein and Schneider:

The lack of substantive underpinning virtually rationalized the unbridled belief in chiropractic that played such a pivotal role in the profession's survival strategy, insulating it from potentially contradictory evidence. True believers need research to "prove chiropractic" about as much as a minister needs the space program to prove the existence of God.[23] (p. 45)

Now, of course, the stakes are much higher, with the ever-present scrutiny of third-party payers and government regulators requiring accountability in the determination of appropriateness, safety, clinical efficacy, and cost-effectiveness of chiropractic procedures. Technology assessment is at the center of many of the decisions made by managed-care administrators. As Mootz et al suggest: "No one (especially an insurance company) wants to pay for clinical procedures that are ineffective, overpriced or unnecessary ... The advent of better technologies to synthesize research, establish professional consensus, and determine appropriateness has offered a reasonable alternative to the arbitrary and proprietary methods of the past."[37]

TA is at ground zero of the equivocal nature of technique systems in chiropractic. It is imperative that private practitioners, college faculties, and advocates of technique systems (often the same individuals) do not fear the results of TA; they must be prepared to modify or reject their practice activities or college curricula as required, irrespective of their entrenched positions. We have heard it said that the constant danger in research is the slaying of beautiful ideas by ugly facts. "Negative results," wrote Cooperstein and Schneider, "are never encouraging to bring back to one's school or alumni, who wonder aloud why the colleges would undermine confidence in their own curricula."[23] (p. 47) However, such studies are best done internally, by researchers who can appreciate and are sensitive to the broad perspectives and contextual differences within the profession.

There is nothing more disturbing to the research community than being handed a mandate to "prove chiropractic." No good researcher would ever accept such a mandate. There is no role for chiropractic patriotism when it comes to TA and outcomes research. The philosophy of chiropractic (not to be confused with ideological principles) is about the search for truth, and should not be used as a tool for the automatic reiteration of dogma, nor a rubber stamp for untested or invalidated technique procedures. Data never come out wrong, and there is no such thing as good or bad data. Data simply *are*, to be interpreted as such. If a diagnostic or therapeutic protocol is found to be ineffective or harmful, it must be discarded, regardless of its historical roots or longevity.

WHAT THE RESEARCH SAYS

SMT is one of the most studied treatments for back pain. In a recent review, Meeker and Haldeman[38] have summarized the results gathered from prospective RCTs. At the time of this writing (Spring, 2003), 73 RCTs of spinal manipulation can be found in the English literature, most of which have been published in the medical and orthopedic peer-reviewed journals. Most studies have been conducted on patients with low-back pain, neck pain, and certain types of headache. Clinical trials have included placebo-controlled comparisons, comparisons of other treatments, and pragmatic comparisons of chiropractic management versus common medical management.[38]

Of the 43 RCTs published on the treatment of low-back pain (acute, subacute, and chronic), 30 reported SMT to be more effective than control or comparison treatments in at least some patient subgroups. The other 13 trials reported no significant differences between treatment groups. It is especially noteworthy that none of these trials have found SMT to be clinically or statistically less effective than other comparison treatments.[9,38]

Of the 11 RCTs investigating the effects of SMT on neck pain, four reported positive results for SMT, with seven being equivocal. Seven of the nine trials investigating SMT on patients with various forms of headache were positive in favor of manipulation. Again, manipulation was not found to be less effective than comparison treatments, or control treatments of either neck pain or head pain. The Quebec Task Force on Whiplash-Associated Disorders, a formal systematic review and multidisciplinary expert consensus initiative, concluded that SMT had at least weak cumulative evidence, and recommended that a short regimen of SMT may be used as a therapeutic trial for neck pain. Similarly, the US Agency for Health Care Policy and Research concluded that SMT was safe and effective for acute low-back pain, finding no other treatment to have stronger evidence. Over the past decade, similar guidelines developed in several countries have recommended SMT for low-back pain, neck pain, and certain types of headache, as well as whiplash.[9,38]

Gatterman et al convened an expert panel to rate specific chiropractic adjustive procedures used in the treatment of common low-back conditions.[32] On the direction of the Panel of Advisors to the ACA Council of Technique (see above), the investigators first identified relevant literature sources found by a systematic search of chiropractic and medical databases. Anticipating a paucity of controlled studies, they did not restrict their survey to RCTs, as did Haldeman and Meeker. To be included in this study, the source had to include an operational definition of the technique procedure used, a diagnosis or source of back pain being treated, and a description of outcome measures (either objectively measured or subjectively assessed). After reviewing the literature, and drawing upon their own clinical experience, the expert panel was then asked to rate the clinical value of the specific adjustive methods for the specific low-back conditions. In addition to assessing clinical effectiveness, the expert panel was also asked to rate the quality of the literature upon which their opinions were partially based.

Using a rating scale from 0 to 10 (with 10 being the highest rating, indicating that a technique is used effectively for a given condition), the expert panel reported the following:[32] for the treatment of acute low-back pain, the most effective technique used was side-posture adjusting (9.5), followed by drop-table adjusting (8.7), and distraction technique (8.7). A similar ranking was found for patients with low-back pain and buttock or leg pain. However, among patients with low-back pain with buttock or leg pain and neurogenic deficits, distraction technique and drop-table assist adjusting both ranked higher than side-posture adjusting (scores of 6.9, 6.1, and 5.9 respectively). All other adjustive techniques consistently scored low in all categories in this study. The expert panel produced similar ratings for both acute and chronic presentations, although the effectiveness ratings tended to be lower for chronic presentations. Literature ratings tended to resemble clinical effectiveness ratings – a very interesting finding worthy of serious thought. Did the expert panel prefer adjustive methods that were well-studied clinically, or did they simply believe that methods which they approved had been well studied?

In a companion study, Cooperstein et al characterized the literature pertaining to which specific type of chiropractic adjustive care is most effective for particular low-back pain across both tissue-specific and functional classifications.[31] This characterization is especially important because most clinical trials do not carefully describe either the actual intervention used or the exact condition being treated: herniated disk, spondylolisthesis, sacroiliac joint dysfunction, posterior joint subluxation, non-specific back pain, back pain with neurological deficits, and so on. Based on their extensive review of the literature, the investigators reported that the procedure with the widest base of evidence support is side-posture manipulation for generic low-back pain. The technique procedure with the next highest level of evidence support was distraction manipulation (Ch. 16), followed by mobilization techniques, mostly studied in medical settings.

While many technique representatives have published an impressive quantity of articles in the peer-reviewed literature, with a few notable exceptions, very little of this literature has to do with clinical outcomes. Cooperstein et al conclude: "those researchers attempting to validate the appropriateness of their favored methods had best focus more on the type of research they do – more on outcomes and less on peripheral matters such as modeling and the reliability of diagnostic procedures."[31] (p. 410)

ISSUES OF SAFETY

We are unaware of particular named studies investigating the safety of technique systems, but there are several studies monitoring the reported adverse effects of chiropractic adjustive procedures in general. These studies, therefore, allow us to draw inferences regarding the safety of technique systems that employ these adjustive methods. A large patient-based survey detailed the frequency and characteristics of side-effects following SMT.[39] This study collected data from 4712 treatments on 1058 patients by 102 Norwegian chiropractors. At least one adverse reaction was reported by 55% of patients at some time during the course of the maximum of six treatments. Of reported reactions, the most common were local discomfort (53%), headache (12%), tiredness (11%), and radiating pain (8%). Reactions were either mild or moderate in 85% of cases, with 64% of adverse reactions appearing within 4 h of treatment, and 74% of cases disappearing within 24 h.[39] The results of a Swedish study were similar.[40]

Although chiropractic care does have a favorable safety record, especially when compared to medical interventions such as drug use and surgery, SMT is not without material risk.[38] However, the best evidence suggests that the most serious risk, stroke following cervical adjustments, is an exceedingly rare event. The RAND group estimates the risk of serious complications from SMT to be 5–10 in 10 million for vertebrobasilar reactions, 3–6 in 10 million for major impairments, and incidence of fewer than 5 fatalities per 10 million manipulations.[41] Other experts place the risk of stroke resulting in serious neurological complications or death following SMT at between 1 million and 3 million adjustments and 1 in 1 million patients.[38]

Three recent articles by Haldeman et al have put the issue of stroke resulting from cervical manipulation into perspective.[41–44] Following an extensive review of the literature, Haldeman and his colleagues concluded that, because the event is so rare, and various details are often lacking from the relatively few documented cases of stroke following SMT that do exist, it is impossible to advise patients or practitioners about how to avoid the risk of stroke during manipulation, or to specify which sport or exercise activity presents the greatest potential risk.[42] Moreover, there are cases of stroke in patients following both minor trauma (yoga, stargazing, prayer) and major trauma (car accidents, being hit by trees).

The misuse of research, combined with unsubstantiated allegations of the dangers of chiropractic care by a small number of antichiropractic zealots, is nowhere more apparent than in an inquest underway at the time of this writing (early 2003) in Ontario. In this case, a 45-year-old woman purportedly died of a stroke in 1996. She had seen her chiropractor 17 days earlier. Despite early decisions not to call for an inquest, it was eventually ruled that an inquest would be held in order to determine what role, if any, the chiropractic treatment had in the death. After several delays, the inquest finally began in April 2002. Early on, important evidence immediately came to light, as one of the original authors of the neuropathological autopsy report testified that he now believed that the deceased died of natural causes, due to advanced atherosclerosis. He further testified that mistakes had been made in the original investigation that had concluded that the death resulted from trauma related to spinal manipulation. "We were wrong," he testified, "in retrospect, our conclusions were erroneous."[45] (p. 1)

THE MISUSE OF RESEARCH

In misleading research, an assumed causative link between two facts is often overstated. For example, in two separate articles, Rupert et al[46] and Coulter et al[47] both reported that older patients under chiropractic maintenance care were more likely to be active in their community, less likely to use prescription medications, more likely to report better health status, and less likely to require nursing care facilities. We have often seen students, and even other scholars (who should know better) assume that a cause-and-effect relationship exists between these reported outcomes and chiropractic treatment, with the obvious goal of wanting to extol the virtues of chiropractic maintenance care. However, these results must of course be interpreted cautiously because it is possible that older persons who seek out chiropractic care may already have these characteristics to begin with (as noted by both Coulter et al[47] and Rupert et al[46] in their respective articles).

Schultz, in a letter to the editor defending his concerns with the Council on Chiropractic Practice guidelines, discussed another possible source of misinformation.[48] Citing an article by Ramsey et al,[49] Schultz reminded us that Food and Drug Administration (FDA) approval of a category I or II device does not guarantee any level of physiological or clinical effectiveness, only that the technical performance of the machine is as stated by the developer. This is in stark contrast to FDA approval accorded to a pharmaceutical, wherein the FDA diligently tests a drug in clinical settings. We note that advocates of diagnostic and therapeutic devices used by chiropractic technique systems sometimes declare their methods "FDA-approved" – which does not mean the device has been found to be clinically effective.

Schultz argued that the assertion in the Council of Chiropractic Practice (CCP) guidelines that FDA approval means the device has been shown to perform the function(s) that is/are claimed by the manufacturer, which may be interpreted by a reader to include clinical effectiveness, only hampers the quality of the CCP guidelines.[48] As Schultz suggested: "The interpretation of the scope and importance of FDA approval within an evidence hierarchy might arguably be the difference between supporting and not supporting the use of a diagnostic technology such as thermocouples."[48] (p. vii)

In a recent article, Grod et al published their findings following a survey of chiropractic patient education and promotional material produced by national, state, and provincial societies and research agencies in Canada and the USA.[50] Of 11 organizations sampled, nine were found to distribute patient brochures. Of these nine organizations, all distributed patient brochures that make claims for chiropractic services that have not been scientifically validated.

EXAMPLES OF BIAS AND IGNORANCE IN MEDICAL REPORTING

Organized medicine has often unfairly attacked the chiropractic profession, making unsubstantiated statements and drawing inaccurate conclusions. Carey and Townsend provide several examples of what they referred to as "bias and ignorance" in medical reporting.[51] They discussed several examples of instances where a medical doctor, during trial testimony or documents offered in evidence, is openly critical of aspects of chiropractic treatment, diagnosis, examination, or standards of care. The seriousness of these allegations is compounded by the fact that in not a single case was there any evidence of any form of communication between the medical doctor and *any* chiropractor. Rather, the medical doctor rendering an opinion more often than not relied solely on the opinion offered by the patient.[51]

Striking a similar theme, Rosner[52] systematically deconstructed the arguments made by some medical scholars in the *British Medical Journal* that speculated that chiropractic might be hazardous to a patient's life. He accurately reviewed the literature with respect to the risk of chiropractic care, as well as pointing out that accusations of the overuse of radiographs by chiropractors often derive from the unsubstantiated commentaries of a few authors who, either consciously or unconsciously, inaccurately describe elements of chiropractic practice.[52] Many medical writers ignore knowledge that contradicts what they already think about chiropractic, leading them to publish erroneous conclusions about its efficacy and cost-effectiveness.

FAILED UNIVERSITY AFFILIATION

Whether chiropractors feel the superabundance of technique systems is a professional asset or liability, it is certain that outsiders looking in are at best confused by the lack of standardization, and, at worst, horrified by it. At the limit, the abhorrence for a few technique systems, not even taught beyond simply being described at the Canadian Memorial Chiropractic College (CMCC), contributed to its losing an opportunity for university affiliation. Starting in the mid-1990s, CMCC had pursued affiliation with York University in Toronto. A letter of intent was signed, and both institutions worked diligently to try and develop an agreement. However, after passing several academic meetings, the affiliation process came to an abrupt end in the spring of 2000, in no small part due to the objections raised by a small but very vocal group of faculty members from within the university.[53] Much of the concern from York University faculty focused on four contentious issues: (1) the subluxation theory; (2) the vaccination question; (3) pediatric chiropractic care; and (4) the eccentric character of some of the technique systems – notably Applied Kinesiology (Ch. 12).[54]

Although we can only guess what it was about Applied Kinesiology that so alarmed the York professors, we must assume it was simply used as a surrogate for any technique system that appeared to them particularly on the fringe of a profession already seen as on the fringes of healthcare. Chiropractors had best take responsibility for their professional image. Every piece of weird jargon devised, every stretch of the physiological imagination, every unsubstantiated claim made is noticed by our detractors (Fig. 38.1). They make sure that the excesses of the one technique are made to count against the many. Likewise, whenever the partisans of one technique system find the procedures of another to be unsafe or ineffective, even despite the lack of supportive evidence, and whatever the reason, the entire profession is made to pay the price.

IN CLOSING

At the present time, the EBC results can inform us that chiropractic care is beneficial for a wide range of conditions, and beneficial results are achieved safely, and in a cost-effective manner. There is still much to learn about which adjustive procedures and case management protocols are most appropriate for specific diagnostic entities, occurring in specific patients, who have different expectations and goals in seeking chiropractic care. In the meantime, we must do our best to stick closely to the evidence base. Some of the

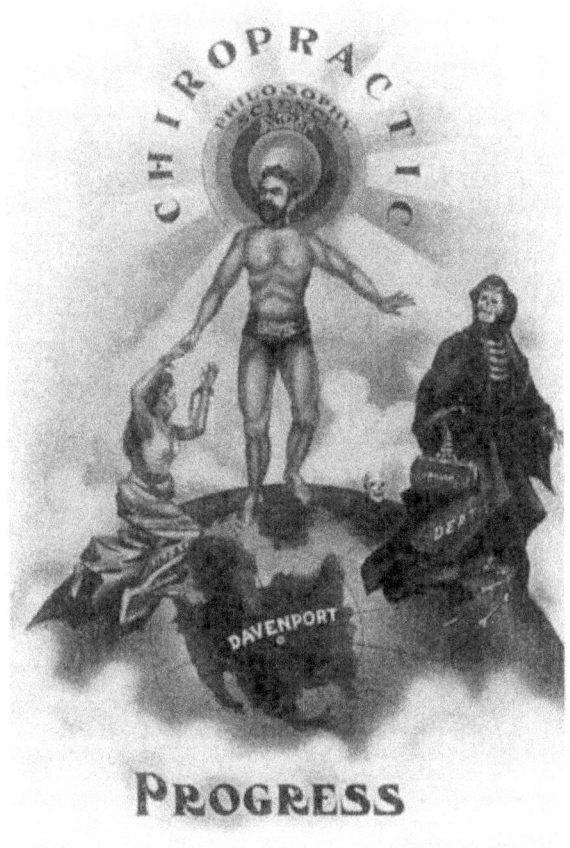

Figure 38.1 A Palmer broadside *c.* 1911 with BJ Palmer, representing chiropractic, warding off disease and death. Courtesy of Palmer College of Chiropractic Archives, Davenport, IA.

unflattering studies in the area of technology assessment are more than offset by the encouraging results of outcome studies, which tend to put chiropractic in its best light. This implies, as suggested by Cooperstein et al, that:[31]

Those who would limit the practice of medicine or chiropractic to those procedures that have been rigorously validated are too quick to jettison the wisdom of the experienced clinician. Those who would defend the clinician's right to practice as he or she sees fit irrespective of the evidence, no matter how limited, assume an equally untenable position. Somewhere in the mix, reasonable people should be able to strike a balance between imperfect knowledge and the exigencies of practice.

Lastly, the importance of the patient should not be lost on clinicians. The value of patient satisfaction, since it directly affects patient compliance (and thus quality of care) cannot be overestimated.[2,54]

Haldeman, during a recent plenary discussion on the philosophy of chiropractic, opined that chiropractic should not be obsessed with either condition-based or subluxation-based care; rather, he suggests, chiropractic clinicians should focus on being patient-centered.[55]

REFERENCES

1. Palmer D D 1914 The chiropractor, p. 10. Beacon Light Press, Los Angeles, CA
2. Bolton J E 2001 The evidence in evidence-based practice: what counts and what doesn't count? (commentary) Journal of Manipulative and Physiological Therapeutics 245: 362–365
3. Sackett D L 1998 Evidence-based medicine (editorial). Spine 23 (10): 1085–1086
4. JNC-VI 1997 The sixth report of the Joint National Committee on prevention, detection, evaluation and treatment of high blood pressure. Archives of Internal Medicine 157: 2413–2446
5. Vernon H 1999 Spinal manipulation for chronic low back pain: a review of the evidence. Topics in Clinical Chiropractics 6 (2): 8–12
6. Goodwin J S 1999 Geriatrics and the limits of modern medicine (commentary). New England Journal of Medicine 340 (16): 1283–1285
7. Rosner A 2003 Fables or foibles: inherent problems with RCTs. Journal of Manipulative and Physiological Therapeutics 26(7): 460–467
8. Philips R B, Adams A H, Sandtur R 1997 Chiropractic research: In: Cherkin D C, Mootz R D (eds) Chiropractic in the United States: training, practice and research p. 91. AHCPR publication 98-N002. US Dept of Health and Human Services, Agency for Health Care Policy and Research, Rockville, MD
9. Meeker W C, Mootz R D, Haldeman S 2002 The state of chiropractic research. Topics in Clinical Chiropractics 9 (1): 1–13
10. Perle S M 2000 Concept paper on chiropractic. Unpublished
11. Keating J C Jr 1997 B J Palmer of Davenport. Association for the History of Chiropractic, Davenport, IA
12. Killinger L Z 1995 A chiropractic case series of seven chronic headache patients. Palmer Journal of Research 2 (2): 48–53
13. Killinger L Z 1995 Chiropractic care in the treatment of asthma. Palmer Journal of Research 2 (3): 43–47
14. Killinger L Z, Azad A 1997 Multiple sclerosis patients under chiropractic care: a retrospective study. Palmer Journal of Research 2 (4): 96–100
15. Killinger L Z, Azad A 1998 Chiropractic care of infantile colic: a case study. Palmer Journal of Research 3 (1): 203–206
16. Hoiriis K T, Burd E, Owens E F Jr 1999 Changes in general health status during upper cervical chiropractic care: a practice based research project update. Chiropractic Research Journal 6 (2): 65–70
17. Hoiriis K T, Owens E F Jr, Pfleger B 1997 Changes in general health status during upper cervical chiropractic care: a practice-based research project. Chiropractic Research Journal 4 (1): 18–26
18. Owens E F Jr, Hoiriis K T, Burd D 1998 Changes in general health status during upper cervical chiropractic care. PBR progress report. Chiropractic Research Journal 5 (1): 9–16
19. Hawk C M 1995 The use of measures of general health status in chiropractic patients: a pilot study. Palmer Journal of Research 2 (2): 39–44
20. Blanks R H I, Schuster T L, Dobson M 1997 A retrospective assessment of Network Care using a survey of self-rated health, wellness and quality of life. Journal of Vertebral Subluxation Research 1 (4): 15–31
21. RAND 1982 Health Sciences Program. RAND 36-item health survey 1.0. RAND
22. Ware J The SF-36 health survey. www.sf-36.com/general/sf.36.html
23. Cooperstein R, Schneider M S 1996 Assessment of chiropractic techniques and procedures. Topics in Clinical Chiropractics 3 (1): 44–51
24. Cooperstein R 1996 Council on technique. Journal of the American Chiropractic Association (July): 37–38, 61
25. ACA council on technic 1984 Minutes of meeting, March. Sunnydale, CA
26. ACA council on technic 1988 Minutes of meeting, September 16–18. St Louis, MO
27. Shrader T L 1983 Technic council sponsors conference on fundamentals. ACA Journal of Chiropractic 20: 52–54
28. Association of Chiropractic Colleges 1996 Position paper 1. ACC
29. Bartol K M 1991 A model for the categorization of chiropractic treatment procedures. Chiropractic Technique 3 (2): 78–80
30. Bartol K M 1992 An algorithm of the categorization of chiropractic treatment procedures. Chiropractic Technique 4 (1): 8–14
31. Cooperstein R, Perle S, Gatterman M et al 2001 Chiropractic technique procedures for specific low back conditions: characterizing the literature. Journal of Manipulative and Physiological Therapeutics 24 (6): 407–411
32. Gatterman M, Lantz C, Perle S, Schneider M 2001 Rating specific chiropractic technique procedures for common low back conditions. Journal of Manipulative and Physiological Therapeutics 24 (7): 449–456
33. Panel of Advisors to the ACA council on technique 1996 Inter-collegiate conference #27, September 12–15. Life Chiropractic College, Marietta, GA

34. Technique Consortium of the Association of Chiropractic Colleges 2000 Minutes of meeting September 14–16. St Louis, MO

35. Kaminsky M 1990 Evaluation of chiropractic methods. Chiropractic Technique 2 (3): 107–112

36. Lawrence D 1989 The challenges of teaching technique. Chiropractic Technique 1 (1): 6–8

37. Mootz R D, Shekelle P G, Hansen D T 1995 The politics of policy and research. Topics in Clinical Chiropractics 2 (2): 56–70

38. Meeker W C, Haldeman S 2002 Chiropractic: a profession at the crossroads of mainstream and alternative medicine. Annals of Internal Medicine 136: 216–227

39. Senstead O, Leboueuf-Yde C, Borchgrevink C 1997 Frequency and characteristics of side effects of spinal manipulative therapy. Spine 22 (4): 435–441

40. Leboeuf-Yde C, Hennius B, Rudberg E et al 1997 Side effects of chiropractic treatment: a prospective study. Journal of Manipulative and Physiological Therapy 20 (8): 511–515

41. Terrett A 1996 Vertebrobasilar stroke following manipulation. National Chiropractic Mutual Insurance, West Des Moines, IA

42. Haldeman S, Kohlbeck F J, McGregor M 1999 Risk factors and precipitating neck movements causing vertebrobasilar artery dissection after cervical trauma and spinal manipulation. Spine 24 (8): 785–794

43. Haldeman S, Kohlbeck F J, McGregor M 2002 Unpredictability of cerebrovascular ischemia associated with cervical spine manipulation therapy. Spine 27 (1): 49–55

44. Haldeman S, Carey P, Townsend M, Papadopoulos C 2001 Arterial dissection following cervical manipulation: the chiropractic experience. Canadian Medical Association Journal 165 (7): 905–906

45. Chiropractic Communication Working Group 2002 Information bulletin. May 9

46. Rupert R, Manello D, Sandefur R 2000 Maintenance care health promotion services administered to US chiropractic patients aged 65 and older, part II. Journal of Manipulative and Physiological Therapy 23: 10–19

47. Coulter I, Hurwitz E, Aranow H et al 1996 Chiropractic patients in a comprehensive home-based geriatric assessment, follow-up and health promotion program. Topics in Clinical Chiropractic 3 (2): 46–55

48. Schultz G 2002 Letter to the editor in reply. Topics in Clinical Chiropractic 9 (2): vi–vii

49. Ramsey S, Luce B, Deyo R, Franklin G 1998 The limited state of technology assessment for medical devices: facing the issues. American Journal of Managed Care 4 (SP): SP188–SP199.

50. Grod J P, Sikorski D, Keating J C Jr 2001 Unsubstantiated claims in patient brochures from the largest state, provincial, and national chiropractic associations and research agencies. Journal of Manipulative and Physiological Therapy 24 (8): 514–519

51. Carey P F, Townsend G M 1997 Bias and ignorance in medical reporting. Journal of the Canadian Chiropractic Association 41 (2): 105–116

52. Rosner A L 1999 Chiropractic: more good than harm or vice versa? (commentary) Journal of Manipulative and Physiological Therapy 22 (4): 250–253

53. Grayson J P 2002 The academic legitimization of chiropractic: the case of CMCC and York University. Journal of the Canadian Chiropractic Association 46 (4): 265–279

54. Gleberzon B J 2003 The academic legitimization of chiropractic: the case of CMCC and York University letter to the editor. Journal of the Canadian Chiropractic Association 47 (1): 61–63

55. Haldeman S 2001 Plenary discussion on the principles and philosophy of chiropractic. Presented during the World Federation of Chiropractic, Sixth Biennial Congress. World Federation of Chiropractic, Toronto, Ontario

Appendices

Appendix 1: Toward a taxonomy of subluxation-equivalents

"When I use a word," Humpty Dumpty said, in rather a scornful tone, "it means just what I choose it to mean – neither more nor less".
"The question is", said Alice, "whether you can make words mean so many different things".
"The question is, said Humpty Dumpty, "which is to be master – that's all".

From Lewis Carroll's Through the Looking Glass and What Alice Found There[1]

THE SUBLUXATION QUESTION

Like Lewis Carroll's fictional character, the chiropractic profession has attempted to create all-encompassing definitions, hoping to satisfy the tenets of all its members and thus achieve professional unity. These oft-repeated attempts, having taken the form of moderated consensus processes, intercollegiate meetings, scholarly articles, whole books on the subject, and debates at professional meetings share but one thing in common: their failure to achieve this desired unification.

There is no reason to herein review chiropractic's long history of professional civil war, but we must acknowledge that much of it has revolved around "Subluxation," both its definition and usage. Conferences and consensus proceedings, aimed at halting the internecine chiropractic fratricide, inevitably center on the word. The renewal of hostilities that has inevitably followed periods of brokered agreement has been, again, all about *Subluxation*. After pointing out that although "there have been several efforts and projects devoted to redefining subluxations," Nelson adds "this movement has not brought clarity and consensus to the subluxation debate but rather obfuscation and confusion".[2]

Pointing toward this or that highly-negotiated and well-publicized definition of Subluxation (we have seen several) does not alter our conclusion: as is usually the case with "united front politics," wherein individuals come together more out of perceived mutual threat rather than shared substantive agreement, the pact is abandoned at whim by any of the participants, whenever political or economic circumstances change. Previous failures notwithstanding, and however byzantine all this must seem to outsiders (who surely must be wondering "what's in a word?"), the chiropractic professions leaders, if not its clinicians, seem to agree that the road to professional unity must pass through agreement on the Subluxation question. But is that true?

We intend to question that assumption. If a considerable majority of chiropractic clinicians, apart from the opinions of their official and sometimes self-appointed spokespeople, tend to approach and treat patients in a broadly consistent manner (and we think they do), then the subluxation question, as it has been heretofore posed, can be seen through the lens of a different perspective. The road to professional unity, rather than passing through endless turmoil regarding "The Subluxation," would rather traverse through better description and professional appreciation of the *different types of clinical practice*. From the practice descriptions, in turn, would come the characterizations of the *types of subluxations* that clinicians purport to treat. (We say "purport" because there remain many unanswered scientific questions, beyond the scope of this article to discuss.)

The chiropractic profession could rid itself of a huge albatross, that Subluxation question hanging around its neck, by retaining indeed, championing the term, but backing off its stubborn insistence that there be an immediate, binding, or permanent consensus on a definition. The last thing chiropractors need are subluxation definitions that tower above them, like Godzilla over Tokyo. Indeed, any meaningful usages should derive from the real world of chiropractic clinical practice. The methodology involved would do for chiropractic terminology what practice-based research has done for the chiropractic clinical research effort: draw its impetus from practicing chiropractic clinics, rather than continuing to proffer the abstractions of chiropractic organizations. (The term "clinics" here should be broadly interpreted to include the chiropractic colleges, which favor a variety of clinical approaches.)

The chiropractic organizations and their spokespersons have been especially demanding in recent years, having put on a protracted series of gargantuan debates, in which the extreme protagonists of allegedly irreconcilable positions have locked horns at a variety of venues, usually research symposia. College presidents, professors, celebrated private practitioners, and attorneys have been asked to line up "for or against" on issues like vaccination, the chiropractor as primary care physician, wellness vs. musculoskeletal paradigms, and yes, the Subluxation. (Imagine being "for" or "against" the Subluxation!) However important the subluxation question may be to chiropractic leaders, of all different stripes and for a variety of reasons, it doesn't follow that it is such a burning question for the clinicians out there, nor for their patients. On the proverbial Monday morning following the conference, little will have changed: the same patients will come in with about the same complaints, and they will be adjusted about the same way.

We would ask the reader, no matter how self-indulgent (or even trite) it may seem to expect people to read yet another article on Subluxation, to regard what follows as something of a fresh

departure. Our goal is not to produce yet another definition, or even rigorous comparison of definitions, but to lay some of the groundwork for an eventual taxonomy of subluxation, the already-written but as yet uncompiled production of many individuals, technique systems, and chiropractic colleges.

PROLIFERATION OF CHIROPRACTIC TECHNIQUES: PREVENTING PROFESSIONAL CONSENSUS

Almost from the beginning[3] chiropractic fragmented into a series of competitive, often mutually exclusive techniques and ideologies, each claiming to be largely self-sufficient for addressing either the totality or an expansive range of human ailments.[4] An interesting aspect of chiropractic history is that when new technique systems are invented, they add to, rather than displace any of the existing techniques. For that reason, Bergmann was able to list many dozens of techniques in use as of 1993,[5] a list which shows no signs of diminishing. Although how this has come about, how it may be changing, and what are the driving forces, is all very interesting, it is beyond our scope here, except insofar as it bears on the subluxation question. The base fact is: each of these several dozen technique systems feels compelled to develop or agree its favored definition or at least usage of a "subluxation-equivalent," a term we discuss below. (See references 6 for a discussion of technique systems in chiropractic.) The practice of science involves knowledge that has been attained through specialized methods of fact-finding, research, and interpretation. The ensemble of such methods warrants the descriptive term "technique," in the sense of a body of technical and conceptual procedures by which the knowledge accrues and the science advances. Any particular scientific profession consists in the tooled knowledge,[7] that establishes its unique professional identity. Chiropractic science, or technique in the expanded sense of the term, is thus a kind of tooled knowledge that has focused historically on "the relationship between structure (primarily the spine) and function (primarily the nervous system) of the human body that leads to the restoration and

Table 1   Super-proliferation of technique systems and ideologies in chiropractic

1. *Development at the margins of society:* It is always at the margins of society that freedom of experimentation commingles with reckless adventurism, that lack of regulation breeds simultaneously bold innovation and abject quackery.
2. *Lack of market penetration:* The frustrations of partial success sow disunity and foster internecine struggle.
3. *Economic advantage of retaining several techniques:* health care providers, just like the vendors of other sorts of goods and services, are subject to market forces that drive them to strive for product diversification and the establishment of brand names.
4. *The chiropractor as generalist:* to distinguish him or herself from another, the chiropractor must emphasize the particular type of technique used, rather than conditions or types of patients treated, since almost all are generalists.
5. *Sensationalist bent of the founders:* The founders, not without consequences for today, were not adverse to lurid advertising claims for the advantages of chiropractic care, for both economic and political reasons related to professional survival.
6. *Lack of knowledge:* Although actual data and substantive research should constitute the best potential check on technique hyperbole, there have been many phenomena germane to chiropractic procedures that have so far defied explanation and resisted investigation.
7. *The quest for "nerve interference":* Since chiropractors have always hung their hat on the hook of "nerve interference," it should be noted that the consequences of a hypothetical subclinical neuropathy, occurring at the histological level, may be extraordinarily difficult to detect.
8. *The allure of brand name techniques*[6]: Chiropractors and chiropractic students remain vulnerable to the exploitation of the technique hawkers, who offer absolute conviction in the value of the technique for sale, who link their particular technique and ideology to a whole set of purely extraneous, unrelated values, such as loyalty to chiropractic, staunch opposition to medical expropriation, quality service to patients, and above all, *the daily accomplishment of miracles.*

preservation of health".[8] Chiropractic has evolved a unique terminology that goes along with this specialized tooled knowledge, the most important item of which is undoubtedly "subluxation."

More amazing than the mind-numbing gaggle of different technique and ideological systems is the mind-boggling success of the chiropractic profession to keep it all under one technique hat. How do so many strange bedfellows get along so well? Probably because no matter how substantively different and even inconsistent the techniques and ideologies may be, the great majority of them seem equally at home among just a few sweeping phrases and organizing principles: Subluxation, Nerve Interference, the Adjustment, the intimate relationship of structure and function. (Alas, the devil is the details!)

It may seem odd at first to emphasize the moderating, harmonizing role of the chiropractic ideological umbrella, given how often we are reminded that "chiropractors have been waging war against themselves for 90 odd years",[9] that "the chiropractic technic wars go on, with 'new' technics coming and going as frequently as woman's fashions".[10] The conventional wisdom at play here fails to appreciate that "technic wars" are not entirely unlike Pepsi vs. Coke confrontations, where both beverage companies have a common long-term interest in promoting cola vs. flavored teas, no matter the short-term

struggle over market share. Likewise, the chiropractic wars are very often largely over infrastructure: scope of practice, terminology, case management, billing practices, relations with allied health professionals, college curricula.

These ideological confrontations stand apart from and may even conceal essential agreement over the basics: chiropractors adjust the spine, which helps the nerves, which promotes health. Two chiropractors who could kill one another over the vaccination issue might be in perfect accord on subluxation detection and correction, while another pair of doctors at odds over manipulative vs. soft-tissue techniques might be willing to live and let live, provided they share the ultimate goal of reducing "nerve interference." Of course, this would not stop either one from claiming his or her own methods would be a better way to achieve the desired end! Table 1, abstracted from ref. 11 , lists some of the reasons chiropractic has developed such a vast array of technique systems and ideologies. As we have previously commented, each of the system techniques advocates one or more versions of subluxation-equivalents.

Subluxation or subluxation?

The word "Subluxation" is and always has been central to most chiropractors, who have adopted the simplifying assumption that patients suffer at root from the same type of disorder, no matter how extreme the differences in manifestation. Our use of the upper case "S" is deliberate, to convey the notion that this term is an umbrella for many other terms, and has a distinctly metaphysical character. Although there are profoundly different definitions from one technique grouping to another, almost all chiropractors who use the term "Subluxation" have in mind that there is something wrong with the spine (sometimes the brain[12]), that has had negative consequences for human health, and is amenable to manual and other conservative treatments. We honestly think *it is* that simple. The term "manipulable lesion" is a very elegant and concise rendering of our thought, although we would prefer the equivalent phrase "adjustable lesion," since chiropractic adjustive care includes more than manipulation; we also wonder if we can do better than the term "lesion," due to its historical association with the osteopathic profession.

The chiropractic profession has drawn some heat over the years for espousing such a "monocausal theory of disease," for having supposed it needed to reduce just about all the symptomatic and non-symptomatic ailments they treat to the common denominator of "Subluxation." We must point out that the chiropractic profession has had no long term monopoly on monocausal theories of disease; witness the various specific etiology theories of disease generated by 19th century medical practitioners. Indeed, Palmer's emphasis on "Subluxation" emanated from the same reductionist *Weltanschauung* as the same period's germ theory of disease (Koch, Pasteur), "inborn errors of metabolism" approach, inherited characteristics approach (De Vries, Muller, Morgan), and Freud's views on the unconscious and repressed libido. Owen quite correctly states "the one cause, one cure concept is so closely associated with chiropractic's model of vertebral subluxation that the vertebral subluxation is in danger of being thrown out with it".[13]

Nonetheless, looking back at the 20th century, while the chiropractors mostly clung to their monocausal outlook, their medical colleagues went on to produce comprehensive textbooks of pathology, with chapters organized by process (general pathology) and by organ system (systemic pathology). By comparison, chiropractic's pathology book mostly consists of one chapter, entitled "Subluxation" with a series of subheadings that amount to subluxation-related conditions. We are not unaware of Gatterman's impressive and useful book on the Subluxation,[14] but it is just that: a book that emerged from a consensus conference on Subluxation, and which assumes all the way through that the various conditions and syndromes from which patients suffer are all manifestations of The Subluxation or a *Subluxation-equivalent*, a term we discuss below.

SUBLUXATION-EQUIVALENTS (SEs)

Although most chiropractors continue to insist upon the primacy of the term, it is not without some obvious misgiving, conscious and unconscious. Much work has gone into the elaboration of increasingly baroque "vertebral subluxation complex" models,[15] lending a polyglot veneer to the monocausality of Subluxation. However, including multiple tissues and poly-hyphenated pathologies in the vertebral subluxation complex doesn't really overcome the monocausal essence of the unadorned Subluxation, nor does it quell the anxiety that fuels endless consensus processes and desperate calls for unity under this or that version of the model definition. The "vertebral subluxation complex" must be considered a Subluxation-equivalent (SE), any word of phrase used by a technique partisan that renders that same reductionist thought and serves the same function as the mere word "Subluxation." We note Rome's list of 296 such SEs,[16] and explore some of the primary ones below.

We believe that the chiropractic profession, in its zeal to construct a United Front on the Subluxation question, is seeking a solution to a problem that is still poorly defined. It's not that there are too many definitions of *Subluxation*, but rather we are unsure what clinical entities are addressed by the various technique procedures, which surely cannot each be having the same impact on patients. It would be useful to categorize, in a taxonomic sense, the various SEs as they are addressed by the described

Table 2   Potential benefits of a taxonomy of subluxation-equivalents

1. Enable appreciation of the context-sensitivity of different definitions and clinical descriptions.
2. Allow allied health professions to better understand the relationship between the individual chiropractor's examination findings and the recommended course of care.
3. Categorize operational descriptions of subluxation-equivalents, so as to go beyond mere compilation of lists.
4. Promote the ascent of evidence-based agreement on subluxation concepts, advancing beyond the more usual ideological level of discourse.
5. Inform and prioritize fruitful areas of research, especially in neuroscience.
6. Advance a more multifactorial perspective on subluxation, increasing the profession's distance from unenlightened, overly-simplistic monocausal views.

treatment approaches. Then, the different system techniques would take on something of the character of chiropractic specialities, treating related but not necessarily identical pathologies; and the load of the monocausal albatross would be considerably lightened. Perhaps refining the fundamental approach to categorizing the clinical perspectives on subluxation could produce an inventory of clinically-based SEs that can better inform the discussion, and beyond that, clinical research. The clinical imperative to discover which adjustive methods work best for which conditions would be much encouraged were we to at least back off, pending more data, the abstract search for common denominators. Table 2 lists some of the potential benefits of a taxonomy of subluxation.

Before proceeding to our focus on SE categorizations, there is still one more matter we must address: the issue of the historical derivation of the word Subluxation. As is well known, the term "subluxation" originated in the medical literature, where it conveys the sense of a minor, or partial joint luxation (misalignment). How important is it that any chiropractor using the term *always* has in mind some sense of misalignment, thus remaining loyal to the original "bone out of place" or rendering? Some would say very important, including some who would prefer *not* to use the word, such as Brantingham, who wants to abandon subluxation as a term denoting a manipulatable lesion because he finds restriction, not misalignment, to best render the sense of the pathology.[17]

Actually, it is very common for biomedical (that includes "biochiropractic") terms to change, and there is no requirement to remain true to original usages. The term "cretin," referring to infantile

hypothyroidism, is derived from the French word *chretién*, meaning Christian or Christ-like, because these simple unfortunates were considered by physicians of times past as being incapable of sinning.[18] Does anyone believe modern definitions of "cretinism" should acknowledge religious antecedents? Similarly, the word "tumor," almost always referring to neoplasm, derives from the Latin word *tumeri*, to swell, with a very different significance. Nothing bars the chiropractor from using the term "subluxation," even when treating spine related problems thought not to include an important element of misalignment, except semantic rigidity. Although it is very important to preserve chiropractic's unique professional identity through the use of entrenched terms like "subluxation" and "adjustment," there is no reason to demand their mummification.

SUBLUXATION-EQUIVALENT TAXONOMY

In discussing the various types of subluxation classifications, we limit (but not quash) our temptation to marshal evidence or advance opinions on which SEs seem to have the most merit and how they may be best interpreted. Leach,[19] Gatterman,[14] and others have reviewed the evidence in great detail. Herein, we are more interested in contributing towards an eventual subluxation taxonomy, a descriptive undertaking in the sense of Linnaeus.

In a Linnaean classification system, there are both hierarchical *categories*, each described in terms of its defining characteristics; and within each category, there are *taxa* (singular: taxon), which are named examples of the category. Table 3

Table 3   Taxonomy of a human: *Homo sapiens*

Category	Taxon	Characteristics
Kingdom	Animalia	Multicellular organisms requiring complex organic substances for food
Phylum	Chordata	Animals with notochord, dorsal hollow nerve cord, gill pouches in pharynx at some stage of life cycle
Subphylum	Vertebrata	Spinal cord enclosed in a vertebral column, body basically segmented, skull enclosing brain
Superclass	Tetrapoda	Land vertebrates, four-limbed
Class	Mammalia	Young nourished by milk glands, skin with hair or fur, body cavity divided by a muscular diaphragm, red blood cells without nuclei, three ear bones (ossicles), high body temperature
Order	Primates	Tree dwellers or their descendants, usually with fingers and flat nails, sense of smell reduced
Family	*Hominidae*	Flat face; eyes forward; color vision; upright, bipedal locomotion
Genus	*Homo*	Large brain, speech, long childhood
Species	*Homo sapiens*	Prominent chin, high forehead, sparse body hair

Table 4   Taxonomy of the Gonstead subluxation-equivalent: Segmental *misalignment*

Category	Taxon	Characteristics
Kingdom	Musculoskeletal	Encompasses primarily musculoskeletal structures, rather than viscera.
Phylum	Full-spine	The SE may occur anywhere in the axial skeleton, unlike in upper cervical techniques.
Class	Nerve int.	The SE includes obligatory nerve interference
Order	Anterior joints	Intervention believed to target the anterior more than posterior zygapophysis.
Genus	*Segmental*	Embraces a motion unit consisting of two vertebra, rather than regions of the spine or full-body spinal distortions.
Species	*Misalignment*	Intervention more informed by vertebral misalignment than motion restriction, although informed by each

illustrates the Linnaean classification of *Homo sapiens*. Eventually, we will classify the major SEs in a similar manner, thus having constructed the obverse of Bartol's classification of adjustive techniques according to their mechanical characteristics.[20,21] Table 4 gives an example of what that may look like, for the primary SE treated (some would say "corrected") by Gonstead adjustive measures. Rather than pause to invent new terminology for the categories, we elected to temporarily retain the standard Linnaean terms: kingdom, division, class, order, family, genus, species.

Clearly, before being able to populate the classification scheme with *taxa*, it is necessary to define the categories. The quantity of stand-alone chiropractic techniques out there boggles the mind, and each of them features in its core an SE. Some of the categorizations developed below transect others, creating in effect a multidimensional matrix of SEs. A fully-elaborated, hierarchical classification scheme would draw out those relationships in detail. Although representative examples are given in some cases, it should be remembered that no shoe ever fits perfectly.

Structural and functional SEs

Until fairly recently the great majority of chiropractors took it for granted that chiropractic clinical intervention fundamentally addressed the *structure* (or form) of the body, which then determined function. This would be unlike architecture, where it is said that "form follows function." It has been further said that chiropractic doctors treat the structural causes of disease, whereas medical doctors treat symptoms, what amounts to the resultant dysfunction. Gonstead practitioners provide a good representative example of a traditional, structurally-based subluxation concept.[22] A very Gonstead-like SE also shows up in an otherwise very different technique, Network Spinal Analysis, in its *Class A subluxation*.[23] It is structural in nature, with elements of fixation, misalignment, and nerve interference, treatable with high-velocity, low-amplitude (HVLA) thrusting.

Nevertheless, there are many reasons to believe that the dynasty of the purely structurally-based SE is over. Looking forward, it would appear that SEs will have to be classified as being primarily functionally or structurally based, and structure should no longer be assumed as primary. One important problem with this is that in most cases, the anatomical cause of the back pain, the actual pain generator, is unknown.[24,25] Moreover, there is a generally poor correspondence of imaging results, including degenerative changes, and patient symptoms.[26-28] On the whole, it is usually very difficult to say whether pain of mechanical origin is primarily related to structural problems (positional fault, architectural changes, etc.) or functional problems (muscle hypertonus, kinetic chains, pain-spasm-pain cycles, failed synergy, muscle hypertonus, etc.). Long term, uncorrected functional derangement is likely to lead to accelerated musculoskeletal breakdown, including spinal architectural degenerative changes. In that situation, it would have to be said that *function has determined structure.*

The growing awareness of the importance of psychosocial factors in spine-related disorders establishes yet another rationale for the increasing respectability of functionally-based SEs. There is nothing *entirely* new about this, DD Palmer having used the term "auto-suggestion" to render the thought,[29] and Carver used the term "suggestion"[30] against the will of BJ Palmer. What does seem to be entirely new is that we now have psychosocial SEs, not the cause or result of an SE, but *the SE itself.* For example, Network Spinal Analysis finds that subluxations contain memory patterns that accumulate in the body,[31] and we find a similar concept, the "semantic event," in Neural Organization Technique.[32] The *semantic event* would be the person's "organism-as-a-whole" response to a word, a situation, or some other stimulus. In Walker's version of this, "Any such response involves intellectual, emotional, and physiological factors," or gut-level responses.[33] Babcock calls them "response semantic reactions".[34]

Finally, the emphasis by some techniques on nutrition and environmental toxins is so extreme, we are forced to conclude, no matter the denial we would expect of their practitioners, that their SE is purely environmental/chemical. For example: despite the claim that "CRA is not a form of treatment or diagnosis, but is simply a method of determining nutritional needs",[35] Contact Reflex

Analysis most certainly diagnoses diseases and prescribes nutritional support for an immense number of conditions and symptoms. We may of course take CRA's claim at face value, that nutritional analysis is an adjunct of some sort to Subluxation-based practice, but it seems more accurate to regard the identification of the nutritional need as a SE, given its central role in the patient-doctor interaction.

Tonal and non-complicated mechanical SEs

DD Palmer spoke of the "tone" of the nervous system, and how it could be impeded by vertebral misalignment. His vertebral subluxation model required four components: (1) vertebra out of normal alignment in relationship with the segments above or below, resulting in (2) occlusion of the foramen (spinal or intervertebral), which (3) applies pressure on corresponding nerves, thereby (4) interfering and interrupting the normal quantity flow of mental impulses.[36] Given the central role of the nervous system, it is clear how this would have adverse consequences for health.

Many current chiropractic technique systems, from Network Spinal Analysis to Hole-In-One upper cervical technique remain very true to Palmer's tonal model, and indeed, it is difficult to find chiropractors who do not claim to find some element of nerve interference to be an obligatory component of their SE. Owens provides an articulate statement of the neurological involvement premise.[13]

When a patient presents with an obvious neurological problem, such as lacking a deep tendon reflex, muscle atrophy, or paresthesia, no one would have any problem attributing a tonal dimension to the SE. Who would balk at understanding any of these to reflect "nerve interference," however defined? On the other hand, lacking any such obvious neurological signs, chiropractors traditionally infer them from more subtle phenomena: leg length inequality, weakness on manual muscle testing, asymmetric thermograms, asymmetric skin electrical conductivity, a limitless number of metaphysiological reflexes, etc. That's where things can get dicey.

The tonally-based chiropractor tends to identify the presence of subluxation by thermography. In this case, a thermographic reading found not to be in flux or changing would be interpreted to mean that the individual is not adapting to his or her environment, is not in homeostasis, is in a state termed "disease." Thus, this practitioner would *infer* the presence of a vertebral subluxation by its resultant manifestations on neurological function.

We suspect many chiropractors (including at least one of the authors) would have no problem, at least in certain cases, diagnosing non-complicated mechanical lesions, adjustable lesions lacking a neurological component; although Owen's would state by definition these chiropractors would not be treating vertebral subluxation.[13] At any rate, in our view the categorization of SEs should not assume an obligatory neurological/tonal parameter for each.

Segmental and regional SEs

Throughout most of its history, starting with the Palmers, chiropractic has emphasized *segmental* subluxations, spinal problems attributed to two adjacent vertebra and the related soft tissues. Of course, this was generalized to include the atlanto-occipital, lumbosacral, and sacroiliac joints as well, and quite often the extremity joints. On the other hand, there has almost always been a *structuralist* tendency as well, probably starting with the work of Dr. Carver,[30] that emphasized spinal regional considerations, and beyond that, the relation of the various spinal regions to one another.

The segmentalist believes that cranial-spinal-pelvic subluxations, however defined in terms of alignment, movement, or other properties, occur at *specific motor units* consisting of two bones. As a general rule, the segment above is characterized with respect to the one below. In this view, a segmental subluxation may result in postural distortions, such as lateral curvature or abnormal sagittal curves, but these postural distortions would be seen as associated or even compensatory consequences of specific motor unit subluxations, not the problems themselves.

Gonstead Technique is the classic example of such a world view, and the Gonstead practitioners take great pride in having custom-designed their interventions to carefully address specific segments.[22,37] Many, but not all, practitioners of so-called Diversified Technique posit a similar SE, as in the work of States[38] and as described by Gitelman.[39] Caution should be exercised in attributing any particular SE to Diversified technique, since the technique exists in a dual capacity as both umbrella for most things chiropractic, and a more narrowly defined system technique parallel to the others.[40]

The structuralist, as described by Montgomery[3] views subluxation as a matter of *postural distortion*, and offers up a language of listings which describes the linear and angular relationship of entire regions of the cranial-spinal-pelvic articulations. (This usage of "structuralist" should not be confused with the distinction of structure and function-based SEs discussed above.) A given motor unit may exhibit more signs and symptoms than another, but this would be the consequence, not the cause, of the primary postural distortion or loss of global range of motion. For example, although the apex of a lateral curvature in the frontal plane may present more clinical problems (pain, osteophytosis, etc.) than the other segments which comprise the curvature, it is the curvature, not the segment, that defines the SE. Harrison[41] and Troyanovich,[42] of the Chiropractic Biophysics Technique, Pettibon[43] of the Spinal Biomechanics Technique, and to some extent Ward of Spinal Stressology[44] describe regionalist SEs. At the limit, Ward and Koren are capable of commenting: "We found the entire spine subluxated".[45] As another example, Bahan points out that a cervical lordosis may appear normal when considered alone, but could be found abnormally situated anterior to the rib cage, thus afflicted with meningeal tension.[46]

The temptation to comment is irresistible. The doctrinaire partisanship of segmentalists and posturalists notwithstanding, a modern clinician should not feel the need to choose between segmentalist and structuralist thinking. It is more likely that given patients are better understood as suffering from either segmental or regional complaints; that a segmental problem is very much affected by the regional environment in which it occurs, just as the regional spinal environment is bounded by segmental components that are likely significant in themselves.

Restriction and misalignment-based SEs

Those who continue to emphasize vertebral misalignment can trace their lineage in virtually every detail straight back to the founder himself, DD Palmer. Bones misalign, partially occlude the intervertebral foramen, produce nerve interference, and eventually disease.[8,19,47] Although throughout most of its history chiropractic emphasized vertebral misalignment as the primary pathology addressed, there has been something of a paradigm shift in the last two decades in which many have come to the conclusion that intervertebral joint function (increased, decreased, or aberrant movement) may be of greater significance. No doubt the two are intimately related, so that vertebral misalignment could result in impaired movement, while impaired movement in turn could lead to misalignment. However, in spite of much speculation and many naive assumptions, no one has been able to produce a chiropractic "Rosetta stone" that would allow us to predict specific misalignments from identified fixations, or predict specific directions of fixation from identified misalignments.

Granted the current renewed interest in movement restriction in chiropractic, the concept itself dates back to 1906, in the text *Modernized Chiropractic* by Smith, Langworthy, and Paxson.[17] The main methodological position of the motion palpation world view is that if all segments of the spine and pelvis are free to move in all their anatomically allowable ranges of motion, then the neuromuscular control mechanism will achieve that organization that maximizes the efficiency of body function.[48,49] At the limit, the disregard for positional relationships is so extreme that it vanishes: even what appears to be a hyperextended segment should be adjusted toward greater extension, if examination shows that to be a direction in which movement is limited. Arguably the most

Table 5 Segmentalist/structuralist dimension intersecting misalignment/fixation dimension

	Segmentalist approach	Structuralist approach
Alignment problem	L3–4 misalignment	Lumbar curvature (scoliosis)
Movement problem	L3–4 fixation	Unilateral reduced lumbar lateral flexion

extensively tested of the chiropractic diagnostic procedures, motion palpation has not been shown to have the reproducibility one would expect of a procedure so dominant at the chiropractic college level. Triano reflects that "Several efforts have been made to critically examine interrater reliability with very troubling results".[50]

In considering how restriction/fixation should be categorized, we note that for some chiropractors, fixation does not so much produce nerve interference, as result from it. Van Rumpt felt that fixation is less a primary problem and more a protective response to nerve insult.[51] Specific correction of all the components of the subluxation would remove the need the body feels to maintain hypomobility. Table 5 illustrates how the segmentalist/structuralist dimension intersects the misalignment/fixation dimension, and gives examples of representative listings.

Anatomico-physiological and metaphysiological SEs

The distinction here has to do with the basic conception of how the body works. Some SEs are essentially physiological, in that the pathophysiology invoked is consistent with mainstream anatomy and physiology; that is, consistent with "normal science." Others invoke "reflexes" of various types, involving for example "neurovascular" or "neurolymphatic" points that are said to affect somatic structures.[52-57] It may be fair to use the term *metaphysiological* to describe such reflexes, to distinguish them from other reflexes (deep tendon reflexes, pathological reflexes, etc.) around which there is no scientific controversy. Not surprisingly, reflex-based SEs are found among reflex techniques: technique systems in which local observations, palpatory contacts, or other maneuvers are thought to provide information about or achieve remote effects at other body locations, even in cases where no known anatomical or physiological connection can be demonstrated.

Among some reflex practitioners, the reflex SE is primary to the subluxation, so that the goal of care is to treat the cause of the subluxation, not the subluxation itself. Nelson took strong exception to the traditional chiropractic emphasis on correcting subluxations, because he felt that this practice ignored physiology, insisting "It is the continually changing internal milieu that changes skeletal muscle that ultimately affects the skeleton".[58] He and other Neurovascular Dynamics practitioners strongly believe that the treatment of internal disorders, primarily though the stimulation of vasomotor reflexes, dietary intervention, and stress reduction, would normalize mechanical function. The idea that mechanical dysfunction is best addressed by normalizing physiology, including muscle tone, shows up in other chiropractic techniques as well, such as Nimmo's *Receptor-Tonus Technique*.[59-61]

In our view, in these techniques the reflexes have become the real SE under care, not some other sort of subluxation. We say this because of their operant role in the doctor–patient interaction; moreover, the goal of care is precisely that of suppressing the reflex, which amounts to what may be called a "metaphysiological subluxation," as an entity unto itself.

Primary and compensatory SEs

Almost all of the system techniques posit some sort of central SE, as we have already stated. Then, other spinal problems (symptomatic or not) are seen as SE-related syndromes. As a variation on the theme, some of the techniques, such as the Gonstead Technique,[22] contrast the *primary* subluxation from *compensatory* subluxations. The primary subluxation would be the focus of care, because it alone is at the core of the patient's problem. The compensatory subluxations are thought to resolve upon the successful correction of the primaries. As another example, Directional Non-Force Technique practitioner John believes

that "distortions" are adaptations or compensations for subluxation. According to John, they are self-correcting when the primary subluxations are corrected, and so should not be treated.[62]

Clearly, some techniques place more emphasis on contrasting primaries from secondaries than others, and some do not seem to feel the need at all. Logan felt that although subluxations could occur anywhere, all would be self-resolving provided the primary sacral subluxation were corrected.[63] Some of the upper cervicalists adopted a similar position, emphasizing atlas in much the same way Logan did the sacrum, but with an important difference: the upper cervical specialists declined to even use the term subluxation for these associated spinal (problems? boo-boos?).[64] BJ Palmer introduced the concept of the primacy of the atlas, and to a lesser extent, the axis subluxation, in the early spring of 1930 (Dye, 1939).

Symptomatic and asymptomatic SEs

To put the matter simply, at one extreme, some chiropractors feel the SE by definition includes symptoms such as pain; whereas at the other extreme, the SE would be a "silent killer".[65] We suspect most chiropractors are somewhere in-between, recognizing that in addition to symptomatic spinal problems, there are spinal conditions presently asymptomatic that could lead to overt problems later on, untreated. The categorization of SEs according to the presence or absence of symptoms will be an especially difficult undertaking, because it must directly confront the large and increasing mass of data on the reliability and validity of chiropractic examination procedures that purport to detect spinal problems in the absence of symptoms.

In presenting a somewhat different approach to this "prefiguring pathology" approach to the asymptomatic subluxation, Owens defines an "objective straight chiropractic," which states there is no inference that vertebral subluxation will necessarily lead to disease *later on*.[13] Owens contrasts the approach of the objective straight chiropractor, who would say the existence of vertebral subluxation means that disability is *already present*, to that of preventive subluxation care, which as the term implies, intends to prevent further disability.

At the Research Agenda Conference V in the year 2000, Reikman distinguished condition-based chiropractic care, aimed at treating diagnosed conditions (e.g., back pain, gastric ulcers, etc.), from subluxation-based chiropractic care, aimed at reducing the severity of biomechanical derangements of the spine (vertebral subluxation), arguing that both have a role to play in the contemporary chiropractic setting. He suggested that chiropractic clinicians attempt to identify and proactively treat such biomechanical derangements before they become symptomatic.

Thoughts such as these provide the rationale for maintenance[66] and preventive care, and clearly posit SEs that would show no symptoms. Meeker voices his concern on the dangers inherent in the concept of asymptomatic subluxation: "There is much concern that the presence of subluxation be the primary outcome of chiropractic care rather than the signs and symptoms of any particular illness or other pathology".[67] No doubt there is much potential for patient abuse in practice scenarios where the SE is cleanly divorced from symptoms, just as there is in practice scenarios where the doctor only addresses spinal problems, perhaps years in the making, that only become manifest after irreversible damage has been done.

Vertebral and extravertebral SEs

In its strictest sense, some chiropractors maintain that a subluxation can exist only among vertebral articulations, whereas other chiropractors would maintain that subluxations may occur wherever two bones meet. (There is an anecdote in which Reggie Gold, asked when he would adjust an extremity, said only in the event that he had found an "extravertebral vertebra" in the joint.) Not surprisingly, those chiropractors who most insist upon an element of neuropathy in the SE are the most likely to restrict it to the spine, whereas those who do not assume their SE includes neurological/tonal complications would have the least problem diagnosing extra-spinal SEs. Of course, it is not hard to develop models in which extremity

SEs indirectly result in spinal dysfunction, leading to neuropathy via that route.

Even among techniques that are very locked into the spinal cord, we see some that have more to do with nerve roots, and others with the spinal cord and meninges. In Network Spinal Analysis (formerly Network Technique) the *Class B meningeal subluxation* is essentially neurological (facilitated), located within the brain or spinal cord.[23] It involves a "multisegmental facilitation of the paraspinal musculature due to adverse cord-brain tension and interference in the cord, brain, and/or dural sleeves".[68] Furthermore, it is a "concussion of forces" on an emotional or chemical level overloads the CNS, and the vertebra displaces secondarily, as an adaptative feature. At some point, Epstein began to prefer the term facilitated subluxation to meningeal subluxation.[69]

We find a similar concept in Sacro-Occipital Technique, whose Category I is said to be "the first level of subluxation to develop," according to Saxon.[70] It involves failed coordination between the sacroiliac and cranial-sacral respiratory mechanisms, normally connected by the dural membranes and the flow of cerebral spinal fluid. Ward's Spinal Stressology, which uses very few traditional chiropractic terms, and even questions the value of the term "subluxation",[71] also invokes a meninges-related SE. The claim is made that stress breaks down the spinal-meningeal unit and may also cause an over-reactive defense mechanism that increases the damage. Ward even suggests that meningeal tension can produce diseases like Alzheimer's.[72]

Morter, leading figure within the Bioenergetic Synchronization Technique, is certainly not committed to an exclusively vertebral SE, believing subluxation can occur in the cerebellum or between the thalamus or the hypothalamus.[73] He states that subluxation is "an interference which shall include, but not be limited to, vertebral disrelationship which alters nerve function."[12] Indeed, Morter credits Toftness with the idea that the primary source of nerve dysfunction is in the brain, rather than the spinal cord or spinal nerves. Morter offers up the "Sensory dominant subluxation," "any recurring vertebral subluxation complex caused by sensory nerve interference," caused in the "high brain" and induced by stress.[74]

As another example of a SE that is brain-related, Toftness and Jenness originally theorized that microwave radiation is abnormally emitted from the body due to sensory overload of the brain.[75] They further speculated that emission of radiation from the body is the result of aberrant nerve impulses called "nerve stress".[75] Other authors have suggested that segmental spinal joint dysfunction, rather than brain overload, causes the microwave emission.[76,77]

CONCLUSION

We think it best that the quest for a universal definition of Subluxation, with which all chiropractors could live, whatever its political and economic benefits, is a diversion from a clinical and research point of view. We think it would be valuable to categorize the various subluxation-equivalents, drawing directly upon the system technique perspective in which so many were hatched. The contextual approach to model building that Mootz offers[78] emphasizes that to best understand perspective how an individual (or group of individuals) perceive a term, situation or concept, it is best to understand it from within that person's (or group of person's) perceptive. The many meanings of "subluxation" should follow from practice, directly from the evaluative and adjustive procedures, and not the other way around.

The adjustive approaches already directly descend from the evaluative procedures, so that the SE should ultimately derive from the patient examination. Bergmann proposed that their P.A.R.T.S. acronym and assessment model (Pain/tenderness; Asymmetry; Range of motion; Tissue tone, texture and temperature; and Special tests) is flexible enough to be utilized by advocates of any technique system,[79,80] but that remains to be seen. Ironically, although many of the components of the P.A.R.T.S. model are very straightforward, several subcomponents lead inexorably to "nerve interference." Again, there is little controversy about the significance of asymmetric or impaired deep tendon reflexes, muscle weakness or wasting, skin sensory abnormalities, etc. It's the

subclinical, inferred neurologicals, based on functional leg length inequality, uneven weight distribution, therapy localization, thermal asymmetry, and the like, that fuel the debates. No doubt pain-spasm-pain cycles, facilitation, complicated reflexes and many other subtle neurologically-mediated mechanisms can figure in the patient's overall symptom picture, but more research in neuroscience is need to validate the suggestion that the SE always involves "nerve inference," however defined.

Nothing is more disturbing to most professional researchers in the chiropractic milieu than the mandate to "prove the subluxation" or perform "subluxation-based" research. New and improved clinical understanding, that leads directly to better patient care, is a more appropriate goal of research. Subluxation taxonomy amounts to an inventory of clinical phenomena, observed over many decades and by countless individuals. This inventory helps inform the lines of inquiry of most potential benefit. Research must never be enlisted to validate an ideology, no matter how carefully word-smithed, and no matter how much blood was spilled attaining consensus. Meeker, approaching the subluxation question from a research point of view, states: "The concept of subluxation also lacks a useful operational definition, compounding the problem of its theoretical relationship to a concept of health. The basic question is, What is a subluxation? *There is no one answer*" (our emphasis).[67] Leboeuf-Yde also develops the research implications of traditional subluxation theory.[81]

Nothing we have written is meant to deny the political and economic importance of having a concise, easily interpreted, and broadly accepted definition of Subluxation to take to legislators, managed care providers, insurers, and other health care constituents. For that purpose, we believe the statement of the Association of Chiropractic Colleges serves well enough: "A subluxation is a complex of functional and/or structural and/or pathological articular changes that compromise neural integrity and may influence organ system function and general health".[82]

Furthermore, nothing we have written is meant to denigrate the contributions that many of the system techniques and individual technique innovators have made to chiropractic. True, we have seen the development of a bewildering array of chiropractic techniques, each claiming to be the legitimate pretender to the medical throne. Yes, much of this spectacle is of little redeeming value, and it is all too easy to point an accusatory finger at the custodians of proprietary technique; they frequently confuse the public, make insupportable claims, and ignore standard scientific method. However, it is equally true that these same technique mavens, past and present, are the ones who have reduced to practice much of what will evolve into the more responsible generic technique just over the horizon. The technique spectacle, past and present, deserves no less than a healthy admixture of constructive and destructive criticism. That starts with accurate description of what is, an *operational* (not a mere list) inventory of subluxation-equivalents.

A subluxation taxonomy, could do much to advance research on adjustable lesions. Meeker continues: "At one level of description, it is easy to get agreement among chiropractors. There is obviously professional desire for agreement on the existence of the broad concept. But, we have a hard time agreeing about how to detect it, or measure the effect of adjustments. Unfortunately, it is at these deeper levels of description, measurement, and explanation that agreement starts to deteriorate into defensiveness and polemics".[67] We would say, it is at this deeper level that the United Front for Subluxation definition falls apart, always.

Refining the fundamental approach to categorizing the clinical perspectives on subluxation could produce an inventory of technique-based SEs that can better inform the discussion. Because the focus of each technique may offer a unique clinical perspective and desired result, the interventions might actually be addressing different, but possibly linked, pathophysiological responses or dysfunctions. Developing a Linnaean taxonomy for a variety of subluxation-equivalents offers several advantages to research efforts, technique development, patient care improvements, and the professional efforts to unify on a substantive basis.

(Reprinted from Cooperstein R, Gleberzon BJ 2001 Toward a taxonomy of subluxation-equivalents. Topics in Clinical Chiropractic 8(1):49–60.)

NOTES

1. Carroll L 1946 Through the Looking Glass and What Alice Found There. London: McMillan and Company
2. Nelson C The subluxation question. Journal of Chiropractic Humanities 1997: 46–55
3. Montgomery P D, Nelson M J 1985 Evolution of chiropractic theories of practice and spinal adjustment, 1900–1950. Chiropractic History 5: 71–77
4. Nelson C F 1993 The cognitive roots of chiropractic theories and techniques. Journal of Chiropractic Humanities 42–55
5. Bergmann T F 1993 Various forms of chiropractic technique. Chiropractic Technique 5 (2): 53–55.
6. Cooperstein R 1990 Brand name techniques and the confidence gap. The Journal of Chiropractic Education 4 (3): 89–93.
7. Schumpeter J A 1954 History of economic analysis. New York: Oxford University Press
8. Gatterman M I 1990 Chiropractic management of spine-related disorders. Baltimore MD: Williams & Wilkins
9. Diggett D M 1987 Commentary: The chiropractic wars. Journal of Manipulative and Physiological Therapeutics 10 (2): 71–77
10. Homola S 1963 Bonesetting, chiropractic, and cultism. Panama City, Florida: Critique Books
11. Cooperstein R 1995 Contemporary approach to understanding chiropractic technique. In: Lawrence D, editor. Advances in Chiropractic Volume 2. Chicago IL: Mosby Year Book, Inc. p. 437–459
12. Morter M T 1985 B.E.S.T. Bioenergetic Synchonization Technique. American Chiropractor 1985 (April): 30–36
13. Owens E F 2000 Theoretical constructs of vertebral subluxation as applied by chiropractic practitioners and researchers. Topics in Clinical Chiropractic 7 (1): 74–79
14. Gatterman M I 1995 Foundations of Chiropractic Subluxation. St. Louis, MI: Mosby-Year Book, Inc.
15. Dishman R W 1988 Static and dynamic components of the chiropractic subluxation complex: a literature review [see comments]. J Manipulative Physiol Ther 11 (2): 98–107
16. Rome P L 1996 Usage of chiropractic terminology in the literature: 296 ways to say "subluxation": complex issues of the vertebral subluxation. Chiropractic Technique 8 (2): 49–60

17. Brantingham J W 1988 A critical look at the subluxation hypothesis [see comments]. J Manipulative Physiol Ther 11 (2): 130–2

18. Cotran R S, Kumar V, Collins T 1999 Robbins pathologic basis of disease. 6th ed. Philadelphia PA: W.B. Saunders Company

19. Leach R A 1986 The chiropractic theories. 2nd. ed. Baltimore, MD: Williams & Wilkins

20. Bartol K M 1992 Algorithm for the categorization of chiropractic technique procedures. Chiropractic Technique 4 (1): 8–14

21. Bartol K M 1991 A model for the categorization of chiropractic treatment procedures. Chiropractic Technique 3 (2): 78–80

22. Herbst A 1980 Gonstead chiropractic science and art: the chiropractic methodology of Clarence S. Gonstead. Mount Horeb WI: Schichi Publications

23. Epstein D M 1984 Network Chiropractic explores the meningeal critical. Part I: anatomy and physiology of the meningeal functional unit. Digest of Chiropractic Economics (January/February): 78–80, 82

24. Giles L G F 1990 Anatomical basis of low back pain. Baltimore MD: Williams & Wilkins

25. Deyo R 1987 Epidemiology of low back pain. Spine 12 (3): 264–268

26. Liebenson C S 1992 Pathogenesis of chronic back pain. Journal of Manipulative and Physiological Therapeutics 15 (5): 299–308

27. Phillips R B, Schultz G D, Howard B, Hoyt T 1993 Posterior osteophytes and low back pain. Chiropractic Technique 5 (1): 32–35

28. Phillips R B, Howe J W, Bustin G, Mick T J, Rosenfeld I, Mills T 1990 Stress x-rays and the low back pain patient. Journal of Manipulative and Physiological Therapeutics 15 (3): 127–133

29. Palmer D D 1914 The Chiropractor. Los Angeles, CA: Beacon Light Printing Company

30. Carver W 1921 Carver's Chiropractic Analysis of Chiropractic Principles as Applied to Pathology, Relatology, Symptomology and Diagnosis. 1st ed. Oklahoma City, Oklahoma

31. Herriot E M 1990 Life-changing chiropractic. Yoga Journal (Sept/Oct): 23–25

32. Ferreri C Neural Organization Technique international. Chiropractic Products 1996(Oct): 18–19

33. Walker S Disobedient vertebrae: are they (neuro) emotionally disturbed? Chiropractic Products 1996(Oct): 22

34. Babcock B 1999 The triangle of health.

35. Versendaal D A 1989 Contact Reflex Analysis and Applied Trophology. Vista, CA: D.A. Versendaal

36. Boone W R, Dobson G J 1996 A proposed vertebral subluxation model reflecting traditional concepts and recent advances in health and science. J Vertebral Subluxation Res 1 (1): 19–30

37. Plaugher G editor 1993. Textbook of clinical chiropractic: a specific biomechanical approach. Baltimore, Maryland: Williams & Wilkins

38. States A Z 1967 Spinal and pelvic techniques. Lombard, Ill.: National College of Chiropractic

39. Gitelman R, Fligg B 1992 Diversified Technique. In: Haldeman S, ed. Principles and practice of chiropractic. 2nd ed. New York NY: Appleton-Century-Crofts; p. 483–501

40. Cooperstein R 1995 Diversified technique, historically considered: core of chiropractic, or "just another technique system"? In: Cleveland III C, Gibbons R, ed. Conference Proceedings of the Chiropractic Centennial Foundation; September 14–16, 1995; Davenport, Iowa: Chiropractic Centennial Foundation; p. 21–22

41. Harrison D D 1994 Chiropractic: The Physics of Spinal Correction. CBP Technique

42. Troyanovich S J, Harrison D D 1996 Chiropractic biophysics (CBP) technique. Chiropractic Technique 8 (1): 30–35

43. Pettibon B R 1989 Pettibon Spinal Bio-Mechanics. Tacoma, WA: Pettibon Bio-Mechanics Institute, Inc.

44. Ward L E 1995 Systemic Chiropractic. 37th ed. Long Beach, CA: Spinal Stress Seminars, Inc.

45. Ward L E, Koren T Spinal column stressology. American Chiropractor 1987(July): 16–21

46. Bahan J R 1991 Spinal column stressology: a concept pioneering its way into the structural health care profession. Digest of Chiropractic Economics (November/December): 46, 98

47. Palmer D D 1910 The chiropractor's adjuster, the science, art and philosophy of chiropractic. Portland, Oregon: Portland Printing House

48. Gillet H, Liekens M 1981 The different types of fixation. In: The Belgian chiropractic research notes. Huntingon Beach, CA: Motion Palpation Institute; p. 13–16

49. Schafer R C, Faye L J 1989 Motion palpation and chiropractic technique. Huntington Beach CA: MPI

50. Triano J J 1990 The subluxation complex: outcome measure of chiropractic diagnosis and treatment. Chiropractic Technique 2 (3): 114–120

51. Van Rumpt R 1977 Directional Non-Force Technique. In: Kfoury PW, editor. Catalog of chiropractic techniques. Logan College of Chiropractic p. 13–16

52. Walther D S 1981 Applied Kinesiology, Volume I. Pueblo, Colorado: Systems DC

53. Bennett T J 1960 A new clinical basis for the correction of abnormal physiology. Burlingame, CA: self-published

54. Goodheart G J 1977 Applied Kinesiology. In: Kfoury PW, editor. Catalog of chiropractic techniques. Logan College of Chiropractic; p. 117–119

55. Goodheart G J Applied Kinesiology – the beginning. Digest of Chiropractic Economics 1989(May/June): 15, 17 20, 22–23

56. Goodheart G J The Applied Kinesiology Technique. Today's Chiropractic 1993; 22(July/August): 56–58.

57. Chaitow L 1988 Soft-tissue manipulation. Rochester, Vermont: Healing Arts Press

58. Nelson W A 1994 Whither now? Chiropractic Technique 6 (3): 104

59. Nimmo R L 1963 The Receptor-Tonus Method. Granbury, Texas: self-published

60. Nimmo R L 1971 Vannerson JF. Specificity and the law of facilitation in the nervous system. The Receptor 2 (1)

61. Schneider M 1994 Receptor-Tonus Technique assessment. Chiropractic Technique 6 (4): 156–159

62. John C Directional Non-Force Technique Seminars. In. Beverly Hills, CA: Christopher F. John; unknown.

63. Logan H B 1950 Textbook of Logan Basic Methods. St. Louis, Missouri: unknown

64. Palmer B J 1934 The Upper Cervical Specific; the Adjustment Specific; and the exposition of the cause of all disease. Davenport, Iowa: Palmer School of Chiropractic

65. Carter J R 2000 Subluxation – the Silent Killer (Commentary). J Can Chiropr Assoc 44 (1): 9–18

66. Koch D 2000 Chiropractic maintenance and wellness care: a clinical research challenge. In: Research PCfC, ed. RAC V: Integrating Chiropractic Theory, Evidence, and Practice; Chicago, IL: Palmer Center for Chiropractic Research p. 19–20

67. Meeker W C 2000 Concepts germane to an evidence-based application of chiropractic theory. Topics in Clinical Chiropractic 7 (1): 67–73

68. Epstein D 1987 The stress connection: gauging the role of the nervous system. Today's Chiropractic 15 (6): 15–7

69. Epstein D 1992 Network Chiropractic: a unified application of chiropractic principles

70. Saxon A 1985 Participant Guide. SOT: A Seminar for Technical Excellence: SORSI; (app)

71. Ward L High risk heart attack and stroke. Part III. Today's Chiropractic 1986(Jan–Feb): 75–81

72. Sehl T, Proetz J F New answers for old stress problems – part 2. An exclusive interview with Dr. Lowell Ward. Digest of Chiropractic Economics 1986(March/April):36, 38–39, 41

73. Morter M T 1982 Bio Energetic Synchronization. American Chiropractor 1982(July/August)

74. Morter M T The Bio-Energetic Synchronization Technique: a breakthrough in subluxation detection. Today's Chiropractic 1993(September/October):68–69

75. Jenness M E, Toftness I Validation of the Toftness/Jenness system of chiropractic. Digest of Chiropractic Economics 1981(Sept/Oct): 22–26, 126–129

76. Gemmell H J, Jacobson B H Comparison of two adjustive indicators in patients with acute low back pain. Chiropractic Technique 1998(Feb.): 8–10

77. Gemmell H A, Jacobson B H 1993 Association between level of acute spine pain and level of sustained pressure used in the Toftness adjustment. Chiropractic Technique 5 (4): 150–151

78. Mootz R D 1995 The contextual nature of manual methods: challenges to the paradigm. Journal of Chiropractic Humanities 28–40.

79. Bergmann T PARTS 1993 joint assessment procedure. Chiropractic Technique 5 (3): 135–136

80. Bergmann T 1997 Toward a reliable, valid method of manual diagnosis. More than the sum of its P.A.R.T.S. Journal of the American Chiropractic Association 34 (10): 24–27

81. Leboeuf-Yde C 1998 How real is the subluxation? A research perspective. J Manipulative Physiol Ther 21 (7): 492–4

82. ACC 1996 Position Paper #1: Association of Chiropractic Colleges; 1996 July

Appendix 2: The special case of Diversified Technique

ON DIVERSIFIED CHIROPRACTIC TECHNIQUE

Not surprisingly, the term "diversified" has been subject to diverse interpretations in the chiropractic milieu, to the point that it is not even clear whether or not the word should be capitalized. For some individuals, "diversified" is an adjective, in the sense of "eclectic," whereas for others, "Diversified" is a noun, representing the name of a specific chiropractic technique system. The issue cannot be explained away as mere semantics, in that the differences in usage underscore divergent historical legacies. The usage of the term "diversified" has ranged from an expansive descriptor of the core of things chiropractic, all the way to a restrictive label for just another named chiropractic technique. *Qua core* of chiropractic, diversified technique is too global to succinctly describe, whereas as a *named technique*, it is too eclectic to distinctly describe. Diversified chiropractic technique is like a close friend with a somewhat fuzzy past, whose true identity must remain unknown until that past is known.

THE EVOLUTION OF *PROTO-DIVERSIFIED TECHNIQUE*

By 1904, DD Palmer's original chiropractic institute had re-emerged as the Palmer School of Chiropractic. Between 1908 and 1911, BJ Palmer introduced, indeed, practically legislated, a number of philosophical and technique innovations, including the "Meric System" of diagnosis, the concept of "Major" and "Minor" subluxations,

the restriction of adjusting to five or six of the "main" vertebrae per visit,[1,2] the recoil method of adjusting, limitation of adjusting to the vertebral column alone, the condemnation of "mixing," the advocacy of "straight chiropractic," the belief that virtually *all* disease is due to vertebral subluxation, and the use of X-ray for diagnostic purposes. Many of these innovations were controversial and engendered opposing viewpoints.

Several schools and individuals vied with BJ Palmer for control of the profession, including his own father, whose 1910 text, *The Science, Art, and Philosophy of Chiropractic*, takes many pages[3] of vitriolic issue with the son. Other competitive chiropractic tendencies became associated with a myriad of schools, the most important of which were the American School of Chiropractic, the National College of Chiropractic, the Carver College of Chiropractic, and somewhat later on the Lincoln Chiropractic College. Loban's break with the Fountainhead and founding of the rival Universal Chiropractic College may have been a reaction to BJ Palmer's introduction of X-ray equipment.[4] In stark contrast with the rigidity and overbearing presence of the Palmer method, these other colleges, somewhat of a loyal opposition, under the circumstances, fostered a more eclectic, broader scope, less dogmatic approach to chiropractic.

BJ Palmer was, of course, incensed by these iconoclastic tendencies, as may be confirmed by Dye's 1939 remarks:[1]

"Of course, in those early days, the principles of Chiropractic ... were very simple. They consisted merely of Locating the 'bumps along the center of the patient's back, over the spinous processes of the vertebrae, and their forcible reduction by a shove, a push, a stiff arm adjustment. No extended or widely diversified [my emphasis] system of instruction was given serious thought at first by the Founder ... [Now we have this] bane of all Chiropractic, new moves ... purloined or taken from osteopathy or even orthopedic surgery. Also the use of other external modalities, treatment adjuncts, sunray lamps, varicolored lamp rays, etc."

The roots of the diversified approach to chiropractic technique lie within a broad-scope, less personalized reaction to the Palmeresque fundamentalism that emanated from the "Fountainhead" during chiropractic's first several decades. Indeed, the philosophies and methodologies of the loyal opposition, primarily Carver, Langworthy, Smith, Forster, Howard, and "the Big Four" (Firth et al), amount to a sort of "proto-diversified" technique, even though the methods associated with these individuals remained either deliberately or accidentally proprietary, not yet truly eclectic and depersonalized. Proto-diversified technique eluded BJ Palmer's attempt to dominate the burgeoning chiropractic profession, many of whose leading individuals did not accept his autocratic position.

Apart from the substantive differences between their methods and those of the Palmer milieu, the loyal opposition conformed to a more mainstream method of accumulating knowledge. Compared to the essentially anti-establishment position struck by Palmer, they stuck closer to, and for the most part declared allegiance to, the existing body of scientific knowledge, which they intended to improve (but not necessarily replace) through the accretion of chiropractic knowledge. Here then, are the roots of diversified technique, not merely a body of clinical practice, but an approach to sustained development. BJ Palmer greatly accelerated the development of competitive schools of chiropractic by demanding in 1924 that all chiropractors adopt the neurocalometer,[3,5] and in the early 1930s that they abandon vertebral adjusting below the level of C2.[6]

Carver and the Carver Schools

Carver stated in his 1936 history of chiropractic, quoted by Wardwell,[7] that "It therefore came about that the Chiropractic profession was constantly disturbed by 'new adjustments ... other inexplicable things, too numerous to record. As a result of the flurrie there were 'The Parker lumbar discovery,' 'The Langworthy Method,' 'The Smith System,' 'The Howard System,' and so on, throughout the list of all those who assumed to conduct schools." Carver's distaste for *proprietary technique*, what Vear has called "technique systems",[8] constitutes an incipient component of the diversified *weltanschauung*. His openness to more broad-scope practices earned him the epithet "mixer," from Palmer's point of view.[9] Carver also objected to BJ Palmer's insistence that "nerve occlusion" takes place only at the spinal level, holding instead that the nerve stimulus may be "occluded from entering the brain ... from transmission through nerve channels ... may be occluded from normal application upon tissue elements at the periphery of nerves".[10] Finally, Carver's *structuralist* point of view (based on body biomechanics),[11] permitted a much more expansive approach to clinical chiropractic than the strictly segmental views of BJ Palmer.

Langworthy, Smith, and the American School

In 1903[a] the American School of Chiropractic and Nature Cure at Cedar Rapids Iowa was founded by DD Palmer's student, Solon Langworthy, soon joined by fellow Palmer graduates Oakley Smith (a former medical student, who did not complete the program) and chiropractor Minora Paxson. Their *Modernized Chiropractic* of 1906,[12] generally credited to be the first textbook of chiropractic, featured elements of gait analysis, motion inspection, nerve tracing, static and motion palpation, extremity adjustment, and postural analysis.[2] Clearly, their approach was inherently more eclectic and especially more *dynamic* than that reflected by BJ's "bone-out-of-place" mindset. *Modernized Chiropractic* adds many technical innovations to the chiropractic armamentarium, including some that BJ Palmer considered tainted by mixing: traction and traction tables, rib maneuvers, long-lever lumbar adjustments, and extremity adjusting.[2] Oakley Smith would go on to found a "naprapathic school" in Chicago in 1906[6,13] or 1905.[14] According to Zarbuck:[14]

"Naprapathy is a drugless system of treating human ailments discovered in 1905. The theory underlying it is that many of the ailments of the human body are due to a tightened or shrunken condition of a ligament; that such a condition is referred to as a ligatight, and where it takes place near a nerve it brings a mechanical tension on that nerve and induces an abnormal function."

Howard, Schulze, and the National School

John A. Howard, who had been a student of BJ Palmer, founded another rival school in 1906, also in Davenport. He was disturbed over Palmer's reluctance to furnish cadavers for the anatomy students to dissect. Moreover, he strongly objected to BJ Palmer's blend of "Specific, Pure and Unadulterated" chiropractic: "He became overzealous. He claimed that all disease is due to subluxations of the vertebrae and that all diseases could be eradicated by adjustment of the vertebrae. He derided all other forms of therapy, and persisted in his original views to the end",[15] quoted by Gibbons.[13] This *National School* (forerunner of today's National College of Chiropractic) moved to Chicago in 1908, and eventually passed into medical hands when Howard formed a partnership with a medical doctor, William Schulze, in 1910. Dissection, physiotherapy, and much more were introduced into the curriculum. In essence, "These inclusions into the chiropractic core curriculum reflected a different teaching philosophy and an increased amount of attention to other therapeutic approaches that, in Howard's and Schulze's opinions, were necessary for a practicing chiropractor".[6] Although BJ Palmer certainly believed that Carver was a mixer,[9] what really touched off the bitter and never-ending mixer–straight debate were the physiotherapeutics introduced by the National College of Chiropractic: electrotherapy, hydrotherapy, muscle techniques, massage and remedies both internally and externally applied.[2]

"The Big Four" and the Lincoln Chiropractic College[6,9,16]

Although BJ Palmer's introduction of the neurocalometer was well-received by many chiropractors, many others found it objectionable, whether on the basis of professional criticism or distaste for what they saw as Palmer's price-gouging marketing practices.[5] Among these critics were some of the Palmer College core faculty, who according to Gibbons[3] were kept in the dark on the neurocalometer research, although Keating feels this was hardly possible.[5] In any case, James Firth left the Palmer school with 3 colleagues in 1926 to found the Lincoln College in Indianapolis, one of the profession's first 4 year schools. The others were Harry Vedder, Stephen Burich, and AE Hendricks. "The educational foundation of Lincoln College was based on *diversity* [emphasis added] of technics of adjusting and the philosophy that interference of innate intelligence could happen, as DD stated, anywhere a subluxation could be found. They placed a heavy influence on also learning the basic sciences".[6]

THE CRYSTALLIZATION OF *DIVERSIFIED TECHNIQUE*

It is safe to say that diversified technique took shape in substance before assuming the appellation "diversified," the origin of which remains appropriately obscure.[17] Nevertheless, the classic expression of diversified technique can be either probably[18] or unequivocally[17] attributed to Joe Janse, D.C. There is no doubt that his 1947 *Chiropractic Principles and Technic*[19] remains diversified technique's crowning achievement. Although the book assumes some fairly revisionist, anti-fundamentalist ideological positions, e.g., "To say that subluxation is the one and only cause of disease is wrong",[19] what really qualifies Janse as the mentor of diversified technique is the tremendous scope of clinical chiropractic procedures he describes. Moreover, of particular importance is *the way he describes them*: Janse was able to present chiropractic diagnostic and therapeutic methods in a generic, non-proprietary manner.

True, Carver, Langworthy, Smith, Howard and others had already advocated broad-scope practice and had taken iconoclastic positions against the purism of the Fountainhead, but it was up to Janse to rescue chiropractic procedures from fruitless quarreling over issues of inventorship, pretended superiority of this or that method. The dedication is very revealing: "To all those that have consecrated and dedicated a liberal share of their lives and fortunes to the advancement and general dissemination of science, and especially to those that have devoted such effort and substance to the dissemination of the science of chiropractic".[19] In Janse's hands, chiropractic is no longer an alternative to medical science, but rather a complementary science (even though he did discount the existence of communicable diseases, therefore rejecting the practice of vaccination).

The sections of spinal analysis, spinal adjustment, and extremity adjustment occupy 62% of the 635 page book. Janse presents both osseous and reflex procedures, the latter ranging from the spondylotherapy of Abrams to the sacral work of Hugh Logan. The emphasis on the sacroiliac area preceded by 45 years the "First Interdisciplinary World Congress on the Low Back Pain and Its Relation to the Sacroiliac Joint".[20] According to Grice and Vernon, "More than 117 procedures were presented including spinal adjustments, peripheral joint adjustments, and sinus and organ techniques. These techniques, with only slight modifications, continue to be used by the majority of chiropractors and often are referred to as 'diversified techniques' ".[2]

That Janse himself most likely endorsed the term "diversified" may be inferred from his introduction to States' 1968 illustrated chiropractic technique manual: "Roentgen studies reveal that no two spines, and their relating lumbosacral and sacroiliac mechanisms, are totally alike. There are variances in the composite and mechanical dispositions, as well as in the symmetry and architecture, of the articular motor beds. These factors alone make *diversification* [emphasis added] of adjusting procedures imperative".[21]

States's *Spinal and Pelvic Technics,* in essence commissioned by Janse while States instructed at the National College, is another generally acknowledged representative work of diversified technique.[18] According to Gitelman, Otto Reinert's *Chiropractic Procedure and Practice* (Reinert is mistakenly identified by Gitelman as "Rheinhard")[22] has also been referred to as a textbook of diversified technique. Although the various authors may not necessarily agree, the recent textbook entitled *Chiropractic Technique* by Bergmann et al[23] may be considered, a contemporary text of diversified technique, in the sense of eclecticism, as could Stonebrink's *Evaluation and Manipulative Management of Common Musculoskeletal Disorders.*[24]

CONTEMPORARY DIVERSIFIED TECHNIQUE

Some contemporary chiropractors and authors regard diversified as a named technique system, parallel to all the others, largely but certainly not exclusively identified historically with the National College of Chiropractic. From this point of view, diversified technique is sometimes seen as a corpus of *moves,* lacking a *distinct* philosophical, ideological, or mechanical foundation as compared with other technique systems. Other contemporaries consider diversified technique to be immense and generic, comprising the totality of chiropractic therapeutic and diagnostic procedures that, by virtue of overwhelming acceptance, have come to comprise the core of chiropractic technique itself. In a way, the two positions are opposite sides of the same coin: as a named technique, diversified technique is too eclectic to distinctly describe, whereas as the core of chiropractic, it is too global to conveniently describe. That the great majority (91%)[25] of chiropractors themselves claim to use "Diversified" is clearly worthy of interpretation. A few representative positions are presented.

Herbert Vear, DC, defines a "System Technique" as follows: "Following procedural directions as laid down and which follow a sequential order not necessarily related to analysis, synthesis and evaluation of the taxonomy of educational objectives".[5] Vear finds that chiropractic technique systems are "not all bad," but as such have not yet progressed through the analytic phase to synthesis and evaluation. Of course, as a chiropractic educator, he is referring less to the history of chiropractic and more to the development of the chiropractic student; but there is little doubt that *chiropractic ontogeny recapitulates chiropractic phylogeny.* Vear[8] situates diversified technique as antithetical to a systems approach:

"First it must be stated that neither general adjustive technique or its alternative, diversified technique, can be classified as system approaches to chiropractic practice. To be highly skilled in adjusting the many vertebral segments of the spine in as many ways as possible, in essence represents the major objective in general adjustive procedures ... the application of spinal adjustment should be preceded by an intellectual analysis of the patient's spine, pelvis, and other articulations, based upon scientific criteria."

Carl S. Cleveland, III, D.C., also views diversified technique as other than a technique system,[26] even if his sense of the latter term is more historical and less theoretical than that of Vear:

"One of the first technique systems to be developed around basic principles of spinal biomechanics is the toggle recoil, meric recoil or, full-spine specific technique. This technique system, developed by DD Palmer and BJ Palmer, served as an early foundation from which a variety of techniques popular in the profession have evolved. Today's typical practitioner most probably uses certain fundamentals of this system in conjunction with a variety of *diversified* [emphasis added] technique procedures."

Ronald Gitelman, D.C., author of a chapter entitled "Diversified Technique" in a chiropractic textbook, clearly states the diversified-as-core-of-chiropractic position:[17]

"It has been said that all techniques are good and all techniques are bad. The question is, When to use which one, and on whom? This is still the credo of the practitioner who practices diversified technique, which has maintained its eclectic approach to the management of functional disorders of the locomotor apparatus ... unlike the system technique approaches, diversified technique ... attempts to apply the most ideal technique within the context of the reality of the clinical procedure ... The incorporation of other technique systems, or of any technique, has had to pass the scrutiny of the diversified rationale, which is based on sound neurobiomechanical-orthopaedic principles."

Richard Stonebrink, D.C., author of what may be considered a textbook on diversified methods[24]

insists that the term "diversified" must apply not only to the range of treatment methods, but in a larger sense to a broad interpretation of the range of *tissues treated.*[27] Clinicians who address only one type of tissue (or even one specific bone) are correspondingly very limited in their scope of treatment procedures. By contrast, those who acknowledge a multiplicity of anatomically-related pathophysiologies would lean towards diversity in treatment methods. When asked by a chiropractic group to describe "diversified technique" procedures, Stonebrink wrote:[27]

"The segmental misalignment or fixation and specific sectional adaptations are evaluated for their specific intrinsic pathophysiologies, and soft tissue and joint manipulations selected and applied that can best reduce them."

A manual on diversified technique that is used in the chiropractic college that this author attended states "Many of the moves are general, almost universal in use while others are moves that have been adapted and are used as part of other named techniques ... ".[28]

Hinz, in his article on diversified technique methods, the Northwestern College, and John B. Wolf,[29] seems to intend by the usage of the term "diversified" all of the following: emphasis on the basic sciences, educational excellence, avoidance of dogmatic debates over technique and scope of practice. According to Hinz, " ... the system advocated an analysis of the patient, using the knowledge obtained through previous courses and experience, in order to utilize the technique or adjuncts which would fit the particular patient's need. This type of teaching was liberal in the sense that the school did not strictly adhere to any one technique, but studied many techniques and utilized the ones that were deemed most beneficial through deduction from the basic sciences and personal clinical experience."

It is necessary to balance all of these favorable, largely idealistic quotations regarding diversified with an eloquent opinion by Dr. David Peterson. He believes that *de facto* Diversified Technique as a system is fairly nondescript, and not particularly thoughtful. He writes:[18]

"It is a collection of adjustive procedures lacking a clear origin, definition or description ... Diversified technique is a procedure searching for an identity. It does not have a clear definition, description or proponent. It lacks any protocols for differentiating and applying specific adjustments. Perhaps diversified techniques is a term that has outlived any meaningful purpose and the procedures contained within it should be considered to fall within the general realm of chiropractic technique and evaluated by their individual characteristics."

DIVERSIFIED: IS YOU IS, OR IS YOU AIN'T, A TECHNIQUE SYSTEM?

Ironically, as the years went by, the body of chiropractic methodology that had originated as a liberating, eclecticizing response to the myriad of narrowly defined and often cultistic technique systems of the day found itself more than just occasionally arranged alongside of, rather than alternative to them, as yet another technique system. However paradoxically, it appears that modern diversified technique is chiefly distinguished from all of the others by its poor distinction from *any one* of them.

The allure of brand-name techniques shows surprising resilience, in that many contemporary practitioners seem to prefer the cookbookishness of a technique system to the clinical freedom of generic technique.[30] How an individual practitioner regards diversified technique may directly reflect how he or she feels about chiropractic technique in general. Someone who prefers eclectic practice might very well endorse the descriptor "diversified," small d, and resist any attempt to have his or her methods characterized from a systems point of view. Conversely, the type of practitioner who professes to practice "Diversified" with a capital D may believe it best to specialize in a particular technique system, and object to having his or her technique defined away into the essence of all things chiropractic.

As a former New Yorker, I can state with conviction that were I to be asked "Is New York a city or a state?" I would assert that New York is both a city AND a state. Unfortunately, when asked "Is Diversified a technique system or a general adjustive technique?" I would have to answer "It is both, but prefers to be neither." Despite being almost 100 years old, "diversified" just hasn't decided what it wants to be when it grows up. Personally, the next time someone asks me what technique I use, which I usually identify as "a little bit of this and a little bit of that," I think I'll just say "Diversified ... sort of."

(Reprinted with permission from Cooperstein R 1995 Diversified technique: core of chiropractic or "just another technique system"? Journal of Chiropractic Humanities 5(1): 50–55)

REFERENCES

1. Dye A A 1939 The Evolution of Chiropractic – Its Discovery and Development. (Reprint of 1969, Richmond Hall, Inc., Richmond Hill, NY ed.) PA: Dye
2. Grice A, Vernon H 1992 Basic principles in the performance of chiropractic adjusting: historical review, classification, and objectives. In: Haldeman S, ed. Principles and practice of chiropractic. Norwalk, Connecticut: Appleton & Lange, 442–458
3. Gibbons R W 1992 Medical and social protest as part of hidden American history. In: Haldeman S, ed. Principles and practice of chiropractic. 2nd. ed. East Norwalk, Connecticut: Appleton & Lange, 15–28
4. Keating J C 1992 Shades of straight: diversity among the purists. Journal of Manipulative and Physiological Therapeutics 15 (3): 203–209
5. Keating J C 1991 Introducing the Neurocalometer: A view from the Fountainhead. Journal of the Canadian Chiropractic Association 35 (3): 165–178
6. Montgomery P D, Nelson M J 1985 Evolution of chiropractic theories of practice and spinal adjustment, 1900–1950. Chiropractic History 5: 71–77

7. Wardwell W I 1992 Chiropractic: History and Evolution of a New Profession. St. Louis MO: Mosby Year Book
8. Year H J 1981 Introduction to Chiropractic Science. Western States Chiropractic College
9. Ferguson A, Wiese G 1988 How many chiropractic schools? An analysis of institutions that offered the D.C. degree. Chiropractic History 8 (1): 27–31
10. Carver W 1921 Carver's Chiropractic Analysis of Chiropractic Principles as Applied to Pathology, Relatology, Symptomology and Diagnosis. (1st ed.) Oklahoma City, Oklahoma
11. Rosenthal M J 1981 The structural approach to chiropractic: from Willard Carver to present practice. Chiropractic History 1 (1): 25–29
12. Smith O G, Langsworthy S M, Paxson M C 1906 Modernized Chiropractic. Cedar Rapids: Lawrence Press
13. Gibbons R W 1980 The Evolution of Chiropractic: Medical and Social Protest in America. Modern Developments in the Principles and Practice of Chiropractic. 1st ed. New York NY: Appleton-Century-Crofts, 3–24

14. Zarbuck M V 1986 A profession for 'Bohemian Chiropractic': Oakley Smith and the evolution of Naprapathy. Chiropractic History 6: 77–82
15. Forster A L 1915 Principles and Practice of Spinal Adjustment. National School of Chiropractic, Illinois
16. Stowell CC 1983 Lincoln College and the 'big four': A chiropractic protest, 1926–1962. Chiropractic History 3 (1): 75–78
17. Gitelman R, Fligg B 1992 Diversified Technique. In: Haldeman S, ed. Principles and practice of chiropractic. 2nd ed. New York NY: Appleton-Century-Krofts, 483–501
18. Peterson D 1987 Diversified technique and short lever specific contact procedures. Proceedings of the Second Annual Conference on Research and Education
19. Janse J, Houser R 1947 Chiropractic Principles and Technic. Lombard, Illinois: National College of Chiropractic
20. Vleeming A, Mooney V, Sniders C, Dorman T, eds 1992. First interdisciplinary world congress on low back pain and its relation to the sacroiliac joint. Rotterdam: ECO
21. States A Z 1968 Atlas of Chiropractic Tecnic: Spinal and Pelvic Technics. (2nd ed.) Lombard, Illinois: National College of Chiropractic

22. Reinert O 1962 Chiropractic procedure and practice. St. Louis: Marian Press
23. Bergmann T, Peterson D H, Lawrence D J 1994 Chiropractic Technique. New York, NY: Churchill Livingstone Inc.
24. Stonebrink R D 1990 Evaluation and manipulative management of common musculoskeletal disorders. Portland OR: Western States Chiropractic College
25. Christensen M G 1993 Job analysis of chiropractic. Greeley, Colorado: National Board of Chiropractic Examiners
26. Cleveland C S I 1992 The High-Velocity Thrust Adjustment. In: Haldeman S, ed. Principles and Practice of Chiropractic. 1st ed. Norwalk, Connecticut: Appleton & Lange, 459–482
27. Stonebrink D R 1993 Description of Diversified Technique
28. Schmidt M J Diversified Technique. Date unknown. Bell D, ed
29. Hinz D G 1987 Diversified chiropractic: Northwestern College and John B. Wolf, 1941–1984. Chiropractic History 7 (1): 35–41
30. Cooperstein R 1990 Brand name techniques and the confidence gap. The Journal of Chiropractic Education 4 (3): 89–93

Glossary

Most, but not all, of the terms that were defined in sections 2 and 3 of the book are gathered here. We excluded a few terms that we deemed worth discussing in individual chapters, but not in this compilation, such as very individualized usage of otherwise generic terms such as "subluxation." This glossary is not designed to replace, but rather supplement more general glossaries of chiropractic terminology, such as may be found in chiropractic technique books, such as *Chiropractic Technique* by Peterson and Bergmann (see Further reading).

KEY

ACT	Activator Methods Chiropractic Technique (Fuhr)
AK	Applied Kinesiology (Goodheart)
ART	Active Release Technique (Leahy)
BEST	Bionergetic Synchronization Technique (Morter)
CBP	Chiropractic Biophysics Technique (Harrison)
CRANIO	Craniopathy
DNFT	Directional Non-Force Technique (Van Rumpt)
DT	Distraction Technique (Cox)
FSS	Full-Spine Specific (Cleveland)
GON	Gonstead Chiropractic Technique (Gonstead)
LC	Leg checking
LOGAN	Logan Basic (Logan)
MT	Muscle testing, manual
NET	Network (Epstein)
NIMMO	Nimmo/Receptor-Tonus Technique (Nimmo)
PAL	Palpation
PETT	Spinal Biomechanics Technique (Pettibon)
PST	Pierce–Stillwagon Technique (Pierce, G. Stillwagon)
SOT	Sacro-Occipital Technique (DeJarnette)
SS	Spinal Stressology (Ward)
TH	Thermography
TOFT	Toftness Technique (Toftness)
TRT	Torque Release Technique (Holder)
TT	Thompson Technique (Thompson)
UCT	Upper Cervical Technique (Palmer)
X-RAY	X-ray

AAI: {ACT} Activator Adjusting Instrument, "a manually manipulatable instrument capable of providing a dynamic thrust that includes a controlled force of adjustment at a precise and specific line of drive at high speed."[1] It has also been described as a handheld, manually assisted, spring-activated device which delivers a maximum of 0.3 J of energy under controlled conditions.[2]

Abductor tendency/adductor resistance: {TRT} an examination procedure that determines the tendency of one or both legs of a prone patient to remain in abduction, and resist being adducted when moved into that direction by the examiner. Thought to be indicative of a C2 subluxation, usually on the side of greater resistance.

Aberrant nerve impulses: {TOFT} also known as nerve stress, meaning essentially nerve interference.[3]

Aberrative foci: {NIMMO} Nimmo's "subluxation-equivalent," as discussed by Cooperstein and Gleberzon.[4]

Accessory joint movements: {PAL} joint movements that cannot be performed voluntarily (unassisted) by a patient. These are necessary for the normal function of joints and may include such actions as rolls, slides, spins, distractions, and compressions.

Activator: the term "activator" originated from the concept that it does not take much force to move a bone; muscles do the work, provided the bone has been "activated" in the correct direction.[5]

Active and passive range of motion: {PAL} the active range of motion is what can be accessed by the unassisted patient, whereas passive motion is the range that can be accessed by the doctor taking the joint some distance beyond this active limit.

Acu-arc: {PST} drafting tool that enables calculation of the radius of curvature of an arc. PST uses this tool to measure the curviness of the spinal regions in the sagittal plane.

AMCT: {NET} Adverse mechanical cord tension. The term is taken from Breig,[6] redefined by Epstein to include Network Spinal Analysis (NSA) ideology.

Anatometer: {UCT} a device used primarily by National Upper Cervical Chiropractic Association (NUCCA) practitioners to measure postural deviations and leg-length inequalities said to result from C1 subluxations.

Anatomical short leg (or structural short leg): {LC} a leg which is demonstrably shorter than the other leg, due to fracture, deformity, or uneven growth rates.

Anterior iliofemoral technique: {SOT} restriction in medial rotation of the hip in the Category II supine patient, corrected by a patient-resisted internal rotation and a lateral-to-medial thrust on the ligament.

Apex contact: {LOGAN} sacrotuberous ligament, opposite side of sacral apex deviation, using 3–6 oz. (84 g) of pressure;[7] halfway between the ischial tuberosity and the sacrococcygeal joint.[7]

Approach, settle-back, turn-in, arch, roll-in, conversion, triceps pull: {UCT} terms referring to the sequence of events, or "phases" in the NUCCA adjustment.

Approximate normal potential rule: {PST} the arc that is traced out by the anterior bodies of the normal cervical lordosis;[8] the gold standard against which hyperlordotic, hypolordotic, and lorphotic cervical curves are rated.

Arm fossa test: {SOT} "A challenge of multiple stimuli calling on the upper motor neuron system to coordinate function with the lower motor neuron function."[9] The examiner exerts mild pressure at either the superior-lateral or inferior-medial aspects of the inguinal ligament, looking for a potential weakening of the shoulder girdle musculature. This weakening, when present, is thought to confirm the presence of a Category II presentation (post-traumatic sacroiliac dysfunction), and instability of the sacroiliac joint.[10]

Atlas subluxation complex (ASC): {UCT} denotes in NUCCA the "extensive and detrimental effects of a C1 subluxation on the CNS (central nervous system) and the spinal column."[11]

Auxiliary contacts: {LOGAN} taken as aids in application of the other contacts, in accordance to the lines of muscle pull.

Basic I and Basic II cranial adjusting: {SOT} the cranial procedures that are associated with treating the Category I and Category II syndromes, respectively.

Bilateral cervical syndrome: {TT} refers to a bilateral occiput fixation. With the patient's knees extended, the head is turned from side to side. In each direction, the leg ipsilateral to the side of head rotation shortens.

Bio: {BEST} Morter's version of the life force.

Blair Toggle-Torque adjustive thrust: {UCT} the Blair adjustment[12] is essentially a toggle-recoil adjustment, minus the recoil.

Blocks: {SOT} padded wedges used as fulcrums to correct intrapelvic torsion in either the prone or supine position.

Brain-Reward Cascade: {TRT} mechanism by which the TRT is thought to operate. The 1997 advertising brochure describes the cascade as: "a scientific model that provides an understanding of the neurophysiological mechanisms of how the meso-limbic system expresses a state of well-being. The vertebral motor unit and the dorsal horn are the common denominators." The absence of a properly maintained Brain-Reward Cascade cycle is said to result in a deficiency in the state of well-being.

Break analysis: {TH} interpretation of a rapid deflection of the device pointer, back and forth, believed to be within one dermatome.

Breakdown factors: {SS} these cause systemic structural collapse, either by trauma or insidiously.

Catastrophe theory: {CBP} Thom's mathematical term, applied to sudden changes in spinal equilibrium.[13] (p. 3)

Category I: {SOT} "A disturbance in the cranial sacral system in its distribution of the cerebral spinal fluid, the tension of its dural membranes and the function of the cranial/sacral structures to promote these qualities."[9]

Category II: {SOT} "A complex of anatomical, physiological and symptomatic findings associated with ligament sprain and laxity, with resultant hypermobility of the Sacro-Iliac joint … [and] a loss of weight-bearing pelvic stability."[14] There is said to be an associated

disturbance of the "cranial weight-bearing sutural systems."[9]

Category III: {SOT} "A lumbar joint failure resulting in discogenic involvement and nerve root compression or stretching … a failure of the pyriformis muscle."[9] "Category III relates to the cartilaginous system of man."[15]

Central skull line, atlas plane line: {UCT} representative terms drawn from the Upper Cervical Technique (UCT) X-ray line-marking system, referring to a vertical line representing head tilt and a horizontal line representing atlas inclination.

Cervical rotation test: {PST} changes in relative leg length as the head is turned from side to side by a prone patient, signifying cervical subluxation.

Cervical stairstep and figure 8 adjusting: {SOT} caudal pressure on the cranium of the supine patient should cause the skull to glide inferoanteriorly in four discrete steps. If this is not the case, the clinician moves the head and neck in a "figure 8" motion at the point of restriction in gliding.

Challenge: {AK} a provocative test applied to a patient, such as pushing on a bone in a specific direction, to see how the strength of a previously strong indicator muscle (PSIM) is affected. Challenges can be physical, mental, or chemical.[16,17]

Challenge: {MT} a challenge amounts to some sort of mild clinical intervention, such as a mild thrust on a spinous process, or placing a nutritional substance under the tongue, in order to assess its effect on the strength of a PSIM. It usually refers to the weakening, but could refer to the strengthening, of a PSIM.

Chiropractic Manipulative Reflex Technique (CMRT): {SOT} SOT specialty that is said to normalize somatovisceral function and somatospinal reflexes.[18] It involves a series of procedures intended to "improve organ circulation and normal vagal impulse conduction"[19] through postganglionic technique, vertebral adjusting, and "manual stimulation of the organs."[9] CMRT supposedly enables identification of visceral problems and thereby enables the prescription of nutritional support for the compromised organs.

Class A subluxation: {NET} structural in nature,[20,21] with elements of fixation, misalignment, and nerve interference. It is the classic chiropractic subluxation, treatable with high-velocity, low-amplitude (HVLA) thrusting.

Class B meningeal subluxation: {NET} Essentially neurological (facilitated) in nature,[20,21] located within the brain or spinal cord. It involves a "multisegmental facilitation of the paraspinal musculature due to adverse cord–brain tension and interference in the cord, brain, and/or dural sleeves."[22] Furthermore, it is a "concussion of forces" on an emotional or chemical level that overloads the CNS. The vertebra displaces secondarily, as an adaptative feature.

Clear-out: {NET} the adjustment process in NCT.[23]

Compensated, uncompensated subluxations: {PET} compensated subluxations are pain-free at the lesion site, while uncompensated or overcompensated subluxations are usually pain-expressive.

Compustress: {SS} computerized disk stress evaluation system that apparently can be installed in doctors' offices.[24]

Computed tomography (CT): {X-RAY} advanced imaging procedure in which cross-sectional pictures or "tomographic slices" of the body are made by X-ray. A series of X-ray beams from many different angles is used to create cross-sectional images of the patient's body, that can be reconstructed by a computer into a three-dimensional picture displaying organs, bones, and tissues in great detail.

Coupling patterns: {CBP} described in 1987,[25] and more carefully covered in a two-part article by Harrison et al,[26,27] coupling patterns are said to occur in six degrees of freedom, and not simply in rotation and lateral flexion, the directions they claim are stressed by other technique systems.

Cranial fault: {CRANIO} misalignment or movement restriction of the cranial bones, where they articulate at the sutures.

Cranial-sacral respiratory mechanism (CSRM): {SOT} "A combination of integrated functions that support, nourish and enhance the performance of the nervous system as it controls bodily functions."[9] According to Getzoff, it involves each of the following entities: cranial motion, sacral weight-bearing motion, dural tension, cerebrospinal fluid (CSF) pulsation and flow, ventricular respiration, and several other functions that relate to cranial development.[9]

Cranial Rhythm (CR): {CRANIO} The pulse wave created by CSF production from the ventricles and pumped under tension through the dura to the sacrum. The ventricles are thought to flex and extend in a motion similar to that of gills, along with associated movements of the sacrum, thus creating the CR. This movement is thought to create a palpable rhythm of 6–12 cycles/min, distinct and separate from either the respiratory or heart rate.

Cranial rhythmic impulse (CRI): {CRANIO} Sometimes also referred to as the "Sutherland wave." The CR provides a force that moves the bones of the cranium, called the CRI, which is palpable at various points of a person's body. The cranial therapist appreciates not merely the rate of the CRI, but also its quality, vitality, and bilateral symmetry. Five separate motions are thought to comprise the CRI.

Cranial sutures: {SOT} hard and soft tissues of adjoining cranial bones, comparable to other joints of the body.[10]

Craniosacral system: {CRANIO} A system composed of the cranial structures, neural elements, and sacrum.

Cranio-Spinal Meningeal Functional Unit (C-SMFU): {TRT} The composite of the brain, spinal cord, meningeal layers, bones of the cranium, vertebral column, and pelvis, thought to function as an integral unit.

Crest sign: {SOT} Relative hypotonus of the erector spinae and quadratus lumborum muscles at the level of L4, that corrects during blocking. The normal contralateral side is called the "crest sign side." It is seen in Category I presentations. Balanced muscles are thought to indicate reciprocal function of the temporal bone and the innominate.[10]

Cumulative injury cycle: {ART} a mechanism used to explain the effect on tissue and subsequent development of fibrous adhesions as the result of injury, repetitive use, or constant pressure.

Fibrous adhesions: {ART} a product of inflammation from overuse or trauma, these are noxious soft-tissue structures that are thought to cling to and diminish the proper function of other soft tissues. In essence, these entities predispose a patient to biomechanical impediments that ultimately lead to syndromes, notably of the peripheral nerve roots.

Law of repetitive motion: {ART} a mathematical formula developed to express the relationship between the characteristics of a repetitive force and injury or insult to tissue.

Defense factors: {SS} these result from overutilization of energy, and can be determined or measured as degenerative changes seen on X-ray.

Derifield leg check: {LC} a prone leg-checking protocol involving two primary components: (1) assessment of relative leg lengths with the knees extended compared to knees flexed to 90°, identifying pelvic syndrome; and (2) assessment of change in relative leg lengths as the head is turned in either direction, identifying cervical syndrome.

Derifield leg check: {TT} the Thompson leg check is patterned after the work of Romer Derifield and others, and is described in Chapter 4. The behavior of the prone subject's legs, with the knees either extended or flexed, as various test conditions are altered, gives rise to Thompson Technique listings.

Derma-Therm-O-Graph (DTG), Visi-Therm: {PST} thermography devices used in PST. The DTG, developed early on, was a dual-probed thermocouple device that was later replaced by the Visi-Therm, an infrared device capable of measuring absolute (as opposed to simply relative) temperatures (and thus cold points) (Ch. 8).

Diaphragm: {CRANIO} in craniopathy, the body is divided into separate regions or diaphragms, predominantly along the lines of fascia orientation. Collectively, the thoracic outlet, respiratory, and urogenital diaphragms are often referred to as the sternal pump.

Distortions: {DNFT} adaptations or compensations for subluxation, that should not be adjusted.

Doctor-initiated and patient-initiated muscle testing: {MT} different physiological mechanisms may be involved according to the timing, depending on whether the test is begun by the examiner first applying force (eccentric testing, doctor-initiated); or the patient first bracing by exerting resistance (concentric testing, patient-initiated).[28]

Dollar signs: {SOT} relative hypotonus of the gluteal muscle (at junction of piriformis, gluteus medius, and gluteus maximus) in an area the size of a silver dollar 3 in. (7.5 cm) inferior and 2 in. (5 cm) lateral to the posterior superior iliac spine (PSIS), that corrects during blocking. The normal contralateral side is the "dollar sign side." It is seen in Category I presentations. The muscle's relative tone is thought to indicate reciprocal function of the sacrum and occiput.[10]

Double AS, double PI ilium: {PST} these listings are not to be understood as bilateral sacroiliac lesions, but rather as descriptors of the position of the PSISs "in space;" that is, either an anterior or posterior tilting of the entire pelvis, relative to its normal position, accompanied by lumbar adaptation.[29]

Dual-probe thermography: {TH} the thermographic device has two sensors that measure the temperature differential between the two points of application. Examples: the Nervo-Scope, the neurocalometer.

Entrainment: {CRANIO} the integration or harmonization of the different oscillators in the body. CRI is said to be the palpable perception of entrainment, the harmonic frequency that incorporates the rhythms of multiple biological oscillators.

Entrainment: {NET} a term also found in cranial therapy, it refers to the harmonizing oscillations of biological systems. Epstein states that "the entrainment contact or impulse is applied to a segmental region of high, free energy in the vicinity of the attachment of the spinal cord ... is non-therapeutic in design. It is not a form of spinal manipulation, nor is it specifically developed to correct fixation, pain, misalignment or subluxation."[30]

Entropic chaos: {SS} temporary worsening of the patient after care begins.[31]

Entrophic, syntrophic: {SS} bad, good, respectively.

Eyes into distortion: {AK} weakening of a PSIM when the patient gazes in a particular direction.

Five factors of the intervertebral foramen (IVF): {AK} when a muscle tests weak, each of the following etiologic factors are considered, all of which supposedly relate to the IVF: the nervous system, the neurolymphatic reflexes of Chapman, the neurovascular reflexes of Bennett, CSF flow, and acupuncture meridian connectors.[32]

Fixation: {AK} lack of normal motion involving three (not the more typical two) vertebrae.

Fixation: {PAL} a state in which a vertebra has become immobilized in a position it could normally occupy during physiological movement, including an aligned position.

Flexion–distraction: {DT} the term "flexion–distraction," although seeming to be generic in one sense, is virtually synonymous with Cox's concept and clinical application, and thus warrants being considered a technique-specific term.

Foot flare: {TRT} foot inversion/eversion [sic], thought to be indicative of torsion of the spinal cord and meninges. (We note that, although foot flare seems synonymous with internal/external foot rotation, that is not what is usually meant by the terms "inversion/eversion.")

Frontal/lateral headweighting: {PET} suspension of a weight from a harness worn around the skull, to sagittal and frontal plane cervical postural distortions.[33]

Full-spine radiograph: {X-RAY} standing plain film, anteroposterior view taken on 14 × 36 (35 × 90 cm) film; sometimes called a scoliogram in orthopedic medicine.

Functional short leg (or physiological short leg, apparent short leg, etc.): {LC} a leg which is actually even in length with the other leg, but which appears shorter due to a postural imbalance that draws up the hip in the non-weight-bearing position.

Hard vs soft end-feel: {PAL} a hard end-feel to passive joint movement is thought to be due to articular (structural) degenerative changes, while a soft end-feel would be associated with contracted muscles and other soft tissues.

Head subluxation, into the kinks subluxation, and against the kinks subluxations: {UCT} typical NUCCA X-ray listings. In the head subluxation, the head is tilted by more than the cervical spine has lost vertical alignment. In the into and against configurations, the head and neck are oblique to the gravity line, on the same side as the gravity line (the into configuration) or the opposite side from the gravity line (the against configuration).[34] The against configuration is said to be the most common of the three.[34,35]

Heat swing: {TH} interpretation of a deflection of the device pointer to the left and right over one or more apparent dermatomes.

Heel tension: {SOT} a Category I indicator, occurring on the short-leg side. It is detected as a unilateral "difference in relative resistance in one of the heels in response to being stretched," with some degree of dorsiflexion, or as tenderness of the Achilles tendon to pinch.[36] When present, it is thought to reflect atlas adaptation to tension in the dura.[10]

HIO: {UCT} acronym for Hole-In-One, a synonym for Palmer Upper Cervical Specific technique. It refers to the idea that a perfect listing, given a perfect thrust, using perfect technique, will clear the atlas subluxation in one stroke (thrust).

HIO listings: {UCT} a typical four-letter listing would be ASRA. The first A stands for atlas, the S refers to an excessively steep atlas plane line in the sagittal plane, the R refers to atlas laterality to the right, and the second A refers to an anterior rotation of the atlas transverse process (relative to the occipital condyles) on the right, the side of atlas laterality.

Hot boxes: {FSS} locations of elevated temperature along the spine, detected either with the back of the fingers or with the neurocalograph, and thought to indicate subluxated vertebrae.[37]

Hypermyotonia: {NIMMO} muscle hypertonus.[38]

Infrared thermography: {TH} (telethermography device) the thermographic device measures infrared radiation (heat) emitted from the body surface, essentially taking a colorized photo of the skin temperature: an example is the Tytron C-3000.

Integrator®: {TRT} a hand held device that can be used to perform adjustments. It is self-releasing (producing a recoiling effect) and can produce clockwise or counterclockwise torque and recoil.

Intermittent force correction (IFC): {SS} procedure in which the patient walks with the shoe on one foot, first on the defense side, then on the breakdown side.

Intersegmental range of motion (IROM) motion palpation: {GON} a type of motion palpation, intended to identify segmental loss of full ROM in any of the six degrees of freedom; it is to be contrasted with the other main type of motion palpation, end-feel or end-play joint assessment.[39]

In the clear: {AK} this term refers to testing a muscle in the absence of any provocative interventions or challenges.

Into the angles, against the angles, head subluxation: {PETT} terms adapted from Upper Cervical work (Gregory), referring to cervical distortion patterns.

Involved side: {TT} the side of the patient ipsilateral to the side of the short leg.

Isolation testing: {ACT} "Prone observations are made of straight and flexed LLs [leg lengths] while the patient's extremities are positioned so as to exacerbate muscular imbalance at specific spinal segments."[40] The isolation test is a specific, active movement of the patient, aimed at detecting of facilitated segments through leg reactivity.

Isoperimetric: {CBP} a mathematical term that refers to "different possible configurations of the same arc length."[13] (p. 19)

Joint play: {PAL} movements not under voluntary control, but necessary to achieve full painless joint function; a springiness and rebound in the joint movement, that occurs at the end of this passive range of motion, thus inaccessible to the unassisted patient.

Lateral wedge, open wedge, "high side of the rainbow": {GON} all of these expressions refer to the convex side of a lateral flexion malposition, thought to result from ipsilateral shifting of the nucleus pulposus.

Leg checking: {LC} procedure usually, but not always, manual and visual, for assessing leg-length inequality.

Leg-length inequality: {LC} (anisomelia, leg-length discrepancy, etc.) asymmetry in distal foot positions, due to anatomic or functional factors.

Level foundation: {GON} the sacrum is considered the base of the spine;[41] vertebrae that begin lateral inclinations of the spine in relation to the sacral level base are considered possible subluxations, whereas those vertebrae that terminate these lateral inclinations by regaining a parallel relationship to the sacral base would be termed "compensations."

Levels of care: {NET} specifically defines the transition from Network Chiropractic to Network Spinal Analysis. Each of the three levels corresponds to a desired outcome of care: basic, intermediate, and advanced care.[42] Each of the five phases within the phasing system occurs within each of the levels of care.

Lines of mensuration: {X-RAY} although the word "mensuration" simply means measurement, it is generally used in the chiropractic profession to refer to roentgenometrics. These include not only special measures unique to chiropractic technique systems, but measures commonly taken by medical radiologists. Common "medical" cervical lines of mensuration include the horizontal line of the atlas, horizontal line of the axis, lordotic curve angle, Chamberlain's line, physiological stress lines, and George's line. Common lumbar lines of mensuration include the angle of curvature, Ferguson's line, George's line, McNabb's line, the lumbosacral disk angle, Ullman's line, and grades of spondylolisthesis.

Liquid crystal thermography: {TH} an elastomeric latex sheet contacts the body, with embedded organic crystals that change color in relation to skin temperature.

Listening station: {CRANIO} a point on the patient's body the therapist contacts in order to assess the CRI.

LLL: {SOT} Category II finding of Lower fossa active, Lateral knee pain, and Long leg on the ipsilateral side to the weak fossa.

Lorphosis: {PST} a cervical spine that has a kyphotic region, either in the upper or lower cervical spine.[43]

Lower angle: {PET} the angle between a line representing the center of mass of the functional cervical spine (center of the neural canal) and a line transversely through the atlas in the frontal plane.

Lower angle, upper angle, into the angles/kinks: {CBP} these and other terms are taken from Upper Cervical X-ray line-marking systems.

Magnetic resonance imaging: {X-RAY} advanced imaging procedure in which a powerful magnetic field and radio signals provide a detailed picture of structures and organs inside the body. It does not require X-rays or the injection of dyes or other substances.

Mean heat line: {TH} slow and gradual drift of the indicator, thought to reflect some degree of normal bilateral thermal asymmetry.

Meningeal critical: {NET} a clinical entity in which the patient is approaching an impending collapse of the nervous system (e.g., disk herniation),[20] and even death.

Meric: {FSS} refers to the "vertemeres" of the spine, the segments of the vertebral column, so that the term "Meric Technique" has to do with segmental specificity.[44]

Meric chiropractic arch: {FSS} refers to the doctor's hand position, with the wrist fully extended with ulnar deviation and flexion of the metacarpal-phalangeal joints to 90°.

MFMA: {ACT} mechanical force, manually assisted, short-lever adjustment.

Mind language: {MT} although developed by Sacro-Occipital Technique practitioners, mind language bears an obvious resemblance to therapy localization as utilized by Applied Kinesiologists. According to DeJarnette,[45] the right arm is used as the testing mechanism and the left index finger as a pointer or finder. The patient touches the point of pain or complaint area while the doctor tests the arm for strength or weakness. Weakness identifies a problem area.

Mind language: {SOT} according to DeJarnette:[45] "We use the right arm as the testing mechanism and the left index finger as the finder, or pointer, finger … We simply contact the point of pain or complaint and test the arm for strength or weakness. Weakness shows that area to be the problem area."

Mirror-image adjusting: {CBP} a procedure in which the patient is prepositioned prior to an adjustive thrust, so as to reverse postural deviations.

Mirror-image rehabilitative exercise: {CBP} patients are taught how to move their "global body parts"[46] into a postural configuration that is the opposite of their postural distortion pattern.

Misalignment: {PAL} refers to a joint in which the contiguous bones are not in normal alignment when the subject is attempting to remain within a neutral position.

Motion palpation: {PAL} (also known as dynamic palpation) somatic structures are assessed for active and passive movement capacity.

Motion segment: {PAL} according to Lantz,[47] the motion segment (previously known as the spinal motor unit, motor segment, functional spinal unit, or basic spinal unit) is the basic unit of spinal mobility. It consists of two adjacent vertebrae, the intervening intervertebral disk, the two posterior joints, and various ligaments (capsules, interspinous, and intertransverse).

Negative Derifield: {TT} The PSIS of the ipsilateral innominate subluxates posterior-inferior, the innominate rotating about an axis through the sacroiliac joint. The prone short leg with the knees extended remains short when the knees are flexed.

Negative ilium: {PST} Derifield leg-check listing in which the knees-extended short leg remains short when the knees are flexed, leading to any number of possible adjustments, depending primarily on X-ray findings and the possible presence of tender points.

Nerve tracing: {FSS} we can do no better than cite the founder, D D Palmer himself: "The chiropractor should trace sensitive, swollen, longitudinally contracted nerves, for the purpose of locating their impingement and tension … There is no better way to locate the cause of disease, or demonstrate to a prospective patient how bones and nerves are related to each other and why such relationship accounts for health and disease, than by palpation and nerve-tracing."[48] (p. 102)

Network: {NET} in one sense, Network has to do with community, in which a "family" of chiropractors and practice members share a dedication to the growth, development, health, and well-being of the individual and the planet. In another sense, Network has to do with sequencing moves drawn from other chiropractic techniques so that the adjustments will be more efficient and lasting. Finally, Epstein is said to believe that the body is "a functional network in which everything is linked to everything else."[23]

Network protocol: {NET} the distinction between Class A and B subluxations leads to the Network protocol.

Neurologic disorganization: {AK} refers to an inability of the nervous system to respond in a coordinated way to stimuli, the "result of afferent receptors sending conflicting information for interpretation by the central nervous system."[49]

Neurolymphatic reflexes: {AK} points on the body originally developed by Chapman, an osteopath, thought to govern lymphatic drainage of the associated body portion, and digitally treated to strengthen muscles made weak by their involvement.

Neurovascular reflexes: {AK} points on the body originally developed by Bennett, a chiropractor, which are thought to govern vascular flow in an associated body portion, and digitally treated for such purposes. Although Bennett described these points as occurring everywhere, Applied Kinesiology practitioners have only been able to incorporate the cranial neurovascular points into their treatment regimen.

Non-linear: {NET} this refers to the phenomenon that a relatively small neurological input, or even light corrective adjustment, may result in a much larger response or reaction in the body.

Non-linear: {TRT} a principle of TRT that informs a practitioner that he or she should not adjust the same vertebral segments in or with the same vector in the same order in any three visits in a row.

Non-mechanistic: {TRT} unlike other techniques such as Diversified, Gonstead, or Thompson that utilize the principles of Newtonian mechanics of force, momentum, acceleration, mass and so on, proponents of TRT state that their technique operates in the realm of quantum mechanics.

Notch contact: {LOGAN} gluteal muscles, inferior sacrum side.

NUCCA: {UCT} an acronym for National Upper Cervical Chiropractic Association; the technique system associated with founder Gregory and that organization.

Occipital fiber analysis: {SOT} SOT practitioners believe that thoracolumbar subluxations are accompanied by both an organ reflex and occipital fiber involvement. Occipital nodules in precisely defined locations are thought to correspond to blockage in either pre- or postganglionic neurons. Occipital fibers are generally involved in Category I patterns and serve as CMRT indicators as well.

Overcompensated cervical syndrome: {TT} this is a condition of spinous process laterality, diminishing from C2 through C7, as seen on X-ray.

Paraphysiological joint space: {PAL} incremental movement beyond the elastic barrier that is attained at the end of passive range of motion, accessed by means of an HVLA thrust.[50]

Pattern system of analysis: {TH} it is believed that, under normal circumstances, the body is able to adapt to its changing environment in such a manner that there is a constant fluctuation of its thermal pattern.

Pelvic deficiency (PD) leg: {ACT} the leg that appears short in performing a prone leg check, or which "gives, shortens or feels soft and spongy" in the prone leg check;[5] not to be confused with an anatomically shortened lower extremity.

Phasing system:[42] {NET} consists of five phases of AMCT, each of which has distinctive palpatory and biomechanical findings and implications for the vertebral level and type of care to be rendered. Once subluxation is determined to exist, the phasing system is then used to determine what levels are to be adjusted.

PI ilium: {PST} a rotational misalignment of the ilium, in which the PSIS moves inferiorward and the symphysis pubis moves superiorly.

Piriformis contact: {LOGAN} a posteriorward pressure applied at the insertion of the piriformis muscle on the greater trochanter.[51]

Plain film studies: {X-RAY} simple use of X-ray, as opposed to advanced imaging (computed tomography, MRI, etc.) methodologies.

Point of critical tension: {NET} This is that segmental spinal region which appears to give rise to a specific area of meningeal and/or cord tension.[30] According to Epstein, this point varies automatically on a given segment, depending on the directional vectors of the tension. It is often located at the occiput, sacrococcygeal, and lower cervical regions (points where the dura attaches). It is often the point of contact for a corrective procedure.

Positive Derifield: {TT} The PSIS of the ipsilateral innominate subluxates posterior-inferior, the innominate rotating about an axis through the hip. The prone short leg with the knees extended crosses over to become the long leg when the knees are flexed.

Positive ilium: {PST} Derifield leg-check listing in which the knees-extended short leg crosses over to become the knees-flexed long leg, leading to the prone adjustment of the posterior-inferior iliac spine.

Posterior iliofemoral technique: {SOT} restriction in medial rotation of the hip in the Category I or Category III patient, corrected by a double thumb thrust on the posterior aspect of the greater trochanter.

Posterior ischium: {TT} The ischium of the ipsilateral innominate subluxates posteriorly, as seen on an X-ray. The innominate rotates about an axis through the sacroiliac joint.

Posteriority: {GON} Gonstead practitioners believe that, with the exception of atlas, a vertebra must subluxate posteriorly in relation to the segment below (for opposing views, see Harrison[52]).

Practice member: {NET} the person formerly known as "the patient," who has graduated to level 3 care – essentially, maintenance care.

Pre- and postganglionic technique: {SOT} preganglionic work is said to address cholinergic vagal function proximal to the ganglion, whereas postganglionic work would address adrenergic vagal function distal to

the ganglion. The preganglionic reflex involves a contact on the sternum, thought by virtue of its marrow functions to be especially important for nerve conduction. The postganglionic work involves a contact on the anterior aspect of the C5 transverse processes, the approximate site of the carotid reflexes.

Pressurestat model: {CRANIO} postulated by Upledger, this model purports that the craniosacral system functions as a semiclosed hydraulic system containing CSF.

Pressure testing: {ACT} this has been described as "light pressure applied in the direction of the correction,"[1] as it determines the result of the leg-checking procedure. It is a brief application of provocative pressure to a body structure under investigation, typically the spinous process of a vertebra. The outcome of the test is determined by responsiveness or lack thereof in relative leg positions.

Prestressing, post-tensioning: {CBP} mechanical engineering terms, applied to spinal structures.[53]

Previously strong indicator muscle (PSIM): {AK} during the procedure of manual muscle testing, the PSIM is established as a muscle that is strong in the clear, when it is not being tested during a challenge procedure of some kind. The PSIM is thus suitable to be used as an outcome measure following a clinical intervention.

Previously strong indicator muscle (PSIM): {MT} the muscle tester, in order to undertake muscle testing as a diagnostic procedure, must first identify a muscle that is strong (of normal strength) when in the clear. This muscle may be any in the body, and is not specifically related to the subluxation or other clinical problem being investigated.

Primary respiratory mechanism: {CRANIO} a system composed of the mutually interdependent brain, CSF, reciprocal tension membranes of the skull, and bones of the skull and sacrum. It does not refer to the pulmonary system, being independent of both cardiac and pulmonary systems, but rather to the motion of the CRI.

Prone leg check: {LC} Leg-checking procedure commonly employed by Full-Spine practitioners, usually thought to identify pelvic torsion, with posterior innominate rotation on the short leg side.

Pulsation synchronization: {BEST} cellular and organismal pulsations or "beats" which produce waves.[54]

R + C factors: {SOT} the letters stand for "resistance" and "contraction," and relate to the fact that DeJarnette felt that each member of a pair of vertebrae could affect each other, and that atlas related to L5, and axis to L4, and so on.[55] This is comparable to the Lovett brothers' relationships, described by the Applied Kinesiologists.[16]

Radiographic series: {X-RAY} a set of plain films considered adequate for the area under investigation, including at least two films taken at right angles.

Range of motion: {PAL} the amount of translatory and rotatory movement available to a joint.

Reactive leg: {ACT} the leg that relatively shortens in response to a provocative, diagnostic procedure.

Reactive leg reflex: {DNFT} refers to Van Rumpt's leg-check procedure, in which a "challenge" into tissue results in the leg pulling up if there is subluxation.[56,57]

Reactive muscle: {AK} a muscle that tests weak only after its related muscle has contracted, that related muscle being termed the primary muscle.

Reactive spinal abnormalities: {SS} compensations.

Reading: {TH} rapid deflection and return of the indicator to the mean heat line.

Rebound challenge: {MT} a muscle which is specifically inhibited by a vertebral

subluxation may strengthen when a challenge is applied that would correct that subluxation; this is called a rebound challenge.

Receptor Tonus Control Method (RTCM): {NIMMO} the treatment of a trigger point using ischemic compression.

Recovery: {NET} Epstein prefers the term "recovery" to healing, describing it as a process in which innate intelligence accepts the adjustment.[22]

Reflex: {MT} the word "reflex" in this context specifically does not refer to the types of reflexes one could read about in an orthopedics or neurology textbook, such as a deep tendon or pathological reflex. It refers to a hypothetical, often unstudied cause-and-effect physiological relationship between two phenomena. As an example, a mild thrust on a spinous process may cause a reflex weakening of a PSIM, or thyroid disease may produce weakness in the infraspinatus muscle by some sort of reflex.

Relatoscope, cephalometer: {UCT} these tools and their descendants are transparent plates with various slots and line markings, used in NUCCA and other Upper Cevical-inspired techniques (e.g., Pettibon's Spinal Biomechanics, Harrison's Chiropractic Biophysics) to perform line marking on the C1 and skull areas, respectively.

Respiratory and somatopsychic waves: {NET} the spontaneous writhing in which Network Chiropractic Technique (NCT)/NSA patients/practice participants typically engage. The respiratory wave is a smooth, rhythmic muscular movement, synchronized with breathing. The somatopsychic wave is a coordinated wave motion of the major muscle groups, gently rocking restricted spinal segments.

Restriction: {PAL} a limitation of joint movement, named by the direction in which the patient exhibits limitation, in either translatory or rotational movement. For example, a patient restricted in left lateral flexion has difficulty bending toward the left. The term "restriction" is currently preferred in situations where the less specific term "fixation" had been formerly used.

Retracing (both emotional and structural): {SS} temporary worsening on the way to recovery.

Reversal syndrome: {TT} following correction of either a positive or negative Derifield syndrome, the postcheck indicates that the patient has reversed to the other syndrome, presumably as a result of a shift in the interinnominate axis of rotation between the hip and the sacroiliac joint.`

Reward deficiency syndrome: {TRT} a lack of state of well-being, resulting from disruption in the Brain Reward Cascade cycle.

Roentgenometrics: {X-RAY} mensuration of X-ray films, either done by hand, or using computerized radiographic digitization procedures.

Sacral Base+ and Sacral Base−: {SOT} with the examiner's thumb placed lightly on the spinous process of L5, the patient gives a light cough. An upward bounce of the thumb indicates SB+, and a cephalad drag SB−. Each situation requires a specific blocking technique to reduce the sacral component of craniosacral subluxation. The findings are indicative of the extension or flexion fixation of the dural system.[10]

Sacral leg check: {TT} the prone patient is asked to extend one leg, then the other, off the table. The side of greater limitation (slower ascent, less elevation, painful or jerky movement) is thought to indicate an anterior–inferior subluxation of the sacral base, with accompanying contralateral deviation of the sacral apex.

Sensory dominant subluxation (SDS): {BEST} "Any recurring vertebral subluxation complex caused by sensory nerve interference," caused in the "high brain" and induced by stress.[58]

Sensory Engrams: {BEST} a learned motor pattern or memory which, once established, is used as a guide for the body to follow in reproducing the pattern of movement.[59]

Sick pattern: {TH} a relatively constant thermographic pattern, seen for 2–3 days, thought to reflect the body's inability to adapt to environmental changes and thus subluxation.

Single-loop feedback control mechanism: {ART} a concept borrowed from aeronautical engineering, it is the characteristic appearance of an object's position over time as a function of the various internal factors.

Single-probe thermography: {TH} the thermographic device has one sensor that measures the temperature at the point of application: an example is the DT-25.

SMFU: {NET} the spinal meningeal functional unit, associated with increased adrenal stress and an impending "set point positive."[22]

Soft-Tissue Regional Orthopedics (STO): {SOT} developed by Mervyn Lloyd Rees, as described in Heese,[60] STO purports to diagnose musculoskeletal and organ dysfunction,[9] as a further development of the temperosphenoidal reflex work discovered by DeJarnette.[36]

SOTO (step out, turn out): {SOT} a method of stretching the piriformis muscle, especially when sciatica is present[36] by abducting and externally rotating the leg, part of the Category I procedure. Getzoff uses it to monitor Category III pelvic distortions,[10] and describes how the SOTO procedure can be used to identify the category that is present, in addition to treating Category III.[61]

Spastic muscular contraction: {TT} also known as contracted muscle, the process by which neurophysiological imbalance results in leg-length inequality. The short leg itself is said to be contracted.

Specific chiropractic: {UCT} confines all adjustments to C1 and C2.[62]

Spinal column-pelvic-meningeal unit: {SS} the subluxation entity treated by Stressology.

Spinal gateway: {NET} the only way to do justice to this term is simply to quote Epstein: "access point for auto-assessment ... a focal area of free or unbound energy ... sensitive to entrained biological fields and to non-local intelligence."[30] The spinal gateway is "an interface between dimensions of tissue, energy and consciousness" and/or "a nexus for interaction between the passive, active, neural control and the emotional subsystems, contributing to spinal and neural integrity." The points of critical tension seem to indicate a spinal gateway for the practitioner to use in order to develop an entrainment pattern, often seen as respiratory or somatopsychic waves.[30]

Spinal set point: {NET} having to do with the fight-or-flight posture that represents a "loss of recovery from a specific postural state,"[22] an adaptation to adrenal exhaustion, in an attitude of flexion that increases meningeal and spinal cord tension.

Spine-In-Motion study: {PST} PST jargon for the Derifield leg check (Ch. 4), which generates the listings positive ilium, negative ilium, and positive cervical rotation test.

Static palpation: {PAL} somatic structures are assessed in their neutral, stationary position.

Steffensmeier board: {SOT} padded platform used to underlie the patient during blocking procedures.

Still point: {CRANIO} a point on the patient's body that, upon palpation by the examiner, would result in the cessation of the CRI. That is, the craniosacral system becomes still or inactive. This activity is thought to be therapeutic; once released, it is believed that the CRI will resume with better symmetry and vitality.

Stress: the rate of wear and tear in a biological organism.

Stress film: {X-RAY} films acquired in which the patient holds a posture at end-range of motion (lateral flexion, extension, forward flexion), taken to identify hypomobility or hypermobility.

Stress test: {ACT} this has been described as "light pressure applied into the direction of the subluxation."[1]

Strong, weak muscles: {AK} used by Applied Kinesiology practitioners, these terms do not have the same connotation that they have in an orthopedic setting. The so-called weak muscle may be weak on manual muscle testing, and yet to be found normal in strength using an objective measuring device such as a dynamometer. The terms "strong" and "weak" muscles have to do with the ability of the nervous system to mobilize a response to the command to "resist," usually when accompanied by a provocative challenge of some kind, such as therapy localization.

Supine leg check: {LC} leg-checking procedure commonly employed by Upper Cervical practitioners, thought to identify atlas subluxation

Survival segmentation: {BEST} the body's response to illness, in which it organizes itself into magnetic zones of opposite polarity, occurring in either an "anteroposterior" or "lateral pattern."

Switching: {AK} refers to right/left functional mix-up, the patient furnishing exactly wrong responses to stimuli, due to neural disorganization.

Sympathetic and parasympathetic nervous systems: {GON} Dr. Gonstead believed that the spinal range C5–occiput and below L5 governed the parasympathetic nervous system, and C6–L5 the sympathetic nervous system.[63] (p. 357)

Synchronicity: {SS} the interconnectedness of all the spinal-pelvic regions.

Syntropy: {SS} ideal process of reorganizing or putting back together.

Stress dominant side: {SS} side of body opposite that of brain dominance, thought to be more prone to breakdown.

Temporal-sphenoidal line: {AK} a line along the temporal sphenoidal suture, discovered by Rees,[64] that purportedly includes points related to muscle and organ function. Walther once stated: "The temporal-sphenoidal line (TS line) is an infallible indicator and valuable diagnostic aid."[64]

Temporal tap: {AK} a method in which tapping on the temporal bone is used to disturb sensory filtering mechanisms in the brain temporarily; this is accompanied by the administration of some other input (auditory, visual, etc.) so as to effect a change in the patient's behavior, or in the results of therapy localization.[16]

Terminal Point®: {TT} refers to the table's drop piece, which is thought to correct vertebral subluxation at the "terminal point" – the endpoint – of its travel distance once having been set into motion.

Therapeutic release: {CRANIO} a specific technique used by craniopaths to release various tissues, such as the cranial bones, diaphragms, meninges, and so on.

Therapy localization: {AK} a testing procedure in which the patient lightly applies a finger to a location of his or her own body, in order to test it for dysfunction, as would be identified by a PSIM weakening.

Therapy localization (TL): {MT} muscle strength may change when a patient touches his or her own hand to a part of the body, indicating a non-specific problem with that part of the body. The muscle tester must then identify the reflex associated with that positive TL.

Thermocouple thermography: {TH} measures skin temperature by direct contact of a thermal sensor composed of dissimilar wires: an example is the Nervo-Scope.

Through the plane line of the disk: {GON} Gonstead practitioners are adamant about adjusting vertebrae posterior to anterior, with a thrust parallel to the disk plane. Herbst goes so far as to suggest that contrary strategies "may have altered the course of our profession by convincing thousands of chiropractors that 'adjusting' a vertebra cannot change its position, does not get people well, and is painful to the patient."[41] (p. 81)

Thrust vs adjustment: {DNFT} a thrust only becomes an adjustment when it "succeeds 100% in correcting the subluxation and removing the nerve interference."[65] An adjustment, by comparison, does succeed in removing the subluxation and all the nerve interference.

Thumb toggle thrust: {DNFT} refers to the type of contact used by the doctor, in which the overlapped thumbs are used to apply a highly accelerated but very light force to the patient, in an overall style that resembles the toggle-recoil thrust minus the recoil.[57]

Tissue memory: {CRANIO} this concept holds that any tissue of the body has stored memories of emotionally charged events in a person's life that can be liberated during cranial therapy. These awakened emotions may indicate unresolved tensions or unconscious memories.

Toftness Radiation Detector (TRD, Sensometer,[66] or Toftness Electromagnetic Radiation Receiver): {TOFT} a tube containing a series of lenses that serve to focus the radiation emitted by the body on a diaphragm that distorts in the presence of said radiation.[3]

Toggle recoil: {UCT} the HIO adjustive style, using a reinforced pisiform applied to either atlas or axis, delivered in a rapidly accelerated thrust, with torque, followed by a so-called recoil. It is believed that the atlas is thus moved with respect to both the segment above and below,[67] provided enough speed is generated.[68]

Toggle-recoil adjustment: {FSS} has a dual sense, involving the recoil of the doctor's contact hand away from the patient after the thrust, and also the transmission of the force through the patient following the impact.

Torque: {CBP} CBP claims to use the term "torque" correctly,[69,70] as compared with many, if not most, other chiropractic techniques; Herzog felt that Harrison et al[70] had also misused the term.[71]

Torque: {TRT} distortion of the neuraxis, as well as the torque component of the adjustment used to correct spinal subluxation.

Trapezius fiber analysis: {SOT} this involves the palpation of seven areas on the trapezius, between the acromioclavicular joint and the spinous process of C7. A palpable nodule is said to indicate a specific vertebral subluxation and point toward a particular CMRT technique that should be performed. Trapezius analysis addresses subluxations not resolved by other procedures, most often as a follow-up in stubborn Category II presentations.

Triceps pull: {UCT} the actual NUCCA adjustment.

Trigger point, tonoplast, noxious generative point, painful nerve mechanism: {NIMMO} a nerve arrangement, myofascial or ligamentous, that generates noxious impulses that bombard the central nervous system, upsetting its balance.[72] (p. 19)

Ulnar contact: {LOGAN} near the apex contact, but using more force in severely fixated cases.

UMS: {SOT} Category II finding of Upper fossa active, Medial knee pain, and Short leg on the ipsilateral side to the weak fossa.

Unilateral cervical syndrome: {TT} with his knees extended, the patient's head is rotated to a given side. If a leg shortens or a previously short leg remains short, the unilateral cervical syndrome is present. Turning in the opposite direction may even the legs, in which case the direction of rotation that evens the legs identifies the side of the syndrome, e.g., "left unilateral cervical syndrome."

Upper angle: {PET} the angle between a line representing the head, which has been "divided" using a special mensuration tool, and a line transversely through the atlas in the frontal plane.

Vasomotor technique: {SOT} following identification of the SB+ or SB− Category I patient, this breathing and traction procedure may evoke blanching over various of the spinous processes. In this case, the involved segments are adjusted using an inferosuperior line of drive.

Vertebral challenge: {AK} a diagnostic method in which a hypothetical thrust is applied to a putatively subluxated bone, whereby a weakening of a previously strong indicator muscle would indicate the appropriateness of that line of drive.

Videofluoroscopy: {X-RAY} technology that permits dynamic motion X-rays, consisting of an X-ray generator capable of operating at low (1/4 to 5) milliamperage settings, an X-ray tube assembly, an image intensifier tube, a television camera, a video tape recorder, and a monitor. The image intensifier tube permits imaging at very low radiation levels, and is used instead of intensifying screens and film as an image receptor.

X-Derifield: {TT} with knees flexed to approximately 90°, the patient's head is rotated to one side. If one of the legs shortens, or a previously short leg remains short, the X-Derifield syndrome is present. Turning in the opposite direction may even the legs, in which case the direction of rotation that evens the legs identifies the side of the syndrome, e.g., a "left X-Derifield."

X-ray line marking: {X-RAY} the practice of marking anatomical landmarks on plain radiographs, in order to measure distances between them, the angles created by intersecting lines connecting these landmarks, or where these landmarks lie in relation to true horizontal or vertical lines.

REFERENCES

1. Fuhr A 1990 Activator Methods: basic manual. Activator Methods chiropractic technique seminars. Activator Methods, Phoenix, AZ
2. Osterbauer P J, Fuhr A W, Hildebrandt R W 1992 Mechanical force, manually assisted short lever chiropractic adjustment. Journal of Manipulative and Physiological Therapeutics 15 (5): 309–317
3. Jenness M E, Toftness I 1981 Validation of the Toftness/Jenness system of chiropractic. Digest of Chiropractic Economics (Sept/Oct): 22–26, 126–129
4. Cooperstein R, Gleberzon B J 2001 Toward a taxonomy of subluxation-equivalents. Topics in Clinical Chiropractic 8 (1): 49–60
5. Fuhr A 1983 Activator Methods. Today's Chiropractic (Jan/Feb): 16–19
6. Breig A 1960 Adverse mechanical tension on the nervous system. John Wiley, New York, NY
7. Webster L L 1987 An overview of the Logan Basic Technique. Today's Chiropractic (July/August): 71, 111
8. Pierce W V 1979 Curves and curvatures. Chirp, Dravosburg, PA
9. Getzoff H 1990 Sacro Occipital Technique (SOT): a system of chiropractic. American Chiropractor (August): 9–10, 41
10. Getzoff H 1999 Sacro-Occipital Technique categories: a systems method of chiropractic. Chiropractic Technique 11 (2): 62–65
11. Gregory R R 1977 The atlas subluxation complex and its correction technique. In: Kfoury P W (ed.) Catalog of chiropractic techniques, pp. 73–77. Logan College of Chiropractic, Chesterfield, MO
12. http://www.chiro.org/LINKS/blair.html
13. Harrison D D 1981 Chiropractic Biophysics phase I. Harrison Chiropractic Seminars, Sunnyvale, CA
14. Buddingh C, Galinis M R 1980 A brief overview of the stubborn low back and category II. Digest of Chiropractic Economics (July/August): 72–73
15. Unger J F 1991 Category II congruency concept. American Chiropractor (April): 10–17
16. Walther D S 1981 Applied Kinesiology, vol. I. Systems DC, Pueblo, CO
17. Goodheart G J 1993 The Applied Kinesiology technique. Today's Chiropractic 22 (July/August): 56–58
18. DeCamp N Jr 1994 The TMJ and dysfunction of the lumbo-pelvic complex. Today's Chiropractic (July/August): 20–25
19. Koffman D M 1984 Technical excellence: the next key to our survival. Digest of Chiropractic Economics (July/August) 53: 128
20. Epstein D M 1984 Network chiropractic explores the meningeal critical. Part I: anatomy and physiology of the meningeal functional unit. Digest of Chiropractic Economics (January/February): 78–80, 82
21. Epstein D 1998 Network Spinal Analysis: a system of health care delivery within the subluxation-based chiropractic model. Journal of Vertebral Subluxation Research 1 (1): 51–59
22. Epstein D 1987 The stress connection: gauging the role of the nervous system. Today's Chiropractic 15 (6): 15–17
23. Herriot E M 1990 Life-changing chiropractic. Yoga Journal (Sept/Oct): 23–25
24. Ward L 1990 A revolutionary new chiropractic development in stress management technology. American Chiropractor 12 (2): 29–34
25. Harrison D 1987 Basic mechanics applied to the spine (part three of three). Today's Chiropractic (Nov/Dec): 35–39
26. Harrison D E, Harrison D D, Troyanovich S J 1998 Three-dimensional spinal coupling mechanics: part I. A review of the literature. Journal of Manipulative and Physiological Therapeutics 21 (2): 101–113
27. Harrison D E, Harrison D D, Troyanovich S J 1998 Three-dimensional spinal coupling mechanics: part II. Implications for chiropractic theories and practice. Journal of Manipulative and Physiological Therapeutics 21 (3): 177–186
28. Schmitt W H Jr, Yanuck S F Expanding the neurological examination using functional neurologic assessment: part II. Neurologic basis of applied kinesiology. International Journal of Neuroscience 97 (1–2): 77–108
29. Clemen M J 1983 Understanding and adjusting bilateral pelvic unit subluxations. Today's Chiropractic (March/April): 22
30. Epstein D 2001 Network Spinal Analysis seminars. Advanced level intensive. Seminar notes
31. Sehi T, Proetz J F 1986 New answers for old stress problems – part 2. An exclusive interview with Dr. Lowell Ward. Digest of Chiropractic Economics (March/April): 36, 38–39, 41
32. Goodheart G J 1977 Applied Kinesiology. In: Kfoury P W (ed.) Catalog of chiropractic techniques, pp. 117–119. Logan College of Chiropractic, Chesterfield, MO
33. http://www.worldchiropracticalliance.org/tcj/2000/jan/jan2000pettibon.htm
34. Nelson C R, De Visscher-Nelson I 1982 Pilot study. Part 2. Deviations in bodily posture and center of gravity as possible indicators of certain upper cervical subluxation complexes. Digest of Chiropractic Economics (July/August): 88–89, 92, 134–135
35. McAlpine J E 1986 Nasium and vertex x-ray survey. Today's Chiropractic (March/April): 37–39
36. Saxon A 1985 Participant guide. SOT: a seminar for technical excellence (date approximate). SORSI
37. http://216.239.33.100/search?q=cache:G0zFjzs_CwwC:www.acol.org/BURCONCHIROPRACTIC/about.html+%22hot+boxes%22+chiropractic&hl=en&lr=lang_en&ie=UTF-8
38. Cohen J H, Gibbons R W, Raymond L 1998 Nimmo and the evolution of trigger point therapy, 1929–1986. Journal of Manipulative and Physiological Therapeutics 21 (3): 167–172
39. Plaugher G 1994 Specific-contact, short-lever-arm articular procedures: advances in the Gonstead technique. In: Lawrence D J, Cassidy D, McGregor M et al (eds) Advances in chiropractic. Mosby-Year Book, St Louis, MO
40. Osterbauer P J, Fuhr A W 1990 The current status of Activator Methods Chiropractic Technique, theory, and training. Chiropractic Technique 2 (4): 168–175

41. Herbst A 1980 Gonstead chiropractic science and art: the chiropractic methodology of Clarence S. Gonstead. Schichi, Mount Horeb, WI

42. Epstein D 1996 Network spinal analysis: a system of health care delivery within the subluxation-based chiropractic model. Journal of Vertebral Subluxation Research 1 (1): 51–59

43. Stillwagon G, Stillwagon K L 1983 The Pierce–Stillwagon technique. American Chiropractor (July/August): 20–23, 28–31, 65

44. Cleveland C S I 1992 The high-velocity thrust adjustment. In: Haldeman S (ed.) Principles and practice of chiropractic, 1st edn pp. 459–482. Appleton & Lange, Norwalk, CT

45. DeJarnette M B 1983 Sacro occipital technic. Self-published, Nebraska City, NB

46. Troyanovich S J, Harrison D D 1996 Chiropractic biophysics (CBP) technique. Chiropractic Technique 8 (1): 30–35

47. Lantz C 1989 The vertebral subluxation complex – part I: an introduction to the model and the kinesiological component. Chiropractic Research Journal 1 (3): 23–36

48. Palmer D D 1914 The chiropractor. Press of Beacon Light, Los Angeles, CA

49. Walther D S 1988 Applied Kinesiology: Synopsis. Systems DC, Pueblo, CO

50. Sandoz R 1976 Some physical mechanisms and effects of spinal adjustments. Annals of the Swiss Chiropractic Association 6: 91–141

51. Moses D E 1991 Studies on Logan Basic piriformis contact. ACA Journal of Chiropractic (December): 35–37

52. Harrison D D 1992 Subluxation: a mechanical engineering definition. In: Harrison D (ed.) Spinal biomechanics: a chiropractic perspective, pp. 11–32. Harrison CBP Seminars, Evanston, WY

53. Harrison D D 1981 Spinal biomechanics and the model, part II. Today's Chiropractic 10 (1): 12–13, 42–47, 58–59

54. Morter T Jr 1998 The theoretical basis and rationale for the clinical application of Bio-Energetic Synchronization. Journal of Vertebral Subluxation Research 2 (1)

55. Blum C 1999 Spinal/cranial manipulative therapy and tinnitus: a case history [sic]. Chiropractic Technique 10 (4): 163–168

56. John C 1992 The Directional Non-Force Technique of chiropractic. American Chiropractor (July/August): 15–16

57. Van Rumpt R 1987 Van – the innate man. American Chiropractor (September): 4–7

58. Morter M T 1993 The Bio-Energetic Synchronization Technique: a breakthrough in subluxation detection. Today's Chiropractic 22 (5): 68–69

59. Morter M T et al 1991 Seminar notes, level I (timing/toxicity), level II (timing/toxicity) and level III (thoughts/toxicity) [seminar manual notes]

60. Heese N 1988 Distortion patterns involving plumb line analysis. American Chiropractor (April): 32–34

61. Getzoff H 1998 The step out-toe out procedure: a therapeutic and diagnostic procedure. Chiropractic Technique 10 (3): 118–120

62. Kale M 1995 Dr. B J Palmer's upper cervical specific: the final test of greatness. Today's Chiropractic (January/February): 28–31

63. Plaugher G (ed.) 1993 Textbook of clinical chiropractic: a specific biomechanical approach. Williams & Wilkins, Baltimore, MD

64. Walther D S 1976 Applied Kinesiology. Systems DC, Pueblo, CO

65. John C 1999 Directional Non-Force Technique seminars. Christopher F John, Beverly Hills, CA

66. Snyder B J 1999 Thermographic evaluation for the role of the Sensometer: evidence in the Toftness system of chiropractic adjusting. Chiropractic Technique 11 (2): 57–61

67. Kale M 1988 Upper cervical chiropractic: who's responsible? Part II. Dynamic Chiropractic (January 1): 20–21

68. Kale M 1989 How the toggle is used in adjusting. Today's Chiropractic (July/August): 54–58

69. Harrison D D (ed.) 1992 Spinal Biomechanics: a chiropractic perspective. Harrison CBP Seminars, Evanston, WY

70. Harrison D D, Colloca C J, Troyanovich S J, Harrison D E 1996 Torque: an appraisal of misuse of terminology in chiropractic literature and technique. Journal of Manipulative and Physiological Therapy 19 (7): 454–462

71. Herzog W 2000 Torque: an appraisal of misuse of terminology in chiropractic literature and technique. Journal of Manipulative and Physiological Therapeutics 23 (4): 298–299

72. Schneider M, Cohen J, Laws S (eds) 2001 The collected writings of Nimmo and Vannerson: pioneers of chiropractic trigger point therapy. Self-published, Pittsburgh, PA

FURTHER READING

Peterson D H, Bergmann T 2002 Chiropractic Technique, 2nd edn. Churchill Livingstone, St Louis, MO

Index

Note: Page references followed by "f" refer to figures and diagrams, those followed by "t" refer to tables and boxed material. Abbreviations used as subentries are defined as main entries and in the glossary on page 361.

www.ingramcontent.com/pod-product-compliance
Lightning Source LLC
Chambersburg PA
CBHW082011230526
45468CB00022B/1840